ENT for

Entrance Exams (EEE)

Fifth Edition

Manisha Sinha Budhiraja MBBS (LHMC, Delhi)

MS (ENT), Safdarjung Hospital
Delhi University
DNB (ENT)

(manisha.budhiraja@yahoo.com)

Editor

Sachin Budhiraja MBBS (UCMS, Delhi)

MD (Medicine), Safdarjung Hospital
Delhi University

(sachin.budhiraja@yahoo.com)

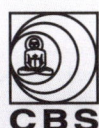

CBS Publishers & Distributors Pvt Ltd

New Delhi • Bengaluru • Chennai • Kochi • Kolkata • Mumbai
Hyderabad • Jharkhand • Nagpur • Patna • Pune • Uttarakhand

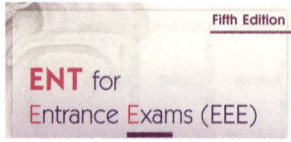

Fifth Edition

ENT for Entrance **E**xams (EEE)

ISBN: 978-93-87964-09-9

Fifth Edition: 2020
   Reprint: 2021
First Edition: 2014
Second Edition: 2015
   Reprint (May): 2016
   Reprint (July): 2016
Third Edition: 2017
   Reprint: 2018
Fourth Edition: 2019
   Reprint: 2020

Published by Satish Kumar Jain and Produced by Varun Jain for

CBS Publishers & Distributors Pvt Ltd
4819/XI Prahlad Street, 24 Ansari Road, Daryaganj, New Delhi 110 002, India
Ph: 011-23289259, 23266861, 23266867 Fax: 011-23243014   Website: www.cbspd.com
                                            e-mail: delhi@cbspd.com; cbspubs@airtelmail.in.
Corporate Office: 204 FIE, Industrial Area, Patparganj, Delhi 110 092, India
Ph: 011-4934 4934   Fax: 011-4934 4935   e-mail: publishing@cbspd.com; publicity@cbspd.com

Branches

- **Bengaluru:** Seema House 2975, 17th Cross, K.R. Road, Banasankari 2nd Stage, Bengaluru 560 070, Karnataka, India
  Ph: +91-80-26771678/79   Fax: +91-80-26771680   e-mail: bangalore@cbspd.com
- **Chennai:** 7, Subbaraya Street, Shenoy Nagar, Chennai 600 030, Tamil Nadu, India
  Ph: +91-44-26680620, 26681266   Fax: +91-44-42032115   e-mail: chennai@cbspd.com
- **Kochi:** 42/1325, 1326, Power House Road, Opp KSEB, Power House, Ernakulam 682 018, Kochi, Kerala, India
  Ph: +91-484-4059061-67   Fax: +91-484-4059065   e-mail: kochi@cbspd.com
- **Kolkata:** 6/B, Ground Floor, Rameswar Shaw Road, Kolkata-700 014, West Bengal, India
  Ph: +91-33-22891126, 22891127, 22891128   e-mail: kolkata@cbspd.com
- **Mumbai:** PWD Shed, Gala No. 25/26, Ramchandra Bhatt Marg, Next to JJ Hospital, Gate No. 2,
  Opposite Union Bank of India, Noorbaug, Mumbai 400 009, Maharashtra, India
  Ph: 022-66661880/89   e-mail: mumbai@cbspd.com

Representatives

Hyderabad	0-9885175004	**Jharkhand**	0-9811541605	**Nagpur**	0-9421945513
Patna	0-9334159340	**Pune**	0-9623451994	**Uttarakhand**	0-9716462459

Printed at Nutech Print Services, Faridabad, India

This book is dedicated to

The Almighty; Who is the all-knowing,
the all-pervading, the protector and the force behind everything.

My son Medhavi who gives meaning to my life.
My husband Sachin for being the light and strength of my life.

My parents Dr ARP Sinha and Mrs Kumud Sinha
because of whom I am all that I am today.

My parents in law Shri KL Budhiraja and Mrs Geeta Rani
whose support has been there always.

My Naani, Naana Ji, Maa and Lala Ji whose blessings will always
be there and who will always remain in my sweet memories.

and
most importantly to all my dear students

STAND UP, BE BOLD, BE STRONG

Take the whole responsibility on your own shoulders, and
know that you are the creator of your own destiny.
All power is within you;
you can do anything and everything.
Believe in that.
"I will drink the ocean" says the persevering soul,
"at my will, mountains will crumble up".
Have that sort of energy, that sort of will,
work hard and you will reach the goal.

—Swami Vivekananda

For queries, valuable feedback and suggestions please write to
manisha.budhiraja@yahoo.com
sachin.budhiraja@yahoo.com

Also join us at
www.facebook.com/groups/manishasachin/
www.facebook.com/groups/sachinmanisha/

Preface to the Fifth Edition

We would like to thank all our students for the overwhelming response they have given to this book. It gives us the enthusiasm to improve this book further.

The key additions in this 5th edition are:

1. It has been thoroughly updated from the most recent edition of all the standard ENT books especially Scott-Brown, 8th edition and Cummings, 6th edition.
2. References to the answers of all questions have been put from the most recent editions of standard ENT books. With the inflow of so many question banks available nowadays, all giving different answers, the students were in a dilemma of which one to follow giving the need for proper reference.
3. Annexures for quick revision have been added.
4. Points to ponder have been added at the end of each chapter to stimulate your mind which will also be of lots of help to quickly revise the chapter before the exams.
5. A large number of pictures has been added keeping in mind the trend of exams these days.
6. All the recent MCQs from various exams have been added.
7. The text has been made further easy and new flowcharts and tables have been added. Whether it be the prefinal year students or the students preparing for the entrance, the key to success is to understand every topic rather than cramming up the facts and answers to the questions. Understanding makes you remember the topics as well as solve the new MCQs asked from the same topics. It also gives you an edge over the others as even the questions that are repeated are not asked in the same manner again.

The text contains everything possible you need to know in every topic in a very simple and easy to grasp language. With the surge of so many question banks, available students are in a fix what all to do! Our sincere advise is that the questions given after every chapter in this book are a must to do and are sufficient for all the exams.

We have tried our best to make this book a one stop book for ENT which will save your precious time from referring many other ENT books. We hope that you will utilise all our efforts and love reading this book as much as we love writing it. Your suggestions for the further improvement of EEE are always welcome.

All the best and God bless!

Manisha Sinha Budhiraja
Sachin Budhiraja

Preface to the First Edition

ENT (Otorhinolaryngology) is an extremely scoring subject in the MBBS curriculum. Being a teaching faculty of ENT for the past 10 years in the various institutes, I have been closely associated with the students preparing for postgraduate entrance exams.

Almost invariably, after every lecture, students would approach me to know which book to read for ENT for the preparation of PG entrance exams, considering the short time available with many subjects to prepare.

It was then, that I realised the need for a one stop book of ENT containing everything relevant to meet the requirement of students so that consulting many books for text as well as MCQs for ENT can be avoided.

It was a difficult decision considering the time that would be required to accomplish it, which would be very difficult to take out from my busy schedule. But with tremendous perseverance and tremendous will and unstinting support of my husband Dr Sachin Budhiraja, this book has grown out of, my years' long experience in teaching.

Each chapter contains an enriched, concise text written in very simple, easy to understand language. I have tried to illustrate the book extensively with simple explanatory line diagrams along side. Several easy to grasp mnemonics have been given throughout the text to make learning easy. All the topics have been thoroughly scrutinized so as to ensure that no stone is left unturned.

Once the text is read and the concepts are clear, the students will be able to answer not only the previously asked MCQs but also the questions likely to come in future exams.

The text is followed by previously asked MCQs in various PG entrance exams across India along with their answers and explanations.

In spite of keeping an eagle's eye, some imperfections are bound to remain. Suggestions for improvement are most welcome.

I hope this book proves to be useful to you and that you enjoy reading it as much as I enjoyed writing it.

Manisha Sinha Budhiraja
MS (ENT), DNB (ENT)
manisha.budhiraja@yahoo.com

Editor's Note

The author, my wife, Dr Manisha Sinha Budhiraja has done a tremendous effort and has finally come up with a very good book on ENT.

The book reflects the vast teaching experience and absolute command of the author over the ENT subject.

She has herself made all the diagrams in Section I and many a diagrams of other sections as well, in the book.

Besides a very good human being and a perfect mother, she is also the best teaching faculty and a great clinician and surgeon. Sometimes I wonder how many qualities a person can have simultaneously!

I am sure that this book *ENT for Entrance Exams* (*EEE*) will be of great help to the students.

I have thoroughly and repeatedly read this book as a student to point-out the areas which require more simplification and further elaboration for better understanding from a student's perspective.

I have thoroughly edited this book with the help of the author and placed tables and added mnemonics wherever required.

I being a consultant in medicine, my expertise in this subject has helped to make the concepts clearer in areas where there is a cross link of ENT with Medicine, for example, vestibular system and stridor, etc.

This is the first of its kind book in the ENT. All the chapters contain an up-to-date, concise text followed by all the possible MCQs available, of various PG entrance exams.

Besides this book being easy to understand and easy to memorise, the other USP of this work is that all the other choices given in the MCQs have been commented upon which will help the students to solve further new questions.

This book will definitely be of help to:

1. All the students preparing for various PG entrance exams.
2. All the undergraduate students, while giving *viva voce* and MBBS professional exams.
3. Postgraduate students for a quick revision and understanding of ENT in the beginning of their course.

Purity, patience and perseverance are the three essentials to success, and above all, love!

All the Best and God Bless!

Sachin Budhiraja
MD (Medicine)
sachin.budhiraja@yahoo.com

Acknowledgements

I owe this effort to many people without whose help this book would have remained just a dream.

Words cannot describe the contribution of my husband Sachin, who besides editor is also the typist of this book and my son Medhavi, my parents, my sisters Rashmi and Swati & Anand for their constant support throughout and not letting me give up at any moment.

I would like to acknowledge the guidance of Prof. Dr VP Venkatachalam, Dr Gul Motwani, Dr NN Mathur, Dr S Mandal, Dr Neena Chaudhary, Dr Himani Lade, Dr S Majhi, Dr Deepak Gupta, Dr Tilak Raj, Dr Naresh Bharadwaj, Dr Niranjan, Dr Vikas all faculty in the department of ENT at Safdarjung Hospital, Delhi and Dr B Gupta (Head, Department of Medicine, Safdarjung Hospital) and Dr Kalpana Uppal (Head of the Department, ABGH, Moti Nagar, Delhi) and all my teachers at Lady Hardinge Medical College, Delhi.

I convey my sincere thanks to Dr Gobind Rai Garg (MD, Pharmacology) for giving his valuable advice whenever needed.

Although it is impossible to acknowledge the contribution of every one individually, I extend my heartfelt thanks to:

- Akarsh, Arjun, Medhavi, Madhav, Raghav, Shivani, Anchit, Dr Kisley Dayal and other family members.
- Dr ARP Sinha (Ex Principal, JNRM Govt. College, Port Blair) for the beautiful diagrams of nose and pharynx sections.
- Ms Rashmi Sethi, a wonderful person, teacher and artist, for the beautiful diagrams of larynx section.
- Mr Sunil, Lakhya Arts for the beautiful diagrams of pharynx.
- My seniors Dr Friji MT, Dr Sanjay Aggarwal, Dr Alok, Dr Kadambari, Dr Sanjeev, Dr Nitin, Dr Dravid.
- My colleagues Dr Bulbul Gupta, Dr Sameer Sethi, Dr Pooja Gambhir, Dr Siddharth, Dr Rajeev, Dr Lalming, Dr Natesh.
- My juniors Dr Priya, Dr Payal, Dr Deepti, Dr Sameer, Dr Dipti, Dr Ashutosh, Dr Sarav Jeet Singh, Dr Arti, Dr Saurabh, Dr Radha, Dr Shveta, Dr Himanshu, Dr Amrita.
- Dr Mukesh Kumar Joon (DM, Cardiologist), Dr Rashmi Joon (MD, Obs & Gynae), Dr Nitin Arora (MD, Paeds), Dr Harpreet Kaur Jassi (MD, Obs & Gynae), Dr Deb Datta Mazumdar (DM, Cardio), Dr Anish Singhal (MD, Medicine), Dr Ratnesh Kanwar (MD, Medicine), Dr Rajeev Singhal (MD, Medicine), Dr Pankaj Tikku (MD, Paeds), Dr Raman Allawadi (MD, Paeds), Dr S P Singh (MD, Skin), Dr Deepali and Anuj Gupta (MD, Paeds), Dr Dinesh Chauhan (MD, Biochemistery), Dr Neelam (MD, Pathology), Dr Swati (MD, Anaesthesia), Dr Ashish Goel (MS, Ortho), Dr Dinesh (MS, Anatomy), Dr Vipin Daga (MD, Radiology), Dr Vipin Nagpal (MS, Surgery), Dr Vineet (MS, Surgery), Dr Rajeev Dhawan (MS, ENT), Dr Deepak Arora (MS, ENT), Dr Vandana (MD, Paeds), Dr Parul and Mrs Shabana Yunus.
- All my students specially Dr Prakriti, Dr Vasu, Dr Sabiya, Dr Afzal who have made the effort to point out the areas which needed further simplification and improvement.

I also owe my sincere thanks to Mr Ganesh, Mrs Janki, Dr Suyog Sahu, Mr Neeraj Salunke, for their cooperation, help and support.

I convey my sincere thanks to Mr SK Jain, CMD, CBS Publishers & Distributors Pvt. Ltd., Delhi, for his unstinted cooperation to bring out this 4th edition.

Thanks to Mr YN Arjuna Senior Vice President Publishing, Editorial and Publicity, Mr SK Verma Vice President, Ms Ritu Chawla General Manager—Production, Mr Vikrant Sharma, Mr Ram Murti, Mr Kshirod Sahoo and Mr Neeraj Prasad for their fresh ideas, unparallel skills and enthusiasm to this venture. I am grateful to all of them for their help and support.

With the blessings of Bhagwan Mahavir, Who are there on every book from CBS Publishers, I hope to reach my goal, i.e. to further the education and provide a foundation for the generations to follow.

Manisha Sinha Budhiraja

List of References

1. Shambaugh—Surgery of the Ear, 6th Edition
2. Scott-Brown's, Otolaryngology, Head and Neck Surgery, 8th Edition
3. Stell and Maran's, Head and Neck Surgery, 5th Edition
4. Current Diagnosis and Treatment Otolaryngology Head and Neck Surgery, 3rd Edition
5. Otolaryngology, Head and Neck Surgery, Cummings, 6th Edition
6. Otolaryngology, M Paparella, 3rd Edition
7. Diseases of Ear, Nose and Throat and Head and Neck Surgery, PL Dhingra, 6th Edition
8. Ear, Nose, Throat and Head and Neck Surgery, P Hazarika, 4th Edition
9. Otorhinolaryngology, Zakir Hussain, 3rd Edition
10. ENT Journals
11. Harrison's Principles of Internal Medicine, 20th Edition
12. Current Medical Diagnosis and Treatment (CMDT), 2020
13. The Neurologic Examination, De Jong's
14. Human Anatomy, BD Chaurasia, 7th Edition
15. Human Embryology, Inderbir Singh
16. Tintinalli's Emergency Medicine, 8th Edition
17. Clinical Audio-Vestibulometry, Anirban Biswas, 5th Edition
18. Exam Preparation in ENT and Head–Neck Surgery with Many Easy to Remember One-lines, JP Purohit

Join us at
www.facebook.com/groups/manishasachin/
www.facebook.com/groups/sachinmanisha/

Contents

Embryology and Anatomy of Ear

EMBRYOLOGY

The ear is comprised of three parts (as we go medially, *see* Fig. 1.1):

1. **External ear** (it has three parts, the pinna, the external auditory canal (EAC) and the lateral surface of the tympanic membrane(TM).
2. **Middle ear** (it is like a cuboid shaped box, extending medially from the TM and has bony ossicles and other structures). Through the Eustachian tube (pharyngo-tympanic tube) middle ear communicates with the nasopharynx.
3. **Inner ear** also called **Labyrinth** (it is comprised of a membranous labyrinth surrounded by a bony labyrinth).

The external ear and the middle ear are situated in petrous, tympanic and mastoid parts of temporal bone.

The whole of the inner ear is situated in the **petrous part** of the temporal bone (*see* Fig. 1. 2). The petrous part of the temporal bone is pyramidal in shape with an anterior and a posterior slant. The anterior slant faces the middle cranial fossa and the posterior slant faces the posterior cranial fossa. On the posterior slant of the petrous part of temporal bone is an opening called the **Internal Acoustic Meatus (IAM)** which connects the inner ear to the posterior cranial fossa.

DEVELOPMENT OF PINNA

The **1st and 2nd branchial arch** mesoderm gives rise to 6 mesodermal thickenings (auricular tubercles) known as "**HILLOCKS of HIS**" which fuse to form pinna.

The 1st Hillock comes from the 1st arch and forms the tragus and adjacent part of helix; the remaining 5 Hillocks come from the 2nd arch and form the rest of the pinna (*see* Figs 1.3 and 1.12).

Developmental Anomalies of Pinna

- The failure of fusion of the 1st and 2nd arch leads to the formation of a sinus in front of the tragus. This is known as "**PRE-AURICULAR SINUS**". This is seen in between the tragus (from 1st arch) and the ascending limb of helix (from 2nd arch) most commonly either above the tragus or at the root of helix.

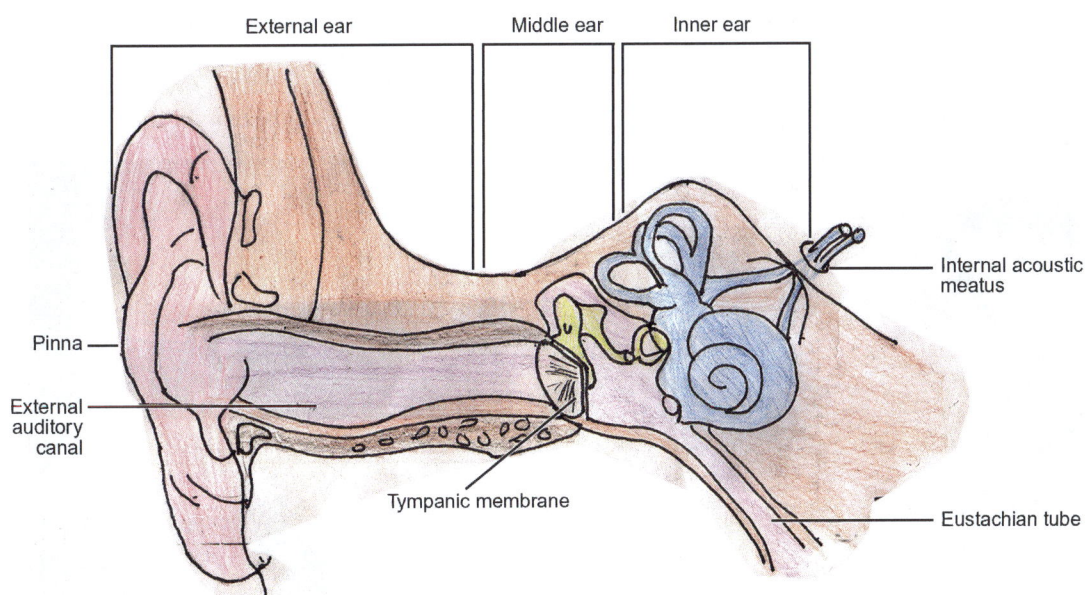

Fig. 1.1: Parts of Ear

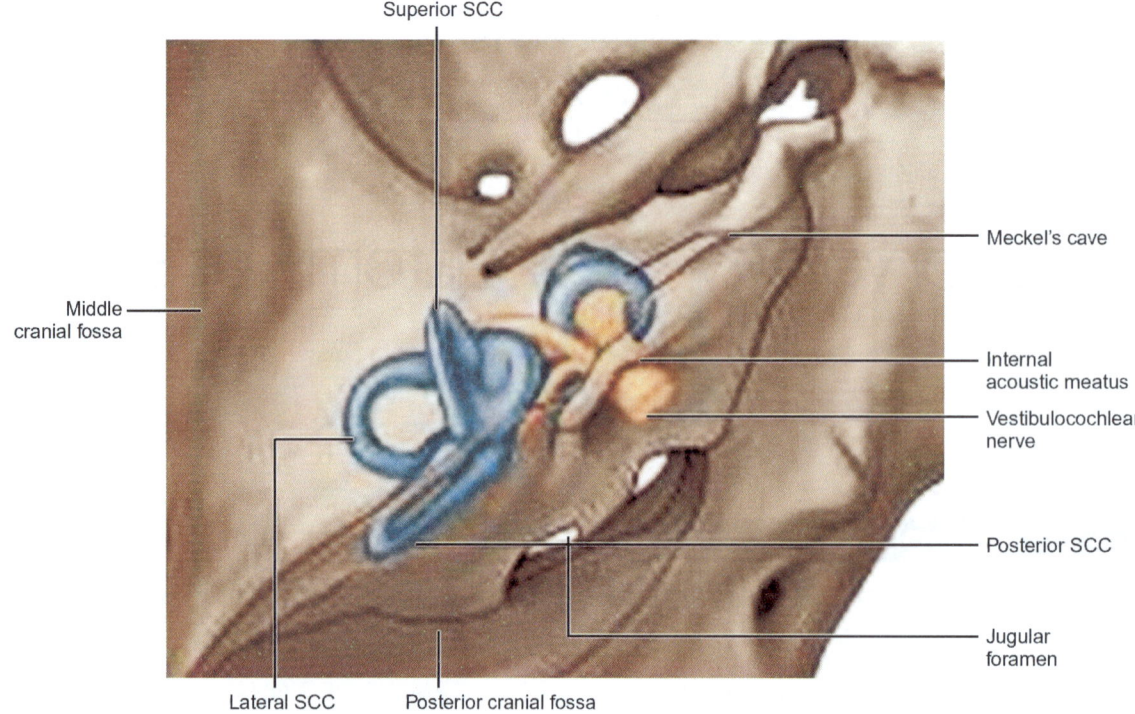

Fig. 1.2: IAM in Petrous part of Temporal bone (left sided). The petrous part of temporal bone separates the middle cranial fossa from posterior cranial fossa and has anterior and posterior slants, the posterior slant having IAM.

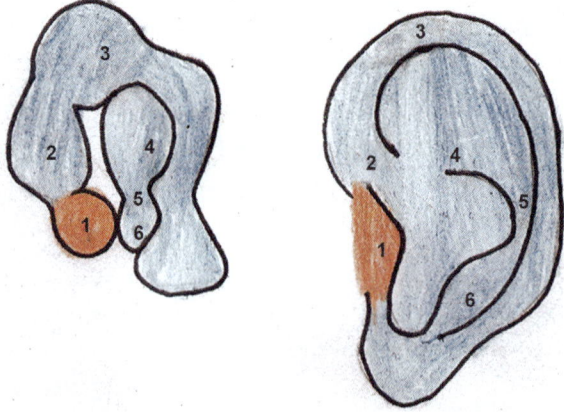

Fig. 1.3: Development of Pinna from "Hillocks of His"

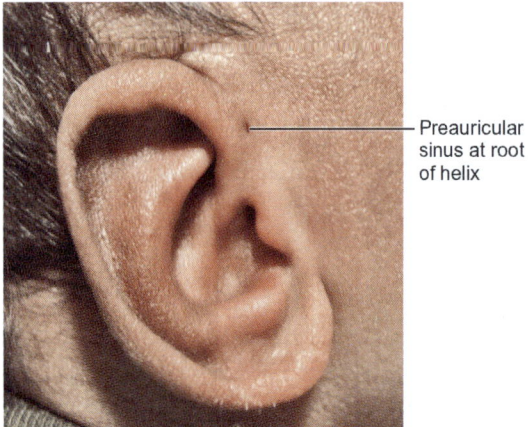

Fig. 1.4: Preauricular Sinus

The preauricular sinus may get infected and discharge on and off. Management is surgical excision.

- Pinna can be malformed, it may be small known as "Microtia" or absent known as "Anotia". In this regard it is important to remember that the surgical **reconstruction of pinna is done at or after 6 years of age for the following 2 reasons:**
  1. Autologous Costal (rib) cartilage is used as graft here. The costal cartilage gets developed enough for this purpose by 6 years of age.
  2. Pinna attains almost the adult size by 6 years. So the side which is to be reconstructed can be compared with the normal side pinna.
- Sometimes as a result of unequal turning in of the helix, in the fetus, develops a thickening on the postero-superior portion of the helix (usually at the junction of upper and middle third). This is known as Darwin's tubercle, shown in the picture below. It can be U/L or B/L.

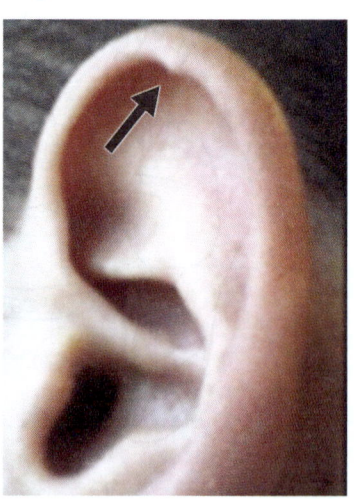

DEVELOPMENT OF EXTERNAL AUDITORY CANAL (EAC)

The dorsal part of **1st ectodermal cleft** (or 1st branchial groove) grows medially and forms the external auditory canal (EAC). **At birth, only the cartilaginous part of EAC is completely developed; the bony part of EAC continues to grow after birth.** Due to this the tympanic membrane is nearly horizontally placed at birth. The completion of the bony part of EAC gives the tympanic membrane its adult angulation by 4–5 years.

Developmental Anomaly of EAC

Normally, the ventral or anterior part of this 1st cleft which connects the EAC to the neck disappears. But if it persists it leads to an abnormal connection between the EAC and the neck. This congenital anomaly is known as **"CALL-AURAL FISTULA"**. The external opening of this Call-aural fistula is in between the angle of mandible and Sternocleidomastoid muscle and internal opening is in the floor of EAC.

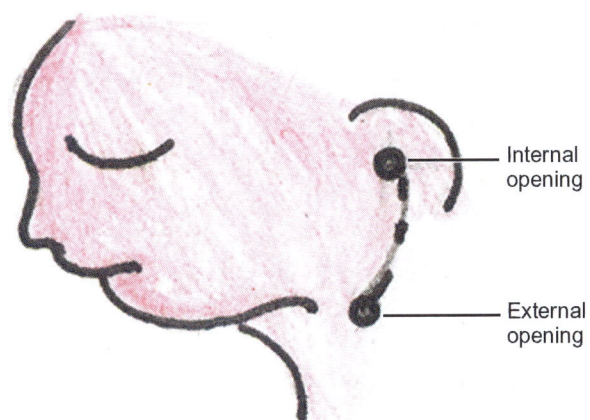

Fig. 1.5: Call-aural fistula

The fistula may get infected and discharge on and off. Management is surgical excision.

DEVELOPMENT OF MIDDLE EAR AND TYMPANIC MEMBRANE

Middle Ear

The **1st endodermal pouch (or 1st visceral pouch) along with a small part of the 2nd pouch forms tubo-tympanic recess** which leads to the formation of Eustachian tube (tubo) and tympanic cavity (tympanic recess), i.e. middle ear cavity along with mastoid antrum (*see* below). Together the Eustachian tube, middle ear and mastoid antrum are called the **middle ear cleft**.

Of the 3 ossicles in the tympanic cavity, **Malleus and Incus develop from 1st arch**. The **supra-structure of stapes,** i.e. its head, neck and the two cruras develop from **2nd arch** (*mnemonic*: S for suprastructure of stapes—Second arch), whereas the **foot plate** of stapes overlying oval window develops from the inner ear bone which is called **"Otic capsule"** or bony labyrinth (*see* below).

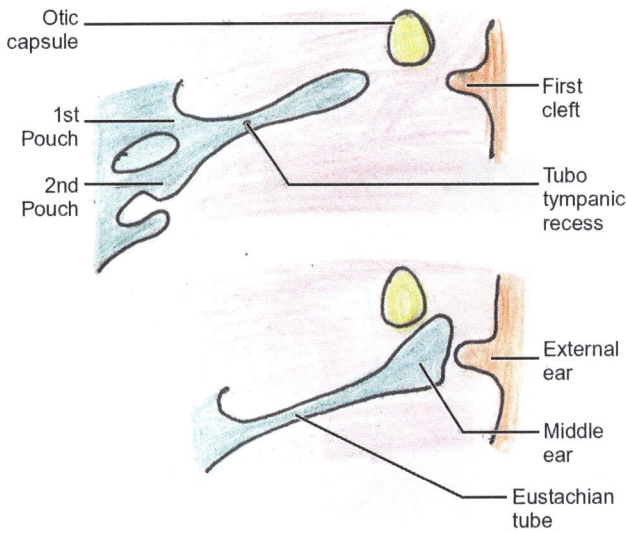

Fig. 1.6: Development of External Auditory Canal, Middle ear and Eustachian tube

The **ossicles** attain **adult configuration by 20 weeks** period of gestation (POG).

Tympanic Membrane (TM)

The 1st cleft meets the 1st pouch with the mesoderm in between them to form the tympanic membrane.

So **the tympanic membrane develops from all the 3 layers**, of embryonic disc; outer epithelial layer from ectoderm, inner endothelial layer from endoderm and in between these two is the fibrous layer from mesoderm. Both the TM and middle ear cavity, like ossicles, are **completely developed at birth**.

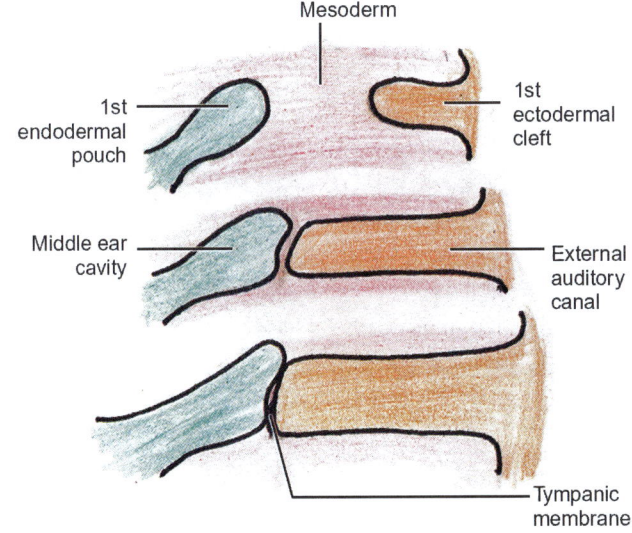

Fig. 1.7: Development of Tympanic membrane

DEVELOPMENT OF MASTOID

Mastoid develops from the superficial squamous and the deep petrous parts of temporal bone. In between the 2 parts is the **petro-squamosal suture** which generally

Section I | **Ear**

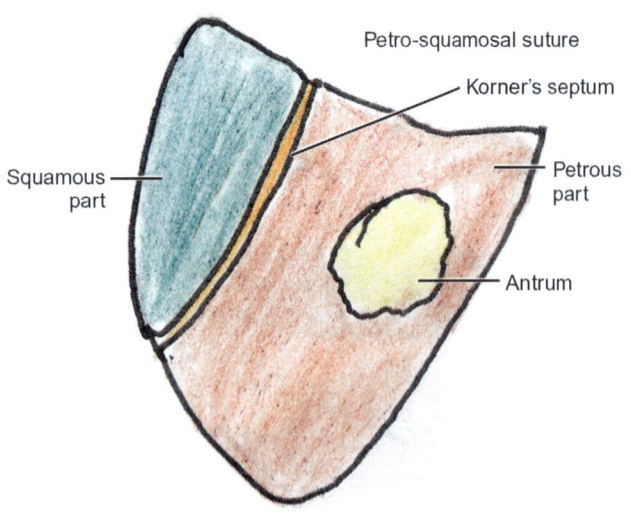

Squamous part

Petro-squamosal suture

Korner's septum

Petrous part

Antrum

Fig. 1.8: Korner's septum

disappears. However, sometimes it persists and is called "**KORNER'S SEPTUM**".

Mastoid is a spongy bone and contains multiple air cells. The mastoid is incompletely developed at birth and continues to develop till 18 years of age. The antrum is the largest and most prominent mastoid air cell which develops from 1st and 2nd pouch (tubo-tympanic recess, *see* above). The **antrum is present at birth and is almost**

of adult configuration. The mastoid antrum lies in the petrous part deep to the Korner's septum. In diseases of mastoid, maximum disease lies in the mastoid antrum.

Surgical Importance of Korner's Septum

While removing disease from mastoid, if the Korner's septum is present, the surgeon might confuse the Korner's septum with medial most wall of antrum, i.e. the boundary which separates the antrum from the posterior cranial fossa. For the fear of entering posterior cranial fossa the surgeon stops the surgery at the Korner's septum, whereas he has not yet entered the mastoid antrum. This will lead to incomplete clearance of disease from the mastoid.

Surgical Importance of Mastoid Tip

The tip of mastoid develops by 2 years of age because of the constant pull by the sternocleidomastoid and the posterior belly of digastric muscle. The facial nerve exits from stylomastoid foramen just below the mastoid tip and turns horizontally towards the parotid gland, in which it gives off motor branches for the muscles of face.

The mastoid tip being absent below 2 years, the facial nerve lies very superficial just below the skin. So in a child below 2 years with post auricular abscess, the incision should be superior and horizontal so as to avoid damage to facial nerve.

To summarise:

Ear part	Embryonic layer	Respective Ectodermal cleft/Mesodermal arch/ Endodermal pouch or other area	Congenital anomaly/ developmental importance
Pinna (cartilage)	Mesoderm	1st and 2nd arch	Pre-auricular sinus, Microtia, Anotia
EAC (epithelium)	Ectoderm	1st cleft/groove (dorsal part)	Call-aural fistula
TM	All the three; Ectoderm, Endoderm and Mesoderm	1st cleft grows medially to join 1st pouch along with the mesodermal layer in between to form the TM	Small TM (congenital Rubella syndrome)
Middle ear cavity along with mastoid antrum and Eustachian tube	Endoderm	1st and 2nd pouch forms Tubo-tympanic recess	Antrum lying deep to Korner's septum (*see* its importance in the text)
Malleus and incus	Mesoderm	1st arch	Rare congenital malformations
Supra structure of stapes	Mesoderm	2nd arch	Rare congenital malformations
Foot plate of stapes	Mesoderm	Enchondral bone formation from Otic capsule	Fixation of stapes is the most common congenital middle ear anomaly
Mastoid	Mesoderm	Squamous and petrous parts of temporal bone	Mastoid tip absent below 2 years leading to superficially lying facial nerve
Membranous labyrinth (*see below*)	Surface Neuro-ectoderm (Otic placode)	Neuro-ectoderm Overlying hind brain	Michel aplasia. Scheibe, Mondini and Alexander dysplasia (*see below*)
Bony labyrinth (*see below*)	Mesoderm	Mesenchymal tissue around the membranous labyrinth	Michel aplasia Scheibe, Mondini and Alexander dysplasia

DEVELOPMENT OF INNER EAR

Development of Membranous Labyrinth

The inner ear consists of a membranous labyrinth surrounded by a bony labyrinth. The membranous part of inner ear also called as membranous labyrinth develops from a specialised area of **surface ectoderm** overlying the developing hind brain. This area of surface ectoderm is called as "Otic Placode". This becomes otic pit and then otic vesicle. This otic vesicle which is like a sac or balloon ultimately forms membranous labyrinth. So the membranous labyrinth is like a designer balloon (designed by God!) and being a **closed sac does not communicate with any other structure.**

When fully developed, the membranous labyrinth has the following parts (*see* Fig. 1.9):

1. **Three semicircular canals:** Lateral (horizontal), posterior and superior (anterior). The semicircular canals are at an angle of 90 degrees to each other. This angle formed among the three semicircular canals is known as **solid angle.**

2. **Utricle:** The three semicircular canals open into utricle by 5 openings (why 5? actually there have to be 6!). This is because one of the crus (crus means an elongated part of an anatomical structure, especially one which occurs in the body as a pair) of the posterior and superior semicircular canals fuse together to form a common crus called **"crus commune"**, which then opens into the utricle.

3. **Saccule:** The utricle is connected to the saccule through a utriculo-saccular duct. This utriculo-saccular duct forms the endolymphatic duct which ends blindly into **Endolymphatic sac.** This endolymphatic sac is situated in between the endosteal and meningeal layer of the dura mater, i.e. in between the dura of the posterior fossa and skull bone (please note: This is not the subdural space which is in between dura and arachnoid).

The **Endolymphatic sac** is responsible for the absorption of endolymph. Endolymph is the fluid that fills the whole of the membranous labyrinth (i.e. the 3 semicircular canals, utricle, saccule and the scala media (*see* below)).

4. **Membranous cochlea:** After the saccule is the membranous cochlea. Saccule is connected with the cochlea by ductus re-unions. The membranous cochlea is also known as "Scala media" or cochlear duct. This Membranous cochlea or scala media is a coiled tube which takes **2 and 1/2 to 2 and 3/4 turns** around a bony axis which is known as "modiolus".

Certain areas of the membranous labyrinth ultimately differentiate into specialised areas of hearing and balance (*see* Fig. 1.10). Hence diseases involving inner ear either present as hearing loss or as imbalance or both.

Sensory end Organ of Hearing

The sensory organ of hearing is known as "**Organ of Corti**". It is situated inside the Scala media/membranous cochlea.

The organ of Corti situated in the **basal turn** of membranous cochlea is responsible for sensing **high frequency** sounds, whereas the organ of Corti situated in the **apical turns** is responsible for sensing **low frequency** sounds (easy to remember basal turn is wider so senses (larger) higher frequency, and apical turn is narrow with less space so senses (smaller) lower frequency sounds).

Therefore diseases affecting the apical turn will lead to low frequency hearing loss, whereas those affecting basal turn will lead to high frequency hearing loss.

In Meniere's disease which is characterised by increase in endolymph, the narrow apical part of scala media experiences the dilatation first therefore affecting low frequency sounds first.

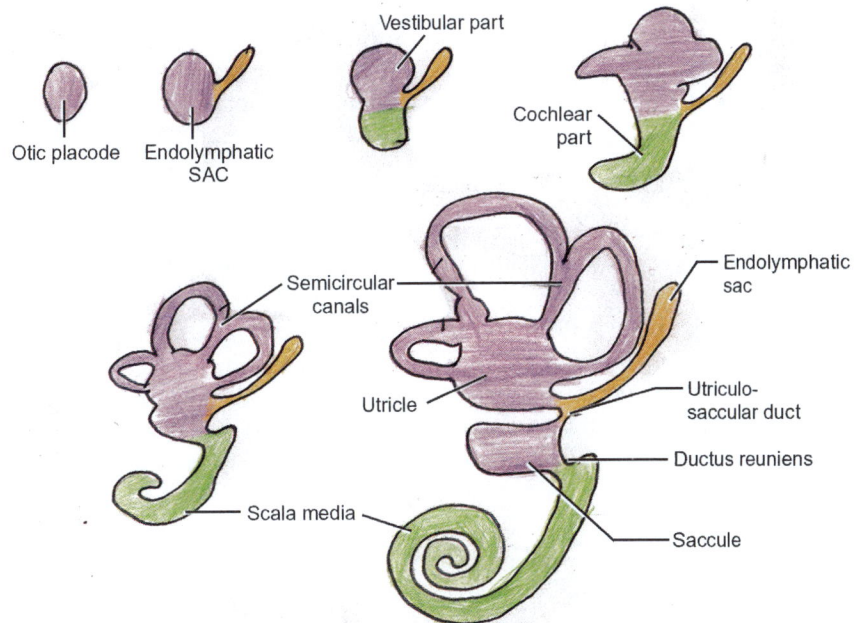

Vestibular part

Cochlear part

Otic placode   Endolymphatic SAC

Endolymphatic sac

Semicircular canals

Utriculo-saccular duct

Utricle

Ductus reuniens

Scala media

Saccule

Fig. 1.9: Development of membranous labyrinth

Section I | Ear

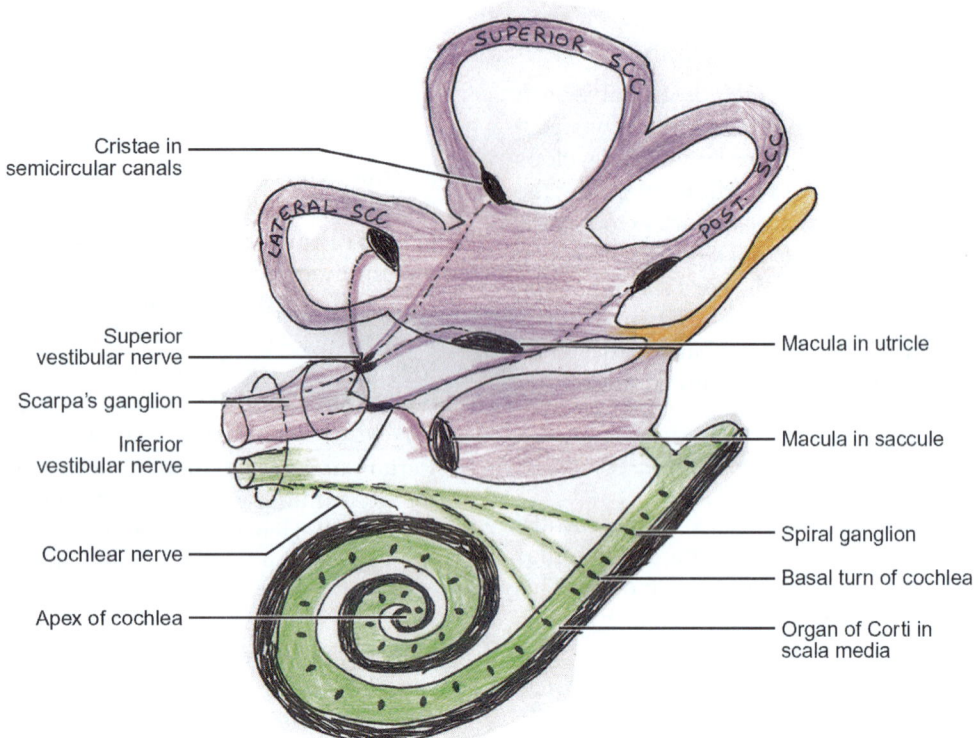

Fig. 1.10: Sensory end organs of hearing and balance

Whereas ototoxic drugs, noise trauma, presbycusis, etc. which involve basal turns first, affect high frequency sounds early.

The organ of Corti is differentiated to such a degree by **20 weeks** POG that the foetus can hear and respond to fluid borne sounds. The organ of Corti approximates the adult structure by 25 weeks (in Mahabharata Abhimanyu heard about the technique of breaking the chakravheu while he was a 5 months fetus).

The whole of the bony and membranous labyrinth gets completely developed at birth.

Structures which are fully developed at birth are:
- TM
- Middle ear cavity with the ossicles
- Mastoid antrum
- Bony and membranous labyrinth

Sensory end Organs of Balance

The sensory end organs of balance are called Cristae and Maculae (*see* Fig. 1.10).

Cristae are present in semi-circular canals (easy to remember C for C). They are responsible for sensing **rotational and angular movements** (again to remember easily, semicircular canals being round (rotational) and are at an angle of 90 degrees to each other (senses angular movements).

Maculae are present in the utricle and saccule and sense **linear acceleration, gravitational** (movement either with or against gravity) and **head tilt movements** and it helps to maintain **static equilibrium** (by facilitating postural, tonic neck and righting reflexes).

Development of Bony Labyrinth

Once the development of membranous labyrinth is complete, the mesenchymal tissue around the membranous labyrinth **condenses to form cartilage.** Later **endochondral bone formation** occurs in this cartilage to form the bony labyrinth (otic capsule).

However, some portions of the bony labyrinth remain cartilaginous, i.e. they retain their activity to divide. One such area is **"Fissula ante fenestrum"** (just anterior to fenestra of oval window). With certain stimuli, it may start dividing and subsequently undergoes endochondral bone formation. Since this area lies anterior to the oval window on which is present the footplate of stapes, this overgrowth extends till foot plate of stapes leading to its fixation. This condition is called otosclerosis.

To summarise **bony labyrinth is derived from mesoderm, whereas membranous labyrinth is formed from surface neuro-ectoderm.**

The following parts of bony labyrinth can be recognised:
1. **Three bony semi-circular canals:** This is the bony labyrinth around membranous semi-circular canals.
2. **Vestibule:** It is the bony labyrinth around utricle and saccule. The bony canal around the utriculo-saccular duct and endolymphatic duct is called **vestibular aqueduct**.
3. **Bony Cochlea, Scala vestibuli and Scala tympani** are the portions of bony labyrinth on the two sides of Scala media (that is why the term media). The Scala vestibuli lies above the Scala media, whereas the Scala tympani lies below it. As discussed above the Scala media is filled with endolymph, whereas

the Scala vestibuli and Scala tympani, along with rest of the bony labyrinth, are filled with perilymph which is an extension of CSF (*see* below). The Scala vestibuli meets the Scala tympani at the apex of Scala media. The area where they meet is called **"Helicotrema"**.

The membranous labyrinth being a closed sac, does not communicate with any other structure, however the bony labyrinth is connected laterally to the middle ear and medially to the cranial fossa.

The **bony labyrinth communicates with middle ear via two openings** present on the common wall between inner ear and middle ear, i.e. the medial wall of middle ear. These are:

1. **Oval window:** This is situated on the bone separating the vestibule (mnemonic; **OV**al–**O**val **V**estibule) from the middle ear, hence it is also known as fenestra vestibuli (*see* Fig. 1.11). The **foot process of stapes** overlies the oval window. Hence the foot plate of stapes develops from the enchondral bone of the bony labyrinth, whereas the rest of stapes is formed from 2nd arch, as discussed above.

   The importance of oval window:

   • The **sound vibrations** are transmitted through the **footplate of stapes** to the oval window and then **through the vestibular perilymph to the Scala vestibuli** and then through helicotrema to the Scala tympani towards the round window. So whenever the stapes foot plate causes the oval window to move in, the round window moves out. This opposite movement leads to deflection of the basilar membrane (which forms the lower boundary of scala media, *see* below) and stimulation of the organ of Corti situated upon it in the Scala media.

• Normally during sound transmission foot plate does not stimulate the utricle and saccule. Therefore a loud sound normally does not cause imbalance. In Meniere's disease which is characterised by the hydrops of utricle and saccule (due to increase in endolymph), the utricle and saccule bulge and come very close to the oval window. The excessive movement of stapes on loud sounds now causes stimulation of utricle and saccule leading to imbalance. Vertigo on loud sounds is known as **"TULLIO'S phenomenon"**. It is seen in Meniere's disease and superior semicircular canal dehiscence (*see* Chapter 12).

• In congenital syphilis where the foot plate of stapes is hyper mobile, external pressure changes in the EAC by tragal pressure or Siegel's speculum lead to excessive movement of the footplate, stimulating the utricle and saccule, causing imbalance. This vertigo, on external pressure changes, is known as **"HENNEBERT'S sign"**.

• The foot plate can become fixed (in otosclerosis) and not allow the sound to go from middle ear to inner ear leading to hearing loss.

2. **Round window:** This connects the Scala tympani with the middle ear. It is also known as fenestra cochleae. The round window is covered by **secondary tympanic membrane** (easy to remember secondary tympanic membrane (STM) over scala tympani (ST)).

   The importance of round window:

   i. The round window is also important in sound transmission: as mentioned in the Ist bullet above.

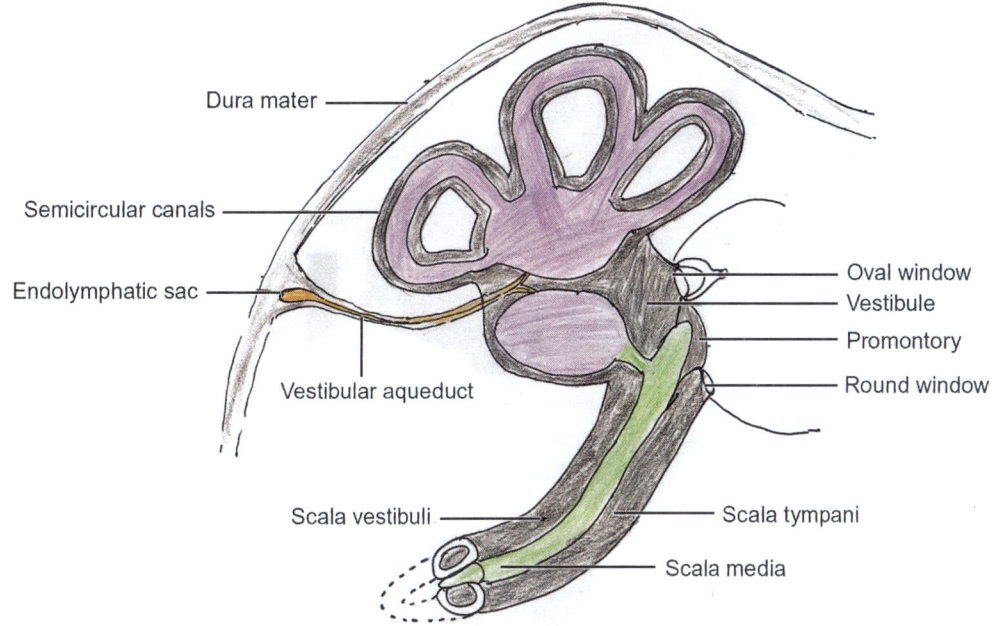

Fig. 1.11: Parts of bony labyrinth

Dura mater

Semicircular canals

Endolymphatic sac

Vestibular aqueduct

Oval window

Vestibule

Promontory

Round window

Scala vestibuli

Scala tympani

Scala media

ii. The electrodes of cochlear implant are **introduced** through this window and **placed** in the scala tympani.

iii. Drugs are given via this window (by continuous infusion by Micro Wick and micro catheter sustained release devices) into the inner ear, e.g. Gentamicin in Meniere's disease and steroids in sudden sensorineural hearing loss of immune aetiology.

The bony labyrinth communicates with the cranium via 2 openingse

1. **Cochlear aqueduct:** This is the connection between the CSF and scala tympani. Via this connection the **CSF** in the subarachnoid space enters scala tympani and becomes **perilymph** which circulates in whole of the bony labyrinth. CSF being an extracellular fluid therefore perilymph is rich in Na^+. So Scala Tympani communicates with middle ear, Scala Vestibuli and subarachnoid space via round window, helicotrema and cochlear aqueduct respectively.

2. **Internal acoustic meatus:** This is the opening connecting the inner ear to the posterior cranial fossa. The 7th and 8th cranial nerves respectively enter and leave the inner ear through the internal acoustic meatus. This is present in the petrous part of temporal bone on its posterior slant (*see* Fig. 1.2).

Any meningeal infection can lead to labyrinthitis or any labyrinthitis can lead to meningitis through these connections between inner ear and cranium.

APLASIA/DYSPLASIAS OF THE INNER EAR

During development there can be certain anomalies of the inner ear, these are:

- **Scheibe's dysplasia:** This is the most common anomaly of the inner ear. It involves dysplasia of the saccule and cochlea, hence it is also known as cochleosaccular dysplasia. It can be managed with cochlear implantation.
- **Mondini's dysplasia:** Here the cochlea has only **1.5 turns**. Hearing rehabilitation with **cochlear implantation can** also **be done** here.
- **Alexander's dysplasia:** It involves deformity of the basal turn of cochlea. High frequency sound is therefore affected here. Again, it can be managed with cochlear implantation.
- **Michel aplasia:** Here there is complete nondevelopment of both bony and membranous labyrinth and the vestibulocochlear nerve. Therefore, cochlear implantation cannot be done here. Michel aplasia is an **absolute contraindication** to do cochlear implantation.

Superior Semicircular Canal Dehiscence (SSCD)

A congenital anomaly involving the bony labyrinth is superior semicircular canal dehiscence.

The bulge of superior semicircular canal is present on the anterior slant of petrous part of temporal bone in the base of skull and is known as **arcuate eminence**. Superior semicircular canal dehiscence is a rare condition where the bone between the Superior semicircular canal and brain area is missing or thin.

This leads to the formation of a 3rd mobile window in the inner ear (the other two being the round and oval window). This SSCD faces the middle cranial fossa.

This dehiscence leads to exposure of inner ear to changes in intracranial pressure as well as external pressure causing symptoms very similar to that of a round or oval window fistula.

For further details *see* Chapter 12 on Meniere's disease and disorders of vestibular system.

🤔 **"For Quick revision"**

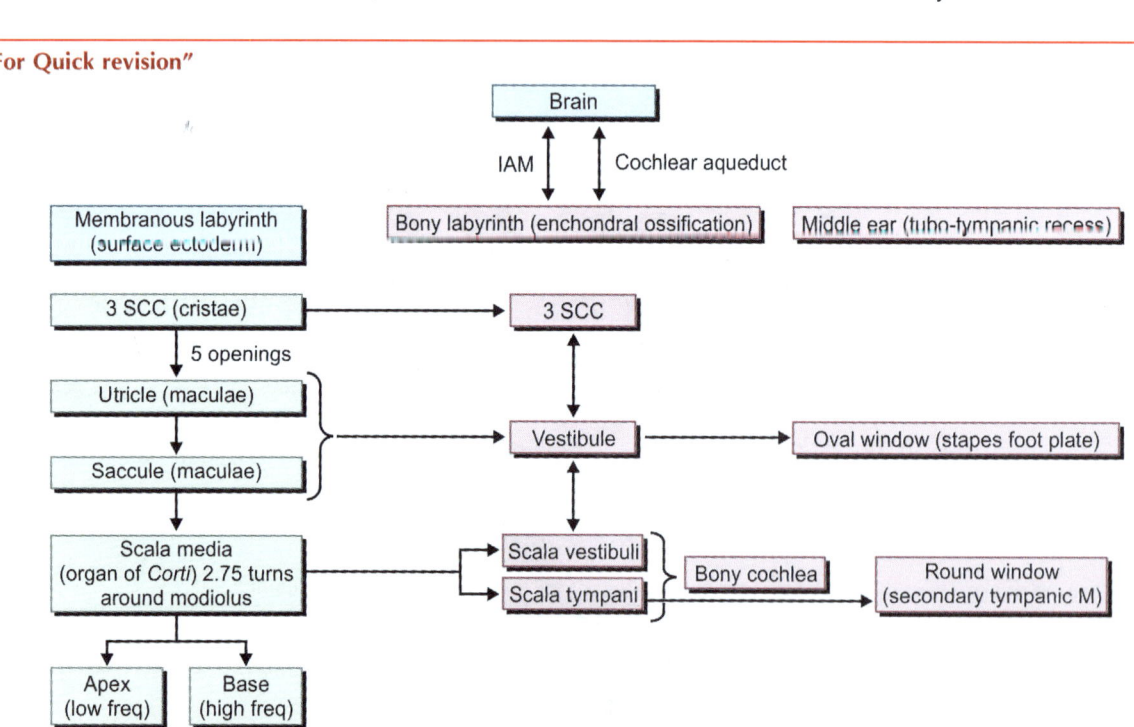

ANATOMY OF EAR

PINNA (AURICLE)

The pinna is made up of a **single** elastic fibrocartilage (formed by the fusion of the "HILLOCKS of HIS").

The Various Parts of Pinna or Auricle are (Fig. 1.12):

Tragus, helix, and lobule—these are the structures at the boundary. Anterior to the helix is the prominence of ante-helix. Just behind the tragus is the opening of external auditory canal (EAC), also called external acoustic meatus (EAM). Just behind the EAM, the part of pinna is called concha. The concha extends anteriorly and superiorly into an area which is called cymba conchae.

The **cymba conchae** is the cartilaginous landmark for mastoid antrum.

Medial to the cymba conchae (on the mastoid process), is a bony landmark for mastoid antrum called "**Macewen's**" **triangle** or suprameatal triangle.

The boundaries of Macewen's triangle are (see Fig. 1.13) superiorly temporal line/supra mastoid crest, anteriorly posterosuperior segment of bony external auditory canal or post-auricular groove and postero-inferiorly by a tangent drawn to meet the above two lines.

- Just anterior to the Macewen's triangle on the mastoid bone is a projection known as **spine of Henle**, which is seen during surgery. It acts as another important bony landmark of mastoid antrum.

These landmarks are important while doing mastoid surgeries in approaching the mastoid antrum.

This is because any other approach to mastoid antrum can be dangerous because mastoid is surrounded all around by important structures (mentioned below) which can be damaged during mastoid surgeries.

Superiorly is the bone separating mastoid from middle cranial fossa; posteriorly is the bone separating mastoid

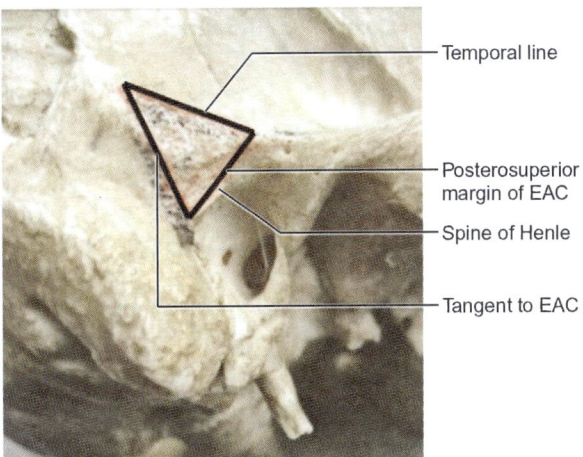

Fig. 1.13: Boundaries of Macewen's triangle

from sigmoid sinus. Inferiorly lies the facial nerve just below the mastoid tip.

- Between the tragus and the ascending crus of helix is an inter-cartilaginous area which is devoid of cartilage (see the development of Pinna, Tragus and adjacent part of helix develops from the 1st arch and rest of the Pinna by 2nd arch). This is called "**INCISURA TERMINALIS**". This is the site where incision is made in "**ENDAURAL**" approach (an approach to tympanic membrane and middle ear through the external acoustic meatus) for various ear surgeries.

- The skin on the lateral side of pinna is more tightly adherent to underlying perichondrium than on medial side, where it is loose. Therefore any condition of the pinna (perichondritis, furuncle, etc.) on its lateral side is more painful than on the medial side.

- The tragal and conchal cartilage can be used for reconstructive surgeries of middle ear (tympanoplasty) and nose (augmentation rhinoplasty for depressed nasal bridge).

EXTERNAL AUDITORY CANAL (EAC)

The EAC in adults is S-shaped and is **24 mm** long. It has 2 parts (see Fig. 1.14):

1. **Cartilaginous part:** This is the **outer 1/3rd,** i.e. **8 mm** long (easy to remember the part of EAC adjoining the cartilaginous pinna is cartilaginous).

At birth, only the cartilaginous part of EAC is completely developed; the bony part of EAC continues to grow after birth. So in comparison to adults the EAC is straight and short in children. In adults the cartilaginous part of EAC courses **upwards, backwards and medially**.

- The skin in this cartilaginous EAC is thick and contains hair follicles, therefore a furuncle is localised only to the cartilaginous part of EAC.

- The skin in this cartilaginous EAC also contains ceruminous glands which are the modified sweat (apocrine) glands so wax is produced in this portion of EAC.

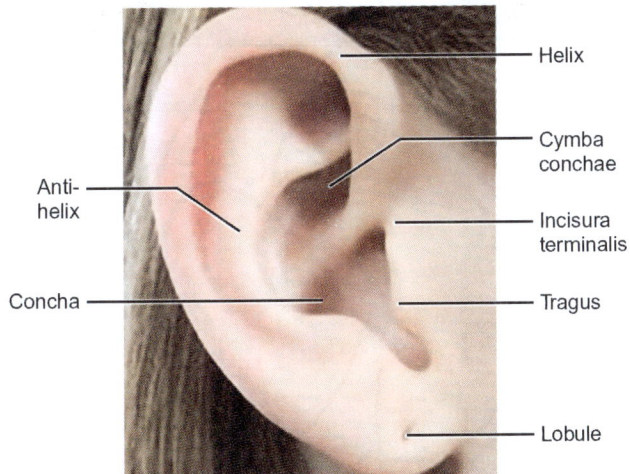

Fig. 1.12: Parts of Pinna

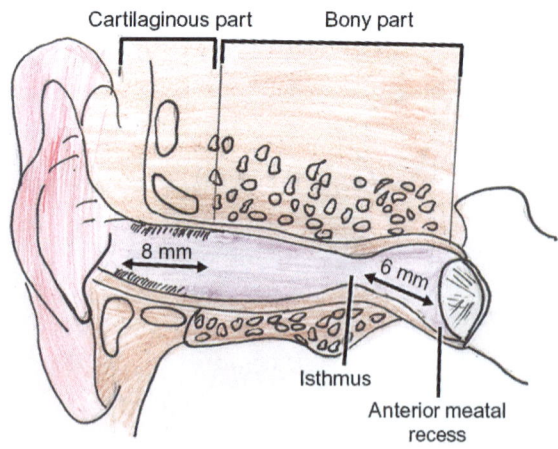

Fig. 1.14: External auditory canal anatomy

- In the antero-inferior part of this cartilaginous portion are deficiencies known as **"fissures of SANTORINI"**.

Through these fissures of Santorini, the EAC communicates with parotid. So parotid infection can track through these fissures and can involve the EAC. Similarly infection in the canal may lead to involvement of parotid.

2. **Bony part:** This is the **inner 2/3rd** portion (i.e. **16 mm** long) of the EAC. This part is not completely developed at birth. This is lined by thin skin which is devoid of hair follicles and ceruminous glands. In adults the bony part of EAC courses downwards, forwards (in contrast to the cartilaginous part which was upwards and backwards, *see* above) and medially. Therefore to see the TM in adults, we have to pull the pinna upwards, backwards and laterally so that the cartilaginous and the bony parts of EAC come in straight line.

   - The narrowest part of EAC called **isthmus** is situated in this bony portion. The isthmus is situated 5 mm lateral to the tympanic membrane.
   - Foreign bodies lodged medial to the isthmus, get impacted and are therefore difficult to remove.

After the narrowing at isthmus, there is a dilatation.

This dilatation in the floor of EAC is called **anterior meatal recess**. Any discharge through middle ear tends to collect in this anterior meatal recess. It is a difficult to access area.

   - Like the cartilaginous portion, the bony part of EAC in the antero-inferior aspect also has a deficiency which is called as **"foramen of HUSCHKE"**. This foramen of Huschke also permits infections to and from the parotid.
   - The bony-cartilaginous junction, fissures of Santorini and foramen of HUSCHKE are the potential paths for the spread of infections and tumours from EAC to the base of skull and parotid.

TYMPANIC MEMBRANE

- The tympanic membrane is present at an angle of **55 degrees** with horizontal. The longest diameter of TM is 10 mm and its shortest diameter is 9 mm.

The approximate **surface area of TM is 90 mm²**. But **the effective vibratory area** of TM is only approx. **55 mm²** (easy to remember same as the angle of TM).

- It is obliquely set; therefore its postero-superior part is more lateral than antero-inferior part which is medial. This orientation makes the posterior part of EAC shorter than its anterior part and also the posterior part of TM more accessible through the EAC.
- The tympanic membrane is **pearly grey** in colour and is translucent.
- The tympanic membrane develops from all the **3 embryonic layers,** therefore, it has an outer epithelial layer in continuation with the epithelium of bony EAC, a middle fibrous layer and an inner mucosal layer in continuation with the lining of middle ear cavity.

The tympanic membrane (TM) is divided into two parts, a lower "pars tensa" and an upper "pars flaccida" (Fig. 1.15).

Pars Tensa

This is so called because it is firm and tense. This is because in its periphery/rim the fibrous layer coalesces to form a fibrous annulus which fits tightly into the surrounding tympanic sulcus, thus tightly anchoring the pars tensa to the surrounding bone. It forms lower 2/3rd of the TM.

In the centre of the TM is attached the tip of the handle of malleus leading to central tenting (the cone of this tent points towards the middle ear contributing to narrowing

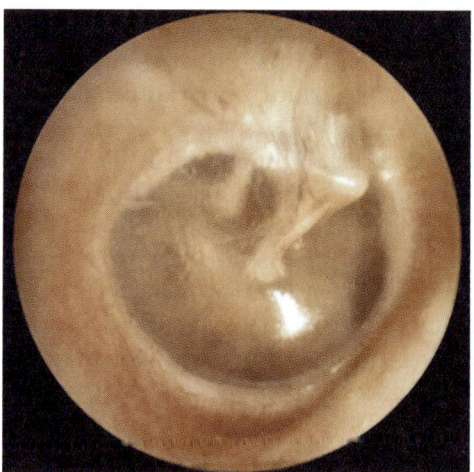

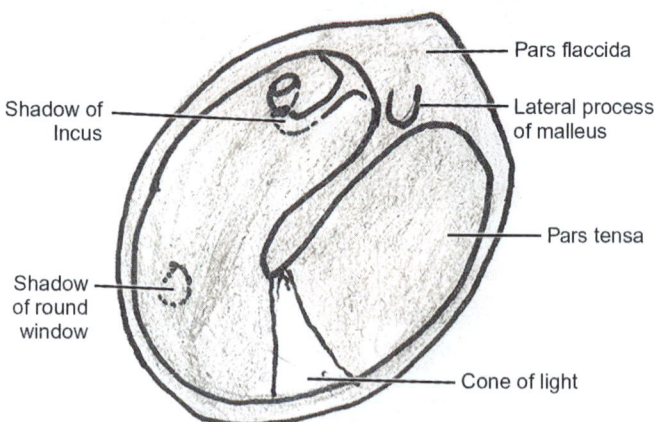

Fig. 1.15: Right tympanic membrane

of the middle ear at mesotympanum (please read below the anatomy of middle ear). This central tented part of TM is called **"UMBO"**. Since the TM is fixed at the centre (where it attaches to the tip of handle of malleus) as well as the annulus, therefore the **paramedian portion of the TM** (on either side of malleus) **is most mobile.**

A **cone of light** extends from the umbo to the periphery of pars tensa in the antero-inferior quadrant. This is the reflection of the handle of malleus due to the obliquity of the tympanic membrane. In right TM the cone of light is on the right side and in left TM, it is on the left side (as shown in Fig. 1. 15). This helps in the identification of the TM drawing.

Pars Flaccida

This is so called because it is loose or flaccid, as the middle fibrous layer here contains more loosely arranged collagen fibrils.

The fibro cartilaginous ring, i.e. the tympanic annulus is deficient superiorly. This deficient area is known as the notch of Rivinus. This notch of Rivinus is the upper attachment of pars flaccida.

Pars flaccida is also known as "**SHRAPNELL'S Membrane"**.

The pars flaccida being flaccid therefore it is more susceptible to retraction whenever pressure in the middle ear cavity becomes negative due to Eustachian tube blockade.

Hence pars flaccida is the most common site of **retraction pocket formation** leading to **primary cholesteatoma** formation (*see* Chapter on unsafe CSOM).

NERVE SUPPLY OF THE EXTERNAL EAR

Pinna or Auricle

The pinna is supplied by the **G**reater auricular nerve, **l**esser **O**ccipital nerve, **A**uriculotemporal nerve and **A**uricular branch of vagus (this is also called **A**rnold's or Alderman's nerve). It also receives some fibres from the facial nerve. Mnemonic to remember the nerve supply of pinna-**G O A A** (*see* Fig. 1.16).

1. Greater auricular nerve (C2, 3) supplies most of the pinna. On the lateral side it supplies the lobule, posterior aspect of helix and ante-helix. It supplies

most of the medial surface except the upper part and the post-auricular groove.

2. Lesser **O**ccipital (C2) supplies only the upper part of the medial surface.

3. **A**uriculotemporal, a sensory branch of the mandibular division of the trigeminal nerve (i.e. V3), supplies tragus and ascending crus of helix and some area of cymba conchae.

4. **A**uricular branch of vagus (X), also called Arnold's nerve supplies the concha on the lateral surface and the postauricular groove medially.

5. Facial nerve (VII) also supplies the concha and the post-auricular groove along with the auricular branch of Vagus.

External Auditory Canal (EAC)

As can be anticipated three nerves supplying the pinna, supply the EAC (the last two As of GO**AA** along with facial nerve).

1. **A**uriculotemporal (V3) supplying the tragus continues inwards to supply the anterior wall and roof of the EAC.

2. and 3. **A**uricular branch of Vagus **(Arnold's nerve)** and Facial nerve supplying the concha continues inwards to supply the posterior wall and floor of the EAC. The cough response caused while cleaning the ear canal is mediated by the vagus which also supplies the larynx.

Tympanic Membrane (TM)

The nerves supplying the external auditory canal supply the lateral surface of tympanic membrane and the nerves supplying the middle ear supply the medial surface of tympanic membrane.

Hence the **nerve supply of the tympanic membrane** is as follows:

1. **Auriculotemporal (V3)** supplying the anterior wall of EAC supply the anterior half of the lateral surface of the TM.

2. **Auricular branch of Vagus (X)** supplying the posterior wall of EAC supplies the posterior half of the TM. Please note: On the TM, Facial nerve does not accompany the Vagus.

3. **Glossopharyngeal (IX):** Tympanic branch of Glossopharyngeal also called Jacobson's nerve, is the sensory nerve of whole of the middle ear (please read Middle ear). Therefore, it supplies the medial aspect of the TM.

Therefore, pain in the ear can be either because of direct involvement of external ear or middle ear or referred pain from the other territories of supply of any of the above nerves.

Pain referred to the ear from:	The common nerve, responsible
TM joint and dental conditions	Auriculotemporal (V₃)
Acute tonsillitis, peritonsillar abscess and carcinoma base of tongue	Glossopharyngeal (IX)
Carcinomas of the larynx and hypopharynx	Vagus (X)

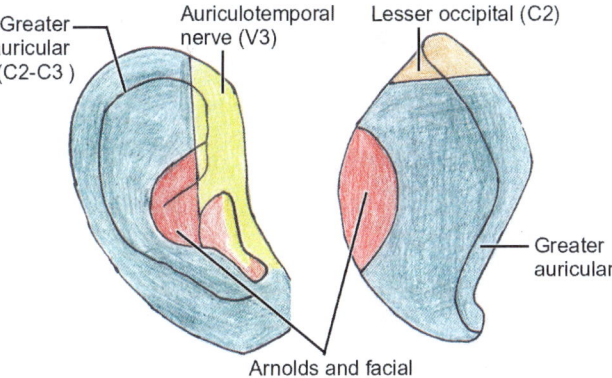

Fig. 1.16: Nerve supply of Pinna (Lateral and Medial surface)

MIDDLE EAR

The middle ear can be assumed to be like a cuboid and therefore has six walls (*see* Fig. 1.17).

1. **Lateral wall:** This is the common wall between external auditory canal and middle ear. This is formed by **tympanic membrane (TM) below and scutum above**. The scutum is the bone above the pars flaccida forming the lateral wall of attic (the attic is the upper part of the middle ear cavity), *see* Fig. 1.18.

2. **Medial wall:** This is the common wall between middle ear and inner ear. The six important structures on this medial wall are:

    i. **Promontory:** This is a bulge in the centre of the medial wall, produced by the **basal turn of cochlea**. On the promontory, tympanic plexus is present (please read below).

    ii. **Processus Cochleariformis:** This is a hook like structure present antero-superiorly on the medial wall. It has the following two significance:

    a. The **tensor tympani** muscle originates from a canal in the anterior wall of middle ear. It then runs medially where its tendon winds around the processus cochleariformis and then turns laterally to get attached to the malleus (just below its neck).

    b. It acts as a **landmark for the first genu** (or turn) of facial nerve. The first genu of facial nerve lies above the processus cochleariformis.

    The facial nerve enters the inner ear through the internal acoustic meatus. After running through the inner ear it enters the middle ear on its medial wall.

Here it takes a turn called the 1st genu and continues horizontally backwards towards the posterior wall of middle ear as the horizontal or tympanic segment. The geniculate ganglion is situated at the first genu. Please also *see* the chapter on facial nerve.

   iii. **Bulge of lateral semicircular canal:** The bulge of lateral/horizontal canal is present on the most posterosuperior portion of the medial wall just above the horizontal or tympanic segment of facial nerve.

   iv. **Oval window:** This lies postero-superiorly on the medial wall, with foot process of stapes overlying it, separating the vestibule from the middle ear. The oval window lies inferior to the horizontal or tympanic segment of facial nerve.

   The bulge of lateral semicircular canal and oval window are important landmarks of the tympanic segment of facial nerve. The tympanic segment of facial nerve runs horizontally in the posterior direction on the medial wall between the bulge of lateral semicircular canal (lying above) and oval window (lying below it).

   v. **Round window:** This lies postero-inferiorly on the medial wall. This is covered by secondary tympanic membrane, separating the middle ear from the scala tympani. See the importance of round window above in the embryology section.

   vi. **Facial nerve:** The facial nerve coming from the inner ear enters the middle ear on its medial wall where it takes a turn called as the 1st genu. It then

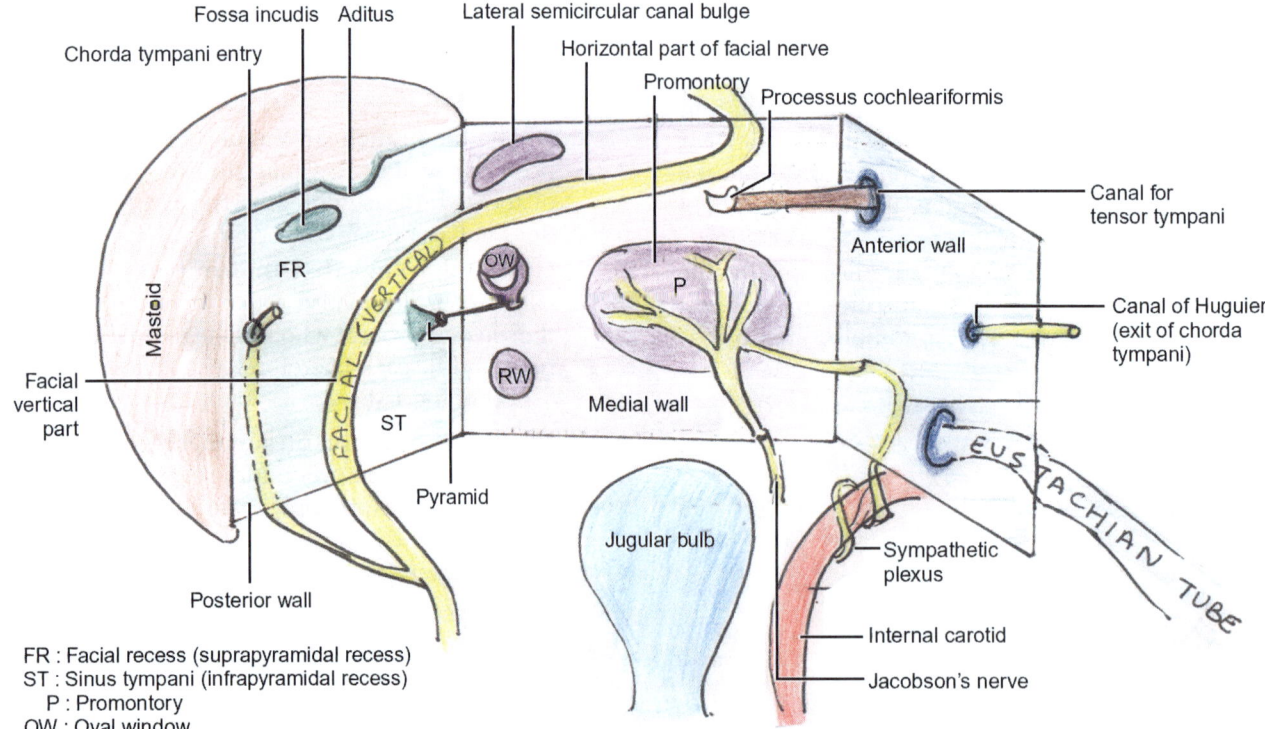

FR : Facial recess (suprapyramidal recess)
ST : Sinus tympani (infrapyramidal recess)
 P : Promontory
OW : Oval window
RW : Round window

Fig. 1.17: Walls of middle ear

continues horizontally backwards towards the posterior wall as the horizontal or tympanic segment. The processus cochleariformis, bulge of lateral semicircular canal and oval window are its important landmarks on the medial wall, as discussed above.

3. **Posterior wall:** This is the common wall between middle ear and mastoid. The seven important structures on this posterior wall are:

   i. **Aditus:** On the upper border of this wall there is an opening known as aditus which connects the attic (the attic is the upper part of the middle ear cavity) to the mastoid antrum.

   ii. **Pyramid:** It is a projection on the posterior wall from which originates the **stapedius muscle**. The stapedius attaches to the neck of stapes. The stapedius muscle, like the suprastructure of stapes, is a second arch derivative and therefore is supplied by the nerve of the 2nd arch, i.e. facial nerve. It mediates an important protecting reflex known as **stapedial reflex**. This reflex protects the inner ear from loud noise. Please refer to chapter on audiometry.

   iii. **Facial nerve:** At the junction of medial and posterior wall, the **tympanic or horizontal segment** of facial nerve takes a lateral turn onto the posterior wall known as the 2nd genu. It then descends vertically down behind the pyramid and here it is named as vertical or descending or mastoid segment of facial nerve.

   iv. **Sinus tympani/Infra pyramidal recess:** It is the area medial to the bulge of vertical/descending or mastoid part of facial nerve bounded above by ponticulus and below by subiculum. The ponticulus and subiculum are respectively the upper and lower bony ridges extending from the promontory to the posterior wall.

   Sinus tympani is considered as the **hidden area** of the middle ear. It is the most common site for residual cholesteatoma, *see* chapter on unsafe CSOM.

   v. **Chorda tympani nerve entry:** The vertical or descending part of facial nerve in the posterior wall of middle ear, i.e. in the mastoid portion of temporal bone ultimately exits the temporal bone through the stylomastoid foramen. Just 4–6 mm before its exit, it gives the chorda tympani nerve which then ascends up and enters the middle ear cavity through an opening on the posterior wall. Passing between the fibrous and mucosal layers of TM, the chorda tympani then runs in between the neck of malleus and the body of incus in the attic (or epitympanum, i.e. the upper part of middle ear cavity, *see* below). It then ultimately exits the middle ear cavity through the **canal of "HUGUIER"** present in the anterior wall of middle ear (*mnemonic*—since chorda is leaving the middle ear it's been given a HUG-here). The chorda tympani

gives taste sensations to the anterior 2/3rd of the tongue.

   vi. **Fossa incudis:** It is a fossa on the posterior wall on which rests the short process of incus.

   vii. **Facial recess/Supra pyramidal recess:** This is an area on the lateral side of the vertical or descending segment of the facial nerve, i.e. on the other side of sinus tympani. The facial recess is limited **superiorly** by the fossa incudis, **laterally** by chorda tympani entry and **medially** by the descending facial nerve segment.

   The surgical importance of facial recess is that, it is the site where opening is made on the posterior wall to access the middle ear cavity through the mastoid, e.g. in **"INTACT CANAL WALL"** surgeries of the ear. Also the **electrodes of cochlear implant** are introduced into the middle ear from the mastoid through the facial recess. This approach of the middle ear through its posterior wall is known as the **posterior tympanotomy approach**, see chapter on unsafe CSOM.

4. **Anterior wall:** It is a thin plate of bone separating the middle ear from **internal carotid** artery. The four important structures on this wall are:

   I. **Opening of Eustachian or pharyngo-tympanic tube:** The Eustachian tube connects the middle ear cavity with the nasopharynx. From the anterior wall of the middle ear cavity starts its **bony part,** which forms the **lateral 1/3rd**, following which the **medial 2/3rd** is **fibro-cartilaginous** (easy to remember the lateral part being in continuation with bony middle ear cavity, is bony). The fibro-cartilaginous portion of the ET is surrounded by a collection of adipose tissue known as ostmann fat pad (read Chapter 6 for the clinical importance of Ostmann pad of fat).

   The fibro-cartilaginous nasopharyngeal opening is present 1–1.25 cm behind and a little below the posterior end of inferior turbinate.

   The length of Eustachian tube is about 36 mm (32–38 mm) out of which the bony part is 12 mm and the cartilaginous part is 24 mm. The narrowest part of Eustachian tube is the junction of the bony and cartilaginous parts and is known as **isthmus**.

   The Eustachian tube is at an angle of 45° with the horizontal.

   The length of Eustachian tube at birth is approximately half the length of adults, i.e. around 13–18 mm. It reaches adult size by 7 years of age. The Eustachian tube in children is wider, shorter, more horizontal and flaccid (containing less of elastin) making children prone to retrograde reflux of nasopharyngeal secretions into the middle ear and thereby increased frequency of nasopharyngeal infections reaching the middle ear. Also the Eustachian tube ventilatory function is less efficient in children than in adults.

Section I Ear

External auditory canal	Eustachian tube
2/3rd part is bony and 1/3rd part is cartilaginous	1/3rd part is bony and 2/3rd part is cartilaginous
Lateral 1/3rd is cartilaginous in continuation with the cartilaginous pinna	Lateral 1/3rd is bony in continuation with the bony middle ear cavity
Total length 24 mm (cartilaginous part 8 mm and bony part 16 mm)	Total length 36 mm (12 mm bony and 24 mm cartilaginous)
Narrowest part (isthmus) is situated in the bony part 6 mm lateral to the TM	Narrowest part (isthmus) is the junction of bony and cartilaginous parts

Eustachian tube normally remains closed and opens intermittently during swallowing, yawning and sneezing. **Tensor palati** plays the major role in opening the tube.

Normally the Eustachian tube opens frequently, stably maintaining the middle ear pressure between +50 mm and –50 mm H_2O.

II. **Canal for origin of tensor tympani muscle:** Tensor tympani originates from a canal in the anterior wall of middle ear. As discussed above, it then runs medially where its tendon winds around the processus cochleariformis and then turns laterally to get attached on the upper part of the handle of malleus (i.e. just below its neck).

The **tensor tympani** muscle like malleus is a **derivative of 1st arch** and is **supplied by** the nerve of the 1st arch, i.e. **mandibular nerve** (through its **anterior or motor branch**).

In response to loud noises, the tensor tympani contracts pulling the neck of malleus medially, thereby decrease the sound conduction, though in this regard the stapedius muscle is more important.

III. **The canal of Huguier:** As stated previously this is the exit site for chorda tympani from middle ear.

IV. **Petro-tympanic fissure (Glaserian fissure):** This is the site of attachment of anterior ligament of malleus and the site for entry of anterior tympanic artery. Sometimes the canal of Huguier opens in the petro-tympanic fissure.

5. **Roof:** The roof of the middle ear is known as "TEGMEN TYMPANI". It contributes to the anterior slant of the petrous part of the temporal bone and separates the middle ear from the middle cranial fossa (temporal lobe), *see* Fig. 1.18 below.

6. **Floor:** It is a thin plate of bone separating the middle ear from the **jugular bulb** along with the 9th and 10th cranial nerves.

The tympanic segment of glossopharyngeal nerve (also known as **"JACOBSON'S NERVE"** enters the middle ear through floor and along with sympathetic plexus (coming into the middle ear from around the internal carotid artery) forms tympanic plexus on the promontory (*see* Fig. 1.17).

This tympanic plexus gives sensory nerve supply to whole of the middle ear cavity, Eustachian tube and medial surface of the tympanic membrane.

MIDDLE EAR CAVITY

The middle ear cavity is divided into 3 parts (*see* Fig. 1.18) by lines drawn from the upper and lower borders of pars tensa. These are:

i. **Epitympanum or Attic:** As the name it is the uppermost part of the middle ear cavity. This is the **widest** part of the middle ear cavity. It lies medial to pars flaccida below and scutum above. It has a width of 6 mm. As can be seen in Fig. 1.18, the **epitympanum contains** the head, neck, anterior and lateral process of malleus and the body and short process of incus (the head of malleus articulates with the body of incus). This **incudomalleolar joint** is a **saddle type** of **synovial joint**. The Chorda tympani nerve (branch of facial carrying taste sensations from anterior 2/3 of tongue) passing in between the neck of malleus and the body of incus also lies in the epitympanum. The space of the epitympanum, lying in between the Shrapnell's membrane or pars flaccida and the neck of malleus is known as "**PRUSSAK'S SPACE**". When a retraction pocket on Pars flaccida (leading to the formation of primary cholesteatoma, *see* chapter on unsafe CSOM) grows medially, it goes into this Prussak's space making this the most common site of primary cholesteatoma.

ii. **Mesotympanum:** As the name it is the middle part of the middle ear cavity. This is the **narrowest** part of middle ear due to the constrictions caused by umbo laterally and promontory medially. The distance between the TM (UMBO) and promontory is **2 mm**.

Mesotympanum contains the handle of malleus, the long process of incus ending in lentiform nodule which articulates with the head of stapes and the whole of the stapes (the head, neck, anterior and posterior crura and footplate). This **incudostapedial joint** is a **ball and socket** type of **synovial joint**.

iii. **Hypotympanum:** This is the lower compartment of middle ear cavity.

It is the **smallest part** of middle ear cavity. It has a width of 4 mm.

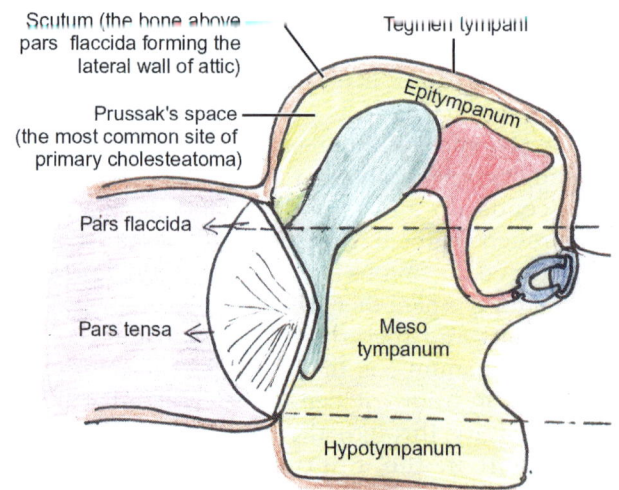

Fig. 1.18: Parts of Middle Ear Cavity

MASTOID

Posterior to the middle ear cavity is the mastoid. The mastoid is a **pneumatic** bone which encloses numerous air cell spaces giving it a honeycomb appearance.

The largest and most prominent air cell is called the mastoid antrum.

Boundaries of Mastoid Antrum
(*see* Figs 1.20 and 1.21)

- **Superiorly** is the base of skull, also known as tegmen antri, which separates it from the dura overlying, the temporal lobe in the middle cranial fossa. Hence tegmen antri is also called as **dural plate**.
- Posteriorly is the base of skull which separates it from the sigmoid sinus (**sinus plate**).

  The sinodural angle formed in between the dural plate superiorly and the sinus plate posteriorly is known as **Citelli's angle**. It is the position where

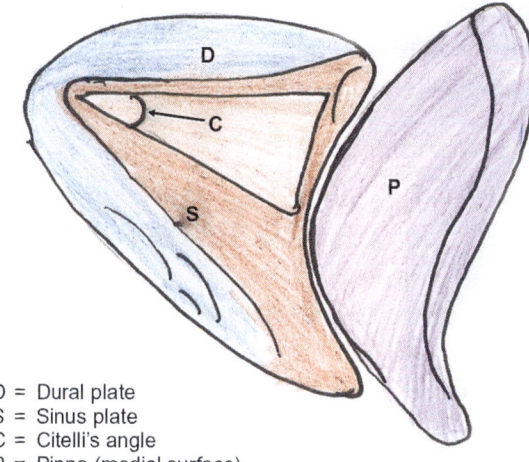

D = Dural plate
S = Sinus plate
C = Citelli's angle
P = Pinna (medial surface)

Fig. 1.21: Showing Citelli's angle

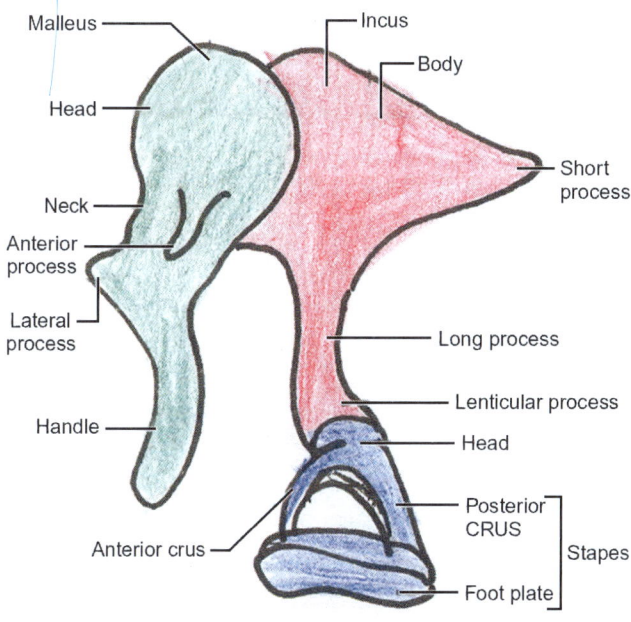

Fig. 1.19: Ossicles and their parts

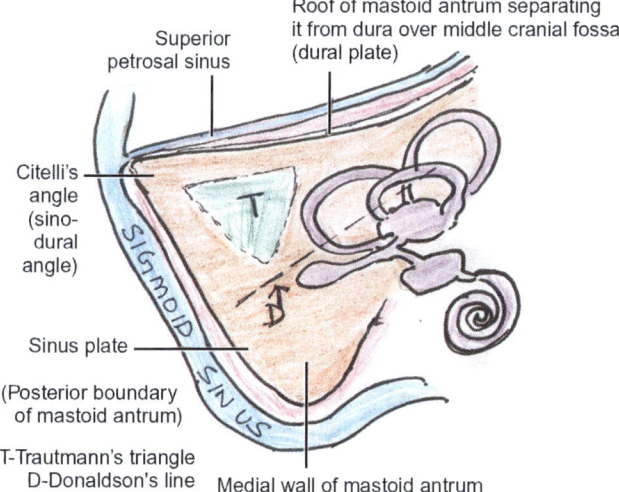

Fig. 1.20: Medial wall of mastoid antrum

superior petrosal sinus enters the sigmoid sinus (superior petrosal sinus joins the sigmoid sinus with cavernous sinus).

- **Medially:** The medial wall of mastoid antrum is related superiorly to the posterior semicircular canal and inferiorly to the base of skull separating it from the endolymphatic sac and posterior cranial fossa.

  The surgical landmark of endolymphatic sac on this wall is an imaginary line, drawn from the lateral semicircular canal bisecting the posterior semicircular canal, known as **"Donaldson's line"**.

  The endolymphatic sac lies inferior to this Donaldson's line, *see* Fig. 1.20.

  A triangular area on the medial wall of mastoid antrum, bounded superiorly by the superior petrosal sinus, posteriorly by the sigmoid sinus and anteriorly by the bony labyrinth is used as a landmark to approach the posterior cranial fossa. This triangular area is known as **Trautmann's triangle**. Since the bone in this area is relatively thin, it is also a potential site for spread of infections from the mastoid to the cerebellum.

- Laterally the antrum is anatomically marked by the **Macewen's triangle** or suprameatal triangle on the outer surface of the skull. The antrum lies approximately 1.5 cm deep to Macewen's triangle (please refer to the development of mastoid and the anatomy of pinna for these landmarks).

- **Anteriorly** the antrum is bounded by the posterior wall of middle ear. The antrum is connected to the attic (epitympanum) through the aditus on the posterior wall of middle ear (please refer to the middle ear anatomy).

Besides antrum, the various other mastoid air cells are also named. These are named according to their anatomical site in the temporal bone. These are:

a. Zygomatic cells (in the zygomatic root)
b. Tegmen cells (in the roof)
c. Perisinus cells (on the sinus plate)
d. Marginal cells (behind the sinus plate)
e. Tip cells (in the mastoid tip)

f. Retrofacial cells (around the facial nerve)

g. Peri-labyrinthine cells (around the labyrinth)

h. Squamosal cells (in the squamous part of temporal bone)

INNER EAR ANATOMY

Most of the anatomy of the inner ear has already been discussed in the section of the embryology of inner ear (*see* Fig 1.22).

Structure of Scala Media

Membranous cochlea or Scala media or cochlear duct is a coiled tube, coiling over a bony axis which is known as "**modiolus**". It takes **2 and 1/2 to 2 and 3/4 turns** around the modiolus.

Osseous spiral lamina or ligament is a bony canal running spirally around the modiolus, within the lumen of the membranous cochlea. Inside this bony spiral lamina is the "**Rosenthal canal**" which contains the 8th nerve ganglion known as the **spiral ganglion**.

The Scala media or cochlear duct is triangular in cross section (*see* Fig. 1.22) and is bounded by:

1. *Basilar membrane:* It separates Scala media or cochlear duct from Scala tympani. The organ of Corti rests on the basilar membrane.
2. *Reissner's membrane:* It separates Scala media from Scala vestibuli.
3. *Stria vascularis:* It is the site for the **production of endolymph**. It plays an important role in cochlear homeostasis by generating the endocochlear potential and maintaining the ionic composition of endolymph.

It contains $Na^+ K^+ 2 Cl^-$ channel (the same channel is present in the loop of Henle in the nephronic tubule on which act the loop diuretics) which is responsible for making the endolymph rich in K^+ leading to the development of an **endolymphatic potential** of + 80 to + 85 mV. As discussed above, in comparison to endolymph the perilymph is rich in Na^+. The Bartter's syndrome (an inherited tubulointerstitial disease of the kidney) is characterised by mutation of the $Na^+ K^+ 2 Cl^-$ channel and as a result one of the manifestations in Bartter's is sensorineural deafness.

Structure of Organ of Corti (*see* Fig. 1.22)

1. **Hair cells:** there are two types of hair cells in the organ of Corti, the inner and the outer hair cells. The hairs of the inner and outer hair cells project into a membrane which is known as **Tectorial membrane**.
2. **Supporting cells:** these support the outer hair cells. They are named as cells of Dieters, Claudius and Hensen (*mnemonic*—DCH).
3. **Tunnel of Corti:** It is formed by the inner and outer rods and contains a fluid called cortilymph.

Difference between inner and outer hair cells of organ of Corti	
Inner hair cell	*Outer hair cell*
These are arranged in a single row, therefore	These are arranged in 3–4 rows, therefore
These are less in number These are more resistant to noise trauma and ototoxic drugs (easy to remember, body's defence strategy-inner cells being less in number so more resistant)	These are much more in number These are less resistant to noise trauma and ototoxic drugs
Nerve supply–mainly afferent	Nerve supply–mainly efferent
Therefore their function is to transmit auditory stimuli	They modulate the function of inner hair cells and generate oto-acoustic emissions (easy to remember outer-oto)

Auditory Pathway

Inner hair cells → afferent nerves which fuse to form the Cochlear nerve → spiral ganglion (this is the cochlear nerve ganglion present in Rosenthal canal inside spiral lamina) → Cochlear nerve exits through the internal acoustic meatus (here it is inferior to the facial nerve–please see below) → dorsal and ventral cochlear nuclei (in the pons).

The mnemonic of further auditory tract is **S L I M.**

From the cochlear nuclei, the fibres go to both ipsilateral and contralateral **S**uperior Olivary complex (S) (the crossing to the contralateral superior olivary complex occurs through "TRAPEZOID Body" → **L**ateral lemniscus (L) → **I**nferior Colliculus (I) → **M**edial geniculate body (M)).

From medial geniculate body, the auditory fibres pass through the **posterior limb of internal capsule to**

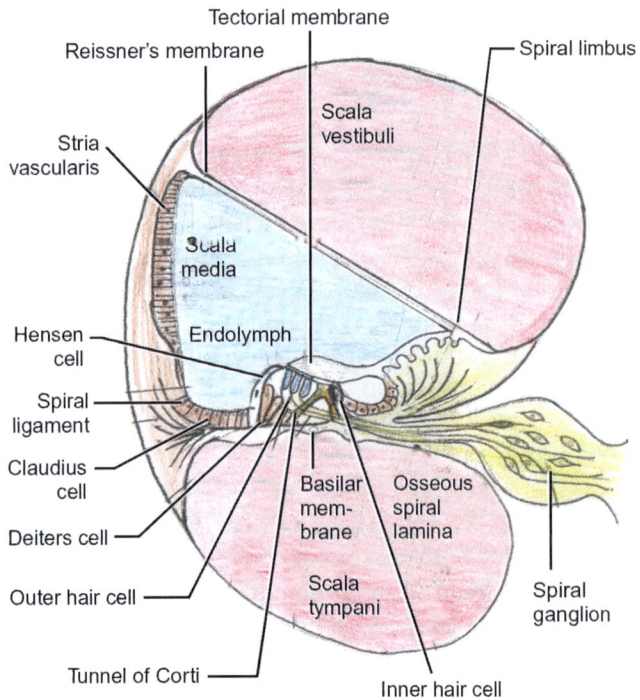

Fig. 1.22

Labels in figure:
- Tectorial membrane
- Reissner's membrane
- Spiral limbus
- Scala vestibuli
- Stria vascularis
- Scala media
- Hensen cell
- Endolymph
- Spiral ligament
- Claudius cell
- Deiters cell
- Basilar membrane
- Osseous spiral lamina
- Outer hair cell
- Scala tympani
- Spiral ganglion
- Tunnel of Corti
- Inner hair cell

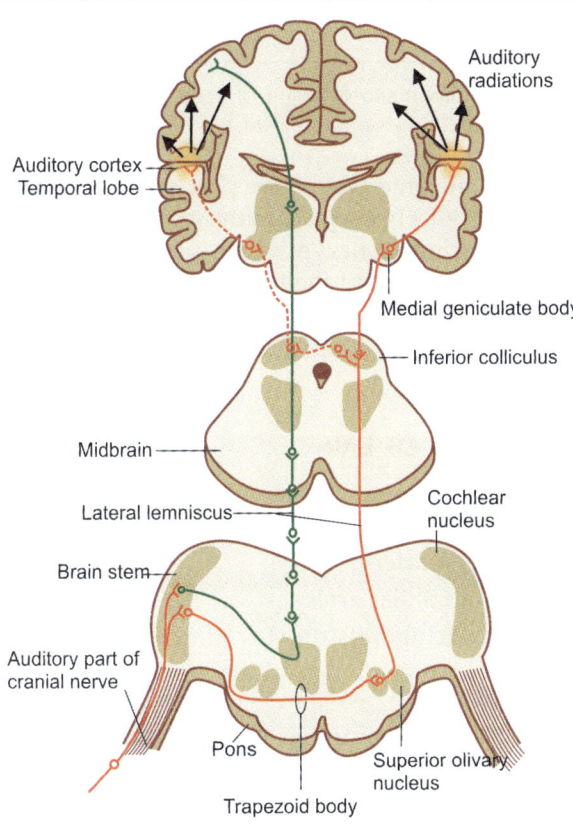

Fig. 1.23: Auditory pathways

Note:

Hair cells in the Organ of Corti, in the Cristae and in the Maculae have cilia emerging from their apical surfaces. There are tiny thread-like connections from the tip of each cilium to non-specific cation channels on the side of the neighbouring cilium. These connections called **"The tip links"** open these channels mechanically due to the **distortion effect** caused by cilliary movement. This then leads to an influx of potassium.

An inward K^+ current then opens voltage-dependent calcium channels. This in turn causes neurotransmitter **(glutamate)** release at the basal end of the hair cell, eliciting an action potential in the dendrites of the VIIIth cranial nerve.

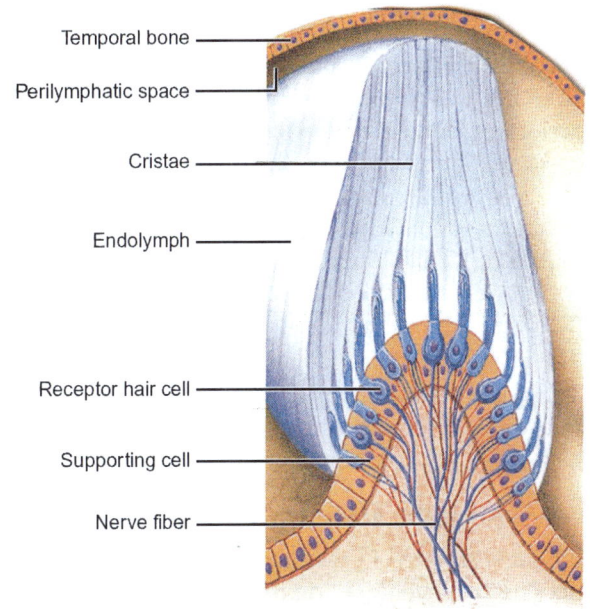

Fig. 1.24: Cristae

transverse temporal gyrus (Auditory cortex- Broadmann area no 41). **Appreciation of sound occurs in the transverse temporal gyrus which is a part of superior temporal gyrus.**

The auditory pathway of both the sides have multiple interconnections because of which sound, even if heard from one ear, is perceived by both the cerebral hemispheres.

There are also interconnections at **superior olivary complex with facial nerve mediating stapedial reflex** (please refer to the audiology section).

The auditory pathways and the **higher auditory centre is responsible mainly for sound localisation and selective listening,** i.e. allowing an individual to listen to one channel of information while blocking out sounds in other competing channels (as hearing in noisy environment).

Structure of Cristae

These are the rotational or angular acceleration sensing structures inside the semi-circular canals.

The cristae contain type 1 and type 2 hair cells which project into a gelatinous matrix known as "**CUPULA**". *See* Fig. 1.24.

Structure of Maculae

These are the linear acceleration sensing structures (*see* above in the embryology section) present in the utricle and saccule. Here again there are two types of hair cells, **type 1 and type 2**. The cilia of these hair cells project into a gelatinous matrix which is covered by calcium carbonate crystals on its top. *See* Fig. 25.

These **calcium carbonate crystals are known as "Otolith or Otoconia"** and together with the gelatinous mass is known as "Otolithic membrane".

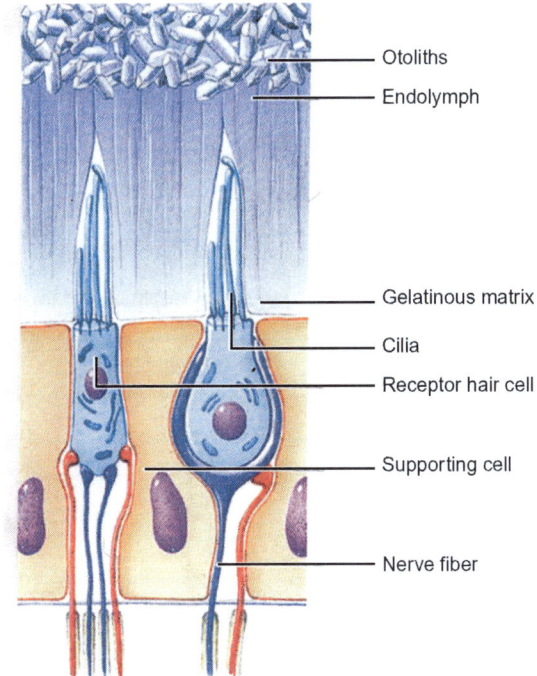

Fig. 1.25: Maculae

Vestibular Pathway

The hair cells of cristae in the **posterior semicircular canal** are **supplied by** the **singular nerve** which is a branch of inferior vestibular nerve (easy to remember si**ngular-in**ferior vestibular nerve). *Mnemonic*—this important fact can be remembered in this fashion; posterior SCC is involved in BPPV (P for P here). BPPV is the single (singular nerve) most common cause of vertigo in clinics, see chapter on Meniere's.

The **inferior vestibular nerve** also **supplies** the hair cells of the **maculae in the Saccule**.

The hair cells of **cristae** in the **superior and lateral semicircular canals** and **maculae in the Utricle** are supplied by the **superior vestibular nerve**.

The ganglion of vestibular nerves is situated in the lateral part of internal acoustic meatus and is called as the **"SCARPA'S GANGLION"**. Finally the inferior and superior vestibular nerves exit the internal acoustic meatus to go to vestibular nuclei in the pons.

The vestibular nuclei of the two sides have inter-connections with each other as well as with Cerebellum, Spinal cord, Medial longitudinal bundle (and through this with 3rd, 4th and 6th ocular nerves), Autonomic nervous system and cerebral cortex.

The above together maintain the body's balance.

These inter-connections also explain the occurrence of several other clinical manifestations along with imbalance (e.g. nystagmus, vomiting, sweating, palpitations, etc.).

Internal Acoustic Meatus (IAM)

The IAM is situated in the petrous part of temporal bone on its posterior slant, facing the posterior cranial fossa.

All the structures that pass from the cranial fossa to the inner ear and vice-versa pass through the IAM.

The IAM is divided into a superior and inferior part by a transverse crest known as falciform crest. The superior part is further divided into anterior and posterior parts by a vertical crest of bone known as **"BILL'S BAR"** *see* Fig. 1.26.

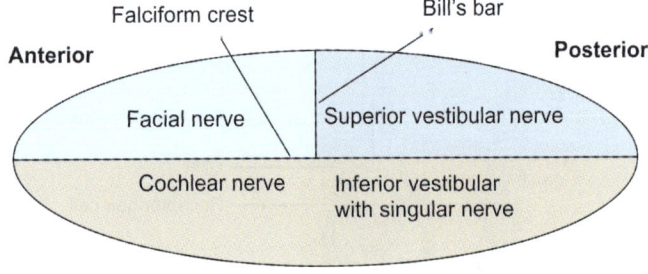

Fig. 1.26: Schematic diagram of IAM (right sided)

 *Note:*_____

The most common site of origin of acoustic neuroma is the inferior vestibular nerve in the IAM.

Through the antero-superior part of IAM passes the facial nerve. Bill's bar separates the facial nerve from the superior vestibular nerve which passes through the postero-superior area of the IAM.

In the inferior part of IAM, Cochlear nerve lies anteriorly and the inferior vestibular along with singular nerve lies posteriorly.

BLOOD SUPPLY OF EAR

External Ear

The external ear is supplied by the two branches of the external carotid artery:

a. Posterior auricular artery

b. Superficial temporal artery.

Middle Ear

The middle ear is supplied by both the internal and external carotid arteries.

From the external carotid:

a. Anterior tympanic artery and middle meningeal artery (middle meningeal artery gives superior tympanic and petrosal branches). Both anterior tympanic and middle meningeal arteries are branches of maxillary artery.

b. Inferior tympanic artery, a branch of ascending pharyngeal artery.

c. Stylomastoid artery, a branch of posterior auricular artery.

From the internal carotid:
Caroticotympanic

Inner Ear

The inner ear is supplied by labyrinthine artery which is a branch of anterior inferior cerebellar artery (AICA) or sometimes basilar artery.

Lymphatic Drainage of Ear

Part of the ear	Draining lymph nodes
Auricle and EAC	Parotid, preauricular, postauricular and upper deep cervical
Middle ear, mastoid and ET tube	Deep jugular and retropharyngeal
Inner ear	No lymphatics

1. **Pinna develops from:**   (*MH 2002, 2014*)
   a. 1st pharyngeal arch
   b. 1st and 3rd pharyngeal arch
   c. 1st and 2nd pharyngeal arch
   d. 2nd pharyngeal arch

2. **True regarding, the marked below is:**
   (*MAHE 2007, 2015*)

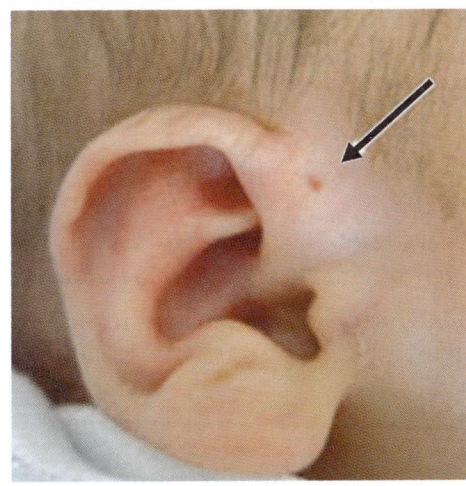

   a. Improper fusion of auricular tubercles
   b. Persistent opening of first branchial arch
   c. Autosomal recessive pattern
   d. First cleft anomaly

3. **External auditory canal is formed by:**
   (*MH 2007, 2015*)
   a. 1st branchial groove
   b. 1st visceral pouch
   c. 2nd branchial groove
   d. 2nd visceral pouch

4. **Call Aural fistula is:**   (*JIPMER 2004, 2010*)
   a. 1st branchial cleft anomaly
   b. 2nd branchial cleft anomaly
   c. 1st branchial pouch anomaly
   d. 2nd branchial pouch anomaly

5. **A newborn presents with bilateral microtia and external auditory canal atresia. Corrective surgery is usually performed at:**   (*AI 2007, 2013*)
   a. < 1 year of age   b. 5–7 years of age
   c. Puberty   d. Adulthood

6. **Eustachian tube develops from:**   (*PGI 97, 2011*)
   a. 2nd and 3rd pharyngeal pouch
   b. 1st pharyngeal pouch
   c. 2nd pharyngeal pouch
   d. 3rd pharyngeal pouch

7. **The proximal part of Tubotympanic recess leads to the formation of:**   (*MH 2014*)
   a. External Ear   b. Pharyngotympanic tube
   c. Middle ear cavity   d. Antrum

8. **The following structure represents all the three components of the embryonic disc:**   (*TN 98, 2010*)
   a. Tympanic membrane
   b. Retina
   c. Meninges
   d. None of the above

9. **Stapes develop from:**   (*AI 2009*)
   a. 1st arch   b. 2nd arch
   c. 3rd arch   d. 4th arch

10. **True regarding development of the ear:**
    (*PGI 2007, 2012*)
    a. Eustachian tube develops from 1st cleft
    b. Eustachian tube opens behind the level of inferior turbinate
    c. Pinna develops from 1st pouch
    d. Growth of organ of Corti is completed by 5th month
    e. Ossicles are adult size at birth

11. **Korner's septum is seen in:**   (*PGI 99, 2013*)
    a. Petrosquamous suture
    b. Temporosquamous suture
    c. Petromastoid suture
    d. Frontozygomatic suture

12. **All of the following are of the size of adult at birth except:**   (*APPG 06, 2011*)
    a. Tympanic membrane
    b. Ossicles
    c. Tympanic cavity
    d. Mastoid

13. **Which of the following attains adult size before birth?**   (*Exam 2013*)
    a. Mastoid   b. Orbit
    c. Ear ossicles   d. Cornea

14. **Which of the following attains adult size before birth?**   (*AI 2007, 2010*)
    a. Ear ossicles   b. Maxilla
    c. Mastoid   d. Parietal bone

15. **Inner ear is present in which bone:** (*PGI 97, 2009*)
    a. Parietal bone
    b. Petrous part of temporal bone
    c. Occipital bone
    d. Petrous part of squamous bone

16. **Inner ear bony labyrinth is:** (*Karnataka 2006, 2011*)
    a. Strongest bone in the body
    b. Cartilaginous bone
    c. Long bone
    d. Membranous bone

17. **Which of the following is not a pneumatic bone?**   (*AP 2009, 2012*)
    a. Ethmoid   b. Sphenoid
    c. Mastoid   d. Malleus

Ear

Section I

18. **Crus commune is a part of:**
    (Jharkhand 2006, 2015)
    a. Cochlea   b. Middle ear
    c. Semicircular canal   d. Vestibule

19. **Endolymphatic duct connects which structure:**
    (Delhi 2005, Exam 2017)
    a. Scala media to subdural space
    b. Scala vestibule to aqueduct of cochlea
    c. Scala tympani to subdural space
    d. Utriculo saccular duct to endolymphatic sac

20. **Not included in bony labyrinth:**
    (AI 2006, Exam 2017)
    a. Cochlea   b. Semicircular canal
    c. Organ of Corti   d. Vestibule

21. **The bony cochlea is a coiled tube making ... turns around a bony pyramid called ____:**
    (MH 2003, Exam 2017)
    a. 2 ¼, modiolus   b. 2 ½, helicotrema
    c. 2 ¾, modiolus   d. 2 ¾, helicotrema

22. **Organ of Corti is situated in:** *(Kerala 98, Exam 2017)*
    a. Scala media   b. S. Tympani
    c. S. Vestibuli   d. Saccule

23. **Foetus starts hearing by what time in intrauterine life:** *(Exam 2011)*
    a. 14 weeks   b. 20 weeks
    c. 32 weeks   d. 38 weeks

24. **Sense organ for hearing:** *(Exam 2017)*
    a. Organ of Corti   b. Cristae
    c. Maculae   d. None

25. **Semicircular canals are stimulated by:**
    (MP 2000, Exam 2013)
    a. Gravity   b. Linear acceleration
    c. Rotation   d. Sound

26. **Horizontal semicircular canal responds to:**
    (UP 2005, Exam 2017)
    a. Horizontal acceleration
    b. Rotational acceleration
    c. Gravity
    d. Head tilt

27. **Angular movements are sensed by:**
    (JIPMER 93, Exam 2013)
    a. Cochlea   b. Saccule
    c. Utricle   d. Semicircular canals

28. **Stapes foot plate covers:**
    (AIIMS May 2003, Exam 2017)
    a. Round window   b. Oval window
    c. Sinus tympani   d. Pyramid

29. **Movement of stapes causes vibration in:**
    (Exam 2002, Exam 2017)
    a. Scala media   b. Scala tympani
    c. Scala vestibuli   d. Semicircular canal

30. **Where is electrode kept in cochlear implant?**
    (Exam 2013, AIIMS 2008)
    a. Round window   b. Oval window
    c. Scala vestibuli   d. Scala tympani

31. **Micro Wick and micro catheter sustained release device are used in** *(AIIMS 2011)*
    a. Drooling of saliva
    b. Frey's syndrome
    c. Control of epistaxis
    d. Delivering drug to round window membrane

32. **Perilymph contains:** *(Exam 2013)*
    a. Na^+ b. K^+
    c. Mg^{++} d. Cl^-

33. **Site where endolymph is seen:**
    (Kerala 97, Exam 2013)
    a. Scala vestibuli   b. Scala media
    c. Helicotrema   d. Scala tympani

34. **Fluid, which has high potassium and low sodium content, is:** *(JIPMER 2003, Exam 2017)*
    a. CSF   b. perilymph
    c. Endolymph   d. Pleural fluid

35. **Cochlear aqueduct:** *(Exam 2017)*
    a. Connects internal ear with subarachnoid space
    b. Connects membranous cochlea with vestibule
    c. Contains endolymph
    d. Connects endolymphatic sac to subarachnoid space

36. **Most potential route for transmission of inner ear infection leading to Meningitis is:**
    (AI 2009, AIIMS 2011)
    a. Cochlear Aqueduct
    b. Endolymphatic sac
    c. Vestibular Aqueduct
    d. Hyrtle fissure

37. **Infection of CNS spreads in inner ear through:**
    (AIIMS 2010, Exam 2013)
    a. Cochlear Aqueduct b. Endolymphatic sac
    c. Scala media   d. Vestibular aqueduct

38. **The commonest genetic defect of inner ear causing deafness is:** *(AIIMS 2010)*
    a. Michel aplasia   b. Mondini dysplasia
    c. Scheibe dysplasia   d. Alexander dysplasia

39. **Skin over pinna is:** *(JIPMER 95, Exam 2017)*
    a. Firm on both sides
    b. Loose on medial side
    c. Loose on lateral side
    d. Loose on both sides

40. **Length of external auditory canal is:**
    (Exam 2013)
    a. 12 mm   b. 24 mm
    c. 36 mm   d. 48 mm

41. Cartilaginous part of external auditory canal is:
(Exam 2017)
   a. Medial 1/3
   b. Lateral 1/3
   c. Medial 2/3
   d. Lateral 2/3

42. Ceruminous glands present in the ear are:
(AIIMS May 2005, Exam 2017)
   a. Modified eccrine glands
   b. Modified apocrine glands
   c. Modified endocrine glands
   d. Modified holocrine glands

43. Dehiscence in the external auditory canal cause infection in the parotid gland via:
(AIIMS 2004, Exam 2017)
   a. Fissure of Santorini
   b. Notch of Rivinus
   c. Petro-tympanic fissure
   d. Retro pharyngeal fissure

44. What is the colour of the normal tympanic membrane:
(CUPGEE 96, Exam 2017)
   a. Pearly grey
   b. Pink
   c. Blue
   d. Red

45. Pars Flaccida of the tympanic membrane is also called:
(MP 2007, Exam 2013)
   a. Reissner's membrane
   b. Shrapnell's membrane
   c. Basilar membrane
   d. Secondary tympanic membrane

46. The most mobile part of the tympanic membrane:
(TN 98, Exam 2017)
   a. Central
   b. Peripheral
   c. Both
   d. None of the above

47. Surface area of tympanic membrane:
(Manipal 2006, Exam 2013)
   a. 55 mm^2
   b. 70 mm^2
   c. 80 mm^2
   d. 90 mm^2

48. The effective vibratory area of the tympanic membrane:
(UP 2005, Exam 2017)
   a. 25 mm^2
   b. 30 mm^2
   c. 40 mm^2
   d. 55 mm^2

49. Which nerve supplies the tragus?
(AIIMS 96, Exam 2017)
   a. Greater auricular
   b. Auriculo temporal
   c. Vagus
   d. Glossopharyngeal

50. Nerve supply for external ear are all except:
(MAHE 2007, Exam 2016)
   a. Greater occipital nerve
   b. Greater auricular nerve
   c. Auriculotemporal nerve
   d. Lesser occipital nerve

51. Arnolds nerve is a branch of: *(AIIMS 99, Exam 2017)*
   a. Vagus
   b. Glossopharyngeal
   c. Auditory
   d. Facial

52. Major part of the skin of pinna is supplied by:
(AP 2000, Exam 2017)
   a. Auriculotemporal nerve
   b. Auricular branch of vagus
   c. Lesser occipital nerve
   d. Greater auricular nerve

53. All of the following nerves, supply Auricle and external auditory canal except: *(TN 2003, Exam 2017)*
   a. Trigeminal nerve
   b. Glossopharyngeal nerve
   c. Facial nerve
   d. Vagus nerve

54. Sensory supply of external auditory meatus is by:
(PGI June 2007, 2013)
   a. Sphenopalatine ganglion
   b. Geniculate ganglion
   c. Facial nerve
   d. Auriculotemporal nerve

55. The cough response caused while cleaning the ear canal is mediated by stimulation of:
(AIIMS Nov 2002, Exam 2013)
   a. The Vth cranial nerve
   b. Innervation of external ear canal by C1 and C2
   c. The Xth cranial nerve
   d. Branches of the VIIth cranial nerve

56. During ear examination, cough occurs due to stimulation of: *(Exam 2013)*
   a. Vagus
   b. Trigeminal
   c. Hypoglossal
   d. Trochlear

57. Nerve supply of the tympanic membrane is by:
(PGI Dec 2002, Exam 2013)
   a. Auriculotemporal
   b. Auricular branch of vagus
   c. Occipital nerve
   d. Great auricular nerve
   e. Glossopharyngeal nerve

58. Sensory nerve supply of middle ear cavity is provided by: *(AI 95, Exam 2013)*
   a. Facial
   b. Glossopharyngeal
   c. Vagus
   d. Trigeminal

59. Which nerve is responsible for referred pain to the ear? *(Exam 2013)*
   a. IX
   b. III
   c. XI
   d. XII

60. Which of the following pain is not referred to ear?
(Rj 2008, Exam 2017)
   a. Pharynx
   b. Tongue
   c. TM joint
   d. Vestibule of nose

61. Referred otalgia can be due to: *(AIIMS 2009)*
   a. Carcinoma larynx
   b. Carcinoma oral cavity
   c. Carcinoma tongue
   d. All of the above

Ear

Section I

62. **In carcinoma base of tongue pain is referred to the ear through:** *(Kerala 2001, Exam 2017)*
    a. Hypoglossal nerve
    b. Vagus nerve
    c. Glossopharyngeal nerve
    d. Lingual nerve

63. **Stapedius is supplied by:** *(JIPMER 92, Exam 2017)*
    a. Maxillary nerve   b. Facial nerve
    c. Auditory nerve   d. Mandibular nerve

64. **Tensor tympani is supplied by:** *(JIPMER 2002, Exam 2017)*
    a. Anterior part of V nerve
    b. Posterior part of V nerve
    c. IX nerve
    d. VII nerve

65. **Promontory seen in the middle ear is related to:** *(AI 98, Exam 2017)*
    a. Jugular bulb   b. Basal turn of cochlea
    c. Semicircular canal   d. Body of incus

66. **Processus cochleariformis is related to:** *(JIPMER 95, Exam 2016)*
    a. Tendon of tensor tympani
    b. Basal turns of cochlea
    c. Handle of malleus
    d. Incus

67. **Stapes foot plate covers:** *(AIIMS May 2003, Exam 2014)*
    a. Round window   b. Oval window
    c. Sinus tympani   d. Pyramid

68. **Secondary tympanic membrane is present over:** *(Delhi 2000, Exam 2017)*
    a. Round window
    b. Oval window
    c. Lateral wall of middle ear
    d. Scala media

69. **Facial recess is bounded by:** *(TN 2003, Exam 2016)*
    a. Medially by the vertical part of VII nerve
    b. Laterally by the chorda tympani
    c. Above by fossa incudis
    d. All of the above

70. **While doing posterior tympanotomy through the facial recess there are chances of injury to the following except:** *(AIIMS 2013, AI 2007)*
    a. Facial nerve horizontal part
    b. Chorda tympani
    c. Dislodgement of short process of incus from fossa incudis
    d. Vertical descending part of facial nerve

71. **All are true about facial recess except:** *(JIPMER 2006, Exam 2017)*
    a. Supra pyramidal recess

b. Medially it is bounded by chorda tympani and laterally by facial nerve
    c. Important in cochlear implant
    d. Middle ear can be approached through it

72. **Eustachian tube opens into middle ear cavity at:** *(UP 2000, Exam 2017)*
    a. Anterior wall   b. Medial wall
    c. Lateral wall   d. Posterior wall

73. **The length of Eustachian tube is:** *(AP 1999/TN 2006, Exam 2017)*
    a. 16 mm   b. 24 mm
    c. 36 mm   d. 40 mm

74. **About Eustachian tube, true is:** *(PGI June 2002, 2010)*
    a. 24 mm in length
    b. Outer 1/3rd is cartilaginous
    c. Inner 2/3rd is bony
    d. Inner 2/3rd is cartilaginous
    e. Opens during swallowing

75. **True about Eustachian tube is/are:** *(PGI June 2001, 2012)*
    a. Size is 3.75 cm
    b. 1/3rd cartilaginous and 2/3rd bony
    c. Opens during swallowing
    d. Nasopharyngeal opening is narrowest
    e. Tensor palati helps to open it

76. **True about Eustachian tube:** *(PGI Nov 2010)*
    a. Length is 36 mm in children
    b. Higher elastin content in adults
    c. Ventilator function of ear better developed in infants
    d. More horizontal in adults
    e. Angulated in infants

77. **Which of the following causes opening of Eustachian tube?** *(MH 2010)*
    a. Salpingopharyngeus
    b. Levator veli palatini
    c. Tensor veli palatini
    d. None of the above

78. **Floor of middle ear cavity is in relation with:** *(AI 2001, Exam 2016, MH CET 2016)*
    a. Internal carotid artery
    b. Bulb of the internal jugular vein
    c. Sigmoid sinus
    d. Round window

79. **Tegmen tympani separates middle ear from the middle cranial fossa containing temporal lobe of brain by:** *(Karnataka 2006, Exam 2016)*
    a. Medial wall of middle ear
    b. Lateral wall of middle ear
    c. Roof of middle ear
    d. Anterior wall of middle ear

80. **The distance between tympanic membrane and medial wall of middle ear at the level of centre is:** *(Exam 2017)*
    a. 3 mm   b. 4 mm
    c. 6 mm   d. 2 mm

81. **Distance of promontory from tympanic membrane:** *(Delhi 2005, Exam 2017)*
    a. 2 mm   b. 5 mm
    c. 6 mm   d. 7 mm

82. **Narrowest part of middle ear is:** *(Exam 2017)*
    a. Hypotympanum   b. Epitympanum
    c. Attic   d. Mesotympanum

83. **Prussak's space is situated in:** *(MAHE 2002, Exam 2017)*
    a. Epitympanum   b. Mesotympanum
    c. Hypotympanum   d. Ear canal

84. **All the following are components of epitympanum except:** *(AI 2002, Exam 2017)*
    a. Body of incus   b. Head of malleus
    c. Chorda tympani   d. Footplate of stapes

85. **What is the type of joint between the ossicles of ear?** *(AI 2008)*
    a. Fibrous joint
    b. Primary cartilaginous
    c. Secondary cartilaginous
    d. Synovial joint

86. **Macewen's triangle is the landmark for:** *(MP 98, Exam 2017)*
    a. Maxillary sinus   b. Mastoid antrum
    c. Frontal sinus   d. None

87. **Macewen's triangle overlies which structure?** *(Exam 2013)*
    a. Mastoid antrum   b. Inner ear
    c. Cochlea   d. Saccule

88. **The suprameatal triangle overlies the:** *(JIPMER 91, Exam 2017)*
    a. Mastoid antrum   b. Mastoid air cells
    c. Antrum   d. Facial nerve

89. **What forms lateral wall of mastoid antrum?** *(Exam 2013)*
    a. Squamous temporal
    b. Tegmen Antri
    c. Posterior semicircular canal
    d. None

90. **All of the following form the boundary of Macewen's triangle except:** *(Delhi 2008)*
    a. Temporal line
    b. Postero-superior segment of bony external auditory canal
    c. Promontory
    d. Tangent drawn to the external auditory meatus

91. **All are false about McEwen's triangle except:** *(AI 2004, Exam 2017)*
    a. Mastoid antrum lies 1.5 cm deep to it
    b. Surgical landmark for facial nerve
    c. Present in preauricular region
    d. It is bounded by suprameatal crest anteriorly

92. **Citelli's angle is:** *(Exam 2013)*
    a. Solid angle   b. CP angle
    c. Sinodural angle   d. Part of Macewen's triangle

93. **Spine of Henle is a land mark for:** *(MH 2003, Exam 2017)*
    a. Eustachian tube
    b. Mastoid
    c. Tympanic membrane
    d. Facial nerve

94. **Organ of Corti is situated on:** *(TN 2006, Exam 2017)*
    a. Basilar membrane   b. Utricle
    c. Saccule   d. None of the above

95. **Endolymph in the ear:** *(AIIMS May 2009, Exam 2013)*
    a. Is a filtrate of blood stream
    b. Is secreted by stria vascularis
    c. Is secreted by basilar membrane
    d. Is secreted by hair cells

96. **In cochlea, endolymph has potential of:** *(Exam 2012)*
    a. +80 mV   b. –80 mV
    c. +20 mV   d. –20 mV

97. **The function of stria vascularis is:** *(AI 2002, Exam 2017)*
    a. To produce perilymph
    b. To absorb perilymph
    c. To maintain electric milieu of endolymph
    d. To maintain electric milieu of perilymph

98. **Primary receptor cells of hearing:** *(Exam 2013)*
    a. Supporting cell
    b. Tectorial membrane
    c. Tunnel of Corti
    d. Hair cell

99. **All of the following are concerned with auditory pathway except:** *(AI 95, Exam 2017)*
    a. Trapezoid body
    b. Medial geniculate body
    c. Genu of internal capsule
    d. Lateral lemniscus

100. **Trapezoid body is associated with:** *(Kerala 2009, PGI 2006)*
    a. Auditory pathway
    b. Visual pathway
    c. Pyramidal pathway
    d. Gustatory pathway
    e. Extra pyramidal system

101. **Higher auditory centre determine:**   (*AIIMS 2009*)
    a. Sound frequency
    b. Loudness
    c. Speech discrimination
    d. Sound localisation

102. **Appreciation of sound occurs in** (*TN 99, Exam 2017*)
    a. Organ of Corti
    b. Basilar membrane
    c. Cochlear nuclei
    d. Transverse temporal gyrus

103. **Otolith organs are concerned with function of:**
                                    (*Exam 2013*)
    a. Hearing   b. Rotatory nystagmus
    c. Linear acceleration d. Angular acceleration

104. **Static equilibrium is due to:**   (*Exam 2013*)
    a. Macula   b. Cupula
    c. End organ of Corti d. Cristae ampulla

105. **All are correctly matched except:**
                            (*TN 2007, Exam 2014*)
    a. Otolith–made up of uric acid crystals
    b. Position of otolith-changes with head position
    c. Otolith–component of maculae
    d. Otolith organs–stimulated by gravity and linear acceleration

106. **Not correctly matched pair is:**
                            (*UPSC 2003, Exam 2017*)
    a. Utricle and saccule–cristae
    b. Oval window–foot plate of stapes
    c. Antrum–Macewen's triangle
    d. Scala vestibuli–Reissner's membrane

107. **Vertical crest of bone in the internal acoustic meatus is:**   (*AIIMS 2011*)
    a. Bill's bar   b. Ponticulus
    c. Cog   d. Falciform crest

108. **Singular nerve is a:**   (*AP 2007, Exam 2017*)
    a. Superior vestibular nerve supplying posterior semicircular canal
    b. Inferior vestibular nerve supplying posterior semicircular canal
    c. Superior vestibular nerve supplying anterior semicircular canal
    d. Interior vestibular nerve supplying anterior semicircular canal

109. **Labyrinthine artery is a branch of:**
                            (*AIIMS 91, Exam 2013*)
    a. Internal carotid artery
    b. External carotid artery
    c. Posterior inferior cerebellar artery
    d. Anterior inferior cerebellar artery

110. **What is scutum?**   (*Exam 2014*)
    a. Lateral wall of attic
    b. Posterior wall of attic
    c. Superior wall of attic
    d. Inferior wall of attic

111. **Eustachian tube:**   (*Exam 2014*)
    a. Connects middle ear to pharynx
    b. Is oblique in infants
    c. Is wider in adults
    d. Opens in oropharynx

112. **In the utricle, tip links in the hair cells are involved in:**   (*MH-CET 2015*)
    a. Formation of perilymph
    b. Regulation of distortion activated ion channels
    c. Depolarisation of stria vascularis
    d. Movements of the basement membrane

113. **Type of joint between malleus and incus is:**
                                    (*Exam 2014*)
    a. Saddle   b. Ball and socket
    c. Hinge   d. Pivot

114. **Site of Darwin's tubercle is:**   (*Exam 2016*)
    a. Postero-lateral part of helix
    b. Tragus
    c. Incisura terminalis
    d. Lobule

115. **Common nerve supplying pinna, TM and EAC:**
                                    (*Exam 2016*)
    a. Glossopharyngeal
    b. Arnolds
    c. Greater Auricular
    d. Occipital

116. **The direction of bony EAC is:**   (*Exam 2016*)
    a. Upwards, backwards, medially
    b. Upwards, backwards, laterally
    c. Downwards, forwards, medially
    d. Downwards, forwards, laterally

117. **Oval window opens into:**   (*Exam 2016*)
    a. Utricle   b. Saccule
    c. Scala tympani   d. Vestibule

118. **Membranous labyrinth develops from:** (*Exam 2016*)
    a. Surface ectoderm
    b. First cleft
    c. Tubo-tympanic recess
    d. Mandibular arch

119. **Complete absence of bony and membranous labyrinth:**   (*Exam 2016*)
    a. Mondini aplasia
    b. Michel aplasia
    c. Cochleo-saccular aplasia
    d. Alexander aplasia

120. **Pinna is made up of how many cartilage/s:**
                                    (*Exam 2015*)
    a. One   b. Six
    c. Five   d. Two

121. **Pain in tonsillitis is referred to the ear through:**
    (Exam 2016)
    a. IX
    b. X
    c. XI
    d. VII

122. **Location of pre-auricular sinus is:** *(Exam 2016)*
    a. Tragus
    b. Ant-tragus
    c. Root of helix
    d. Anti-helix

123. **Not seen on the medial wall of the middle ear:**
    (Exam 2016)
    a. Promontory
    b. Oval window
    c. Facial recess
    d. Lateral semicircular canal bulge

124. **Nerve supply of Auricle and EAC are all except:**
    (Exam 2016)
    a. Arnold's
    b. Auriculotemporal
    c. Jacobson's
    d. Lesser Occipital

125. **Skin of the lower one-third of the auricle is supplied by the nerve** *(MH CET 2016)*
    a. Lesser occipital
    b. Greater occipital
    c. Greater auricular
    d. Auriculotemporal

126. **Sensory supply of the marked area is:**
    (Practice question by Author)

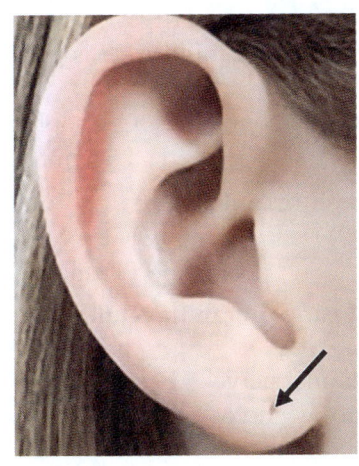

    a. Auriculotemporal nerve
    b. Lesser occipital nerve
    c. Greater auricular nerve
    d. Facial nerve

127. **Chorda tympani passes between which layers of tympani membrane:** *(Exam 2014)*
    a. Outer and middle
    b. Middle and inner
    c. Epithelial layer
    d. None of the above

128. **Suprameatal triangle is the external marking of:**
    (Exam 2014)
    a. Aditus
    b. Chorda tympani
    c. Mastoid antrum
    d. Facial nerve

129. **The angle of TM with the horizontal is:** *(Exam 2016)*
    a. 35 degrees
    b. 55 degrees
    c. 75 degrees
    d. 90 degrees

130. **The significance of the marked structure is in the given picture:** *(Practice question by Author)*

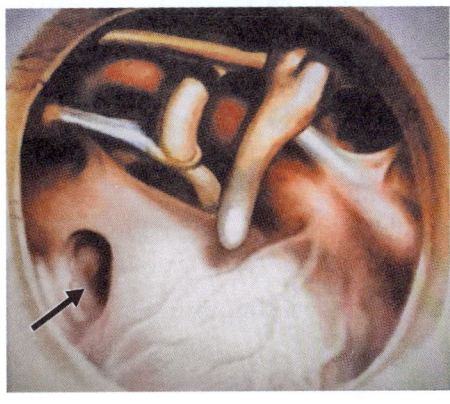

    a. Stapes foot plate is present on it
    b. Intact canal wall surgery is done through it
    c. It ventilates the middle ear
    d. Cochlear implant electrodes are introduced through it

131. **Encircled area is:** *(AIIMS May 2016)*

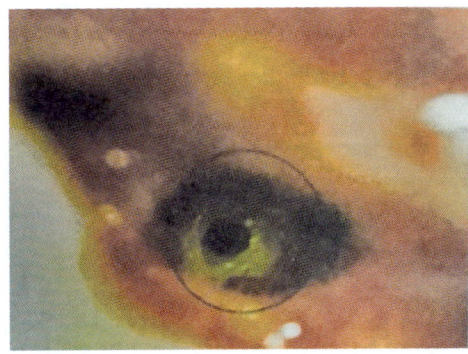

    a. Facial recess
    b. Fossa incudis
    c. Sinus tympani
    d. Pyriform fossa

132. **True about the marked area in the given picture:**
    (Practice question by Author)

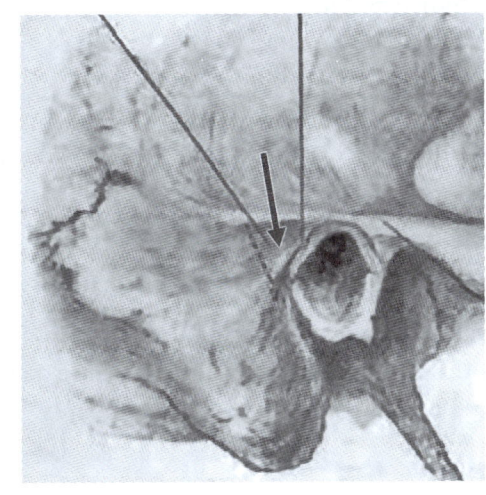

    a. It is the landmark for antrum
    b. It is known as Trautmann's triangle
    c. The Prussak's space is being depicted
    d. It is the site for approach while doing myringotomy

133. Find the incorrect pair. :   (*Bihar PGMAT 2014*)
    a. Tympanic membrane: malleus
    b. Helicotrema: apex of cochlea
    c. Basilar membrane: cochlea
    d. Otoliths: semicircular canals

134. A 5-year-old child develops parotitis following otitis externa. This could have happened through: (*WB PG 2016*)
    a. Cochlear aqueduct   b. Fissures of Santorini
    c. Isthmus   d. Foramen of Morgagni

135. Cranial nerve passing through internal auditory meatus: (*PGI MAY 2013*)
    a. 7th cranial nerve   b. 9th cranial nerve
    c. 10th cranial nerve   d. 11th cranial nerve
    e. 12th cranial nerve

136. Stria vascularis is present in: (*Exam 2016*)
    a. Cochlea   b. Saccule
    c. Utricle   d. Semi-circular canals

137. Otoconia is seen in: (*Exam 2016*)
    a. Utricle
    b. Superior semicircular canal
    c. Lateral semicircular canal
    d. Cochlea

138. Feature of Scheibe's dysplasia is: (*Exam 2016*)
    a. Semicircular canal fistula
    b. Abnormality in bony labyrinth
    c. Dysplasia of cochlea and saccule
    d. Middle ear anaomaly

139. Endocochlear potential is: (*Exam 2016*)
    a. +45 mV   b. – 45 mV
    c. +60 mV   d. +85 mV

140. Facial nerve exits the skull through: (*Exam 2016*)
    a. Stylomastoid foramen
    b. Jugular foramen
    c. Foramen Lacerum
    d. Foramen Rotundum

141. Where is the auditory cortex located inside the brain?   (*Exam 2016*)
    a. Superior temporal gyrus
    b. Inferior temporal gyrus
    c. Area 31
    d. Cingulate gyrus

142. Inferior and vertical postauricular incision in children less than 2 years old may cause damage to which cranial nerve?   (*Exam 2016*)
    a. VIII   b. VII
    c. VI   d. V

143. Which of the following helps in detection of horizontal movement of head and body?   (*Exam 2016*)
    a. Cristae   b. organ of Corti
    c. Utricle   d. Endolymphatic sac

144. Facial nerve lies with which nerve in internal auditory meatus?   (*Exam 2016*)
    a. Trigeminal nerve
    b. Abducent nerve
    c. Vestibulocochlear nerve
    d. Hypoglossal nerve

145. All of the following are parts of the bony labyrinth except: (*Exam 2016*)
    a. Vestibule   b. Cochlea
    c. Utricle   d. Semicurcular canals

146. Length of external auditory canal is: (*Exam 2016*)
    a. 2.4 cm   b. 4.2 cm
    c. 5 cm   d. 7 cm

147. Korners septum arises from: (*Exam 2016*)
    a. Petro squamous suture
    b. Petrotympanic suture
    c. Tympanomastoid suture
    d. Tympanosquamous suture

148. Tensor tympani is attached to: (*Exam 2016*)
    a. Malleus
    b. Stapes neck
    c. Processes cochleariformis
    d. Incus

149. Sensory supply of middle ear is provided by: (*Exam 2016*)
    a. Facial   b. Glossopharyngeal
    c. Vagus   d. Trigeminal

150. Endolymph resembles: (*Exam 2016*)
    a. CSF   b. ICF
    c. ECF   d. Plasma

151. Referred ear pain can travel through all except: (*Exam 2016*)
    a. Trigeminal nerve   b. Glossopharyngeal nerve
    c. Abducens nerve   d. Vagus nerve

152. Citelli angle is: (*Exam 2016*)
    a. Solid angle   b. CP angle
    c. Sinodural angle   d. Part of Macewen's triangle

153. Cone of light is seen in which part of TM: (*Exam 2016*)
    a. Anterosuperior   b. Posterosuperior
    c. Posteroinferior   d. Anteroinferior

154. True about Eustachian tube is: (*Exam 2016*)
    a. Bony part measures 24 mm
    b. Lateral part is cartilaginous
    c. Valsalva manoeuvre opens ET
    d. Tensor veli palatini closes ET

155. Muscle originating from pyramid of middle ear: (*Exam 2016*)
    a. Tensor tympani   b. Stylohyoid
    c. Stapedius   d. Levator palatini

156. **Most common congenital middle ear abnormality:** *(AIIMS Nov 2015)*
    a. Absent footplate of stapes
    b. Fixation of footplate of stapes
    c. Oval window abnormality
    d. Absent long process of incus

157. **Volume of middle ear and mastoid antrum:** *(Exam 2011)*
    a. 2 ml   b. 6 ml
    c. 12 ml   d. 15 ml

158. **Ostmann pad of fat is related to:** *(Exam 2018)*
    a. Ear lobule   b. Buccal mucosa
    c. Eustachian tube   d. Tip of nose

159. **Not a part of middle ear cleft:** *(Exam 2018)*
    a. Semicircular canal   b. Mastoid antrum
    c. Eustachian tube   d. Tympanic cavity

160. **The structures marked in the given picture:** *(Exam 2017, 2018)*

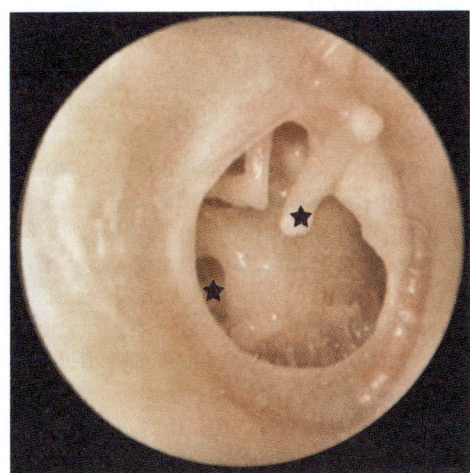

    a. Malleus and round window
    b. Incus and round window
    c. Stapes and oval window
    d. Promontory and aditus

161. **Following is true about the given picture:** *(Exam 2017)*

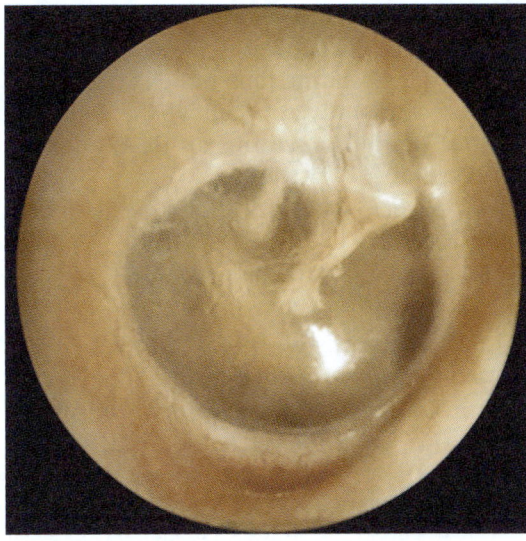

    a. It is the left TM
    b. Posterior part is more easily assessible
    c. Develops from 1st arch
    d. Shrapnells membrane more tense

162. **Inner hair cells of organ of Corti releases which excitatory neurotransmitter:** *(JIPMER 2018)*
    a. Glycine
    b. Glutamate
    c. GABA
    d. Acetylcholine

ANSWERS AND EXPLANATIONS

1. **(c) 1st and 2nd pharyngeal arch** (*Ref. Scott Brown, 8th ed., Vol 2, page 541*)
2. **(a) Improper fusion of auricular tubercles** (*Ref. Cummings, 6th ed., 2827*)
   - The failure of fusion of 1st and 2nd arch leads to the formation of the "PRE-AURICULAR SINUS". This is seen in between the tragus (from 1st arch) and the ascending limb of helix (from 2nd arch) most commonly either above the tragus or at the root of helix (*see* the clinical photo in the question).
3. **(a) 1st branchial groove** (*Ref. Scott Brown, 8th ed., Vol 2, page 541*)
4. **(a) 1st branchial cleft anomaly** (*Ref. Scott Brown, 8th ed., Vol 2, page 541*)
5. **(b) 5–7 years of age (please refer to text)** (*Ref. Cummings, 6th ed., 3000*)
6. **(b) and (c) 1st pharyngeal pouch, 2nd pharyngeal pouch** (*Ref. Scott Brown, 8th ed., Vol 2, page 540*)

Pharyngeal pouch	Structure develops
1st and a small part of 2nd (also called as tubo-tympanic recess)	Middle ear cleft, i.e. Eustachian tube, tympanic cavity and mastoid antrum.
2nd	Tonsil
3rd	Inferior parathyroids and the thymus
4th	Superior parathyroids and some part of the thyroid

7. **(b) Pharyngotympanic tube** (*Ref. Shambaugh, 6th ed., page 7*)
8. **(a) Tympanic membrane** (*Ref. Scott Brown, 8th ed., Vol 2, page 540*)
   - The 1st cleft grows and meet 1st pouch medially to form the tympanic membrane.
   - So the tympanic membrane is made from all the 3 layers, outer epithelial layer from ectoderm and inner endothelial layer from endoderm and in between these is the fibrous layer from mesoderm.
   - Retina develops from neuro-ectoderm.
   - Dura mater is derived from mesoderm. Pia and arachnoid are derived from neural crest.
9. **(b) 2nd arch** (*Ref. Scott Brown, 8th ed., Vol 2, page 540*)
10. **(b), (d), (e) are true** (please refer the text) (*Ref. Scott Brown, 8th ed., Vol 2, page 540*)
11. **(a) Petrosquamous suture** (*Ref. Shambaugh, 6th ed., page 32*)
12. **(d) Mastoid** (*Ref. Shambaugh, 6th ed., page 5*)
    - The mastoid is incompletely developed at birth and continues to develop till 18 years of age.
    - The largest air cell of mastoid called as mastoid antrum is present at birth and is of adult configuration.

Note:

The bony part of EAC and the mastoid tip are not present at birth.

   - The middle and inner ear structures attain adult size well before birth.
   - TM is also of adult size but, in the absence of bony part of EAC, is horizontally placed.
13. **(c) Ear ossicles** (*Ref. Shambaugh, 6th ed., page 5*)
    - The tympanic membrane, middle ear and the inner ear structures are fully developed and are of adult size at birth.
    - Orbital structures continue to grow after birth.
14. **(a) Ear ossicles** (*Ref. Scott Brown, 8th ed., Vol 2, page 540*)
    - Maxilla and Parietal bone continue to grow after birth.
15. **(b) Petrous part of temporal bone** (*Ref. Shambaugh, 6th ed., page 32*) (*see* the explanation below)
16. **(b) Cartilaginous bone** (*Ref. Scott Brown, 8th ed., Vol 2, page 542*)
    - Cartilaginous bones ossify from a cartilage model (endochondral bone formation), e.g. Bony labyrinth also called as Otic capsule
    - In contrast to cartilaginous bone, membranous bone also called as dermal bone does not form from cartilage that then calcifies. Dermal bone is formed within the dermis and grows by accretion only–the outer portion of the bone is deposited by osteoblasts. Examples of membranous or dermal bones are clavicle and patella.
    - Inner ear bony labyrinth is present in the petrous part of temporal bone. It is known as petrous (which means rock like) as it is one of the densest bones of the body, though not the strongest. The strongest bone of the body is the femur.
17. **(d) Malleus** (*Ref. Scott Brown, 8th ed., Vol 2, page 538*)
    - Pneumatic bones are those bones which contain an air filled cavity within them which make them light in weight. In humans, they are seen in relation to the nasal cavity, and enclose the paranasal sinuses. Besides making the skull light in weight, they also help in resonance of sound and act as air conditioning chambers for the inspired air.
    - Pneumatic bones are–maxilla, frontal bone, sphenoid and ethmoid.
    - The mastoid is also most commonly a pneumatic (air filled) bone which encloses numerous air cell spaces giving it a honeycomb appearance. However in some people the mastoid may be diploic (marrow filled) or sclerotic (solid bone without air).
18. **(c) Semicircular canal** (*Ref. Shambaugh, 6th ed., page 42*)
    - The posterior and superior semicircular canals fuse together to form a common crus called as

"crus commune" which opens into the utricle. Because of this the three semicircular canals open into utricle by five openings instead of six.

19. **(d) Utriculo saccular duct to endolymphatic sac,** please *see* the text. (*Ref. Shambaugh, 6th ed., page 42*)

20. **(c) Organ of Corti (it is a part of membranous labyrinth)** (*Ref. Shambaugh, 6th ed., page 42*)

21. **(c) 2 ¾, modiolus** (*Ref. Shambaugh, 6th ed., page 42*)

22. **(a) Scala media** (*Ref. Shambaugh, 6th ed., page 73*)

23. **(b) 20 weeks** (*Ref. Shambaugh, 6th ed., page 11*)

24. **(a) Organ of Corti** (*Ref. Shambaugh, 6th ed., page 73*)

25. **(c) Rotation** (*Ref. Shambaugh, 6th ed., page 113*)
    - Semicircular canals contain cristae which sense angular or rotational acceleration.
    - Gravitational movements, head tilt and linear acceleration are sensed by maculae in the utricle and saccule.
    - Sound is sensed by organ of Corti present in the scala media, situated on the basilar membrane.

26. **(b) Rotational acceleration** (*Ref. Shambaugh, 6th ed., page 113*)
    - The horizontal/lateral semicircular canal along with posterior and superior semicircular canal contains cristae which sense angular or rotational acceleration.
    - Horizontal acceleration, i.e. linear acceleration, gravitational movements and head tilt movements are sensed by maculae in the utricle and saccule.

27. **(d) Semicircular canals** (*Ref. Shambaugh, 6th ed., page 113*)

28. **(b) Oval window** (*Ref. Shambaugh, 6th ed., page 38*)
    - The Oval window is covered by the footplate of stapes.
    - The Round window is covered by secondary tympanic membrane.
    - The part of middle ear medial to the descending part of facial nerve is called sinus tympani.
    - Pyramid is the projection on posterior wall from which originates the stapedius muscle.

29. **(c) Scala vestibuli,** please refer the text (*Ref. Cummings, 6th ed., 1997*)

30. **(c) Scala tympani** (*Ref. Shambaugh, 6th ed., page 599*)
    - The electrodes of cochlear implant are placed into the Scala tympani by passing through the round window.

31. **(d) Delivering drug to round window membrane** (*Ref. Scott Brown, 8th ed., Vol 2, page 580*)

32. **(a) Na⁺** (*Ref. Shambaugh, 6th ed., page 79*)
    - Perilymph is the fluid which fills the bony labyrinth.
    - Perilymph is actually an extension of CSF which enters from the subarachnoid space into the scala tympani through Cochlear aqueduct.

- CSF being an extracellular fluid therefore perilymph is rich in Na^+.
- Endolymph filling the membranous labyrinth and secreted from stria vascularis is rich in K^+.

33. **(b) Scala media** (*Ref. Scott Brown, 8th ed., Vol 2, page 545*)
    - Endolymph is present in the membranous labyrinth, whereas perilymph is present in the bony labyrinth.
    - Hence scala vestibuli, scala tympani and their interconnection helicotrema, which are parts of bony labyrinth, are filled with perilymph.
    - Scala media, utricle, saccule and semicircular canals, which are parts of membranous labyrinth, are filled with endolymph.

34. **(c) Endolymph** (*Ref. Scott Brown, 8th ed., Vol 2, page 545*)
    - Rest are extracellular hence have more of sodium.

35. **(a) Connects internal ear with subarachnoid space** (*Ref. Scott Brown, 8th ed., Vol 2, page 545*)
    - The internal ear communicates with the cranium via two openings:
      1. Cochlear aqueduct: via this CSF in the subarachnoid space enters scala tympani and becomes perilymph which circulates in the bony labyrinth.
      2. Internal acoustic meatus
    - Membranous cochlea is a part of membranous labyrinth which is a closed sac and is not connected to vestibule which is a part of the bony labyrinth.
    - Endolymphatic sac is a blind pouch responsible for absorption of endolymph and is situated in between the endosteal and meningeal layer of the dura mater.

36. **(a) Cochlear Aqueduct** (*Ref. Cummings, 6th ed., 2992*)
    - Endolymphatic sac is a closed sac. It does not communicate with CSF.
    - The bony canal around the utriculo-saccular duct and endolymphatic duct is called vestibular aqueduct
    - Hyrtle fissure is a tympanomeningeal fissure which obliterates by 26 weeks period of gestation. If persistent it can lead to a connection between CSF and middle ear.

37. **(a) Cochlear Aqueduct** (*Ref. Cummings, 6th ed., 2992; 2169*)

38. **(c) Scheibe dysplasia** (*Ref. Cummings, 6th ed., 2982*)

39. **(b) Loose on medial side** (*Ref. Scott Brown, 8th ed., Vol 2, page 526*)
    - The skin on the lateral side of pinna is firmly attached because of which any inflammatory condition on the lateral side is more painful.

Section I | **Ear**

40. **(b) 24 mm** (*Ref. Scott Brown, 8th ed., Vol 2, page 527*)
41. **(b) Lateral 1/3** (*Ref. Scott Brown, 8th ed., Vol 2, page 527*)
42. **(b) Modified apocrine glands** (*Ref. Shambaugh, 6th ed., page 30*)
    - Ceruminous glands are modified sudoriferous glands (sweat glands) located subcutaneously in the external auditory canal. They are apocrine glands, i.e. while discharging the secretions their cell's apical parts are shed off.
    - Eccrine or merocrine glands secretions are thrown out of the cells by a process of exocytosis, the cell remaining intact, e.g. sweat glands.
    - In some glands the entire cell disintegrates while discharging its secretion. These are said to be holocrine glands, e.g. sebaceous glands.
    - Apocrine, merocrine and holocrine are the descriptions of exocrine glands i.e. the glands which pour their secretions on to an epithelial surface directly or through ducts.
    - Endocrine glands pour their secretions into blood.
43. **(a) Fissure of Santorini** (please *see* the text) (*Ref. Cummings, 6th ed., 1981*)
    - The notch of Rivinus is the upper attachment of pars flaccida.
    - Petro-tympanic fissure is present on the anterior wall of middle ear, on which attaches the anterior malleolar ligament.
    Retropharyngeal fissure does not exist.
44. **(a) Pearly grey** (*Ref. Scott Brown, 8th ed., Vol 2, page 923*)

Condition of the ear	Colour of TM
Normal	Pearly grey
Glue ear or SOM	Blue
ASOM	Red (congested)
Active otosclerosis	Flamingo pink

45. **(b) Shrapnell's membrane** (*Ref. Shambaugh, 6th ed., page 380*)
    - Reissner's membrane separates Scala media from Scala vestibuli in the inner ear.
    - Basilar membrane separates Scala media or cochlear duct from Scala tympani in the inner ear. The organ of Corti rests on the basilar membrane.
    - Secondary TM overlies the round window in the middle ear.
46. **(b) Peripheral** (*Ref. Scott Brown, 7th ed., page 3180*)
    - Peripheral is the best answer here (please refer to the text).
47. **(d) 90 mm²** (*Ref. Dhingra, 6th ed., page 14*)
48. **(d) 55 mm²** (*Ref. Dhingra, 6th ed., page 14*)
49. **(b) Auriculotemporal** (*Ref. Scott Brown, 8th ed., Vol 2, page 526*)
50. **(a) Greater occipital nerve** (*Ref. Shambaugh, 6th ed., page 30*) (does not supply pinna, please see text for the nerve supply of external ear).

51. **(a) Vagus** (*Ref. Shambaugh, 6th ed., page 30*)
52. **(d) Greater auricular nerve** (*Ref. Shambaugh, 6th ed., page 30*)
53. **(b) Glossopharyngeal nerve** (*Ref. Shambaugh, 6th ed., page 30*)
    - Glossopharyngeal does not supply auricle and external auditory canal. It gives sensory supply to middle ear.
54. **(c) and (d)** (*Ref. Current Diagnosis and Treatment Otolaryngology, Lalwani, 3rd ed., 600*)
    - Sphenopalatine ganglion is the largest parasympathetic ganglion responsible for lacrimation, nasal secretion and palatine secretion.
    - The greater superficial petrosal nerve originates from the geniculate ganglion of facial nerve. It then joins with the deep petrosal nerve to form the vidian nerve and then through the sphenopalatine ganglion supplies lacrimal, nasal and palatine glands. See chapter on the anatomy of nose.
55. **(c) The Xth cranial nerve** (*Ref. Shambaugh, 6th ed., page 45*)
    - The Xth cranial nerve also supplying the larynx leads to cough on cleaning the ear canal.
56. **(a) Vagus** (*Ref. Shambaugh, 6th ed., page 45*)
57. **(a), (b) and (e)** (*Ref. Scott Brown, 8th ed., Vol 2, page 529*)
58. **(b) Glossopharyngeal** (*Ref. Scott Brown, 8th ed., Vol 2 page 535*)
    - The sensory supply of the middle ear is by the tympanic plexus which is formed by the Jacobson's nerve which is the tympanic branch of Glossopharyngeal (IX) along with sympathetic plexus from around the internal carotid.
59. **(a) IX nerve, i.e. the glossopharyngeal nerve** (*Ref. Scott Brown, 8th ed., Vol 2, page 535*)
    The rest of the nerves do not supply the ear.
60. **(d) Vestibule of nose** (*Ref. Shambaugh, 6th ed., page 45*)
    - Vestibule of nose is supplied by the maxillary nerve which does not supply the ear.
    - Pharynx is supplied by the pharyngeal plexus formed by the vagus and Glossopharyngeal, both of which also supply the ear.
    - Tongue is supplied by the lingual branch of mandibular, Glossopharyngeal and vagus, all of which also supply the ear.
    - TM joint is supplied by the Auriculotemporal nerve which also supplies the ear.
61. **(d) All of the above** (*Ref. Shambaugh, 6th ed., page 45*)
    - Larynx is supplied by the vagus which also supplies the ear.
    - Tongue and oral cavity is supplied by the lingual branch of mandibular, Glossopharyngeal and vagus, all of which also supply the ear.

62. **(c) Glossopharyngeal nerve** (*Ref. Shambaugh 6th ed., page 45*)
    - The base of tongue is mainly supplied by the glossopharyngeal nerve which also supplies the ear.

 Note:

- Anterior 2/3rd of the tongue is supplied by lingual nerve (a branch of mandibular). Auriculotemporal nerve also a branch of mandibular nerve supplies the ear so in carcinoma anterior 2/3rd of tongue pain is referred to ear through mandibular nerve.
- Posterior 1/3rd, i.e. the base of the tongue is mainly supplied by glossopharyngeal nerve and the posterior most part of this posterior 1/3rd tongue is supplied by vagus, both of which also supply the ear, so in carcinoma of this part of tongue, pain will be referred to ear through both glossopharyngeal and vagus.
- But since glossopharyngeal supplies most of the base of the tongue so in pathologies of base of tongue the pain is referred to the ear mainly through the glossopharyngeal nerve.

63. **(b) Facial nerve** (*Ref. Scott Brown, 8th ed., Vol 2, page 580*)
    - The stapedius muscle is a second arch derivative and therefore is supplied by the nerve of the 2nd arch, i.e. facial nerve.

64. **(a) Anterior part of V nerve** (*Ref. Shambaugh, 6th ed., page 38*)
    - The tensor tympani muscle is a derivative of 1st arch and is supplied by the nerve of the 1st arch, i.e. mandibular nerve (anterior or motor branch).

65. **(b) Basal turn of cochlea** (*Ref. Shambaugh, 6th ed., page 39*)
    - Promontory is a bulge in the centre of the medial wall of middle ear, produced by the basal turn of cochlea. On the promontory, tympanic plexus is present
    - Lateral semicircular canal bulge is present on the most postero-superior portion of the medial wall of middle ear just above the horizontal or tympanic segment of facial nerve.
    - Jugular bulb is below the floor of the middle ear
    - Body of incus is present in the epitympanum of middle ear cavity.

66. **(a) Tendon of tensor tympani** (*Ref. Shambaugh, 6th ed. page 38*)
    - Processus Cochleariformis is a hook like structure present antero-superiorly on the medial wall of middle ear.
    - The tensor tympani muscle originating from a canal in the anterior wall of middle ear runs medially where its tendon winds around the processus cochleariformis and then turns laterally to get attached on the upper part of the handle of malleus (i.e. just below its neck).

67. **(b) Oval window** (*Ref. Shambaugh, 6th ed., page 38*)
    - Round window is covered by secondary TM.

- Sinus tympani is the area on the posterior wall of mesotympanum medial to the bulge of vertical part of facial nerve.
- Pyramid is a projection of bone on the posterior wall from which originates the stapedius muscle.

68. **(a) Round window** (*Ref. Scott Brown, 8th ed., Vol 2, page 580*)

69. **(d) All of the above** (*Ref. Cummings, 6th ed., 509; 2192*)
    - Facial recess is an area on the posterior wall of middle ear. The facial recess is limited superiorly by the fossa incudis, laterally by chorda tympani entry and medially by the descending/vertical facial nerve segment.
    - The facial recess is the site where opening is made on the posterior wall to access the middle ear cavity through the mastoid in "INTACT CANAL WALL" ear surgeries. This is known as the posterior tympanotomy approach. See chapter on unsafe CSOM

70. **(a) Facial nerve horizontal part** (*Ref. Cummings, 6th ed., 509; 2192*)

71. **(b) Medially it is bounded by chorda tympani and laterally by facial nerve** (*Ref. Cummings, 6th ed., 509*)
    - Medially the facial recess is bounded by facial nerve and laterally by chorda tympani

72. **(a) Anterior wall** (*Ref. Shambaugh, 6th ed., page 245*)
73. **(c) 36 mm** (*Ref. Shambaugh, 6th ed., page 245*)
74. **(d) and (e)** (*Ref. Scott Brown, 8th ed., Vol 2, page 537*)
    - The total length of Eustachian tube is about 36 mm (32–38 mm), the lateral or outer 1/3rd, i.e. 12 mm is bony, whereas the medial or inner 2/3rd, i.e. 24 mm is cartilaginous.
    - Eustachian tube normally remains closed and opens intermittently during swallowing, yawning and sneezing.

75. **(a), (c) and (e)** (*Ref. Shambaugh, 6th ed., page 245*)
    - The length of Eustachian tube is 32–38 mm, i.e. 3.2–3.8 cm.
    - Its 1/3rd part is bony and 2/3rd part is cartilaginous, just the opposite of EAC.
    - Eustachian tube normally remains closed and opens intermittently during swallowing, yawning and sneezing.
    - Tensor palati plays the major role in opening the tube
    - The narrowest part of Eustachian tube is the junction of the bony and cartilaginous parts known as isthmus.

76. **(b) Higher elastin content in adults**, refer the text (*Ref. Cummings, 6th ed., 2028*)

77. **(c) Tensor veli palatini** (*Ref. Shambaugh, 6th ed., page 245*)

78. **(b) Bulb of the internal jugular vein** (*Ref. Cummings, 6th ed., 1983*)
    - The floor of middle ear cavity is a thin plate of bone separating the middle ear from jugular bulb below.

- Internal carotid artery is in relation to the anterior wall of middle ear.
- Sigmoid sinus is not related directly with middle ear cavity. It lies posterior to the mastoid antrum.
- Round window lies postero-inferiorly on the medial wall of middle ear.

79. **(c) Roof of middle ear** (*Ref. Cummings, 6th ed., 1983*)
- The roof of the middle ear is known as "TEGMEN TYMPANI". It separates the middle ear from the middle cranial fossa.

80. **(d) 2 mm** (*Ref. BD Chaurasia, Human Anatomy 6th ed., Vol 3, page 277*)

Part of the middle ear cavity	Distance from lateral to medial wall
Epitympanum	6 mm (widest)
Mesotympanum (centre)	2 mm (narrowest)
Hypotympanum	4 mm

81. **(a) 2 mm** (*Ref. BD Chaurasia, Human Anatomy 6th ed., Vol 3, page 277*)
- The promontory is present in the centre of medial wall of middle ear. Its distance from umbo is the narrowest part of the middle ear, i.e. about 2 mm.

82. **(d) Mesotympanum–2 mm** (*Ref. BD Chaurasia, Human Anatomy 6th ed., Vol 3, page 277*)
- Epitympanum or attic is widest–6 mm
- Hypotympanum–4 mm

83. **(a) Epitympanum** (*Ref. Cummings, 6th ed., 1983*)
- The space of the epitympanum, lying in between the Shrapnell's membrane or pars flaccida and the neck of malleus is known as "PRUSSAK'S SPACE".
- When the retraction pocket on Pars flaccida grows medially, it goes into this Prussak's space making this the most common site of primary cholesteatoma.

84. **(d) Foot plate of stapes** (it is in mesotympanum) (*Ref. Cummings, 6th ed., 1983*)

Epitympanum contains	Mesotympanum contains
1. Head, neck, anterior and lateral process of malleus	Handle of malleus
2. Body and short process of incus	Long process of incus
3. Incudomalleolar joint (the head of malleus articulates with the body of incus)	Incudostapedial joint and the whole of the stapes
4. The Chorda tympani nerve	—
5. Prussak's space	—

- The hypotympanum does not contain anything.

85. **(d) Synovial joint** (*Ref. Scott Brown, 8th ed., Vol 2 page 533*)
- The head of malleus articulates with the body of incus. This incudomalleolar joint is a saddle type of synovial joint.
- The long process of incus ends in a lentiform nodule. This lentiform nodule of incus articulates with the head of stapes. This incudostapedial joint is a ball and socket type of synovial joint.

86. **(b) Mastoid antrum** (*Ref. Shambaugh, 6th ed., page 32*)
- Macewen's" triangle or suprameatal triangle is a bony landmark for mastoid antrum. It is important while doing mastoid surgeries in approaching the mastoid antrum.

87. **(a) Mastoid antrum** (*Ref. Shambaugh, 6th ed., page 32*)

88. **(a) Mastoid antrum** (*Ref. Shambaugh, 6th ed., page 32*)

89. **(a) Squamous temporal** (*Ref. Scott Brown, 8th ed., Vol 2, page 543*)
- Tegmen Antri forms the roof of antrum.
- The medial wall of mastoid antrum is related to the posterior semicircular canal, which lies in its superior aspect.

90. **(c) Promontory** (refer the text) (*Ref. Shambaugh, 6th ed., page 32*)

91. **(a) Mastoid antrum lies 1.5 cm deep to it** (*Ref. Shambaugh, 6th ed., page 32*)
- It is a surgical landmark for the mastoid antrum, lying in the postauricular area. It is bounded superiorly by temporal line/supra mastoid crest which is the posterior extension of suprameatal crest.
- The suprameatal crest is the superior root of the zygomatic process.

92. **(c) Sinodural angle** (*Ref. Shambaugh, 6th ed., page 775*)

93. **(b) Mastoid** (*Ref. Shambaugh, 6th ed., page 773*)

94. **(a) Basilar membrane** (*Ref. Shambaugh, 6th ed., page 73*)
- Organ of Corti rests on the Basilar membrane which separates Scala media from Scala tympani.
- Utricle and Saccule contain the sensory end organ of balance for linear acceleration known as maculae.

95. **(b) is secreted by stria vascularis** (*Ref. Scott Brown, 8th ed., Vol 2, page 583*)
- Endolymph is the fluid that fills in whole of the membranous labyrinth (i.e. the three semicircular canals, utricle, saccule and the scala media).
- It is secreted by stria vascularis.
- It is absorbed by the endolymphatic duct.

96. **(a) +80 mV** (*Ref. Shambaugh, 6th ed., page 79*)
- The endolymph is rich in K^+ which leads to the development of an endolymphatic potential of + 80–85 mV.

97. **(c) To maintain electric milieu of endolymph** (*Ref. Scott Brown, 8th ed., Vol 2, page 561*)

98. **(d) Hair cell** (*Ref. Scott Brown, 8th ed., Vol 2, page 558*)

99. **(c) Genu of internal capsule** (*Ref. Cummings, 6th ed., 1991*)
- Genu of internal capsule is not concerned with auditory pathway; it is the posterior limb of internal capsule through which ultimately the fibres pass through and reach the auditory cortex.

100. **(a) Auditory pathway** (*Ref. Cummings, 6th ed., 1991*)

101. **(d) Sound localisation** (*Ref. Cummings, 6th ed., 1991*)

102. **(d) Transverse temporal gyrus** (*Ref. Cummings, 6th ed., 1991*)

103. **(c) Linear acceleration** (*Ref. Shambaugh, 6th ed., page 113*)

104. **(a) Macula** (*Ref. Shambaugh, 6th ed., page 113*)
   - Maculae sense linear acceleration, gravitational (movement either with or against gravity) and head tilt movements and they also help to maintain static equilibrium (by facilitating postural, tonic neck and righting reflexes)

105. **(a) Otolith– made up of uric acid crystals** (*Ref. Shambaugh, 6th ed., page 113*)
   - Otolith is made up of calcium carbonate.
   - They are present in the maculae and stimulated by gravity, linear acceleration and head tilt movements.

106. **(a) Utricle and saccule–cristae** (*Ref. Shambaugh, 6th ed., page 113*)
   - Utricle and saccule contain maculae.
   - Cristae are present in the semicircular canal.
   - Foot plate of stapes overlies oval window.
   - Macewen's triangle or suprameatal triangle is the bony landmark of mastoid antrum.
   - Scala vestibuli is separated from scala media by Reissner's membrane.

107. **(a) Bill's bar** (*Ref. Shambaugh, 6th ed., page 42*)
   - Ponticulus is a ridge which runs from the oval window to the sinus tympani forming its superior extent.
   - Cog is a bony projection from the roof of middle ear, i.e. tegmen tympani to the processus cochleariformis, serving as an approximate landmark for the facial nerve.
   - Falciform crest divides the internal acoustic meatus into a superior and inferior part.

108. **(b) Inferior vestibular nerve supplying posterior semicircular canal** (Please refer the text) (*Ref. Shambaugh, 6th ed., page 45*)

109. **(d) Anterior inferior cerebellar artery** (*Ref. Shambaugh, 6th ed., page 47*)
   - The inner ear is supplied by Labyrinthine artery which is a branch of Anterior inferior cerebellar artery or sometimes the basilar artery.

110. **(a) Lateral wall of attic** (*Ref. Scott Brown, 8th ed., Vol 2, page 529*)

111. **(a) Connects middle ear to pharynx** (*Ref. Cummings, 6th ed., 2028*)

112. **(b) Regulation of distortion activated ion channels** (*Ref. Scott Brown, 8th ed., Vol 2, page 554*)

113. **(a) Saddle** (*Ref. BD Chaurasia, Human Anatomy, 6th ed., Vol 3, page 280*)

114. **(a) Postero-lateral part of helix** (*Ref. Scott Brown, 8th ed., Vol 2, page 525*)

115. **(b) Arnolds** (*Ref. Shambaugh, 6th ed., page 30*)

116. **(c) Downwards, forwards, medially** (*Ref. Scott Brown, 8th ed., Vol 2, page 527*)

117. **(d) Vestibule** (*Ref. Scott Brown, 8th ed., Vol 2, page 531*)

118. **(a) Surface ectoderm** (*Ref. Shambaugh, 6th ed., page 9*)

119. **(b) Michel aplasia** (*Ref. Cummings, 6th ed., 2983*)

120. **(a) One** (*Ref. Scott Brown, 8th ed., Vol 2, page 526*)

121. **(a) IX** (*Ref. Shambaugh, 6th ed., page 45*)

122. **(c) Root of helix** (*Ref. Scott Brown, 8th ed., Vol 2, page 541*)

123. **(c) Facial recess** (*Ref. Scott Brown, 8th ed., Vol 2, page 531*)

124. **(c) Jacobson's nerve** (*Ref. Shambaugh, 6th ed., page 30*)

125. **(c) Greater auricular** (*Ref. Shambaugh, 6th ed., page 30*)

126. **(c) Greater auricular nerve** (*Ref. Scott Brown, 8th ed., Vol 2, page 526*)

127. **(b) Middle and inner** (*Ref. Scott Brown, 8th ed., Vol 2 page 530*)

128. **(c) Mastoid antrum** (*Ref. BD Chaurasia, Human Anatomy, 6th ed., Vol 3, 281*)

129. **(b) 55 degrees** (*Ref. Scott Brown, 8th ed., Vol 2, page 529*)

130. **(d)** (*Ref. Shambaugh, 6th ed., 599*) The middle ear is seen here. The marked structure is the round window, through which the cochlear implant electrodes are introduced into the inner ear.
   - Stapes foot plate is present on the oval window, which is seen in the picture above the round window opening
   - Intact canal wall surgery is done through the facial recess present on the posterior wall of the middle ear, not visible in the picture
   - ET tube ventilates the middle ear which is present on the anterior wall, not visible in the picture

131. **(a) Facial recess** (*Ref. Cummings, 6th ed., 2192*)
   - In the given picture, the encircled area is the facial recess through which the round window opening is visible, also see the schematic picture below.

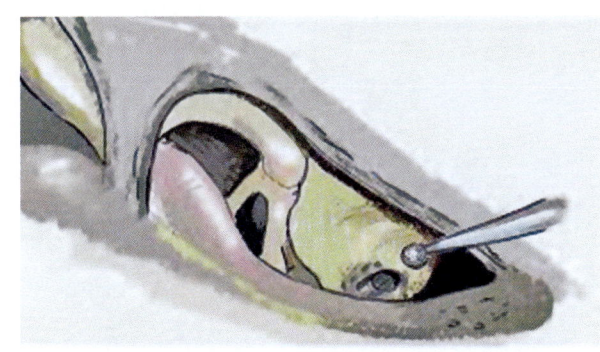

   - Facial recess is used to approach the middle ear through the mastoid, e.g. in cochlear implantation and in intact canal wall surgeries of the mastoid.

   Schematic picture of facial recess, through which a drill is pointing towards round window:

132. **(a) It is the landmark for mastoid antrum** (*Ref. Shambaugh, 6th ed., page 32*)

  - The marked area is the Macewen's or suprameatal triangle. It is the landmark for mastoid antrum.
  - Trautmann's triangle is present on the medial wall of mastoid antrum and is the landmark to approach posterior cranial fossa.
  - Prussak's space is a space in the epitympanum lying medial to pars flaccida, please see the text.
  - Myringotomy is making an opening on the TM to remove fluid or pus from the middle ear. Mastoid is not opened while doing myringotomy.

133. **(d) Otoliths: Semicircular canals** (*Ref. Cummings, 6th ed., 2014*)

134. **(b) Fissures of Santorini** (*Ref. Cummings, 6th ed., 1981*)

135. **(a) 7th cranial nerve** (*Ref. Scott Brown, 8th ed., Vol 2, page 539*)

136. **(a) Cochlea** (*Ref. Shambaugh, 6th ed., page 73*)

137. **(a) Utricle** (*Ref. Cummings, 6th ed., 2014*)

138. **(c) Dysplasia of cochlea and saccule** (*Ref. Cummings, 6th ed., 2982*)

139. **(d) +85 mV** (*Ref. Scott Brown, 8th ed., Vol 2, page 545*)

140. **(a) Stylomastoid foramen** (*Ref. Cummings, 6th ed., 1985*)

141. **(a) Superior temporal gyrus** (*Ref. Cummings, 6th ed., 1991*)

  - **The middle and inferior temporal gyrus are involved in cognitive processes, semantic memory, language process, visual perception and integrating information from different senses.**

142. **(b) VII** (*Ref. Cummings, 6th ed., 1985*)

143. **(c) Utricle** (*Ref. Cummings, 6th ed., 2014*)

144. **(c) Vestibulocochlear nerve** (*Ref. Scott Brown, 8th ed., Vol 2, page 539*)

145. **(c) Utricle** (*Ref. Shambaugh, 6th ed., page 42*)

146. **(a) 2.4 cm** (*Ref. Scott Brown, 8th ed., Vol 2, page 527*)

147. **(a) Petro squamous suture** (*Ref. Shambaugh, 6th ed., page 32*)

148. **(a) Malleus** (*Ref. Scott Brown, 8th ed., Vol 2, page 535*)

149. **(b) Glossopharyngeal** (*Ref. Scott Brown, 8th ed., Vol 2, page 531*)

150. **(b) ICF** (*Ref. Scott Brown, 8th ed., Vol 2, page 545*)

  - **Endolymph resembles intracellular fluid as it has more of K⁺.**
  - **Perilymph resembles intracellular fluid as it has more of Na⁺.**

151. **(c) Abducens nerve** (*Ref. Shambaugh, 6th ed., page 45*)

152. **(c) Sinodural angle** (*Ref. Shambaugh, 6th ed., page 775*)

153. **(d) Anteroinferior** (*Ref. BD Chaurasia, Human Anatomy, 6th ed., Vol 3, 276*)

154. **(c) Valsalva manoeuvre opens ET** (*Ref. Scott Brown 8th ed., Vol 2, page 537*)

155. **(c) Stapedius** (*Ref. Scott Brown, 8th ed., Vol 2, page 535*)

156. **(b) Fixation of footplate of stapes** (*Ref. Scott Brown, 8th ed., Vol 2, page 108*)

  - **According to Teunissen and Cremers classification, the most common congenital anomaly of the middle ear is fixation of footplate of stapes.**

157. **(a) 2 ml** (*Ref. Scott Brown, 8th ed., Vol 2, page 538*)

158. **(c) Eustachian tube** (*Ref. Cummings 6th ed., 2031*)

159. **(a) Semi-circular canal** (*Ref. Scott Brown, 8th ed., Vol 2, page 529*)

160. **(a) Malleus and round window** (*Ref. Scott Brown, 8th ed., Vol 2, page 531*)

161. **(b) Posterior part is more easily assessible** (*Ref. Scott Brown, 8th ed., Vol 2 page 529*)

162. **(b) Glutamate** (*Ref. Scott Brown, Vol 2, page 756*)

Physiology of Hearing and Audiology

PHYSIOLOGY OF HEARING

Whenever a sound is picked up by the pinna, it goes through the following pathway:

Pinna → EAC → TM → Ossicular chain → foot plate of stapes (oval window) → organ of Corti → 8th nerve → Auditory pathway → Auditory cortex (area no. 41).

- From pinna to foot plate of stapes occurs the conduction of sound. So this is the conductive pathway and any defect here will lead to a **conductive deafness**.
- In the organ of Corti **transduction** of sound occurs, i.e. sound energy gets converted to electrical impulses. Since organ of Corti is the sensory apparatus for hearing, any defect here is known as **sensory or Cochlear hearing loss**.
- Any defect of the nerves of the auditory pathway beyond the cochlea will lead to a **retro-cochlear or neural hearing loss**.
- Together the sensory and the neural hearing loss is known as sensorineural hearing loss.
- A defect involving both the conductive and sensorineural pathway is known as **mixed hearing loss**.

MECHANISM OF HEARING (TRANSFORMER ACTION OF MIDDLE EAR)

Whenever a sound passes from the external and middle ear to the inner ear there is a **change in medium** from air (external and middle ear) to liquid (inner ear).

Due to this change 99.9% of the sound gets reflected back.

To overcome this and **match the impedance** (resistance to flow of sound) of the middle ear (low impedance) with the inner ear (high impedance), the middle ear acts as a transformer. By this transformer action of middle ear there occurs an increase in the force of any sound that enters the middle ear, so that more of sound can now enter the inner ear rather than most of it getting reflected back.

This function of the middle ear to **convert sound of greater amplitude and lesser force to lesser amplitude and greater force** so that more of sound can enter the inner ear is known as **transformer action** of middle ear.

The middle ear acts like a transformer in the sense that it steps up the intensity of sound during normal hearing. Similarly it steps down the intensity when there is a loud noise (i.e. a sound 70–100 dB above the hearing threshold) with the help of stapedius and tensor tympani muscles (please refer to stapedial reflex).

STEP UP PHENOMENON OF MIDDLE EAR

The step up of the transformer action occurs by the following:

Areal ratio (or hydraulic ratio): The total area of tympanic membrane is 90 mm². But the whole of it does not vibrate effectively to conduct sound.

The **effective vibratory area of TM is 55 mm²**. The area of the foot plate of stapes is just 3.2 mm².

When sound gets concentrated from a large area to a small area (as occurs during its transmission from the tympanic membrane to footplate of stapes), the force of sound gets increased (depending upon the ratio of the two areas).

The ratio of these two areas is called as **Areal ratio. 17:1** (55 mm²/3.2 mm²).

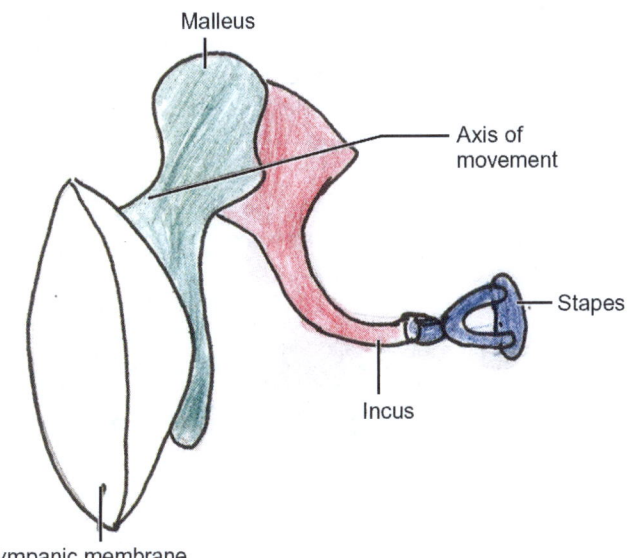

Fig. 2.1: Transformer Action of Middle Ear

Lever ratio: Additionally the handle of malleus is 1.3 times longer than the long process of incus because of which the incus moves 1.3 times more than the handle of malleus. This increases the force of sound 1.3 times so that this lever ratio is **1.3:1**.

So the **total transformer ratio** becomes Areal ratio × lever ratio, i.e. 17 × 1.3 = 22.

Hence the transformer action increases the sound pressure, applied to the inner ear by the stapes footplate, approximately 18–22 times than the sound pressure at the tympanic membrane. This compensates for the loss of sound energy because of change of medium.

Other minor factors contributing to the transformer action (step up phenomenon) are:

i. **Curved membrane effect/Catenary lever:** Since the TM is more mobile at the periphery than at the centre where it is attached to the handle of the malleus, this adds on to the force of sound. This curved membrane effect leads to a **twofold** amplification of the sound pressure.

ii. **Phase difference:** The sound from the TM is passed to the oval window through the ossicular chain and also to the round window through the middle ear air. The latter pathway being slow, so the sound does not reach the two windows simultaneously.

So when there is sound at the oval window there is compression (moving in) in the area of inner ear next to it and at the same time since the sound has not yet reached the round window, there occurs rarefaction (moving out) here and vice versa.

Hence **there is a difference in phase when the sound reaches both the windows**. This phase difference leads to effective transmission of the sound to the inner ear fluids.

Thus the sound waves cause the oval and round windows at the base of the cochlea to move in opposite directions (*see* Fig. 2.2). This causes the basilar membrane to be displaced. Also this starts a travelling wave in the basilar membrane that sweeps from the base toward the apex of the cochlea.

This is known as **travelling-wave theory**. This was given by George Von Bekesy. The theory states that a sound impulse sends a wave sweeping along the basilar membrane. As the wave moves along the membrane, its amplitude increases until it reaches a maximum, then falls off sharply until the wave dies out. That point at which the wave reaches its greatest amplitude is the point at which the frequency of the sound is detected by the ear. And as Helmholtz had postulated, Bekesy found that the **high-frequency** tones were perceived near the **base** of the cochlea and the **lower frequencies** toward the **apex**. For his studies of the travelling wave, **George von Bekesy** received the **Nobel Prize** in 1961.

iii. **Natural resonance of external and middle ear:** Each part of the external and middle ear has a resonating frequency of its own. Whenever a sound of the same frequency passes through that part of the ear, its transmission is accentuated. The natural resonating frequency of different parts of the ear are as follows:

External auditory canal: 3000 Hz

Tympanic membrane: 1000–3000 Hz

Middle ear: 1000–3000 Hz

Ossicles: 500–2000 (these are the normal speech frequencies)

To summarise:

Table 2.1	
Part of the external or middle ear	*Contributing factors for the effective transmission of the sound to the inner ear fluids*
Pinna	Collects and concentrates the sound
EAC	i. Narrowness of the canal causes increase in sound wave velocity ii. Natural resonance 3000 Hz
TM	i. Much larger area than foot plate of stapes (Areal ratio–17:1) ii. Curved membrane effect/ Catenary lever iii. Natural resonance 1000–3000 Hz
Ossicles	i. Handle of malleus longer than long process of incus (Lever ratio 1.3 : 1) ii. Natural resonance 500–2000 Hz
Middle ear	i. Total step up transformer ratio (areal × lever ratio = 22:1) ii. Natural resonance 800 Hz
Oval and round window	Sound does not reach simultaneously causing phase difference which in turn leads to the formation of travelling wave

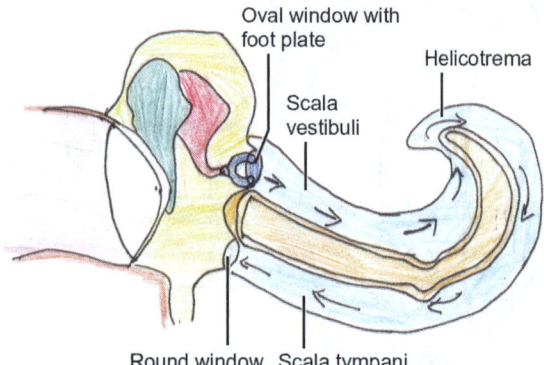

Fig. 2.2: Phase Difference between Oval and Round Windows

AUDIOLOGY

TUNING FORK TESTS

These are the most preliminary tests done (i.e. done initially in the ENT OPD itself) in patients presenting with the complaint of reduced hearing.

The following are the routinely done tuning fork tests:

1. Rinnes test
2. Weber test
3. Absolute bone conduction (ABC) test
4. Schwabach's test
5. Bing test
6. Gelle's test

The tuning fork tests help in finding out the site of lesion. They also provide a rough estimate of the degree of hearing defect.

The tuning fork tests are **most commonly** done with the **512** Hz frequency because it is **better heard**. In contrast to check the vibration sensation in neurology we typically employ 126 Hz tuning forks for they produce more of vibration sense.

Frequencies more than 512 Hz dampen very fast so these tuning forks are less commonly used.

The tuning fork is activated by striking it lightly against the elbow. It should not be struck against a hard solid object as it produces overtones which interferes with the pure tone generated by the tuning fork.

By the tuning fork tests we test the Air conduction (AC) and the Bone conduction (BC).

Air conduction: To test the Air conduction (AC) the vibrating tuning fork is placed 2 cm in front of the pinna.

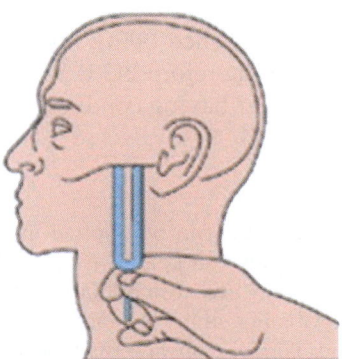

Air conduction

Sound vibration → Pinna → EAC → TM → Ossicular chain → foot plate of stapes (oval window) → organ of Corti → 8th nerve → Auditory pathway → Auditory cortex (area no. 41).

Any sound that enters our ears from the air outside will have to traverse the above pathway to be heard.

Hence **Air conduction (AC) is a measure of all the three pathways,** i.e. conductive, sensory as well as neural.

To test the Bone conduction (BC) the vibrating tuning fork is placed over the mastoid.

Bone conduction: Vibrating tuning fork → vibrates skull → cochlear fluid moves → stimulates organ of Corti →

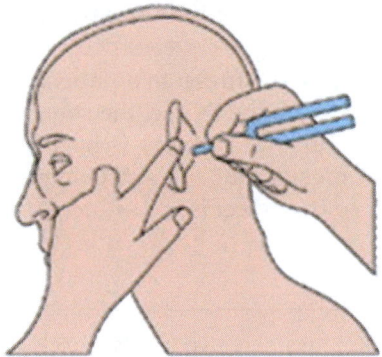

Bone conduction

8th nerve → auditory pathway → auditory cortex (area no. 41).

Hence **Bone conduction (BC) is a measure of** the latter two pathways, i.e. the **sensory and the neural pathway**.

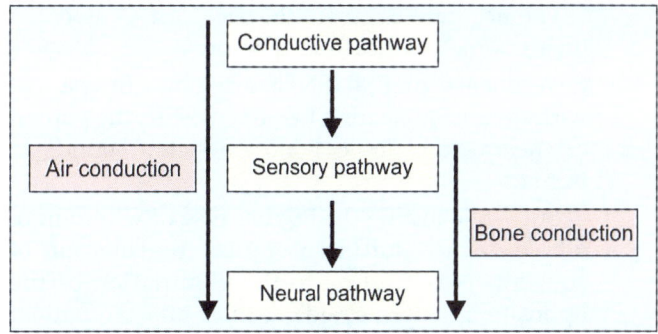

The sensory and the neural pathway are common for both AC and BC.

In both air conduction and bone conduction, there is change of medium but the AC sound passes through the middle ear where the transformer action is occurring. Hence **AC is louder and heard for longer duration than the BC in normal ears.**

1. Rinne's Test

Here we test the AC and BC and compare the two in the same ear.

The Rinne test can be positive or negative.

- When AC > BC Rinne is said to be **positive**.
- When BC > AC Rinne is said to be **negative**.

1. When AC > BC, i.e. **Rinne is positive**, there can be two possibilities:
   a. **Normal ear:** Here as stated above air conduction is more than the bone conduction.
   b. **Sensorineural deafness:** Here since the common pathway, i.e. the sensorineural pathway is defective, both AC and BC will decrease. But since in AC pathway the sound passes through the middle ear where transformer action is taking place so ultimately more sound reaches the defective inner ear than the sound reaching the defective inner ear directly as in BC. Therefore here too air conduction is more than the bone conduction.

Therefore **Rinne is positive in a person having normal ear and also in sensorineural deafness.**

Section I   Ear

2. When BC > AC, i.e. **Rinne negative**, there are again two possibilities:

   a. **Conductive deafness:** In a patient with decreased hearing when the BC, i.e. the sound going directly to sensorineural pathway is heard better than the AC, it means that the sensorineural pathway is good, so the defect is in conductive pathway.

*Note:*_____

Rinne is not a very sensitive test as it picks up conductive hearing loss only if the loss is more than 15–20 dB, i.e. it comes **negative only if the hearing loss is more than 15–20 dB.**

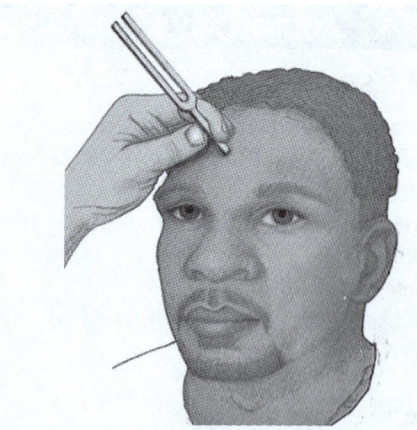

If Rinne is negative with 256, 512 and 1024 Hz tuning forks, there is respectively an approximate hearing loss of 15 dB, 30 dB and 45 dB respectively.

The accurate degree of hearing loss is assessed on audiometry (please read below).

   b. **Severe sensorineural (SN) hearing loss:** In a patient with severe SN hearing loss of one side, the patient can hear neither air nor bone conduction sounds on this side.

But while testing the BC, because of vibration of whole of the skull, transcranial transmission of sound occurs leading to the stimulation of the opposite, i.e. normal side cochlea and the patient hears from the opposite or normal ear. So here patient responds to bone conduction but not to air conduction, i.e. BC > AC or Rinne negative. But here since the BC of the involved ear is actually not better than AC, this negative Rinne is a **false negative Rinne**.

Hence **Rinne is negative in conductive deafness, whereas in severe sensorineural deafness it is falsely negative.** This false negative Rinne in severe SN hearing loss is very important to remember because he can be mistaken to be having conductive deafness. Thus the diagnosis of severe SNHL gets delayed to such an extent that it becomes no longer reversible with the usual steroid treatment. Often these sudden severe SNHL patients are young and therefore it is very important to diagnose them early or else unfortunately they will loose this important sensory organ of hearing due to our negligence.

To confirm whether the **Rinne** is a **true negative or false negative**, we do **Weber's test**.

2. Weber Test

In this test the vibrating tuning fork is placed over the forehead/vertex or teeth (incisors) and the lateralisation of the sound is asked for (i.e. in which ear the sound is heard louder).

Weber is a very sensitive test as it shows lateralisation even with **5 dB difference** between the ears.

In Weber we are checking the BC only and comparing the BC on the two sides.

In a normal person it is heard equally in both the ears.

1. **SN hearing loss:** Here the Weber's is **lateralised towards the better ear,** i.e. the sound is reported to be heard well in the better ear. Since in Weber's test we test the bone conduction and BC is a measure of SN pathway so in SN hearing loss of one ear the BC is decreased in affected ear, i.e. BC is heard better in the ear with normal SN pathway.

   In mild to moderate SN loss as well as in severe SN hearing loss Weber's shows lateralisation towards the better ear.

2. **Conductive hearing loss:** Here the Weber's is **lateralised to the worst ear**, i.e. the patient hears the bone conduction sound better in the worst ear. This is because the ambient noise entering through the AC route ultimately goes through the SN pathway and interferes with the bone conduction sound transmission via the same SN pathway in the normal ear.

   This interference being absent in conductive hearing loss therefore BC is better in the affected ear, i.e. the ear having conductive defect.

*Note:*_____

- The same principle can be applied in a patient with a conductive hearing loss condition e.g. SOM, Otosclerosis, etc. He hears his own voice louder (because when one speaks the vibration of the jaw directly stimulates the bone conduction, i.e. SN pathway). As a result he has low tone speech (this is in contrary to SN hearing loss where the patient is not able to hear his own voice and therefore speaks loudly e.g. presbycusis in elderly).

- **Weber's is lateralised to** the **W**orst ear in **C**onductive hearing loss and **B**etter ear in **S**ensorineural hearing loss. (Mnemonic **We C**reate–**B**est **S**tudents).

3. Absolute Bone Conduction (ABC) Test

This should be remembered as absolutely the bone conduction test as this test is for testing only or absolutely the bone conduction, i.e. SN deafness.

In this test the BC of the patient is compared with the examiner, provided the examiner's hearing is normal. Here both the patient and the examiner are given conductive hearing loss by pressing the tragus and thereby occluding the external auditory canal while testing. Hence it is a test for diagnosing only SN hearing loss.

The vibrating tuning fork is placed 1st over the patient's mastoid while occluding the EAC. When the patient stops hearing, the same tuning fork is placed over the examiner's mastoid.

If the examiner still hears it, this indicates that the patient's BC is decreased, i.e. the patient has SN hearing loss.

So in SN hearing loss ABC (of the patient as compared to the Doctor) is shortened.

4. Schwabach's Test

It is done exactly in the same way as the ABC except that the meatus is not occluded so that we can also test the conductive pathway.

Considering the examiner's hearing as normal if the BC of the patient is less (i.e. shortened) than the examiner's, it means SN pathway of the patient is affected and patient has SN hearing loss.

If the patient's BC is same as examiner, it means that the patient's hearing is normal like the examiner.

If the patient hears the BC for longer duration than the examiner (i.e. his BC is lengthened), it means that the patient has conductive hearing loss. The BC is lengthened here because this sound is not being interfered with the ambient noise entering through the AC route as the AC is defective here due to the pathology in conductive pathway.

So Schwabach's test is shortened in SN hearing loss and lengthened in conductive hearing loss (Mnemonic; **S**tudents **L**et's **C**onclude and **S**tudy **S**ummary → **S**chwabach's is **L**engthened in **C**onductive and **S**hortened in **S**ensorineural hearing loss).

5. Bing test

In this test a vibrating tuning fork is applied to the bone overlying the mastoid. At the same time the meatus is alternately left open and occluded and the patient is asked to judge whether the tone is louder with the ear occluded or patent.

If the patient already has conductive hearing loss there will be no change in hearing whether the ear is open or occluded (Bing negative).

If the patient's hearing is normal or if he is having SN deafness, he hears the sound louder when the ear is occluded as the masking by outer ambient noise is absent in occluded ear (Bing positive). So like Rinne, Bing test is negative in conductive deafness.

6. Gelle's Test

In this test a Siegel's speculum is put in the EAC and at the same time a vibrating tuning fork is placed on the mastoid. When the pressure in the EAC is increased, the TM is pushed medially leading to decreased mobility of ossicles and increased hearing (the increase in hearing occurs because by imparting a conductive hearing loss here upon increased pressure, there occurs masking of ambient noise).

When the pressure is released the ossicular chain and the TM mobility is regained and the hearing becomes normal. This change in hearing on changing the pressure of the external auditory canal is Gelle's positive.

But if the ossicular chain is already fixed there will be no change in hearing with pressure changes. This is Gelle's negative and will be seen in any ossicular chain fixity, e.g. Otosclerosis.

 Note:

In Rinne, Bing and Gelle's same findings in normal and SN deafness.

AUDIOMETRIC TESTS

The earliest audiometric test was "Bekesy" audiometry invented by Von Bekesy who became the Nobel Prize winner in ENT for his travelling wave theory, though it is no more done now.

Pure Tone Audiometry (PTA)

Here the AC and BC are tested with the help of an electronic device known as audiometer (*see* the PTA being done in a sound proof room below).

Test	Normal	SN Deafness	Conductive deafness
Rinne	Positive (AC>BC)	Positive (AC>BC) or False negative in severe SN deafness	Negative (BC>AC)
Weber	Equal in both ears, i.e. not lateralised	Lateralised to better ear (**B**est **S**tudents)	Lateralised to worst ear (**W**e **C**reate)
ABC	Same as examiner's	Shortened as compared to examiner's	Same as examiner's
Schwabach	Same as examiner's	Shortened as compared to examiner's (**S**tudy **S**ummary)	Lengthened as compared to examiner's (**L**et's **C**onclude)
Bing test	Louder (when occluded)	Louder (when occluded)	No effect (Bing negative)
Gelle's test	Increased hearing after increasing pressure	Increased Hearing after increasing pressure	Hearing does not alter with pressure changes (Gelle's negative)

Table 2.2: Summary of tuning fork tests

Section I | Ear

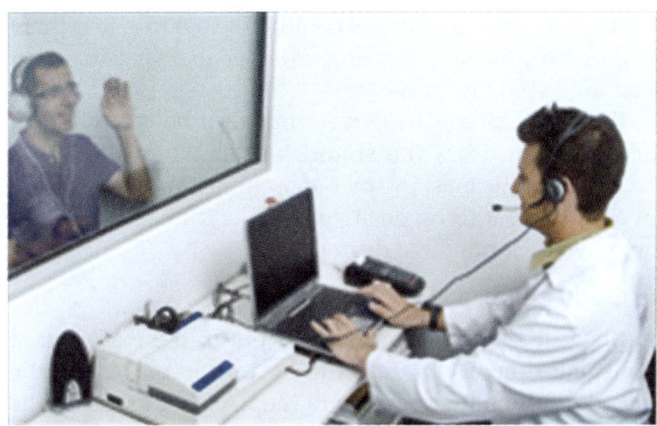

The benefits of PTA over tuning fork tests:

1. It **confirms the type of hearing loss** (i.e. conductive, SN or mixed)

2. The **degree of hearing loss can be measured accurately**. This can also give us an approximate idea of the site of defect in the ear, *see* Table 2.3.

The intensity of sound is expressed as decibel (dB).

$dB = 20 \log SPL_o/SPL_R$ where SPL_o is sound pressure level of observed sound and SPL_R is sound pressure level of reference sound.

If the observed sound is the same as reference sound: $dB = 20 \log 1$. Since $\log 1 = 0$, $20 \times 0 = 0$ dB.

Hence 0 dB loudness is when the loudness is equal to the reference level and should not be considered as complete silence.

If the observed sound is 10 times louder than the reference sound the equation becomes:

$dB = 20 \log SPL_o/SPL_R$, i.e. $20 \log 10 = 20 \times 1$ (as log 10 is 1) = 20.

Hence **20 dB sound means** that the sound is **10 times** louder than the reference sound. Similarly **40 dB** sound means that the sound is **100 times** louder than the reference sound. ($dB = 20 \log 100 = 20 \times 2$ (as log 100 is 2) = 40

So a sound of 40 dB is 10 times louder than a sound of 20 dB and so on.

3. **A large number of sound frequencies can be checked.**

Ear is sensitive to frequencies from 20 Hz to 20,000 Hz.

In conventional audiometry the AC is measured for sound frequencies from 125 Hz to 8000 Hz, whereas the BC is measured for 250 Hz to 4000 Hz.

High frequency audiometry tests sound frequencies from 8000–20,000 Hz, read below.

Since most of the human speech ranges from 500–2000 Hz, these frequencies (500, 1000 and 2000 Hz) are known as **speech frequencies.**

Degree of hearing loss:

While doing PTA, **AC threshold** (i.e. when the patient first recognises the sound) of **up to 15 dB** is considered to be normal and **BC threshold of up to 25 dB is considered to be normal**. Beyond this, hearing loss is categorised by American Speech-language Hearing Association (ASHA)and in a slightly different way by WHO as follows:

The result of PTA is plotted in the form of a graph which is called "audiogram".

The various symbols used while plotting the audiogram are given in Table 2.5.

Right ear is marked in Red and left ear in Blue (*mnemonic:* R for R).

Masking

Whenever a sound is presented to an ear through the air conduction route it gets transmitted to the other ear also via air. During this transmission of sound from one ear to the other (through air), a loss, i.e. interaural attenuation of approximately 40 dB occurs. For, e.g. a sound of 60 dB presented to the right ear will be heard as 20 dB in the left ear.

If the patient has hearing loss of more than 50 dB in an ear and a sound of 50 dB is presented to this ear, he will not hear through this ear, but he will hear 10 dB sound in the other ear and respond. This will give a false result. Therefore masking, which is preventing the better ear to take part in hearing test while testing the worst ear, is

Table 2.3	
Pathology	*Approximate hearing loss*
Complete obstruction of the ear canal	40 dB
Perforation of TM	10–40 dB
Ossicular interruption with intact TM	54 dB
Ossicular interruption with perforated TM	38 dB (lesser loss than above because some sound reaching directly to the foot plate through the perforation)
Complete fixation of foot plate	60 dB

Table 2.4	
Hearing loss	*dB*
ASHA:	
Mild	26–40
Moderate	41–55
Moderately severe	56–70
Severe	71–91
Profound	>91
WHO:	
Mild	26–40
Moderate	41–60
Severe	61–80
Profound	≥81

*Note:*

In Table 2.4 as per ASHA there is increment of 15 dB, except in severe loss where the range is 20 dB so that AC or BC detected above 91dB is considered to be profound hearing loss, whereas as per WHO guidelines there is a change in the degree of hearing loss at every 20 dB and AC or BC detected at or above 81dB is considered to be profound hearing loss. In ASHA there is one extra category of moderately severe hearing loss.

done when there is a difference between the two ears is minimum 40 dB in the air conduction threshold.

In bone conduction the interaural attenuation is 0 dB, thus masking of better ear should be done in all bone conduction sounds.

Masking is done by presenting a complex noise to the ear.

Important Pure Tone Audiograms

Figure 2.3 audiogram shows that the patient hears the various frequencies of sound in BC at 5 dB loudness which is in normal range (0–25 dB). For the same frequencies to be heard in AC the loudness has to be increased to 40dB (approximately).

So here BC (i.e. SN pathway) is normal but AC is defective meaning that the patient has conductive hearing loss.

Since the BC is normal and AC is decreased there is a gap between the AC and BC curves.

So in **conductive hearing loss** (e.g. Wax, Meatal atresia, TM perforation, Ossicular dislocation, otosclerosis/any other cause of ossicular fixation) the audiogram has an **Air –Bone gap,** i.e. a gap between AC and BC curves of **more than 15–20 dB** (AC decreased and BC normal).

In Fig. 2.4 audiogram the patient hears BC in left ear at 35 dB so it is decreased (normally it being detected at up to 25 dB). AC is heard at 40 dB so it is also decreased.

Both AC and BC will be decreased when the common pathway, i.e. SN pathway is affected.

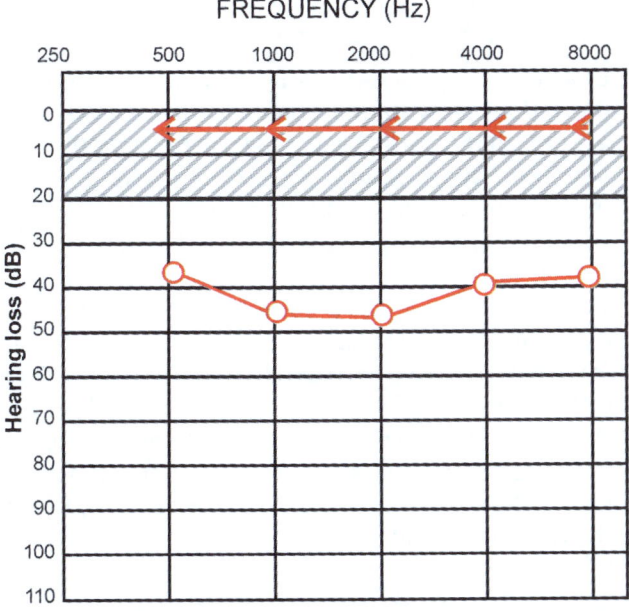

FREQUENCY (Hz)

Fig. 2.3: Audiogram

Table 2.5: Symbols used while plotting the audiogram		
Condition	Symbol for right ear (in red)	Symbol for left ear (in blue)
AC (unmasked)	O	×
AC (masked)	Δ	□
BC (unmasked)	<	>
BC (masked)	[	]
Not-Responding	℔	↘

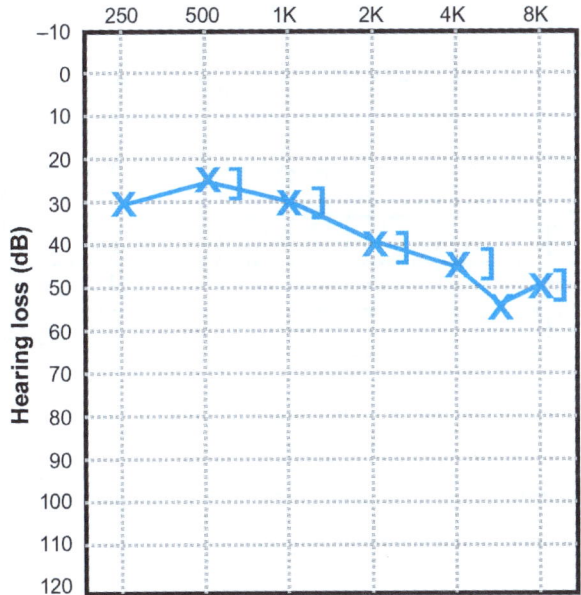

Fig. 2.4: Audiogram

So this audiogram depicts a SN hearing loss (e.g. Meniere's, Presbycusis, ototoxicity, acoustic neuroma, noise trauma, etc.).

Here since both AC and BC are decreased because of defect in the common pathway **the air bone–gap in SN hearing loss is not more than 15–20 dB.**

- Another finding to be noted in the audiogram is that it is a **downsloping/descending audiogram** which means that the high frequencies are affected more. **D**own sloping audiogram is seen in **P**resbycusis, **O**totoxicity, **N**oise induced trauma (*Mnemonic-PON D*).
- Similarly an **up sloping/ascending audiogram** indicates, low frequencies are affected more and is seen in early stages of Meniere's, *see* Chapter 12.
- Diseases causing SN hearing loss involving the speech frequencies, i.e. mid frequency hearing loss leads to a **U shaped/Trough shaped/cookie bite** (a cookie that has been bitten) audiogram. Here the patients have good perception of high and low frequency sounds but find it difficult to follow a conversation. It is seen in **congenital hearing loss** and in **cochlear Otosclerosis.**
- A characteristic dip in both AC and BC at 4000 Hz is seen in noise trauma called **acoustic dip,** *see* Chapter 12.
- A characteristic dip at 2000 Hz in the bone conduction curve is seen in Otosclerosis called as **Carhartz notch** (Please see chapter on Otosclerosis).

In Fig. 2.5 audiogram both AC and BC are decreased which means there is a defect in the common SN pathway. Here the AC is much more decreased than the bone conduction, so there is an additional air-bone gap also present.

So the Fig. 2.5 audiogram depicts **mixed hearing loss,** e.g. unsafe CSOM, Otosclerosis with cochlear involvement, etc. (please refer to chapter on unsafe CSOM).

Ear

Section I

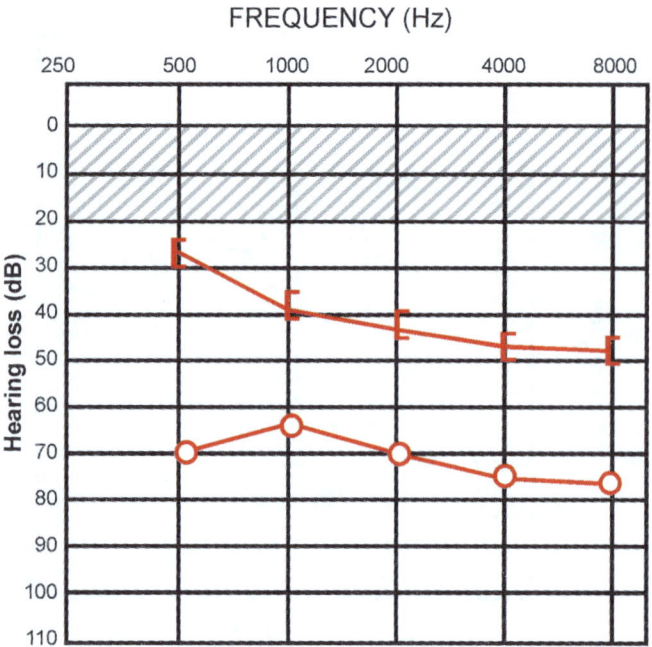

Fig. 2.5: Audiogram

STEPS TO READ ANY AUDIOGRAM

1. Find out if the given audiogram represents only the right or left or both the ears and also identify the AC & BC curves (as per the symbols given in Table 2.5)
2. If AC and BC curves are less than 25 dB – the ear is normal (please note that if only AC curve is given and it is normal, i.e. < 25 dB, the ear is considered to be normal as AC is a measure of both conductive and sensorineural pathway, so BC curve which is a measure of sensorineural pathway only is not needed here).
3. If AC/BC curve is more than 25 dB it is abnormal.
4. Look for the AB gap:
   - If AB gap is present, i.e. > 15 dB – it is conductive hearing loss (CHL).
   - If AB gap is absent or < 15 dB – it is sensorineural hearing loss (SNHL).

 *Note:*

If the AC curve is abnormal and the BC curve is either normal or not given (then presume it to be normal)-it is CHL.

5. See the shape of the curves – upsloping, down sloping, U shaped, Carhartz notch, Acoustic dip etc. to ascertain the underlying aetiologies, as discussed above.

CALCULATING HEARING IMPAIRMENT AND DEGREE OF HANDICAP

To calculate the percentage of hearing impairment, the following procedure is followed:
- *Step 1:* Take the average of hearing threshold of frequencies 500, 1000 and 2000 Hz (i.e. speech frequencies) from the audiogram.
- *Step 2:* Deduct 25 dB from this average (since uptill 25 dB, the hearing is considered as normal).

- *Step 3:* Multiply the result with 1.5 to get the percentage. *Example:* Hearing threshold in frequencies 500, 1000 and 2000 Hz is 30 dB, 45 dB and 60 dB respectively. So average (30 dB + 45 dB + 60 dB)/3 = 45 dB. Then 45 dB – 25 dB = 20 dB. So percentage hearing loss = 20 × 1.5 = 30%.

To calculate the total handicap of hearing, the following procedure is followed:
- (% hearing impairment of the better ear × 5) + (% hearing impairment of the worse ear) divided by 6.

HIGH FREQUENCY AUDIOMETRY

Conventional audiometry tests frequencies between 250 Hz and 8000 Hz, whereas high frequency audiometry tests frequencies in the region of 8000 Hz–20,000 Hz.

It is used to **detect early ototoxicity and noise induced hearing loss** as these lead to high frequency hearing loss and if detected early, involvement of lower frequencies especially speech frequencies can be prevented or minimised.

IMPEDANCE AUDIOMETRY

The importance of impedance audiometry lies in the fact that it is an objective test as compared to tuning fork and PTA which are subjective. In impedance audiometry we have two tests:
1. Tympanometry
2. Stapedial reflex/Acoustic reflex

Tympanometry: This **test is a measure of the condition of the middle ear with intact tympanic membrane**, at the level of TM. It measures the impedance (resistance) to flow of sound energy through the middle ear on pressure changes in the external auditory canal.

In tympanometry a probe with three channels is passed into the EAC.
1. Through one channel **a sound of 226 or 220 Hz is delivered to the TM**. In infants and neonates, a high frequency probe tone of 1000 Hz is used due to resonant differences in small ear canals.
2. Whenever a sound strikes the TM some of it gets absorbed and the rest is reflected back, depending upon the condition of middle ear. The 2nd channel picks up the reflected sound.

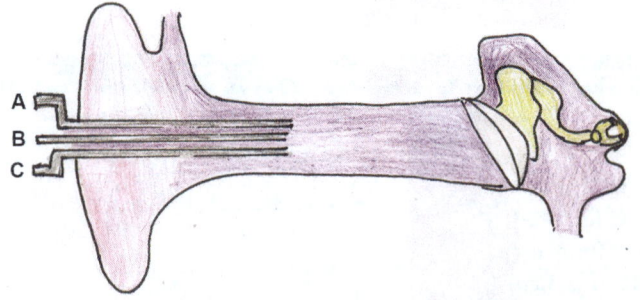

Fig. 2.6: Tympanogram probe with three channels

3. The 3rd channel **changes the pressure of EAC from + 200 to –400**. When the pressure of EAC and middle ear becomes equal, maximum mobility of TM happens and therefore the maximum flow of acoustic energy or sound occurs to the middle ear.

In tympanometry we measure two factors:

i. **Compliance:** Compliance is the ease of mobility of tympanic membrane. The less the impedance (resistance), the more is the compliance. Hence in any ossicular discontinuity **compliance (TM mobility)** is increased and in any ossicular fixation or fluid in middle ear, the compliance is reduced.

ii. **Middle ear pressure:** While changing the pressure of the external auditory canal, when the pressure of the EAC matches that of the middle ear, one gets the maximum compliance, i.e. movement of tympanic membrane. So suppose the tympanic membrane moves maximum when the pressure of EAC is –200 mm of H_2O, this indicates that the middle ear pressure is also –200 mm of H_2O.

The pressure of the middle ear is regulated by the Eustachian tube. The normal pressure of middle ear is the same as the ambient atmospheric pressure, i.e. it is between –50 and + 50 mm of H_2O/da Pa (deca Pascal) in adults. In children the middle ear pressure is –150 to + 50 mm H_2O or da Pa. If the middle ear pressure is negative beyond the normal range, it signifies Eustachian tube blockade.

• In a patient with **reduced compliance** if the **middle ear pressure is also negative**, it signifies Eustachian tube blockade leading to fluid collection in the middle ear, e.g. in Serous Otitis Media **(SOM)**.

• Whereas in a patient with **reduced compliance** if the **middle ear pressure** is **normal**, indicating that the Eustachian tube is normal, the reduced compliance is due to ossicular fixity (e.g. in **otosclerosis**).

The result is plotted as a graph which is called as the "tympanogram".

The X-axis of the tympanogram represents pressure and the Y-axis represents compliance.

Types of patterns on the tympanogram:

1. *Type A:* It indicates normal middle ear pressure and normal compliance. It is seen in **normal middle ear**. Mnemonic 3 idiots movie—**A**ll is well (i.e. normal).

2. *Type A_S:* Here the compliance is decreased but since the Eustachian tube function is normal, middle ear pressure remains normal.

In AS the subscript S, stands for stiffness. This is seen most commonly in Otosclerosis or any other **ossicular fixation**. It can also be seen in tympanosclerosis and tumours of middle ear like glomus jugulare.

3. *Type A_D:* Here the compliance is increased, i.e. the TM moves excessively but again the middle ear pressure is normal, i.e. the Eustachian tube function is normal. This type of curve is seen in **ossicular discontinuity** (subscript D stands for discontinuity) and also in thin and lax TM. It is also seen in post stapedectomy ear.

4. *Type C:* This indicates negative middle ear pressure due to **Eustachian tube closure** (**C** for **C**losure but normal **c**ompliance, read ahead), which is of short duration, i.e. not enough for fluid to collect, hence normal compliance. This is seen in early stages of Eustachian tube obstruction (closure).

5. *Type B:* When the Eustachian tube remains blocked (**B**) for prolonged period, the secretions in the middle ear gets collected (*see* Chapter 6) leading to decreased compliance. The blocked Eustachian tube leads to negative middle ear pressure. This leads to a dome shaped curve (reduced compliance), i.e. with no sharp peak. This is seen in serous Otitis media (SOM) and adhesive otitis media (a sequelae of SOM). Mnemonic SOM may be considered as **B**locked (Eustachian tube) Otitis media (type B curve).

When the secretions or fluid, fill the middle ear cavity completely, leading to no movement of TM, a flat (*Mnemonic:* **FFF**- **F**luid **F**ill completely-**F**lat curve) curve results.

• **In TM perforation**, Tympanometry cannot be done as it is not possible to do pressure changes on the TM, hence a **flat curve** is obtained (*Mnemonic*—in Hindi perforated TM means **F**atta TM- **F**lat curve). So flat curve- in late SOM (middle ear completely fluid filled) and TM perforation.

• However, Tympanometry can be used to test Eustachian tube function in tympanic membrane perforation. The ear canal is sealed with a probe and a positive or negative pressure of +200 or –200 mm of H_2O is created. The patient is now asked to swallow five times in 20 seconds. If the Eustachian

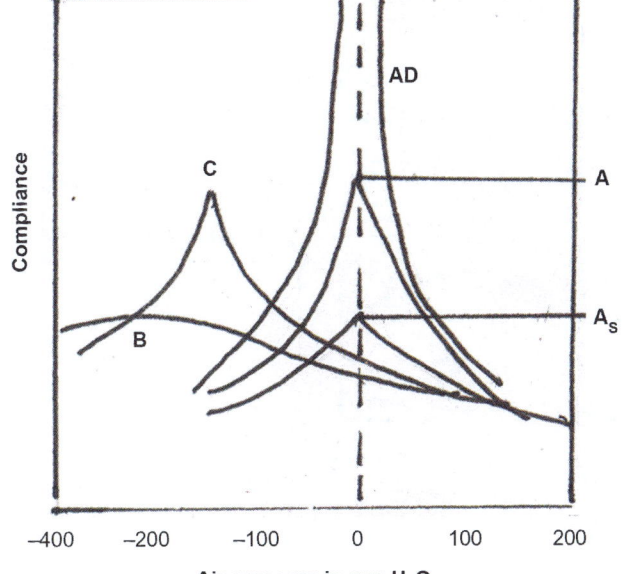

Fig. 2.7: Types of Tympanograms

tube is functioning normally, the pressure gets equilibrated to atmospheric pressure following the swallows (*see* Chapter 6 for other tests of assessment of Eustachian tube functioning).

ACOUSTIC/STAPEDIAL REFLEX

Whenever a loud sound of 70–100 dB above the hearing threshold is presented to one ear, the stapedius muscle of both the ears contract, decreasing the mobility of stapes and thus protecting the inner ear from noise trauma. This is known as stapedial or acoustic reflex.

- It is clear from the below Flowchart 2.1 that the **afferent of the Stapedial reflex is the 8th nerve** and the **efferent is the 7th nerve** and also that it is a **bilateral reflex**. Hence the presence of stapedial reflex implies that there is no lesion in the afferent, central interconnections or the efferent part of this stapedial reflex arc.
- In **afferent palsy Stapedial reflex is absent on both sides** (ipsilateral and contralateral), whereas in **efferent palsy (facial nerve palsy) Stapedial reflex is absent only on the side of lesion** (ipsilateral side).
- The inner ear is protected from loud noise by "acoustic/stapedial reflex", but there is a delay in onset of this reflex of approx. 100–200 ms.

When a high intensity noise >140 dB is subjected to the ear suddenly, it reaches the cochlea before acoustic reflex is activated leading to permanent hearing loss.

Clinical Significance of the Stapedial/Acoustic Reflex

1. **To identify Malingerers:** If a person says that a particular ear is totally deaf but the stapedial reflex is normal in the so called deaf ear on ipsilateral stimulation, it indicates that the ear is not completely deaf. This is because presence of normal Stapedial reflex means all the parts of afferent pathway, central interconnection and efferent are functioning. Since the pathway of the stapedial reflex consists of multiple areas (i.e. EAC, middle ear, organ of Corti, Cochlear nuclei, Superior Olivary complex and Facial) any defect in any part of afferent, central interconnection or efferent will affect the stapedial reflex.

2. **To differentiate cochlear and retrocochlear hearing loss:** In a normal ear the acoustic reflex threshold is between 70 and 100 dB above the pure tone hearing threshold level. In Cochlear lesions because of recruitment (meaning abnormal rapid growth of loudness, read below) this reflex is present much earlier, i.e. at 60 dB above the pure tone hearing threshold level. In retrocochlear lesions the threshold of Stapedial reflex is increased or it can be even absent.

3. **Acoustic reflex decay test:** (please read Tone decay test below) In this test, around 10 dB above the acoustic reflex threshold, a sound (of frequency of 500 and 1000 Hz) is given for a duration of 10 seconds. The acoustic reflex amplitude is measured. If this amplitude falls to less than 5% within 5 seconds, then it is considered as abnormal decay of acoustic reflex. It means that if a loud sound is presented to the ear continuously the Stapedial reflex which should be present continuously, dies out early. It indicates nerve fatigue and is suggestive of retrocochlear pathology.

4. **Identification of the site of lesion in facial nerve palsy:** If the stapedial reflex is present in a patient with facial palsy, it means the injury is beyond the nerve to stapedius, see chapter on facial nerve palsy. Injury of

Flowchart 2.1

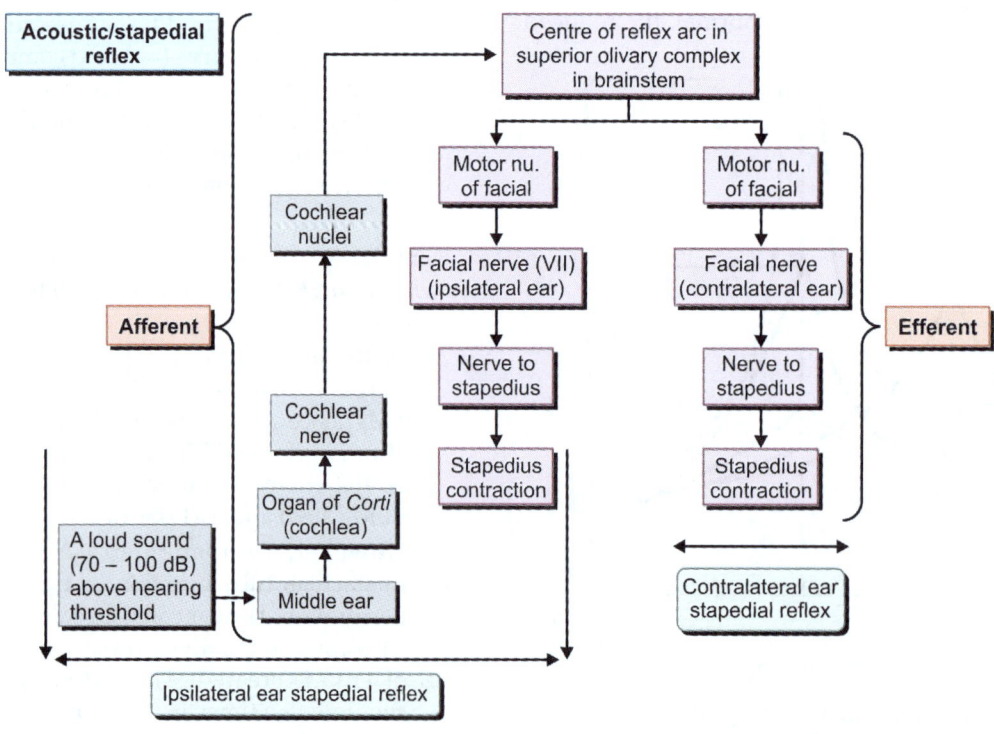

the facial nerve before the origin of the nerve to stapedius will lead to the absence of Stapedial reflex. This leads to normal sounds being heard as loud and painful. This is known as **hyperacusis**.

RECRUITMENT

It is the **abnormal growth of loudness** so that the worse ear which does not hear sounds of low intensity starts hearing greater intensity sounds either equal to or may be even louder than the normal ear.

This phenomenon of recruitment is **seen in cochlear pathology**.

The presence of recruitment can be tested by "ABLB" and "SISI" tests:

1. **ABLB:** This is Alternate Binaural Loudness Balance test. This test can be done in unilateral cochlear lesions.

    In the patient (Fig. 2.8B) a particular frequency sound is heard in the left ear, which is the normal ear, at 0 dB loudness (please note that the 0 dB loudness means that the loudness of the presented sound is equal to the reference sound level), whereas for the same sound to be heard in the defective right ear the loudness has to be increased to 30 dB. But as we go on increasing the loudness of sound we see that an 80 dB sound in the left normal ear which should be heard at 110 dB in the abnormal right ear is actually heard at 80 dB only.

    So in the right ear (Fig. 2.8B) which is the worse ear, because of recruitment, there is abnormal growth of loudness at higher intensities of sound so that it starts hearing a high intensity sound equal or even better than the normal ear. So the patient (Fig. 2.8B) has right sided cochlear deafness.

    Figure 2.8A indicates a patient with conductive hearing loss, in right ear, of 20 dB which is maintained throughout all the sound intensities.

2. **SISI:** Short Increment Sensitivity Index (SISI) is the ability of the recruiting ear to identify short increments of sound.

A normal ear cannot differentiate between 25 dB and 26 dB or between 40 dB and 41 dB, i.e. any increment of 1 dB cannot be identified by a normal ear.

But in a recruiting ear (i.e. in cochlear lesions) such small increments of 1 dB can be differentiated.

SISI test is started 20 dB above the hearing threshold of the patient and 20 increments of 1 dB are given at every 5 second intervals. The total number of increments which the patient is able to identify is noted.

If the patient is able to identify 70–100% of the increments, it is suggestive of a cochlear lesion.

So a SISI score of **70–100%** suggests a **cochlear** lesion, whereas a SISI score of **0–20%** suggests **normal or retrocochlear** lesion.

TONE DECAY

Tone decay is a **function of nerve fatigue** like acoustic reflex decay, discussed above.

Here a tone of particular frequency is given continuously for 1 minute, 30 dB above the PTA threshold of the patient.

If the patient can hear the sound continuously for 1minute, his nerves are normal. If the nerves are fatigued the patient stops hearing the sound before the completion of 1 minute.

The loudness of the sound is then increased till the patient can hear the sound continuously for 1 minute. For the patient to hear the sound continuously for 1 minute, if we have to increase the loudness by **more than 30 dB**, it is suggestive of **retrocochlear** hearing loss.

ELECTROCOCHLEOGRAPHY (ECO G)

Eco G is an objective test in which we record the **electrical activity of the cochlea and auditory nerve** in response to auditory stimuli.

It is a useful test for diagnosing Meniere's.

Here the recording electrode is passed through the TM to rest over the promontory.

Three parameters are recorded on the graph paper:

1. *Cochlear microphonic (CM):* This is the electrical activity from the hair cells.
2. *Summating potential (SP):* This is the sum of all the electrical activity in the cochlea.
3. *Action potential (AP):* It is the electrical activity in the distal part of auditory nerve. This corresponds to the wave I of BERA, read below.

Normally the AP is larger than SP and ratio between the amplitude of SP to the amplitude of AP (SP/AP) is less than 45%. In diseases of cochlea, e.g. **Meniere's SP/AP ratio is more than 0.45 or 45%**.

OTO ACOUSTIC EMISSIONS (OAEs)

This is an objective test. Due to the biological activity of the **outer hair cells** (easy to remember **Oto** AEs from **outer**), some sound is generated. This sound is known as

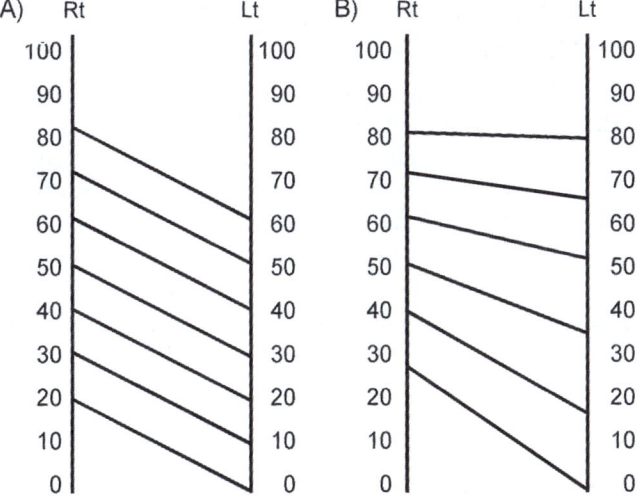

Fig. 2.8: ABLB Test for Recruitment

Ear

Section I

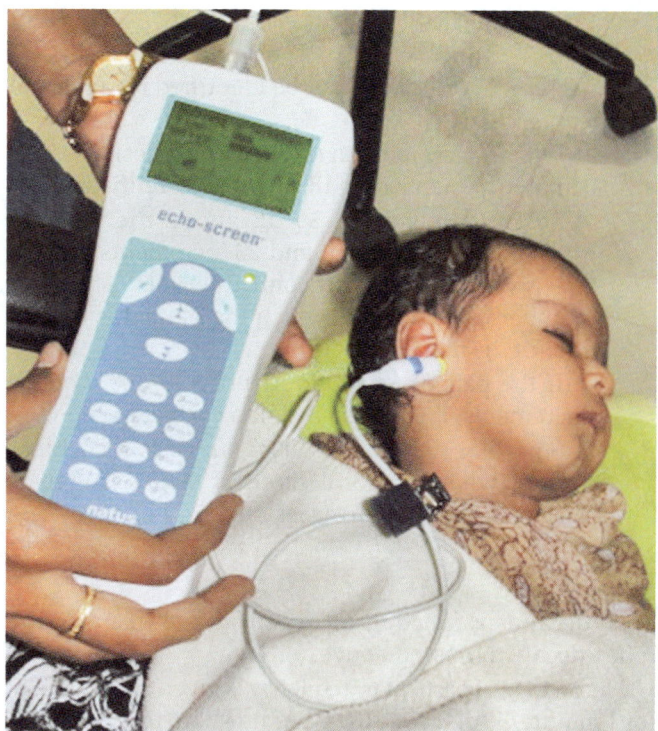

OAE and can be picked up and recorded by placing a microphone deep in the external auditory meatus (provided there is no significant external auditory canal or middle ear pathology). Hence if there is any EAC or middle ear pathology causing a hearing loss of greater than 35 dB, Transient evoked OAEs (*see* below) will most often be absent. Likewise, when the hearing loss in all the pure-tone hearing thresholds are greater than 40 dB, both Transient evoked OAEs and Distortion product OAEs (*see* below) are always absent.

The OAEs are of two types:

1. **Spontaneous:** They are generated spontaneously, i.e. they do not require any external stimulation for being produced. They are found only in 50% of normal hearing people.
2. **Evoked:** They are produced in response to a sound stimulus. They are present in all individuals with normal hearing; hence we test the evoked OAEs by giving click stimuli.

They are also known as **"Kemp"** echoes or cochlear echoes. They are again divided into two types:

a. Transient evoked OAEs (TEOAEs); if the acoustic stimulus consists of a transient sound (click or tone pip), the resulting emission is termed as transient evoked oto-acoustic emission. Click sounds are a mixture of multiple frequencies and stimulate a very large area of the basilar membrane and hence the response gives information of the whole cochlea.

b. Distortion product OAEs (DPOAEs); when two pure tones of separate frequencies (F 1 and F 2) are presented to the ear simultaneously, the resulting emission is a continuous tone of a frequency (which is calculated as: 2 F 1 minus F 2) and is termed as distortion product Oto-acoustic emission. Since

specific frequencies are given here the response gives information about those frequencies. Hence frequency specific hearing can be tested here.

Uses of OAE

1. Since OAE is easy to test, non-invasive, less time consuming, cost effective and results are available immediately, therefore it is used to screen hearing in large population and is considered to be **the best audiometric test to screen hearing in well neonates, infants and small children**. (Please note that in neonates who are in ICU, BERA is done for initial screening, read below). Transient evoked OAEs (TEOAEs) is used more commonly in these well babies. If the response falls within acceptable parameters, it is labelled **"Pass"**. When the response falls outside the permissible parameters, it is labelled as **"Refer"**, which indicates the need for BERA. The term "Fail" is avoided, here, as it has negative impact on the parents.

   Absent OAEs indicate cochlear lesions. If OAEs are absent, the child is taken up for BERA for confirmation, *see* below.

2. **To differentiate cochlear and retro-cochlear hearing loss:** In a patient with SN hearing loss if OAEs are present, it indicates that cochlea is normal, so the person is having a retro-cochlear hearing loss. The patient can then be taken up for BERA to find out the exact site of lesion.

3. It is useful in the **early detection of noise induced hearing loss:** The outer hair cells are more prone to damage by noise trauma and ototoxicity. Since the OAE are produced by outer hair cells, the absence of OAE can be an early indication of noise trauma and ototoxicity. Hence OAE has been used effectively to monitor cochlear function in patients undergoing treatment with potentially ototoxic medication, e.g. cisplatin in chemotherapy. Distortion product OAE is used here. Subsequently high frequency audiometry can confirm and also tell the degree of hearing loss.

BRAINSTEM EVOKED RESPONSE AUDIOMETRY/ AUDITORY BRAINSTEM RESPONSE (BERA/ABR)

Like OAEs BERA is an **objective test**. But unlike OAEs which measure the spontaneous electrical activity from the cochlea (outer hair cells of the organ of Corti), **BERA tests the electrical activity occurring in the auditory pathway** (situated in the brainstem that is why the name) within 10 millisecond in response to a sound stimulus.

In a normal person 5–7 electrical waves are recorded in the form of a graph with latency (i.e. time in milli-second taken for the wave to appear after the stimulus sound is given) on the x-axis and amplitude on the y-axis. These waves come from the different areas of the auditory pathway.

The wave V is the most prominent and easily identifiable and hence the most important wave of BERA.

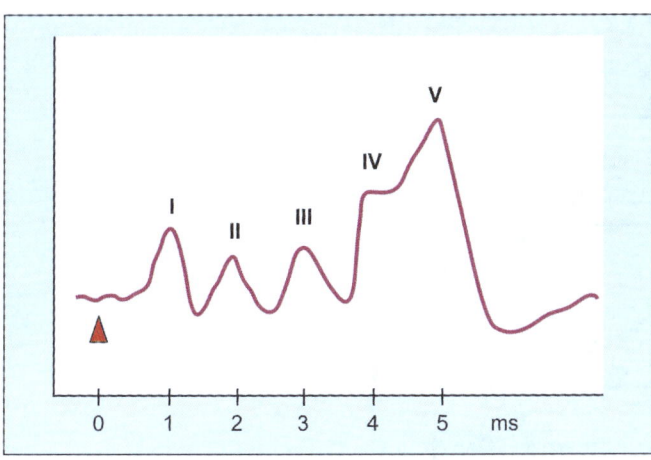

Fig. 2.9: Graph of BERA

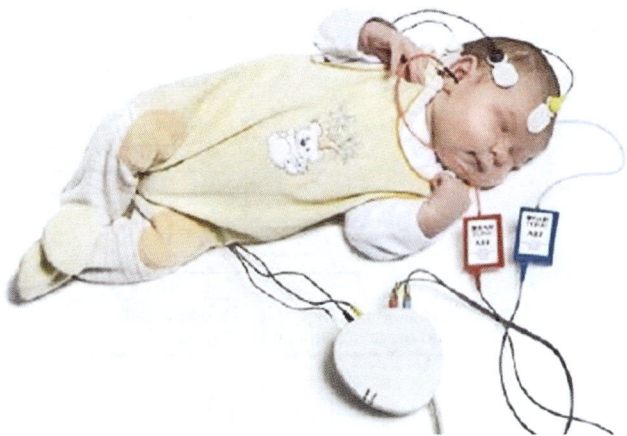

The sites of origin of these waves are:

1. Wave I distal part of cochlear nerve (in the inner ear)
2. Wave II proximal part of cochlear nerve near the brainstem
3. Wave III cochlear nucleus

   The remaining waves come from the **S L I of S L I M** (please refer to the auditory pathway above).

4. Wave IV superior olivary complex **(S)**
5. Wave V lateral lemniscus **(L–Largest and most consistent wave)**
6. Wave VI and VII inferior Colliculus **(I)**

Interpretation of BERA

- **Wave I delayed but inter-peak latency of I–V is normal:** Defect is before Wave I (distal part of cochlear nerve), i.e. in the cochlea or middle ear suggesting conductive or cochlear pathology.
- **Wave I present, rest of the waves absent:** Retrocochlear pathology.
- **Increased inter-peak latency of wave I–V:** It is suggestive of pathology between cochlear nerve and lateral lemniscus. It is one of the diagnostic findings of acoustic neuroma.
- **Increased inter-aural latency of wave V of > 0.2 msec:** Waves normally appear at same time in both the ears, i.e. they have same latency in both ears. Interaural latency difference is the difference of time interval of appearance of same wave in the two ears (in normal ear it is appearing at normal time and in the affected ear it is appearing late). Difference in the latency of wave V in the two ears of > 0.2 msec suggests retrocochlear pathology in the ear with increased latency. This is the most diagnostic finding on BERA in acoustic neuroma.

Uses of BERA

1. **To find hearing threshold:** Wave V appears 10 dB above PTA hearing level. So the PTA hearing threshold can be found by subtracting 10 dB from where wave V is just identified.

2. It is the **best audiometric test to confirm hearing loss in neonates and infants** and mentally retarded patients (please note OAEs is the best screening test in this regard, however in neonates who are in ICU for more than 48 hours BERA is employed as a screening test. This is because these neonates are more likely to have hearing loss and BERA is a more sensitive and specific test).

3. It is the **best** audiometric test for **non-organic hearing loss, i.e. malingering.**

4. It is the **best test to differentiate cochlear and retro-cochlear** hearing loss. Apart from knowing whether the defect is cochlear or retrocochlear, the exact site of lesion can be found out by noting the latency and amplitude of the affected wave.

5. It is the **best audiometric test for acoustic neuroma.**

6. It is used to study central auditory disorders.

   - **Note:** Patients with severe to profound hearing loss do not have a measurable response on BERA. Their hearing should be assessed by ASSR, read below.
   - Though it is possible to record BERA in premature infants as young as 27 weeks, there is a progressive improvement in the detection of waves I, III, and V of BERA with increasing gestational age due to maturation of auditory pathway. The wave forms of BERA are of adult configuration by 18 months to 3 years of age. *See* Flowchart 2.2, next page.

The following are the Neonates and infants who are at high risk of developing hearing loss and are tested periodically with behavioural observation audiometry even if the pass TEOAE at birth:

   i. H/o in utero infection like CMV, herpes, Rubella, syphilis and toxoplasmosis
   ii. H/o use of ototoxic drugs in the mother during pregnancy
   iii. Postnatal infections like bacterial meningitis and encephalitis
   iv. Severe hyperbilirubinemia in the neonate
   v. Neonates with craniofacial anomalies
   vi. Any syndrome with associated component of hearing loss, e.g. Down's. Treacher–Collins, etc.
   vii. Family history of early childhood deafness

Section I | **Ear**

Flowchart 2.2

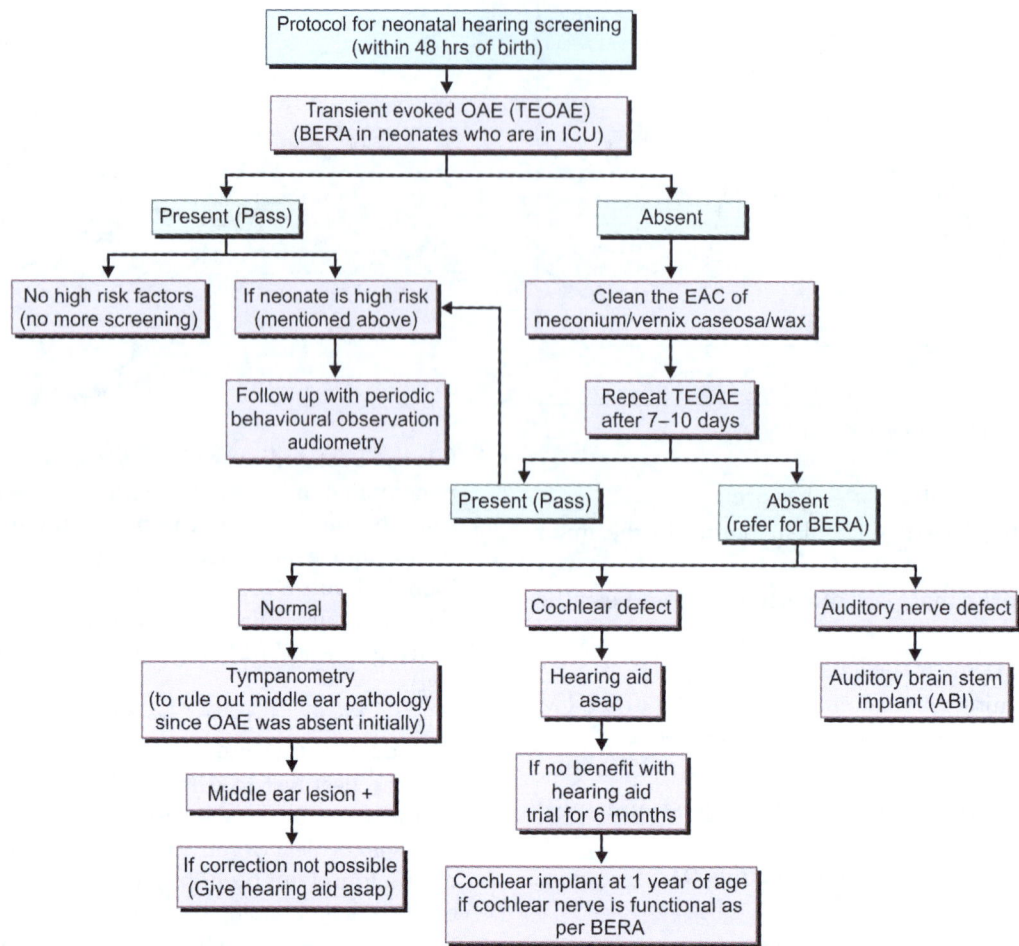

Clinical Assessment of Hearing Loss in Children (Behavioural Observation Audiometry)

The tests for clinical assessment of hearing are age specific depending upon the development of response to sound stimuli at various ages as follows:

1. Birth – 4 months (child is startled by loud sounds):
   i. Startle reflex (sudden movement of the body on loud sound)
   ii. Auro-palpebral reflex (blinking of eyelids in response to loud sounds)
   iii. Arousal reflex (sudden arousal of a sleeping child on sudden loud sound)
2. 5–24 months (child starts to localise sounds and turns head towards sound source)
   i. *Free field audiometry:* The child is placed in between two caliberated loud speakers in the sound treated room. Whenever the child hears sound from one loud speaker he looks at it.
   ii. *Visual reinforcement audiometry:* This is the extension of free field audiometry as children loose interest to sound and do not cooperate after some time. A moving toy is placed over the loud speaker. When the child turns his head towards loudspeaker in response to sound the toy is played for a short time. This reinforces the child to immediately turn his head towards the sound.

3. 2 years–5 years (child develops some vocabulary and follows simple instructions)
   - Play audiometry
   - The child is taught here to carry out a play response (e.g. putting a ball in the bowl) on hearing sound
   - If the response to the above behavioural tests (as per the age group of the child) are inconclusive, the child is subjected to OAE followed by BERA.

AUDITORY STEADY STATE RESPONSE (ASSR)

This test is similar to BERA except that it is tested with steady state pure tone signals instead of transient clicks. It involves recording of the EEG (electroencephalogram) activity in response to acoustic stimulus. If the listener hears the acoustic signal his EEG activity will increase and decrease periodically following the slow modulations in signal. Hence here we can **record frequency specific hearing thresholds**. ASSR has also been used to measure hearing in patients with severe to profound sensorineural hearing loss, who do not have measurable response on BERA.

SPEECH AUDIOMETRY

In this audiometric test the hearing sensitivity for speech is assessed (i.e. patient's ability to hear and understand speech is assessed). It is nowadays used particularly to assess the candidacy and outcome of hearing aid or hearing implants. It consists of two tests:

1. **Speech reception threshold (SRT):** It is the threshold at which the patient is able to identify 50% of the spoken words (two syllable spondee words, e.g. arm chair, ear drum, etc.) correctly.

   SRT is generally **within 10 dB of PTA**. Any difference more than this indicates that the patient is malingering, *see* below.

2. **Speech discrimination score (SDS)/Word recognition score and Roll Over Phenomenon:** It is an assessment of a patient's ability to identify and repeat single syllable words given at suprathreshold level. Here phonetically balanced words (e.g. pin, tin, sin, etc.) are given 30 dB above the SRT. The percentage of correctly identified words is noted.

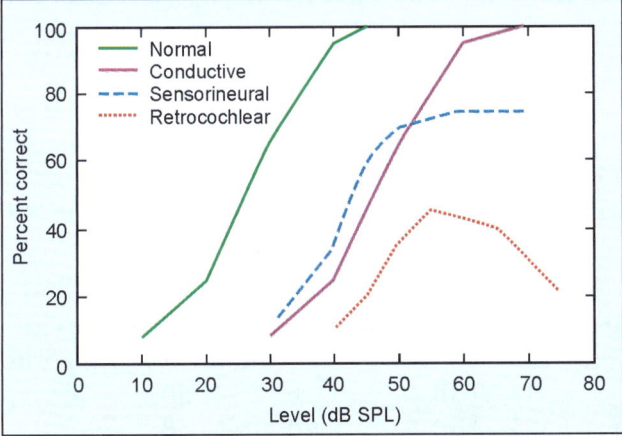

When increasing intensities of sound are given, the percentage of words identified increases till it reaches a plateau in cochlear lesions, see the graph below. But in retrocochlear lesions with the increase in speech intensity above a particular level the percentage of words identified falls down instead of maintaining a plateau, this is known as Roll over phenomenon. This occurs due to nerve fatigue and is suggestive of retrocochlear lesions.

It helps to differentiate between cochlear and retrocochlear lesions. The SDS is normally between 90 and 100%. **It is reduced in cochlear lesions** but in **retrocochlear** or neural lesions it is **very poor** and out of proportion with the hearing loss. Among retrocochlear lesions, it is **worst in cortical deafness** (i.e. involvement of auditory area no. 41).

NONORGANIC HEARING LOSS (NOHL)

Nonorganic hearing loss means that there is no organic cause of hearing loss, i.e. the patient is malingering.

The following are some important tests used to find out NOHL:

1. **Stenger test:** The principle behind this test is that if two tones of different intensities are presented to both the ears simultaneously only the ear which receives the tone of greater intensity will hear it.

   In Stenger test the patient is blind folded. It can be done with tuning fork or with audiometer. When two tuning forks of the same frequency are kept at equal distance (25 cm), the patient will hear it only in the normal ear. When we bring the tuning fork on the side of the alleged deaf ear nearer to the ear (8 cm), the patient should continue to hear in the normal ear.

   But in a patient who is feigning to be deaf in one ear, when the tuning fork is brought nearer to the deaf ear because of increased intensity of sound he starts hearing only in this ear. Since he has claimed that this ear is deaf he says he hears nothing though he should continue to hear in the normal ear.

2. **Stapedial reflex:** It tests the whole of the pathway of hearing along with its central interconnections with facial nerve. If the stapedial reflex is normal, it means the whole of the pathway is normal. So if the patient claims that he is deaf in a particular ear and stapedial reflex in this ear (upon giving a loud sound to this claimed deaf ear) is present, it means he is malingering.

3. **Speech audiometry:** Speech reception threshold is generally within 10 dB of pure tone audiometry threshold. Any difference more than this indicates that the patient is malingering.

   Inconsistencies on repeating PTA and speech audiometry also points to malingering.

4. **BERA:** It is the best audiometric test for non-organic hearing loss.

Cochlear vs Retrocochlear Pathology

If the patient is detected to have SN hearing loss on tuning fork tests which has been subsequently confirmed with PTA, the following table summarises the various tests to differentiate cochlear and retrocochlear pathology:

Test	Cochlear pathology	Retrocochlear pathology
Recruitment, i.e. abnormal growth of loudness (ABLB test)	Present	Absent
SISI score, i.e. ability to identify short increments (1 dB) of sound	70–100%	0–20%
Acoustic reflex threshold	Decreased due to recruitment	Increased
Tone decay (nerve fatigue)	Absent	Present
Acoustic reflex decay (Nerve fatigue)	Absent	Present
OAEs	Absent	Present
BERA (best test)	Delayed wave I, but remaining waves normal	Only wave I is present, rest are absent or affected
Speech discrimination score (SDS) or word discrimination score	Reduced. Roll over phenomenon absent	Very poor. Roll over phenomenon present

Section I | **Ear**

PREVIOUSLY ASKED QUESTIONS

1. Bones of middle ear are responsible for the following except: *(MH 2008)*
   a. Protecting the inner ear
   b. No alteration of sound intensity
   c. Reduction of impedance to sound transmission
   d. Amplification of sound intensity

2. Function of ear ossicles is: *(Exam 2013, 2018)*
   a. Impedance matching
   b. Transduction of sound
   c. Equilibrium
   d. None

3. Lever ratio is: *(UP 2001, Exam 2017)*
   a. 14:1
   b. 1.3:1
   c. 18:1
   d. 1.5:1

4. Ratio of tympanic membrane to oval window is: *(Exam 2013)*
   a. 17:1
   b. 22:1
   c. 50:1
   d. 25:1

5. Impedance matching occurs due to: *(Exam 2013)*
   a. Difference of surface area of tympanic membrane and foot plate
   b. Semicircular canal fluid
   c. Utricle and Saccule
   d. None

6. Scientist who worked on conduction in inner ear: *(PGI 2008)*
   a. Young
   b. Helmholtz
   c. Bekesy
   d. Malcom Ritter
   e. Friesch

7. Conductive deafness occurs in: *(UP 2007, Exam 2017)*
   a. Travelling in an aeroplane
   b. Trauma to labyrinth
   c. Stapes abnormal at oval window
   d. High noise

8. All are causes of sensorineural deafness except: *(Exam 2013)*
   a. Old age
   b. Cochlear otosclerosis
   c. Loud sound
   d. Rupture of tympanic membrane

9. Resonance of tympanic membrane: *(Exam 2012)*
   a. 500–800
   b. 1000–3000
   c. 4000–5000
   d. None

10. Ear ossicles efficiently transmit sound of which frequency: *(AI 2003, Exam 2017)*
    a. 3000–5000 Hz
    b. 300–500 Hz
    c. 500–2000 Hz
    d. 5000–20000 Hz

11. All are tuning fork tests except: *(UP 2002/Exam 2002, Exam 2017)*
    a. Schwabach's test
    b. Grants test
    c. Rinne test
    d. Weber's test

12. Tuning fork of 512 FPS is used to test the hearing because it is: *(Karnataka 2006, Exam 2017)*
    a. Better heard
    b. Better felt
    c. Produces over tones
    d. Not heard

13. Tuning fork frequency used most commonly in ENT is: *(Exam 2013)*
    a. 256 Hz
    b. 512 Hz
    c. 1024 Hz
    d. 2048 Hz

14. Rinne test is negative in: *(AIIMS 2004, Exam 2017)*
    a. Sensorineural deafness
    b. Acoustic neuroma
    c. Tympanosclerosis
    d. Meniere's disease

15. Rinne test negative is seen in: *(JIPMER 2002, Exam 2017)*
    a. Presbycusis
    b. CSOM
    c. Labyrinthitis
    d. Meniere's disease

16. Rinne test is negative if minimum deafness is: *(SRMC 2002, Exam 2017)*
    a. 15–20 dB
    b. 25–30 dB
    c. 35–40 dB
    d. 15–50 dB

17. Positive Rinne test indicates: *(Exam 2013)*
    a. AC>BC
    b. BC>AC
    c. BC=AC
    d. None

18. Positive Rinne test is seen in: *(JIPMER 2001, Exam 2017)*
    a. Otosclerosis
    b. CSOM
    c. Impacted Wax
    d. Presbycusis

19. Rinne test is positive in: *(AIIMS 91, Exam 2017)*
    a. CSOM
    b. Normal individual
    c. Otomycosis
    d. Wax in ear

20. Weber test is best elicited as: *(AI 2002, Exam 2017)*
    a. Placing the tuning fork on the mastoid process and comparing the bone conduction of the patient with that of the examiner
    b. Placing the tuning fork on the vertex of the skull and determining the effect of gently occluding the auditory canal on the threshold of low frequencies
    c. Placing the tuning fork on the mastoid process and comparing the bone conduction in the patient
    d. Placing the tuning fork on the forehead and asking him to report in which ear he hears it better

21. What should be the least hearing loss for Weber test to lateralize? *(Rj 2004, Exam 2016)*
    a. 5 dB
    b. 10 dB
    c. 15 dB
    d. 20 dB

22. In the right middle ear pathology, Weber's test will be: *(AI 2004, Exam 2013)*
    a. Normal
    b. Centralised
    c. Lateralised to right side
    d. Lateralised to left side

23. Weber test in conductive deafness: *(CUPGEE 96, Exam 2013)*
    a. Sound louder in normal ear
    b. Sound louder in diseased ear
    c. Heard with equal intensity in both ear
    d. Inconclusive test

24. Threshold for bone conduction is normal and that for air conduction is increased in disease of: *(AP 96, Exam 2016)*
    a. Middle ear
    b. Inner ear
    c. Cochlear nerve
    d. Temporal nerve

25. Gelle's test is done in: *(JIPMER 98, Exam 2017)*
    a. Senile deafness
    b. Traumatic deafness
    c. Otosclerosis
    d. Serous Otitis media

26. In Bing test on alternately compressing and relaxing the tragus the sound increases and decreases. This indicates: *(JIPMER 2002, Exam 2017)*
    a. SN deafness
    b. Adhesive otitis media
    c. Otosclerosis
    d. CSOM

27. A 38-yr-old male presented with a suspected diagnosis of suppurate labyrinthitis. A positive Rinne test and positive fistula test was recorded on initial investigation. The patient refused treatment and returned to the emergency department after 2 weeks complaining of deafness in the affected ear. On examination, fistula test was observed to be negative. What is the likely expected finding on repeating the Rinne test: *(AI 2009)*
    a. True positive Rinne test
    b. False positive Rinne test
    c. True negative Rinne test
    d. False negative Rinne test

28. One man had 30 dB deafness in left ear with Weber test showing more sound in left ear and BC more on left side and normal hearing in right ear, his test can be summarized as: *(AIIMS 2002, Exam 2016)*
    a. Weber's test left lateralised, Rinne-right positive, BC>AC on left side
    b. Weber's test right lateralised, Rinne-left positive, AC>BC on right side
    c. Weber's test left lateralised, Rinne-false positive on right side, BC>AC on left side
    d. Weber's test left lateralised, Rinne-equivocal, BC>AC on right side

29. A middle aged woman presented with right sided hearing loss, Rinne test shows positive result on left side and negative result on right side. Weber's test showed lateralisation to left side, diagnosis is: *(AIIMS 2000, Exam 2017)*
    a. Right sided conductive deafness
    b. Right sided severe sensorineural deafness
    c. Left sided sensorineural deafness
    d. Left sided conductive deafness

30. A 38-year-old gentleman reports of decreased hearing in the right ear for the last 2 years. On testing with a 512 Hz tuning fork, the Rinne test is negative on the right ear and positive on the left ear. With the Weber's test the tone is perceived as louder in the left ear. Most likely, the patient has: *(AIIMS 2002, Exam 2017)*
    a. Right conductive hearing loss
    b. Right severe sensorineural hearing loss
    c. Left sensorineural hearing loss
    d. Left conductive hearing loss

31. In a patient, Rinne test positive in both ears, Weber's lateralizes to the right. Next step: *(Exam 2013, AIIMS 2016)*
    a. No intervention as both the ears are normal
    b. Remove wax from right ear
    c. Repeat Rinnes test
    d. Do Schwabach test

32. In pure tone audiogram the symbol X is used to mark: *(JIPMER 2002, Exam 2016)*
    a. Air conduction in right ear
    b. Air conduction in left ear
    c. Bone conduction in right ear
    d. No response in air conduction in right ear

33. The "O" sign in pure tone audiogram indicates: *(AP 2005, Exam 2017)*
    a. Air conduction of right ear
    b. Air conduction of left ear
    c. Bone conduction of right ear
    d. Bone conduction of left ear

34. High frequency audiometry is used in: *(AIIMS May 2009)*
    a. Otosclerosis
    b. Ototoxicity
    c. Non-organic hearing loss
    d. Meniere's disease

35. Ear is sensitive to: *(Jharkhand 2003, Exam 2017)*
    a. 500–3500 Hz
    b. 20–20,000 Hz
    c. 300–5000 Hz
    d. 5000–8000 Hz

Section I Ear

36. According to WHO classification, severe degree of impairment of hearing is at: (*TN 2004, Exam 2017*)
    a. 26–40 dB   b. 41–60 dB
    c. 61–80 dB   d. ≥81 dB

37. Threshold for moderate hearing loss (*Exam 2013*)
    a. 26–40 dB   b. 56–70 dB
    c. 41–55 dB   d. >91 dB

38. 40 dB compared to 20 dB is: (*Exam 2001, Exam 2017*)
    a. Double   b. 10 times
    c. 100 times   d. 1000 times

39. After rupture of tympanic membrane the hearing loss is: (*AI 2003, Exam 2017*)
    a. 10–40 dB   b. 60 dB
    c. 30 dB   d. 300 dB

40. Which of the following conditions causes maximum hearing loss: (*AI 2004, Exam 2017*)
    a. Ossicular disruption with intact tympanic membrane
    b. Ossicular disruption with tympanic membrane perforation
    c. Partial fixation of the stapes footplate
    d. Otitis media with effusion

41. In a patient audiogram shows a hearing loss of 54 dB. Most probable condition in his ear is: (*AI 2006, Exam 2017*)
    a. Ossicular disruption with intact tympanic membrane
    b. Ossicular disruption with tympanic membrane perforation
    c. Complete fixation of the stapes footplate
    d. Otitis media with effusion

42. Hearing loss is maximum in: (*Exam 2013*)
    a. Tympanic membrane perforation
    b. Complete destruction of ossicular chain
    c. Complete closure of oval window
    d. Complete obstruction of EAC

43. Trough shaped curve in audiometry is seen in: (*Exam 2013*)
    a. Congenital SNHL
    b. Otitis media with effusion
    c. Ototoxicity
    d. Meniere's

44. Impedance audiometry is for the pathology of: (*UP 2004, Exam 2013*)
    a. External ear   b. Middle ear
    c. Mastoid air cell   d. Inner ear

45. Which of the following test assesses resistance in middle ear? (*MAHE 2000, Exam 2017*)
    a. Pure tone audiometry
    b. Impendence audiometry
    c. Caloric test
    d. BERA (Brainstem evoked response audiometry)

46. Impedance audiometry is done using frequency probe of: (*Delhi 2007 Exam 2012*)
    a. 226 Hz   b. 550 Hz
    c. 440 Hz   d. 1000 Hz

47. True statement on the TM is/are: (*PGI 2007*)
    a. Tympanosclerosis increases compliance
    b. Ossicular disruption with intact TM reduces compliance
    c. Fluid in the middle ear cavity increases compliance
    d. Otosclerosis reduces compliance
    e. Flat curve in TM perforation

48. Dome-shaped graph in tympanogram is found in: (*RJ 2003, Exam 2017*)
    a. Otosclerosis
    b. Ossicular discontinuity
    c. TM perforation
    d. Middle ear fluid

49. B-type tympanogram is seen in: (*Bihar 2004, Exam 2013*)
    a. Serous Otitis media
    b. Otosclerosis
    c. Ossicular discontinuity
    d. All of the above

50. In a patient of TM perforation Tympanometry shows which curve (*AIIMS 2001, Exam 2017*)
    a. Flat   b. As curve
    c. Ad curve   d. C type

51. Flat tympanogram is a feature of: (*PGI 2000*)
    a. Ossicular discontinuity
    b. Serous Otitis media
    c. Perforation of ear drum
    d. Otosclerosis
    e. Safe CSOM

52. In Osteogenesis Imperfecta, the tympanogram is: (*DNB 2003, Exam 2013*)
    a. Flat
    b. Non-compliance
    c. High-compliance
    d. Low-compliance

53. A young man presents with loss of hearing in right ear following an accident. On otoscopic examination the tympanic membrane was normal. Pure tone audiometry shows an air bone gap of 55 dB in the right with normal cochlear reserve. Which of the following will be the likely tympanometry finding: (*AI 2009*)
    a. As type tympanogram
    b. Ad type tympanogram
    c. B type tympanogram
    d. C type tympanogram

54. Post head injury, the patient had conductive deafness and on examination, tympanic membrane

was normal and mobile with increased compliance on impedance. Likely diagnosis is: (*AIIMS 2006*)

a. Distortion of ossicular chain
b. Hemotympanum
c. Tympanosclerosis
d. Otosclerosis

55. **Regarding stapedial reflex which of the following is true:** (*AI 2000, Exam 2017*)

a. It helps to enhance the sound conduction in middle ear
b. It is a protective reflex against loud sound
c. It helps in masking the sound waves
d. It is unilateral reflex

56. **Stapedial reflex is mediated by:** (*JIPMER 92, Jharkhand2006, AP 2007*)

a. V and VII nerves
b. V and VIII nerves
c. VI and VII nerves
d. VII and VIII nerves

57. **Hyperacusis is defined as:** (*AIIMS 2003, Exam 2017*)

a. Hearing of only loud sounds
b. Normal sounds heard as loud and painful
c. Completely deaf state
d. Ability to hear better in noisy surroundings

58. **Stapedial reflex is absent in:** (*Karnataka 2001, Exam 2017*)

a. VIth nerve lesion
b. Xth nerve lesion
c. VIIIth nerve lesion
d. Vth nerve lesion

59. **In facial nerve palsy of right side Stapedial reflex is absent on:** (*AIIMS 2000, Exam 2017*)

a. Right side   b. Left side
c. Both sides   d. Not absent

60. **Tone decay test is done for:** (*Manipal 2001, Exam 2017*)

a. Cochlear deafness
b. Neural deafness
c. Middle ear problem
d. Otosclerosis

61. **Electrocochleography is:** (*Exam 2012*)

a. Probe, stimulation of outer hair cells only.
b. Summation of microphonics.
c. AP of cochlear nerve.
d. Evoked potential generated in cochlea and auditory nerve.

62. **In neonates most sensitive audiometric screening is:** (*AI 2008*)

a. Electrocochleography
b. OAEs
c. BERA
d. Tympanometry

63. **Initial screening test for newborn hearing disorder:** (*Exam 2013, AIIMS 2012, AIIMS May 2014*)

a. ABR–Auditory brainstem response
b. Otoacoustic emissions (OAE)
c. Free field audiometry
d. Visual reinforcement audiometry

64. **Otoacoustic emissions arise from:** (*AIIMS 2005, AI 2008, Exam 2013*)

a. Inner hair cells
b. Outer hair cells
c. Both inner and outer hair cells
d. Maculae

65. **True about Otoacoustic emissions:** (*PGI June 2009*)

a. Are by-product of outer hair cell
b. Are by-product of inner hair cell
c. Used as a screening test of hearing in newborn infant
d. Useful in ototoxicity monitoring
e. Disappear in 8th nerve pathology

66. **Which is the investigation of choice in assessing hearing loss in infants:** (*AIIMS 2011*)

a. Impedance audiometry
b. Brainstem evoked response audiometry (BERA)
c. Free field audiometry
d. Behavioural audiometry

67. **To distinguish between cochlear and post-cochlear damage, the test done is:** (*AIIMS 2002, Exam 2010*)

a. BERA
b. Impedance audiometry
c. Pure tone audiometry
d. All of the above

68. **In normal adult, wave V is generated from:** (*J&K 2005, Delhi 2008, Exam 2013*)

a. Cochlear nucleus
b. Superior olivary complex
c. Lateral lemniscus
d. Inferior Colliculus

69. **Brainstem evoked response audiometry true is:** (*PGI June 2009*)

a. Can differentiate cochlear and retrocochlear lesion
b. Cannot differentiate the site of lesion in sensori-neural hearing loss
c. Can differentiate barbiturate poisoning from other causes of coma
d. As a screening procedure for infants
e. To diagnose brainstem pathology in a patient of deafness

70. **A 9-month-old baby was brought to ENT OPD with complaints of not responding even to loudest sounds. Hearing assessment was done which**

Ear

Section I

showed OAE waves were present but no wave on BERA. This condition can be:

(AI 2006, Exam 2017)

a. Absent cochlea
b. Auditory neuropathy
c. Malformed cochlea
d. Low IQ

71. **Test for detecting damage to cochlea except:**

(MH 2000/2005, Exam 2017)

a. Caloric test b. Weber test
c. Rinne test d. ABC test

72. **All are subjective tests for audiometry except:**

(AI 2004, Exam 2016)

a. Tone decay
b. Impedance audiometry
c. Speech audiometry
d. Pure tone audiometry

73. **Subjective test of hearing is:** *(Exam 2013)*
a. Pure tone audiometry
b. Oto acoustic emission
c. BERA
d. Impedance audiometry

74. **Which one of the following test is used to detect malingering?** *(TN 2007, Exam 2017)*
a. Stenger test b. Bing test
c. Weber test d. Rinne test

75. **Rinne test was negative in right ear and positive in left ear. Which is true?** *(AIIMS May 2014)*
a. 40 dB SNHL in left ear with right ear normal
b. 40 dB conductive hearing loss (CHL) in left ear with right ear normal
c. 40 dB CHL in both ears
d. Profound SNHL in right ear, left ear normal

76. **True about the given test:**

(Practice question by Author)

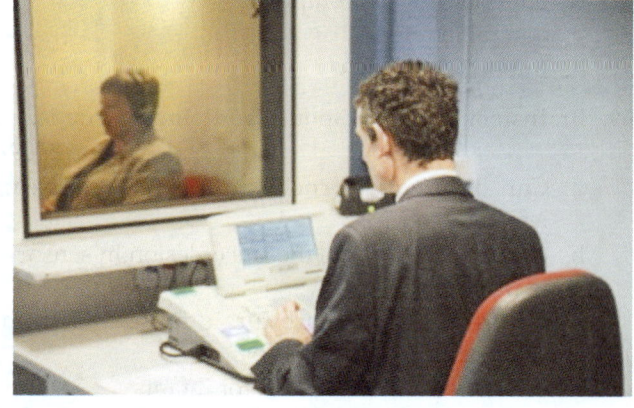

a. X denotes air conduction for right ear
b. It is an objective test
c. It needs sound proof room
d. Frequency detection of 2000–12, 000 Hz is done conventionally

77. **If OAE are absent, the result is mentioned as:**

(Exam 2016)

a. Pass b. Fail
c. Absent d. Refer

78. **Reaction time for stapedial reflex is:** *(TN 2012)*
a. 10–20 msec
b. 100–200 msec
c. 200–350 msec
d. 400–600 msec

79. **Patient complains of decreased hearing in the left ear. His audiogram is given below. What would have been the tuning fork test in his left ear:**

(Practice question by Author)

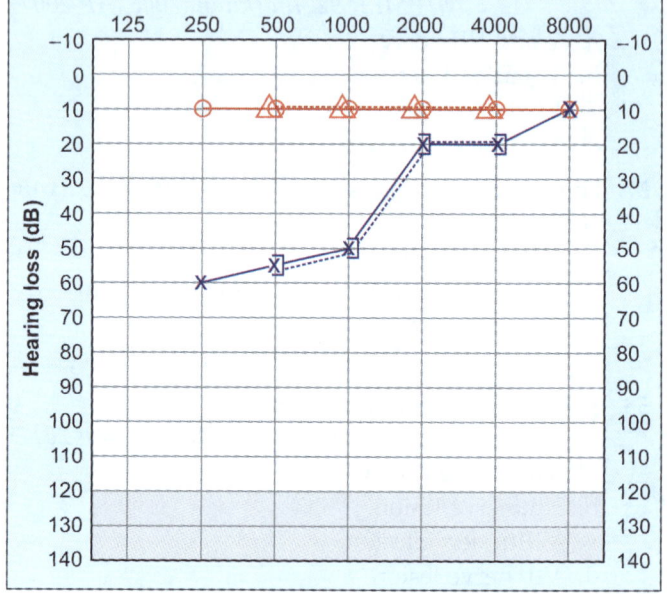

a. Left ear Rinnes +ve; Weber's lateralised to right
b. Left ear Rinnes – ve; Weber's lateralised to right
c. Left ear Rinnes +ve; Weber's lateralised to left
d. Left ear Rinnes – ve; Weber's lateralised to left

80. **Negative Rinne test indicates:** *(Exam 2016)*
a. Meniere's disease
b. CSOM
c. BPPV
d. Sensorineural hearing loss

81. **Most reliable test for Eustachian tube dysfunction:**

(AIIMS 2015)

a. Politzerisation
b. Tympanometry
c. Valsalva
d. Rhinomanometry

82. **All of the following are involved in conductive deafness except:** *(Exam 2016)*
a. Auricle
b. Vestibulocochlear nerve
c. Middle ear
d. External auditory meatus

83. Shown below is an audiometry report. Interpret the audiogram and arrive at the most probable diagnosis: *(AIIMS 2016)*

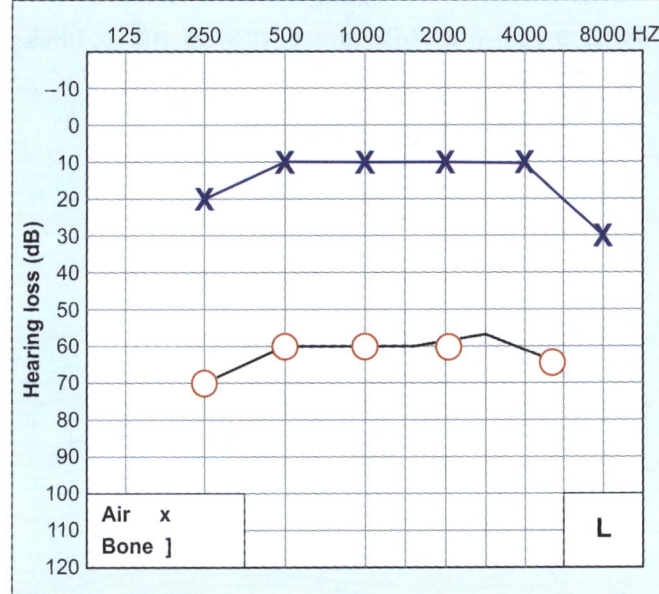

a. Conductive hearing loss right ear
b. Conductive hearing loss left ear
c. SN hearing loss right ear
d. SN hearing loss left ear

84. The centre for stapedial reflex is: *(AIIMS 2016)*
a. Superior olivary complex
b. Medial geniculate body
c. Superior Colliculus
d. Lateral lemniscus

85. Which of the following belongs to profound hearing loss according to WHO? *(AIIMS 2016)*
a. > 71 dB in the better ear
b. >101 dB in the better ear
c. >81 dB in the better ear
d. >91 dB in the better ear

86. What is the intensity in decibel of normal conversation in humans? *(Exam 2016)*
a. 30 dB   b. 60 dB
c. 90 dB   d. 150 dB

87. Sound intensity of whispering is: *(Exam 2014)*
a. 30 dB   b. 90 dB
c. 2 dB   d. 120 dB

88. Maximum hearing loss is caused by: *(Exam 2016)*
a. Ossicular chain damage
b. Tympanic membrane perforation
c. Obliteration of oval window
d. Blockade of ear canal

89. Recruitment is seen in: *(Exam 2016)*
a. Cochlear sensorineural hearing loss
b. Retrocochlear sensorineural hearing loss

c. Conductive hearing loss
d. Mixed hearing loss

90. All of the following are features of cochlear hearing loss except: *(Exam 2016)*
a. SISI test is positive
b. Speech discrimination is highly impaired
c. Otoacoustic emissions absent
d. Damage to inner and outer hair cells

91. Recruitment phenomenon is seen in: *(Exam 2016)*
a. Meniere's disease   b. Otosclerosis
c. Acoustic neuroma   d. Unsafe CSOM

92. Objective method of hearing test: *(Exam 2016)*
a. Tuning fork test   b. Pure tone audiometry
c. Tympanometry   d. Speech audiometry

93. Screeing test for neonate in ICU: *(AIIMS 2016)*
a. Transient evoked OAE
b. Distortion product OAE
c. Automated OAE
d. BERA

94. C-shaped curve on tympanometry is seen in: *(Exam 2016)*
a. Serous otitis media
b. Otosclerosis
c. TM perforation
d. Early Eustachian tube obstruction

95. Hearing loss at 65 dB, what will be the grade of deafness? *(Exam 2016)*
a. Mild   b. Moderate
c. Moderately severe d. Severe

96. Stenger test is used in diagnosis of: *(Exam 2014)*
a. Conductive hearing loss
b. SN hearing loss
c. Non-organic hearing loss
d. Mixed hearing loss

97. SISI is specific for: *(Exam 2014)*
a. Acoustic tumour
b. Otosclerosis
c. Meniere's disease
d. Facial nerve paralysis

98. Otoacoustic emissions are absent when the following is damaged: *(Exam 2016)*
a. Outer hair cells
b. Reissner's membrane
c. Inner hair cells
d. Otolithic membrane

99. All the following are features sensorineural hearing loss except: *(Exam 2016)*
a. Rinnes positive
b. Weber's lateralised to better ear
c. Schwabach test–lengthened
d. ABC-reduced

Section I   Ear

100. **True statement about Oto-acoustic emissions:**
    (Exam 2016)
    a. Spontaneous OAE is absent in 50% normal individuals
    b. Absent in retrocochlear lesions
    c. Absent in hearing loss < 30 dB
    d. All the above

101. **Which of the following does not show negative Rinnes test in the right ear?** *(Exam 2016)*
    a. Sensorineural hearing loss of 45 dB in left ear and normal right ear
    b. Profound hearing loss in the right ear
    c. Conductive hearing loss of 40 dB in both ears
    d. Conductive hearing loss of 40 dB in right ear and left ear normal

102. **Raise of pressure from middle ear to inner ear (the ratio of (air) pressure across the tympanum during transmission of sound) is:** *(Exam 2016)*
    a. 1.3:1   b. 14:1
    c. 17:1   d. 22:1

103. **True about BERA findings in acoustic neuroma:**
    (Exam 2016)
    a. Latency of wave V increased in the affected ear
    b. Latency of wave I increased in the affected ear
    c. No waves on BERA
    d. No change in BERA

104. **In infants hearing loss above 80 dB can be tested by:** *(Exam 2016)*
    a. BERA
    b. Electrocochleography
    c. Auditory steady state response (ASSR)
    d. SISI

105. **Catenary lever provides _____ gain in sound pressure at the level of the malleus.**
    (Kerala PGMEE 2015)
    a. 4 times   b. 3 times
    c. 6 times   d. 2 times

106. **BERA is most accurate at:** *(Jipmer 2014)*
    a. 28 wk   b. 30 wk
    c. 32 wk   d. 34 wk

IMAGE BASED QUESTIONS BY AUTHOR

107. **Not true about the given test is:**

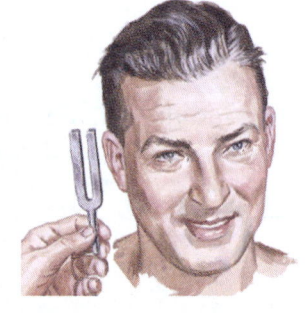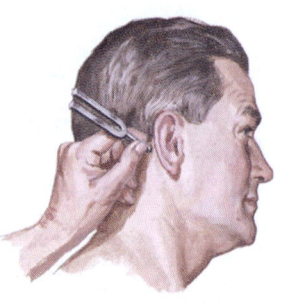

a. In normal ears AC > BC
b. In SN hearing loss AC > BC
c. In severe SN hearing loss AC > BC
d. In conductive hearing loss BC > AC

108. **A 5-year-old child presents with B/L painless hearing loss for the past 10 days. O/E the TM appears dull. His tympanogram finding is given below. Most probable diagnosis is:**

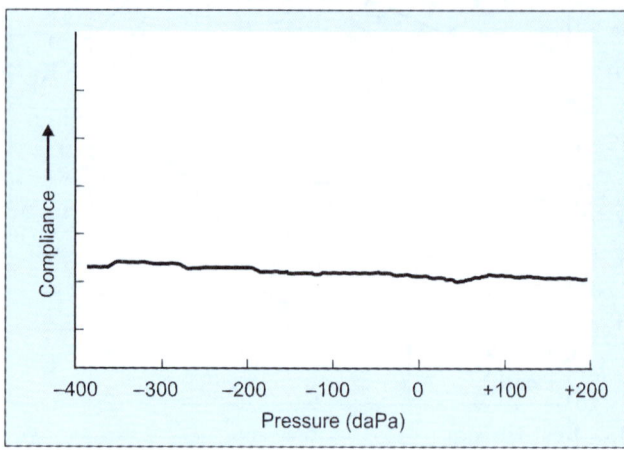

a. Incudostapedial dislocation
b. SOM
c. ASOM
d. Fixation of foot plate of stapes

109. **Not true about the test shown below is:**

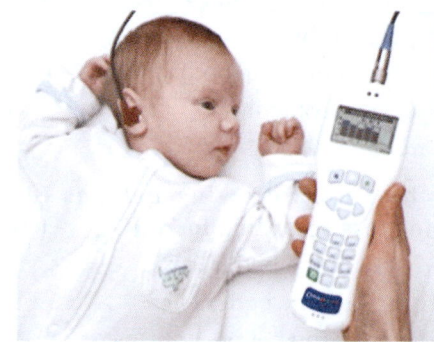

a. Is a by product of outer hair cell
b. Used as a screening test of hearing in neonates
c. Disappear in cochlear pathology
d. Disappear in 8th nerve pathology

110. **A 6-month-old child developed labyrinthitis following meningitis. He was subjected to the test shown below.**

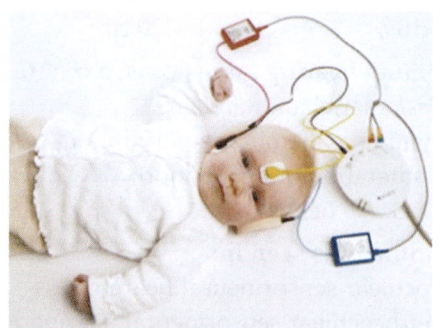

What is this test being performed?

a. OAE   b. BERA

c. Tympanometry   d. PTA

111. **A large perforation in the tympanic membrane can cause sound waves to reach the oval and round windows at the same time. This will cause hearing deficit due to loss of:**   (*Exam 2016*)

a. Travelling wave

b. Hydraulic lever action

c. Transduction

d. Phase differential between the two windows

112. **A patient presents with U/L hearing loss. Right ear Rinnes is positive and left ear Rinnes is negative. Weber's is lateralised to right. What is the diagnosis?**   (*Exam 2018*)

a. Left SN hearing loss

b. Left severe SN hearing loss

c. Right conductive hearing loss

d. Both ears normal

113. **Best time for hearing assessment in an infant:**   (*Exam 2017*)

a. During 1st month

b. 3 – 6 months

c. 6 – 9 months

d. 9 – 12 months

114. **Earliest age for doing BERA:**   (*Exam 2017*)

a. In utero

b. At birth

c. 3 months

d. 6 months

115. **The given audiogram shows:**   (*Exam 2017*)

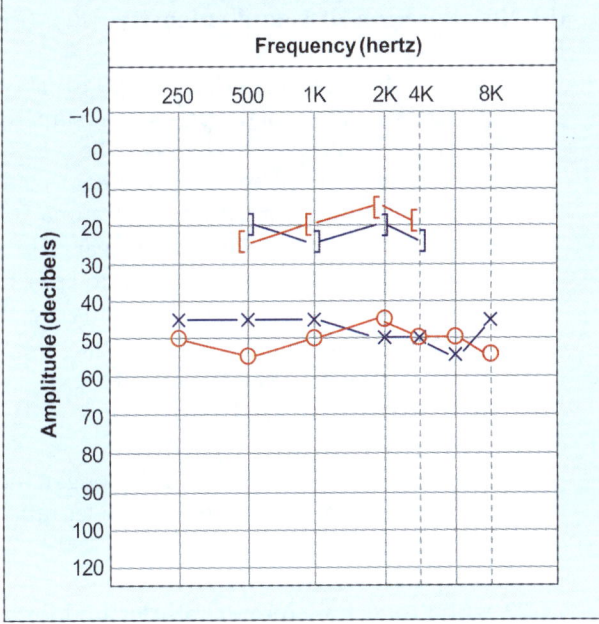

a. U/L CHL   b. U/L SNHL

c. B/L CHL   d. B/L SNHL

116. **Average hearing at 500, 1000 and 2000 Hz is 45 dB in the left ear. Percentage hearing loss in the left ear is:**   (*JIPMER 2014*)

a. 45%   b. 30%

c. 20%   d. 55%

117. **Thick TM as seen in tymapanosclerosis gives rise to which tympanogram:**   (*Exam 2017*)

a. A_s b. A_d

c. B   d. C

ANSWERS AND EXPLANATIONS

1. **(b) No alteration of sound intensity.** (*Ref. Scott Brown, 8th ed., Vol 2; 578*)
    *   Whenever there is a sound of 70–100 dB above the hearing threshold of the person, the stapedial reflex gets activated which does not allow a high intensity sound to damage the inner ear thereby protecting the inner ear from noise trauma.
    *   The transformer action of the middle ear reduces the impedance (resistance) and increases the admittance of sound, thereby amplifying the sound intensity during normal hearing.

2. **(a) Impedance matching (Please refer to text)** (*Ref. Scott Brown, 8th ed, Vol 2; 578*)

3. **(b) 1.3:1** (*Ref. Cummings, 6th ed., 1996*)
    *   The handle of malleus is 1.3 times longer than the long process of incus so that the lever ratio is 1.3:1.
    *   17: 1 is the **Areal ratio**
    *   22 is the **total transformer ratio** of middle ear (Areal ratio × lever ratio), see the text

4. **(a) 17:1** (*Ref. Dhingra, 6th ed., 14*)

5. **(a) Difference of surface area of tympanic membrane and foot plate** (*Ref. Scott Brown, 8th ed., Vol 2; 578*)

6. **(b) and (c) Helmholtz and Bekesy** (*Ref. Cummings, 6th ed., 1997, 2201*)
    *   Bekesy evolved his travelling-wave theory for which he received the Nobel Prize.
    *   Helmholtz detected the sound amplifying effect of the eardrum and the auditory ossicles. Furthermore, he developed the resonance–theory of the perception of pitch in the inner ear. This theory postulates that specific frequencies are displayed on definite locations of the cochlea of the inner ear (place theory of pitch perception). This was replaced by the travelling wave theory by Georg v. Békésy

7. **(c) Stapes abnormal at oval window** (*Ref. Scott Brown, 8th ed., Vol 2; 1063*)
    *   From pinna to foot plate of stapes occurs the conduction of sound. So this is the conductive pathway and any defect here will lead to a conductive deafness.
    *   While travelling in an aeroplane, sudden changes in pressure during descent, leads to forceful closure of the Eustachian tube and tympanic membrane retraction leading to temporary conductive hearing loss and earache. This can be overcome by Valsalva manoeuvre.
    *   Trauma to labyrinth will lead to SN hearing loss.
    *   Noise induced hearing loss is associated with pathological changes in cochlea leading to SN hearing loss.

8. **(d) Rupture of tympanic membrane (leads to conductive deafness).** (*Ref. Cummings, 6th ed., 2201*)

    *   Old age (presbycusis) leads to SN hearing loss.
    *   Loud noise induced hearing loss is associated with pathological changes in cochlea leading to SN hearing loss. Noise trauma, presbycusis and ototoxic drugs involve basal turns of cochlea first; thereby affect high frequency sounds early.
    *   Cochlear otosclerosis leads to sensory hearing loss.

9. **(b) 1000–3000** (*Ref. Scott Brown, 8th ed., Vol 2; 578*)

10. **(c) 500–2000 Hz** (*Ref. Dhingra, 6th ed., 15*)

11. **(b) Grant's test** (*Ref. Scott Brown, 8th ed., Vol 2; 927*) **(there is no entity in ENT called Grant's test)**

12. **(a) Better heard** (*Ref. Cummings 6th ed., 2202*)
    *   The tuning fork tests are most commonly done with 512 Hz (or FPS, i.e. frequency per second) sound frequency producing forks because these are better heard.
    *   Tuning forks with frequency less than 512 have more of vibration sense and those with frequency above 512 dampen very fast because of which comparison is not possible.

13. **(b) 512 Hz** (*Ref. Cummings, 6th ed., 2202*)

14. **(c) Tympanosclerosis** (*Ref. Cummings, 6th ed., 2203*)
    *   Tympanosclerosis being a conductive pathology so BC > AC so Rinne will be negative.
        All the other options being SN deafness so AC > BC so Rinne will be positive.

15. **(b) CSOM** (*Ref. Cummings, 6th ed., 2203*)
    *   CSOM being a conductive pathology so BC > AC so Rinne will be negative.
        All the other options being SN deafness so AC > BC so Rinne will be positive.

16. **(a) 15–20 dB** (*Ref. Cummings, 6th ed., 2203; Anirban Biswas, 5th ed., 27*)

17. **(a) AC>BC** (*Ref. Shambaugh, 6th ed., 181*)

18. **(d) Presbycusis** (*Ref. Shambaugh, 6th ed., 181*)
    *   Presbycusis being a SN pathology so AC > BC so Rinne will be positive.
        All the other options being conductive deafness so BC > AC so Rinne will be negative.

19. **(b) Normal individual** (*Ref. Shambaugh, 6th ed., 181*)
    *   Rinne is said to be positive when AC > BC.
    *   In normal ear air conduction is more than the bone conduction due to the transformer action of the middle ear.
        All the other options are conductive deafness conditions so BC > AC, i.e. Rinne will be negative.

20. **(d) Placing the tuning fork on the forehead and asking him to report in which ear he hears it better** (*Ref. Scott Brown, 8th ed., Vol 2; 927*)

21. **(a) 5 dB** (*Ref. Cummings, 6th ed., 2213*)

22. **(c) Lateralised to right side** (*Ref. Scott Brown, 8th ed., Vol 2; 928*)
    *   Middle ear pathology indicates conductive deafness so Weber will be lateralised to the right

side in the right ear pathology, i.e. towards the worst side.

- **Weber is lateralised to** the **W**orst ear in **C**onductive hearing loss and **B**etter ear in **S**ensorineural hearing loss. (**Mnemonic**: **W**e **C**reate–**B**est **S**tudents).

23. **(b) Sound louder in diseased ear.** (*Ref. Scott Brown, 8th ed., Vol 2; 928*)

24. **(a) Middle ear** (*Ref. Scott Brown, 8th ed., Vol 2; 927*)
    - Threshold for bone conduction is normal means that the sensorineural pathway is normal.
    - Threshold for air conduction is increased means conductive hearing loss.
    So this is indicative of middle ear disease.

25. **(c) Otosclerosis (Gelle's is negative in Otosclerosis)** (*Ref.Anirban Biswas, 5th ed., 49*)

26. **(a) SN deafness** (*Ref. Scott Brown, 8th ed., Vol 2; 927*)
    The other options being conductive pathologies so show no change in hearing.

27. **(d) False negative Rinne test** (*Ref. Scott Brown, 6th ed., Vol 2; 2/5/4*)
    - In a patient of suppurative labyrinthitis, positive Rinne means SN hearing loss.
    - Positive fistula test, *see* chapter on vestibular system, suggests that there is a fistula on the medial wall of middle ear probably this is the cause of labyrinthitis.
    - The fistula test becoming negative after two weeks in the absence of treatment suggest that the ear has become dead and therefore non-responsive (false negative fistula). So Rinne here will be false negative because of severe SN hearing loss.

28. **(a) Weber's test left lateralised, Rinne-right positive, BC>AC on left side** (*Ref. Scott Brown, 6th ed., Vol 2; 2/5/4*)
    In this patient there is 30 dB deafness in left ear, the right ear is normal (so right Rinne positive) and Weber's is lateralised to the left ear indicating conductive pathology of the left ear (BC > AC on left side).
    In left ear the Rinne will be negative.

29. **(b) Right sided severe sensorineural deafness** (*Ref. Scott Brown, 6th ed., Vol 2; 2/5/4*)
    Here the patient has right sided hearing loss. In the right ear Rinne is negative so there can be 2 possibilities:
    (a) Conductive hearing loss of right ear
    (b) Severe SN loss of right ear (false negative Rinne) Weber's will help us to differentiate between the two. Since it shows lateralisation to left side which is the better side it means that there is severe SN hearing loss on the right side.

30. **(b) Right severe sensorineural hearing loss** (Explanation same as above) (*Ref. Scott Brown, 6th ed., Vol 2; 2/5/4*)

31. **(d) Do Schwabach test** (*Ref. Dhingra, 6th ed., 22*)
    With Rinne test positive in both ears means either the hearing is normal or there is SN hearing loss in other words there is no conductive hearing loss. Since here the Weber lateralizes to the right means that the left ear has a SN hearing loss as it cannot be the conductive hearing loss of the right side, Rinne being positive here. So the diagnosis is left SN deafness and Schwabach can confirm this.

32. **(b) Air conduction (AC) in left ear** (*Ref. Cummings, 6th ed., 2203*)
    - Symbol X or □ is used to mark air conduction in left ear in unmasked and masked condition respectively (mnemonic; **cross sign** indicating (crucifixion of) Jesus Christ, (though that is made differently, we all know) Who will always be in our heart (unhidden, i.e. unmasked), and the heart being on **left** side.
    - After His crucifixion on the day now called Good Friday (also called God's Friday/Black Friday), His earthly body was kept in a linen with spices in a coffin (□ symbol can be considered for coffin) and finally 3 days later, on Easter Jesus Christ rose from death). So easy to remember X or □ is used for showing AC in left ear in unmasked and masked conditions respectively.
    - Air conduction in right ear is marked by symbols 0 (mnemonic; zero sign because the above happening was not at all righteous and therefore we pray to God on Good Friday for our sins to The Jesus Christ and vow to become good human beings) and ∆ in unmasked and masked conditions respectively.
    - Another mnemonic, for people who do not believe in God, right is right so left will be wrong (X) → simple and clear! (unmasked left AC). For masked (left AC) let's change this symbol to (□), by rearranging the four limbs of X. Now as in a maths equation, right ear being equal to left ear, left being wrong (zero marks) so right is 0 (zero), clear, nothing hidden! (unmasked)
    - Bone conduction in right ear will be marked by symbols < or [in unmasked and masked condition respectively and BC in left ear is marked by > or] (same but opposite symbols, the opening being towards the respective hand).
    - No response in air conduction in right ear and left ear will be marked as arrow beneath the respective symbols.

33. **(a) Air conduction of right ear** (*Ref. Cummings 6th ed., 2203*)

34. **(b) Ototoxicity** (*Ref. Anirban Biswas, 5th ed., 27*)
    High frequency audiometry:
    - Conventional audiometry tests frequencies between 250 Hz–8000 Hz, whereas high frequency audiometry tests frequencies in the region of 8000 Hz–20,000 Hz.

Section I   **Ear**

- It is used to detect early ototoxicity and early noise induced hearing loss as these lead to high frequency hearing loss initially and therefore if detected early these conditions can be prevented or minimised.

35. **(b) 20–20,000 Hz** (*Ref. Shambaugh 6th ed. 50*)

36. **(c) 61–80 dB** (*Ref. Scott Brown, 8th ed., Vol 2; 76*)

37. **(c) 41–55 dB** (*Ref. Scott Brown, 8th ed., Vol 2; 76*)

    If WHO not given go with ASHA categories. Please note for moderately severe it is 56–70 dB. Easy to remember **MMS–M**oderate and **M**oderately **S**evere; 41–70 dB.

38. **(b) 10 times** (*Ref. Cummings, 6th ed., 1995*) please refer the text

39. **(a) 10–40 dB** (*Ref. Cummings, 6th ed., 2201*) (refer the table in the text. Please note in this table, the hearing loss is in a range in TM perforation only, whereas in other conditions it is a stat value).

40. **(a) Ossicular disruption with intact tympanic membrane** (54 dB-*See* the Table in the text) (*Ref. Cummings, 6th ed., 2201*)
    - Ossicular disruption with perforated tympanic membrane will have rather less hearing loss (38 dB) because some sound is able to enter the windows directly through the perforated TM.
    - In Otitis media with effusion the hearing loss is never more than 40 dB.
    - In otosclerosis the hearing loss increases with increasing fixation of foot plate and reaches a maximum conductive hearing loss of 60 dB in complete fixation.

41. **(a) Ossicular disruption with intact tympanic membrane** (*Ref. Cummings, 6th ed., 2201*)

42. **(c) Complete closure of oval window** (it means complete fixation of foot plate) (*Ref. Cummings, 6th ed., 2201*)

43. **(a) Congenital SNHL** (*Ref. Scott Brown, 8th ed. Vol 2; 712*)
    - Trough shaped or U shaped or cookie bite curve is seen in congenital SN hearing loss and in cochlear otosclerosis.

44. **(b) Middle ear** (*Ref. Cummings, 6th ed., 2203*)
    - In impedance audiometry we do tympanometry which is a measure of the condition of the middle ear at the level of TM.

45. **(b) Impendence audiometry** (*Ref. Cummings, 6th ed., 2203*)
    - Pure tone audiometry tests the threshold of hearing at various frequencies. It tells about the type and degree of hearing.
    - Caloric test is a test of vestibular function.
    - BERA tests the peripheral and central auditory pathways.

46. **(a) 226 Hz** (*Ref. Shambaugh, 6th ed., 196*)

47. **(d) and (e) Otosclerosis reduces compliance, Flat curve in TM perforation** (*Ref. Cummings, 6th ed., 2055*)

48. **(d) Middle ear fluid causes dome shaped /type B curve on tympanogram.** (*Ref.Anirban Biswas, 5th ed., 98*)
    - In Otosclerosis A_s type curve is seen.
    - In ossicular discontinuity A_d type curve is seen.
    - In TM perforation Tympanometry cannot be done as it is not possible to do pressure changes hence a flat curve is obtained.

49. **(a) Serous Otitis media** (due to **B**lockade of Eustachian tube) causes type **B** curve on tympanogram. (*Ref. Cummings, 6th ed., 2203*)

50. **(a) Flat** (*Ref. Cummings, 6th ed., 2055*)

51. **(b), (c) and (e) Serous Otitis media, Perforation of ear drum and Safe CSOM**
    - In Serous Otitis media when the fluid is so much that the tympanic membrane cannot move at all, a B type curve with no peak (flat curve) is obtained.

52. **(d) Low-compliance** (*Ref. Shambaugh, 6th ed., 201*)
    - Osteogenesis Imperfecta an autosomal dominant condition is characterised by recurrent fractures due to brittle bones, blue sclera, dental abnormalities and progressive hearing loss due to Otosclerosis. Therefore, As type of curve, which is a low compliance and normal pressure, is seen.

53. **(b) Ad type tympanogram** (*Ref. Cummings, 6th ed., 2201*)

    Hearing loss with intact TM and normal inner ear (cochlear reserve) following accident suggests that the defect is in middle ear.
    - 55 dB AB gap suggests ossicular discontinuity. Hence Ad type of curve on tympanogram.

54. **(a) Distortion of ossicular chain** (*Ref. Cummings, 6th ed., 2055*)
    - Intact TM with increased compliance on impedance suggests distortion of ossicular chain.
    - Hemotympanum is a possibility following head injury leading to conductive deafness but here TM compliance will be reduced.
    - Tympanosclerosis and otosclerosis do not follow head injury and Tympanometry shows reduced compliance.

55. **(b) It is a protective reflex against loud sound** (*Ref. Cummings, 6th ed., 2055*)
    - Whenever there is a loud sound 70–100 dB above the hearing threshold of a person, the Stapedial reflex gets activated and protects the inner ear from noise trauma. It is a bilateral reflex.

56. **(d) VII and VIII nerves** (*Ref. Cummings, 6th ed., 2055*)
    - The afferent of the Stapedial reflex is the 8th nerve and the efferent is the 7th nerve.

57. **(b) Normal sounds heard as loud and painful is known as hyperacusis.** (*Ref. Cummings, 6th ed., 2343*)
    - It is because of absence of stapedial reflex in facial nerve palsy.

- Ability to hear better in noisy surroundings is Paracusis wilisii phenomenon seen in otosclerosis, *see* Chapter 10.

58. **(c) VIII nerve lesion** (*Ref. Anirban Biswas, 5th ed. 118; Cummings, 6th ed., 2055*)
    - In VIII nerve lesion Stapedial reflex is absent in both ipsilateral and contralateral ears as it is the afferent of the reflex.

59. **(a) Right side** (*Ref. Cummings, 6th ed., 2055*)
    - Since facial nerve forms the efferent of stapedial reflex, in facial nerve palsy of right side Stapedial reflex is absent on the right side only.

60. **(b) Neural deafness** (*Ref. Anirban Biswas, 5th ed. 56*)
    - Tone decay is a function of nerve fatigue.
    - If the nerves are fatigued the patient stops hearing a sound given to him continuously before the completion of 1 minute.
    - A tone decay of more than 30 dB is suggestive of retrocochlear or neural deafness

61. **(d) Evoked potential generated in cochlea and auditory nerve** (refer the text) (*Ref. Cummings, 6th ed., 2057*)

62. **(b) Otoacoustic emissions (OAEs).** (*Ref. Cummings, 6th ed., 2074*)
    - OAE is considered to be the best audiometric test to screen hearing in neonates. Absent OAE indicate cochlear lesions.
    - For screening purposes the test has to be easy to do, less time consuming, results should be available immediately and cost effective.
    - For these reasons OAE is better than BERA for screening hearing in neonates and children.
    - If OAEs are absent, the child is taken up for BERA for confirmation.
    - Electrocochleography is an invasive test. It is done for Meniere's, which is not the pathology, at this age.
    - Tympanometry is used to detect middle ear lesions which are also unusual at this age.
    - Developmental anomalies of the cochlea are to be ruled out at this age, if found, the child can be taken up for cochlear implantation as early as one year of age for proper speech development.

63. **(b) Otoacoustic Emissions (OAE)** (*Ref. Scott Brown, 8th ed., Vol 2; 60*)

64. **(b) Outer hair cells** (*Ref. Cummings, 6th ed., 2071*)
    - Maculae are for balance and not for hearing

65. **(a), (c), (d) Are by-product of outer hair cell, Used as a screening test of hearing in newborn infant, Useful in ototoxicity monitoring.** (*Ref. Cummings, 6th ed., 2074*)
    - Otoacoustic emissions disappear in cochlear pathology.

66. **(b) BERA** (*Ref. Cummings, 6th ed., 2078*)
    - Since BERA is an objective test and it tests the electrical activity occurring in the whole of the auditory pathway, it is the investigation of choice here.
    - Impedance audiometry is also objective but it is limited to middle ear pathologies which are usually not the cause of deafness at this age.
    - In Free field and behavioural audiometry auditory signals are presented to infants and children and their change in behaviour is observed.

67. **(a) BERA** (*Ref. Cummings, 6th ed., 2063*)
    - Impedance and pure tone audiometry test the middle ear.

68. **(c) Lateral lemniscus** (*Ref. Cummings, 6th ed., 2063, 2076*)
    - The wave V is the most prominent and easily identifiable and hence the most important wave of BERA. Wave V is generated from lateral lemniscus.
    - Cochlear nucleus gives wave III
    - Superior olivary complex gives wave IV
    - Inferior Colliculus gives waves VI and VII

69. **(a), (e) Can differentiate cochlear and retrocochlear lesion, to diagnose brainstem pathology** (*Ref. Cummings, 6th ed., 2063*)
    - With BERA the exact site of lesion in SN hearing loss can be found out by noting the latency and amplitude of the affected wave.
    - Complete blood cell count (CBC), electrolytes, BUN, creatinine, and glucose estimations are done to distinguish barbiturate poisoning from metabolic causes of coma. Serum Phenobarbital levels will confirm barbiturate poisoning.
    - OAE is the screening hearing test in infants

70. **(b) Auditory neuropathy** (since OAEs are present so pathology is retrocochlear) (*Ref. Cummings, 6th ed., 2065*)

71. **(a) Caloric test is for vestibular assessment** (*Ref. Scott Brown, 8th ed., Vol 2; 795*)
    - Rinne, Weber and ABC are tests of hearing, to find out conductive and sensorineural hearing loss.

72. **(b) Impedance audiometry** (*Ref. Scott Brown, 6th ed., Vol 2; 2/12/1*)
    - Impedance audiometry is an objective test. It does not require the cooperation of patient.
    - Other objective audiometry tests are; OAEs, Electrocochleography and BERA

73. **(a) Pure tone audiometry** (*Ref. Scott Brown, 6th ed., Vol 2; 2/12/1*)
    Rest are objective.

74. **(a) Stenger test** (refer to the text) (*Ref. Cummings, 6th ed., 2067*)
    - Bing, Weber and Rinne tests are for the detection of conductive and SN hearing loss.

75. **(d) Profound SNHL in right ear, left ear normal** (*Ref. Scott Brown, 6th ed., Vol 2; 2/5/4*)
    Please refer to the text.

76. **(c) It needs sound proof room** (*Ref. Cummings, 6th ed., 2203*)

77. **(d) Refer, see text** (*Ref. Cummings, 6th ed., 2973;* Anirban Biswas, 5th ed., 263)

78. **(b) 100–200 msec** (*Ref. Scott Brown, 8th ed., Vol 2; 76; Anirban Biswas, 5th ed., 126*)

79. **(a) Left ear Rinnes +ve; Weber's lateralised to right** (*Ref. Scott Brown, 6th ed., Vol 2; 2/5/4*)

80. **(b) CSOM** (*Ref. Cummings, 6th ed., 2203*)

81. **(b) Tympanometry** (*Ref.Anirban Biswas, 5th ed., 114*)

82. **(b) Vestibulocochlear nerve** (*Ref. Scott Brown, 6th ed., Vol 2; 2/12/2*)

83. **(a) Conductive hearing loss right ear** (*Ref. Cummings, 6th ed., 2053*)

    In the left ear the AC is 10 dB (average of speech frequencies) which is normal. Since AC is a measure of both conductive and SN pathway and it being normal, both conductive and SN pathway are normal. In the right ear AC is 60dB. Had it been a SN hearing loss in the right ear, the BC would have been worse than AC and would have been shown in the audiogram. Since it is not shown here, it should be presumed that it is normal in the right ear. So the audiogram is showing conductive hearing loss of the right ear.

84. **(a) Superior olivary complex** (*Ref. Anirban Biswas, 5th ed., 119*)

85. **(c) >81 dB in the better ear** (*Ref. Scott Brown, 8th ed., Vol 2; 76*)

86. **(b) 60 dB** (*Ref. Scott Brown, 8th ed., Vol 2; 926*)
    - The intensity of sound at 1 metre, in various human conversations are as below:
        i. Whisper–30 dB
        ii. Normal conversation–60 dB
        iii. Shout–90 dB
            There occurs Discomfort in the ear at 120 dB and pain in the ear at a loudness of 130 dB

87. **(a) 30 dB** (*Ref. Scott Brown, 8th ed ., Vol 2; 926*)

88. **(c) Obliteration of oval window** (*Ref. Cummings, 6th ed., 2201*)

89. **(a) Cochlear sensorineural hearing loss** (*Ref. Scott Brown, 8th ed., Vol 2, 629*)

90. **(b) Speech discrimination is highly impaired** (*Ref.Anirban Biswas, 5th ed., 63*)

91. **(a) Meniere's disease** (*Ref. Scott Brown, 8th ed., Vol 2; 629*)

92. **(c) Tympanometry** (*Ref. Shambaugh, 6th ed., 196*)

93. **(d) BERA** (*Ref. Scott Brown, 8th ed., Vol 2; 60; Cummings, 6th ed., 2975*)

94. **(d) Early Eustachian tube obstruction** (*Ref. Cummings, 6th ed., 2055*)

95. **(c) Moderately severe** (*Ref. Scott Brown, 8th ed., Vol 2; 60*)

96. **(c) Non-organic hearing loss** (*Ref.Anirban Biswas, 5th ed., Vol. 1, 46*)

97. **(c) Meniere's disease** (*Ref.Anirban Biswas, 5th ed., 63*)

98. **(a) Outer hair cells** (*Ref. Cummings, 6th ed., 2074*)

99. **(c) Schwabach test–lengthened 1)** (*Ref. Dhingra, 6th ed., 22*)

100. **(a) Spontaneous OAE is absent in 50% normal individuals** (*Ref. Cummings, 6th ed., 2074*)

101. **(a) Sensorineural hearing loss of 45 dB in left ear and normal right ear** (*Ref. Scott Brown, 6th ed., Vol 2; 2/5/4*)

102. **(d) 22:1** (*Ref. Dhingra, 6th ed., 14*)

103. **(a) Latency of wave V increased in the affected ear** (*Ref.Anirban Biswas, 5th ed., Vol 1, 197*)

104. **(c) Auditory steady state response (ASSR)** (*Ref. Cummings, 6th ed., 2081*)

105. **(d) 2 times** (*Ref. Cummings, 6th ed., 2201*)

106. **(d) 34 wk** (*Ref. Scott Brown, 8th ed., Vol 2; 655*)

    Prenatally there is a progressive improvement in the detection of waves I, III, and V of BERA with increasing gestational age due to maturation of auditory pathway. Since the maximum age given among the options is 34 wks so this is the best answer. The wave forms of BERA are of adult configuration by 18 months.

107. **(c) In severe SN hearing loss AC > BC** (*Ref. Cummings, 6th ed., 2203*)

108. **(b) SOM** (*Ref. Cummings, 6th ed., 2203*)

109. **(d) Disappear in 8th nerve pathology** (*Ref. Cummings, 6th ed., 2074*)

110. **(b) BERA** (*Ref. Cummings, 6th ed., 2076, 2975*)

111. **(d) Phase differential between the two windows** (*Ref. Cummings, 6th ed., 2202*)

112. **(b) Left severe SN hearing loss** (*Ref. Scott Brown, 6th ed., Vol 2; 2/5/4*), Refer to the text

113. **(a) During 1st month. It is done within 48 hours of birth.** Refer to the text. (*Ref. Anirban Biswas, 5th ed., 202*)

114. **(a) In Utero.** Refer to the text. (*Ref. Anirban Biswas, 5th ed., 203*)

115. **(c) B/L CHL** (*Ref. Scott Brown, 8th ed., Vol 2; 639*)

116. **(b) 30%** (*Ref. Dhingra, 6th ed., 39*)

117. **(a) A_s** (*Ref. Cummings, 6th ed., 2205*)

Vestibular Physiology and Assessment of Vestibular Function

VESTIBULAR SYSTEM

The vestibular system is responsible for equilibration, coordination and orientation in space.

The anatomy of vestibular system comprises of:

1. The inner ear: It contains the **receptor organs** in the semicircular canals (cristae), utricle and saccule (maculae).

2. The **superior and inferior vestibular nerves** (cranial nerve VIII). The superior vestibular N carries impulses from cristae of superior and lateral SCC and maculae of utricle whereas the inferior vestibular N carries impulses from cristae of posterior SCC (singular N) and maculae of saccule. These sensory nerves carry the information from these areas to the vestibular nuclei in the brain stem in the floor of the fourth ventricle. The cell bodies of these (Sup & inf vestibular N) 1st order neurons lie in the Scarpa's ganglion in the inner ear just lateral to the IAM.

3. **Vestibular nuclei.** The 2nd order neurons from here go to:

   a. **Medial longitudinal bundle** or fasciculus (and through this connect with 3rd, 4th & 6th ocular nerves nuclei). The 3rd order neurons from here are the motor neurons and supply the ocular muscles. This completes the reflex arc for the vestibulo-ocular reflex (VOR). Defect in this pathway can be assessed by studying the kind of nystagmus, read below.

   b. Anterior horn cells of the spinal cord through **vestibulo-spinal** and other pathways. The 3rd order neurons from here are motor to the postural muscles of neck, trunk and limbs. This completes the reflex arc for the **vestibulo-colic** reflex. One of the ways by which the defect in this pathway can be assessed is by doing c VEMP studies, read below.

4. Also from the vestibular nuclei there occurs to and fro (afferent as well as efferent) flow of information to the cerebellum (via **vestibulo-cerebellar pathway**), cerebral cortex and reticular activating system. These upper or central connections, like elsewhere in neurology, are predominantly inhibitory to the contralateral vestibular nuclei. So lesions here will lead to a hyper active response on the contralateral side leading to vertigo which is labelled as central.

However lesions of the inner ear receptors, vestibular nerves and the vestibular nuclei will lead to a hypo active response on the ipsilateral side leading to vertigo which is labelled as peripheral. These two can be distinguished by studying the kind of nystagmus, read below.

 Note:

Please note that though vestibular nuclei are classified anatomically as part of the central vestibular system, functionally their lesions will be like lesions of inner ear receptors and vestibular nerves. Therefore in all the further discussions below they are being considered in the peripheral vestibular system.

VESTIBULAR PHYSIOLOGY

The **receptor organ** consists of the following (also *see* chapter on anatomy of ear):

1. **Maculae** containing otolith (for sensing linear movements, gravitational and head tilt movements) within the utricle and saccule.

2. **Cristae** containing cupula (for sensing angular movements) within the semicircular canals.

The receptor organs, detect the position and movement of the head in space. This information is converted into electrical signals that travel along the vestibular nerve to the vestibular nuclei in the brainstem. As mentioned above the vestibular nuclei receive the signals and send messages to the following:

i. To the spinal cord via the **vestibulo-spinal tract** for the regulation of muscle tone of the neck and limbs and thereby facilitating postural and righting reflexes.

ii. To the eyes via the medial longitudinal fasciculus (**vestibulo-ocular tract**) to control the eyeball movement (with cranial nerves III, IV, and VI). This helps one's gaze to get fixed on one object (i.e. the image keeps falling on the most sensitive part of the retina, i.e. Fovea) as the head moves. This is called vestibulo-ocular reflex. It can be tested by caloric test and head impulse test, read ahead.

  iii. To the cerebellum via the **vestibulo-cerebellar** tract to maintain coordination of the eyes, neck, body, and limbs in relation to position and movements of the head.

  iv. To the reticular formation in the brainstem and thereby preparing the autonomic nervous system.

  v. To the cerebral cortex via the thalamus for conscious perception of position.

Under normal circumstances, the impulses reaching the brain from all the above systems from both the sides are **equal and opposite** and help to maintain the balance of a person. However, any mismatch in the impulses reaching the brain (from these systems) can lead to vertigo.

VERTIGO AND ASSOCIATED SYMPTOMS

Vertigo or dizziness is the sensation of movement (most commonly rotational) and is often accompanied by feeling of loss of balance. When the vertigo is severe it may be accompanied by autonomic manifestations, e.g. nausea, vomiting, sweating and palpitations. In most instances vertigo is also accompanied by spontaneous nystagmus, *see* below. All these clinical manifestations can be easily understood as per the central connections of the vestibular system as discussed above.

Vertigo can occur either due to a peripheral vestibular pathology (inner ear receptor, vestibular nerves, vestibular nuclei) or a central vestibular pathology (involving the vestibular interconnections with cerebellum, cortex and reticular activating system).

LOCATING THE CAUSE OF VERTIGO (PERIPHERAL/CENTRAL)

To locate the pathology causing vertigo (peripheral or central), the following are done:

1. **To Look for Spontaneous Nystagmus:** Nystagmus is involuntary oscillatory movement of eyeball.

Spontaneous nystagmus means movement of the eyes without a cognitive, visual or vestibular stimulus. This nystagmus occurs due to the difference in the normal **equal and opposite** activity of the vestibular systems of the two sides, as discussed above. If nystagmus is present spontaneously, it indicates an organic lesion. So spontaneous nystagmus is also called pathological nystagmus.

Nystagmus may be of two types:

  a. **Jerk or biphasic** (more common): Here rhythmic eye oscillation is characterized by a slow drift of the eyes in one direction that gets repeatedly corrected by fast movements in the reverse direction, i.e. jerk nystagmus has a **slow component followed by a fast component.** Conventionally the **direction** of the nystagmus is described as per the direction of its **fast component.**

  b. **Pendular** (less common): It is a sinusoidal eye oscillation with equal velocity in each direction.

*As discussed previously pathologic or **spontaneous jerk nystagmus**, which is also an accompaniment to vertigo* is due to an **acute asymmetry in vestibular activity, either peripheral or central.** By the characteristic of nystagmus we can have an idea whether the cause is peripheral or central, *see* Tables 3.1 and 3.3.

So a spontaneous nystagmus with fixed direction, which has an additional superimposed rotatory component and which disappears with visual fixation is due to peripheral vestibular pathology. The direction of this nystagmus is important as it helps in finding the nature of pathology of the peripheral vestibular system (which may be irritative or destructive), *see* below.

The significance of the direction of jerk nystagmus: Under normal circumstances, the vestibular system of the right side pushes the eyeball to the left, whereas the vestibular system of the left side pushes the eyeball to the right. If the **right peripheral vestibular system becomes hypoactive due to any destructive/paretic pathology**, then due to unopposed action of the left vestibular system, the eyeball tends to slowly move to the right. Subsequently due to corrective central compensatory mechanism (the brainstem mechanism involving the medial longitudinal fasciculus), the eyeballs quickly return to their initial location, i.e. towards the left (fast phase).

This goes on repeatedly resulting in nystagmus.

In the above example, the fast component being towards the normal side (left), so we should remember that a destructive peripheral pathology of one side vestibular system leads to a nystagmus towards the opposite (normal) side.

Whereas if the **right vestibular system becomes overactive, due to any irritative pathology**, it will lead to excessive pushing of the eyeball towards the left (slow phase). Again Due to central compensation the eyeballs quickly return to their initial location, i.e. towards the right (fast phase).

This leads to nystagmus (fast component) towards the side of irritative lesion.

As mentioned in Table 3.1, in the above examples, there is an additional torsional component besides horizontal movements.

To summarise: The slow component of nystagmus is by virtue of disease. The fast component is the corrective phase to bring the eyeball back to midline. Direction of nystagmus is named after the direction of the fast component as the fast component is more obvious on clinical examination.

By the direction of the nystagmus in peripheral pathologies we can have an idea of the cause:

  i. In **irritative lesions (overstimulation)** of the labyrinth like serous labyrinthitis, fistula of labyrinth, etc. the nystagmus is towards the ipsilateral side, i.e. the side of the lesion (easy to remember **I** for **I**; Irritative – Ipsilateral).

  ii. In destructive or **paretic lesions**, e.g. purulent labyrinthitis, trauma to labyrinth, section of vestibular nerve, etc. the nystagmus is towards the

Table 3.1: Important differentiating features between peripheral and central nystagmus include the following (*see* Table 3.3 for further differentiating features)

Characteristic of spontaneous nystagmus	Peripheral vestibular	Central vestibular
Form (further elaborated in Table 3.2)	Torsional (i.e. rotatory movement of the eye globe about its anteroposterior axis) component superimposed on a horizontal (left or right movement) or vertical (downbeat or upbeat) nystagmus.	Pure horizontal, pure vertical or purely torsional nystagmus.
Direction	Direction-fixed, i.e. unidirectional nystagmus. The nystagmus becomes more pronounced with gaze towards the side of the fast component.	Direction changing, i.e. bidirectional. Here the direction of the fast component gets directed towards the side of gaze (e.g. left-beating in left gaze and right-beating in right gaze).
On visual/optic fixation	The nystagmus disappears with visual fixation. On removing the visual fixation, the nystagmus reappears. If the nystagmus is very fine, i.e. difficult to be seen by naked eye, then Frenzel glasses, which are strong convex glasses, are used. These glasses allow the examiner to see the patient's eyes greatly magnified. These glasses at the same time remove visual fixation, by blurring the patient's vision, thereby making the nystagmus apparent.	The nystagmus, does not disappear with visual fixation, indicating loss of inhibition
Associated features	Unilateral Tinnitus and deafness is often present, but without any other cranial nerve and cerebellar involvement.	Besides tinnitus and deafness (indicating the involvement of 8th nerve), involvement and deficits of **cranial nerves III to XII** which are closely associated with the brainstem are often present. Also cerebellar manifestations (e.g. ataxia, dysarthria, etc.) may be seen.
Common causes	BPPV, Labyrinthitis, Vestibular neuronitis, Meniere's, Labyrinthine fistula and damage by ototoxic drugs	Vertebrobasilar insufficiency and other central vascular conditions, Demyelinating illnesses and Tumours.

opposite side, i.e. normal side (easy to remember **P** for **P**; **P**aretic–**opp**osite).

Each semicircular canal (SCC) has a synergistic canal on the opposite side lying approximately parallel to it. The horizontal canals act as a pair, while each superior canal is paired with posterior canal on the opposite side. The above example of right vestibular irritative/paretic pathology was with regard to involvement of right sided horizontal (lateral) SCC, also note the nystagmus in the lesions involving superior and posterior SCC in Table 3.2.

2. Induced nystagmus:

If spontaneous nystagmus is not present then nystagmus can be induced for evaluating the cause of vertigo (peripheral or central). This can be done by:

I. **Caloric test:** Thermal changes in the EAC can induce convection currents in the horizontal (lateral) SCC (bulge of which is present on the medial wall of middle ear). Caloric test is a clinical test of the vestibulo-ocular reflex (head impulse test also studies this reflex, read below) by thermal stimulation of the lateral SCC.

The lateral or horizontal SCC is maximally responsive when it is in the vertical position. It can be placed in vertical position by seating the patient

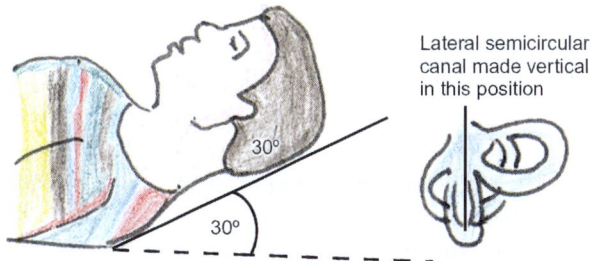

Fig. 3.1: Position of caloric test

with head tilted 60 degrees backward or raising the head 30 degrees forward in supine position.

In this test we can test the vestibular system of each ear separately. However since only the lateral SCC is being stimulated here so only the superior vestibular nerve which supplies it (*see* Chapter 1), can be tested.

There are two types of caloric tests:

a. *Modified Kobrak test:* This is also known as minimal cold stimulation test because this test is done initially with 5 ml ice cold water. With this minimal ice cold water the patient's ear is irrigated after seating the patient with head tilted **60 degrees backwards**.

Table 3.2: The different form and direction of spontaneous nystagmus in various central and peripheral pathologies

Form and direction of nystagmus	Peripheral irritative lesion	Peripheral destructive/ paretic lesion	Central
Horizontal with torsion	Horizontal (lateral) canals, nystagmus towards ipsilateral side	Horizontal (lateral) canals, nystagmus towards opposite side	—
Vertical upbeat with torsion	Posterior semicircular canal (in BPPV), read below	Superior semicircular canal	—
Vertical downbeat with torsion	Superior semicircular canal	Posterior semicircular canal	—
Pure torsional	—	—	Medullary lesions
Pure vertical upbeat	—	—	Medullary lesions
Pure vertical downbeat	—	—	Vertebrobasilar insufficiency, Craniocervical anomalies (Arnold-Chiari Malformation) and drug intoxications
Pure horizontal	—	—	Unilateral disease of the Cerebral hemispheres
Pendular	—	—	Brainstem or Cerebellar dysfunction

Normally nystagmus towards opposite ear is seen with 5 ml of ice cold water. If no response occurs even with 40 ml ice cold water it indicates dead labyrinth.

If response is seen with increased quantities of water between 5 and 40 ml, labyrinth is considered hypoactive.

b. *Fitzgerald Hallpike test:* This test is also known as **bi-thermal caloric test** because it is tested with **cold (30°C)** as well as **warm (44°C)** water, i.e. 7 degrees below and above the normal body temperature of 37°C. The procedure is done in the following order with each irrigation lasting for 40 seconds:

Right warm → left warm → right cold → left cold

An interval of 8 minutes is given in between each irrigation for the temperature to come back to normal.

Here the patient lies supine with head raised **30 degrees forward** to make lateral (or horizontal) semicircular canal vertical in which it is maximally responsive and the ears are irrigated with 30 and 44 degree Celsius water for 40 seconds with a gap of 8 minutes in each in the order mentioned above.

Here the normal response is *C O W S*, i.e. with **C**old water (cold water makes the labyrinth hypoactive/ **p**aretic) nystagmus is towards the **O**pposite side and

with **W**arm water (warm water makes the labyrinth hyperactive/**i**rritative), it is towards the ipsilateral, i.e. **S**ame side. The normal response in a caloric vestibular test is symmetric in the two ears.

Utility of caloric test:

i. Each labyrinth can be tested separately. This test can tell us unilateral paretic/dead or irritative labyrinth.

In **paretic/dead labyrinth no response** is seen, whereas in irritative lesionsan exaggerated response is seen.

ii. The following characteristics of the nystagmus (in addition to those mentioned in Table 3.1), elicited by the caloric test, help to distinguish between a peripheral and central vestibular pathology. Since the central pathways have an inhibitory control on the peripheral vestibular system therefore with central lesions there is loss of inhibition leading to such characteristics, e.g. no latency, no fatigability, no disappearance with visual fixation and prolonged duration of the nystagmus.

Table 3.3		
	Peripheral nystagmus	Central nystagmus
Latency (It is the time taken for the nystagmus to start while testing for it).	2–20 seconds	No latency
Duration	Less than 1 minute	More than 1 minute
Fatigability (It is the inability to elicit nystagmus on repeating the test again and again).	Fatigable	Non-fatigable

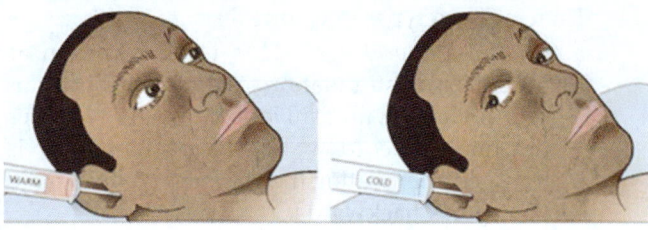

iii. Since the caloric test assesses the vestibulo-ocular reflex arc and the vestibular and ocular nuclei are lying in the brain stem, therefore absent caloric test is a very useful bed side test to look for brain death in comatose patients so that their organs can be used for transplantation.

II. **Cold air caloric text:** In patients with TM perforation where irrigation with water cannot be done, cold air is blown into the ear by passing ethyl chloride through a coiled copper tube known as Dundas Grant tube.

III. **DIX-Hallpike manoeuvre:** This is a manoeuvre to rule out **BPPV** (benign paroxysmal positional vertigo) which is the most common cause of peripheral vertigo.

BPPV is a condition in which dislodged otoconia/debris, moves from the utricle most commonly into the **posterior semicircular canal**.

Movement of these particles in head positions, which make the posterior semicircular canal to come in dependant position, stimulates the cupula of the **posterior semicircular canal** leading to vertigo.

This vertigo disappears when the debris settles down in 10–20 seconds.

These vertigo attacks reappear with change of head position making the posterior SCC dependant again.

To diagnose BPPV the positional test or **Dix Hallpike** manoeuvre is done.

As shown, the patient's head is turned 45 degrees right while sitting on the examination table and then the patient is made to lie supine with his head hanging 30 degrees below the horizontal. The test is repeated with head turned to left.

If while doing this manoeuvre, **vertical upbeat nystagmus with outwards torsion, i.e. upbeating geotropic-torsional nystagmus (upon head tilt towards right or left the torsion will be outwards towards the ground hence the term geotropic),** with the typical features of peripheral pathology as mentioned in Tables 3.1 and 3.3 above,

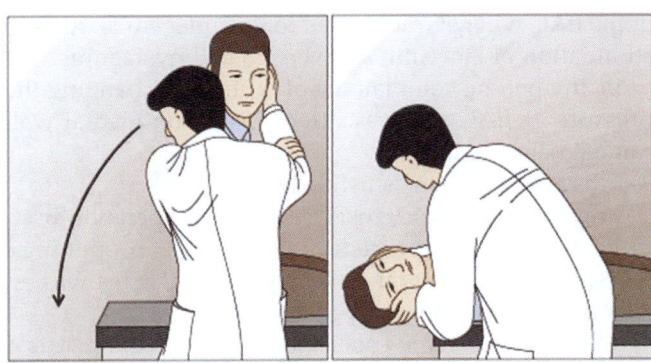

appears then it is reported to be positive, i.e. the patient has BPPV.

TREATMENT OF BPPV

The treatment of BPPV is the canalith repositioning manoeuvre known as **Epley's manoeuvre**.

As shown, in this manoeuvre the patient's head is moved into different positions in a sequence that will move the debris from the semicircular canal back into the utricle. Also see BPPV in Chapter 12 on "Meniere's disease and disorders of vestibular system".

OTHER TESTS TO ASSESS VESTIBULAR FUNCTION
Fistula Test

Whenever pressure changes are done in EAC by pressing and releasing the tragus alternately or by using Siegel's speculum, this pressure change is transmitted to the middle ear through the TM but not to the inner ear.

But whenever there is an abnormal communication (fistula) on the medial wall of middle ear connecting the middle ear to inner ear, e.g. promontory cochlear fistula, erosion of lateral semicircular canal, fistula on the oval window, round window rupture, etc. the change in pressure

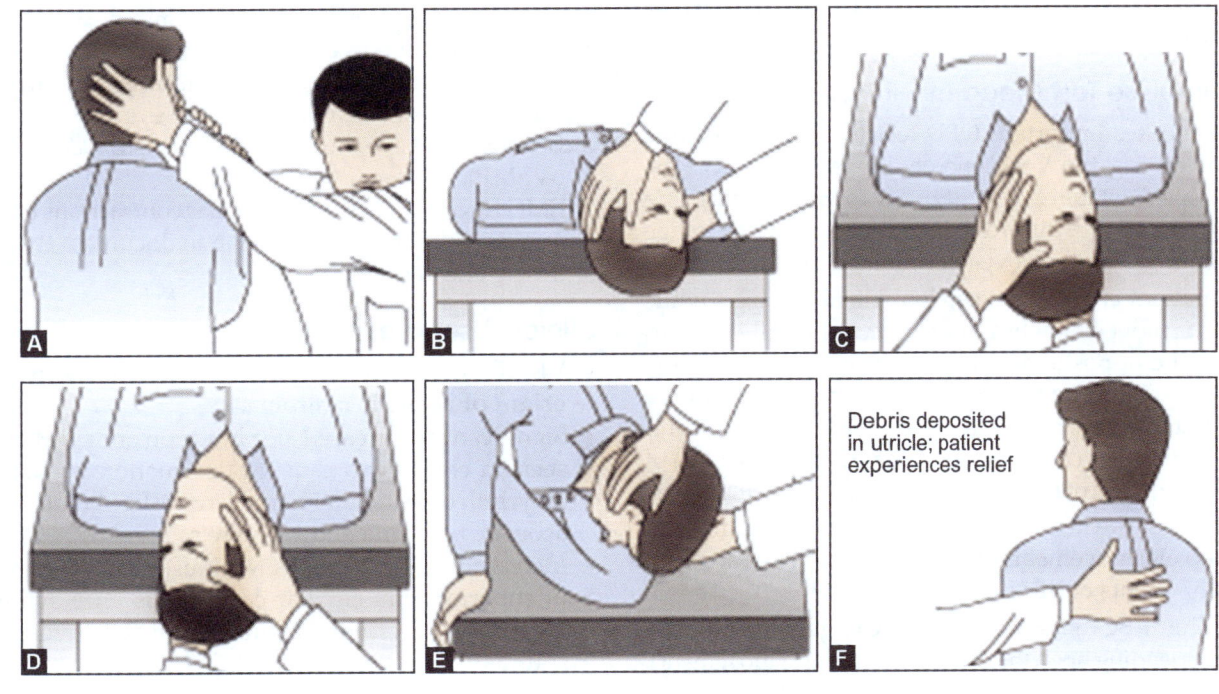

A | B | C

D | E | F

Debris deposited in utricle; patient experiences relief

of the EAC will get transmitted to the inner ear leading to stimulation of labyrinth and vertigo and nystagmus.

In any patient complaining of vertigo on changing the pressure of EAC the presence of fistula on medial wall can be diagnosed.

This test is known as fistula test.

Previously in otosclerosis fenestration operation used to be done. It is a procedure of making an opening/fenestra over the lateral semicircular canal. This was an **iatrogenic cause of positive fistula test**.

Another iatrogenic cause of positive fistula test is a fistula over the oval window that may follow stapedectomy done for otosclerosis.

Hence **fistula test is positive in ears with fistula on the medial wall of middle ear and negative in normal ears**.

False negative fistula test: If the fistula test is negative in spite of a fistula on the medial wall it is known as false negative fistula test. The causes of false negative fistula test are the following:
a. If the fistula on the medial wall is **covered by cholesteatoma** so that pressure is not transmitted to inner ear.
b. **Inner ear is dead** and does not respond to pressure change in spite of presence of fistula.

False positive fistula test/Hennebert's sign: If the fistula test (vertigo on changing the pressure of EAC) is positive in spite of no fistula on the medial wall it is known as false positive fistula test or Hennebert's sign. The causes of false positive fistula test are the following:
a. If the **footplate of stapes is hypermobile** as in congenital syphilis, the footplate moves excessively on pressure changes and even stimulate the utricle and saccule, leading to vertigo and nystagmus.
b. In **25% cases of Meniere's**, fibrous adhesions form between stapes footplate and utricle and saccule. The pressure changes of EAC will now get transmitted to these leading to vertigo and nystagmus (Hennebert's sign).
c. In Superior semicircular canal dehiscence (SSCD), *see* Chapter 12.

Head Impulse Test (Head Thrust Test)

This is another important OPD test (besides the caloric test) for testing the Vestibulo-ocular reflex (VOR). The VOR helps to stabilise our gaze on to an object during head movements in different directions, so that the image keeps falling over the Fovea of retina.

The patient is asked to keep looking at an object while his head is moved briskly and abruptly. Normally the eyes move in the opposite direction at the same speed as the head movement and will appear to remain fixed on the target. In the absence of VOR the eyes will lag behind and there will be jerky catch up movement (called saccades) of the eyes at the end of the head movement to reach the target.

In this test the head is moved briskly 10–15 degrees in steps and eye movements are noted for catch up saccades. The components of this reflex are:
   i. The 6 SCCs (a particular SCC gets stimulated depending upon the direction of the head movement),

   ii. Superior and inferior Vestibular nerve, and
   iii. The medial longitudinal bundle/fasciculus

So a defect at any of the above 3 sites can be picked up by this test. The head impulse/thrust test has an advantage over the caloric test in the sense that it can test each of the 6 SCCs separately, whereas in the caloric test only the 2 lateral (horizontal) canals can be tested.

Galvanic Test

In Galvanic vestibular stimulation test, electric current is delivered transcutaneously to the vestibular afferent nerves through electrodes placed over mastoid bones.

Here the **nerve endings** in all the semicircular canals, on one side, are **stimulated directly** by the current and not through the receptors, i.e. cupula.

Therefore in patients in whom the caloric test, which tests the peripheral receptors, is negative, a response on galvanic stimulation indicates normally functioning vestibular nerves.

Vestibular Evoked Myogenic Potential (VEMP)

It is a test of the otolithic organs (utricle & saccule) and vestibulo-spinalpathway. This is in contrast to the caloric and head impulse test which involve SCCs and vestibulo-ocular pathways.

VEMPs are electromyographic (EMG) responses evoked by loud sounds.

Loud sounds cause strong movements of the oval window. Because of the close proximity of the oval window to the utricle and saccule, this strong movement stimulates the saccule and utricle also. From the **saccule** the impulses are then carried by the **inferior vestibular nerve** to the vestibular nucleus and then through the vestibulo-spinal tract to the sternocleidomastoid muscle. This reflex to stabilise the head on the shoulders by contraction of neck muscles whenever there is vestibular stimulation is known as vestibulo-collic reflex. The EMG recording of the sternocleidomastoid muscle with the help of surface electrode is called cervical VEMP or cVEMP.

Similarly from the utricle the impulses are carried by the superior vestibular nerve to the eye muscles (EMG recording in the eye muscles will be called Ocular VEMP or oVEMP).

EMG recording of these muscular contractions (cVEMP and oVEMP) enables the clinician to document the status of utricle and saccule.

Clinical Usefulness of VEMP

- VEMP is an important test to find out the **nerve of origin of acoustic neuroma**.
- Significantly decreased amplitude on one side has been seen in conditions causing destruction of vesibular labyrinth or vestibular nerve like vestibular neuronitis, acoustic neuroma and Meniere's.
- Increased amplitude of VEMP is useful in the diagnosis of superior semi-circular canal dehiscence syndrome where the labyrinth becomes more sensitive to loud sounds.

PREVIOUSLY ASKED QUESTIONS

1. **True about central nystagmus:**
   (Kerala 2001, Exam 2017)
   a. Duration not limited
   b. Direction fixed
   c. Latency present
   d. Suppressed by visual fixation

2. **Peripheral nystagmus true is:** *(Exam 2013)*
   a. Duration not limited
   b. Direction fixed
   c. No latency
   d. Vertigo not present

3. **Nystagmus is associated with all except:**
   (AP 2003, Exam 2017)
   a. Cerebellar disease
   b. Vestibular disease
   c. Cochlear disease
   d. Arnold-Chiari malformation

4. **Spontaneous pure vertical nystagmus is seen in the lesion of:** *(Kolkata 2005, Exam 2017)*
   a. Medulla   b. Labyrinth
   c. Middle ear   d. Cochlea

5. **Destruction of right labyrinth causes nystagmus to:**
   (DPG 2009)
   a. Right side
   b. Left side
   c. Pendular nystagmus
   d. No nystagmus

6. **Stimulation of posterior semicircular canal produces:**
   (Exam 2013)
   a. Horizontal nystagmus
   b. Pure vertical nystagmus
   c. Pendular nystagmus
   d. Torsional vertical nystagmus

7. **Vertigo of peripheral vestibular origin are all except:**
   (Exam 2013)
   a. Meniere's disease
   b. BPPV
   c. Vertebrobasilar insufficiency
   d. Vestibular neuronitis

8. **Vestibular function is tested by:**
   (PGI 2002, 2013)
   a. Acoustic reflex
   b. Fistula test
   c. Impedance audiometry
   d. Cold caloric test
   e. Gelle's test

9. **Vestibular function is tested by:**
   (PGI Dec 2002, 2014)
   a. Galvanic stimulation test
   b. Acoustic reflex
   c. Fistula test
   d. Impedance audiometry
   e. Cold caloric test

10. **Cold caloric test stimulates:** *(AP 2008)*
    a. Cochlea
    b. Lateral semicircular canal
    c. Posterior semicircular canal
    d. All of the above

11. **At what angle is Hallpike thermal caloric test done:**
    (AP 2006, Exam 2016)
    a. 15°   b. 30°
    c. 45°   d. 60°

12. **Fitzgerald's caloric test uses temperature at:**
    (JIPMER 92, Exam 2016)
    a. 30° and 44°   b. 34° and 41°
    c. 33° and 21°   d. 37° and 41°

13. **Caloric test has:** *(Delhi 96, Exam 2016)*
    a. Slow component only
    b. Fast component only
    c. Both slow and fast components
    d. Mainly slow component and fast component occasionally

14. **In cold caloric stimulation test, the cold water induces movement of the eyeball in the following direction:** *(AI 99, Exam 2013, Exam 2018)*
    a. Towards the opposite side
    b. Towards the same side
    c. Upwards
    d. None of the above

15. **In Fitzgerald and Hallpike differential caloric test, cold water irrigation at 30° centigrade in the left ear in a normal person will produce:** *(DPG 2008)*
    a. Nystagmus to the right side
    b. Nystagmus to the left side
    c. Direction changing nystagmus
    d. Positional nystagmus

16. **Which of the following is not true of caloric test?**
    (MH 2005, Exam 2016)
    a. Induction of nystagmus by thermal stimulation
    b. Normally cold water induces nystagmus to opposite side and warm water to same side
    c. In canal paresis there is no nystagmus
    d. None

17. **If cold water caloric test is done in both the meatus simultaneously the nystagmus will be:**
    (Exam 2012)
    a. Vertical upbeat with slow component downwards
    b. Vertical downbeat with slow component upwards
    c. Horizontal to right
    d. No nystagmus

Ear

Section I

18. **Dunda's grant apparatus used in:**
                              (*DPG 2003, Exam 2017*)
    a. Cold air caloric test
    b. Fitzgerald Hallpike's test
    c. Bithermal caloric test
    d. Rinne test

19. **Fistula test following fenestration operation stimulates:** (*AI 2003, Exam 2017*)
    a. Lateral semicircular canal
    b. Posterior semicircular canal
    c. Anterior semicircular canal
    d. Cochlea

20. **False positive fistula test is associated with:**
                              (*TN 2005, Exam 2017*)
    a. Perilymph fistula
    b. Malignant sclerosis
    c. Hypermobile foot plate of stapes
    d. Cholesteatoma

21. **Hennebert's sign is a false positive fistula test when there is no evidence of middle ear disease causing fistula, it is seen in:** (*Exam 2011, Exam 2016*)
    a. Congenital syphilis   b. Stapedectomy
    c. Fenestration surgery   d. Cholesteatoma

22. **A positive fistula test during Siegelization indicates:**
                              (*AIIMS 95, Exam 2017*)
    a. Ossicular discontinuity
    b. Erosion of lateral semicircular canal
    c. CSF leak through the ear
    d. Fixation of stapes bone

23. **On otological examination all of the following will have positive fistula test except:**
                              (*AI 2002, Exam 2017*)
    a. Dead ear
    b. Labyrinthine fistula
    c. Hypermobile stapes footplate
    d. Following fenestration surgery

24. **Positional vertigo is due to stimulation of:**
                              (*UP 2001, Exam 2016*)
    a. Lateral semicircular canal
    b. Superior semicircular canal
    c. Inferior semicircular canal
    d. Posterior semicircular canal

25. **DIX-Hallpike manoeuvre is done for assessing:**
                              (*Exam 2002*)
    a. Vestibular function b. Corneal test
    c. Cochlear function   d. Audiometry

26. **What is the treatment for benign positional vertigo:**
                              (*APPG 2006, Exam 2018*)
    a. Vestibular exercises
    b. Vestibular sedatives
    c. Antihistamines
    d. Canalith repositioning procedure

27. **Latest treatment in BPPV is:**
                              (*Kerala 2003, Exam 2018*)
    a. Intralabyrinthine streptomycin
    b. Intralabyrinthine steroids
    c. Valsalva manoeuvre
    d. Epley's manoeuvre

28. **Epley's manoeuvre:**   (*Exam 2013*)
    a. Positional vertigo   b. Otosclerosis
    c. ASOM   d. CSOM

29. **Vestibular Evoked Myogenic Potential (VEMP) in sternocleidomastoid muscle detects lesion of:**
                              (*AIIMS 2012*)
    a. Cochlear nerve
    b. Superior vestibular nerve
    c. Inferior vestibular nerve
    d. Inflammatory myopathy

30. **True about Hennebert's Sign is:**   (*Exam 2016*)
    a. Fistula test positive without fistula
    b. Fistula test positive with fistula
    c. Fistula test negative without fistula
    d. Fistula test negative with fistula

31. **In cold caloric stimulation test, the cold water induces movement of the eyeball in the following direction:**   (*Exam 2016*)
    a. Towards the opposite side
    b. Towards the same side
    c. Upwards
    d. Downwards

32. **Dix Hallpike manoeuvre is used to:**   (*Exam 2016*)
    a. Diagnose benign paroxysmal positional vertigo
    b. Differentiate cochlear and retrocochlear deafness
    c. Assess neonatal hearing loss
    d. Assess patency of Eustachian tube

33. **A person has vertigo without central involvement. Causes can be all except:**   (*Exam 2016*)
    a. Perilymph fistula   b. Vestibular neuritis
    c. Meniere's disease   d. Multiple sclerosis

34. **The given manoeuvre is used to:**
                              (*Practice question by Author*)

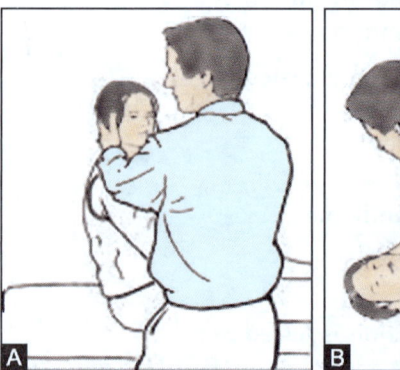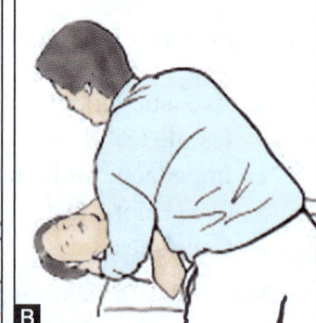

    a. Assess vestibular function
    b. Differentiate cochlear and retrocochlear deafness

c. Assess cerebellar function

d. Find out Lateral semicircular canal fistula

35. Destruction of one semicircular canal leads to:
(Exam 2016)

a. Ataxia and dysarthria

b. Spinning of world around sensation

c. Cranial nerve VI deficit

d. None of the above

36. What is being done in the following image:
(APPG 2015)

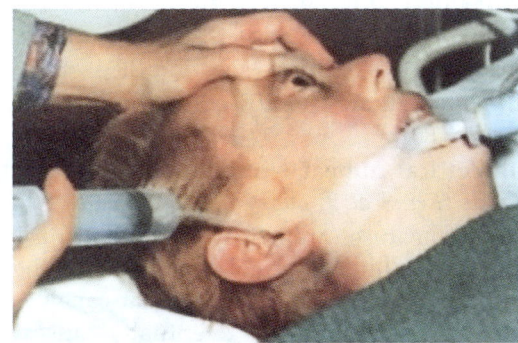

a. Syringing of the ear in a patient with CSOM and meningitis

b. Testing vestibulo-ocular reflex by injecting cold water

c. Politzerization (ventilation of the middle ear in children who cannot perform Valsalva maneuvre)

d. Determining Eustachian tube patency

37. Not true about benign paroxysmal positional vertigo:
(Exam 2016)

a. Hearing loss is often present

b. Hallpike manoeuvre is helpful in diagnosis

c. Epley's manoeuvre is used for treatment

d. Disorder of posterior semicircular canal

IMAGE BASED PRACTICE QUESTIONS BY THE AUTHOR

38. The following procedure is done for the management of:
(Exam 2016, 2019)

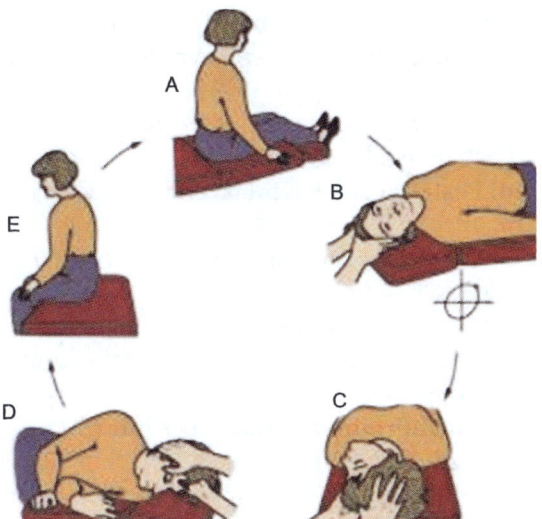

a. Meniere's disease

b. Perilymph fistula

c. BPPV

d. Superior semicircular canal dehiscence

39. Which of the following is not true of the following test:
(MH 2005, Exam 2017)

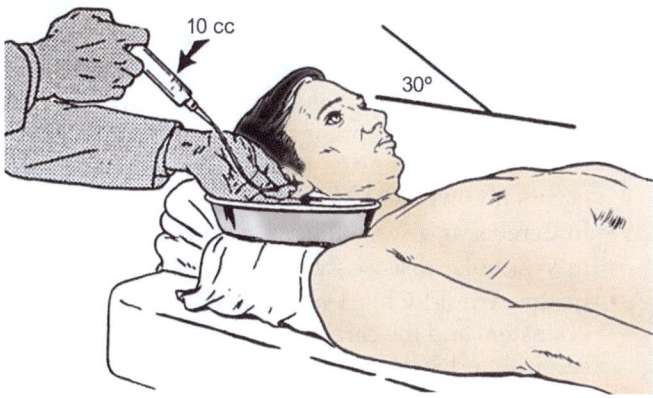

a. Induction of nystagmus by thermal stimulation

b. Normally cold water induces nystagmus to opposite side and warm water to same side

c. In canal paresis there is no nystagmus

d. Stimulates posterior semicircular canal

40. Positive head impulse test is suggestive of:
(Exam 2016)

a. Injury to SCC and vestibulo-cerebellar tract

b. Injury to SCC and vestibulo-spinal tract

c. Injury to SCC and vestibulo-ocular tract

d. Injury to organ of corti and auditory pathways

41. When a patient was administered cold water in the right ear the nystagmus was seen towards the left. Which of the following is the correct interpretation of the test:
(Exam 2018)

a. Fast component is to left

b. Slow component is to left

c. Disease is towards the left

d. Direction of the nystagmus is to the right

Ear

Section I

ANSWERS AND EXPLANATIONS

1. **(a) Duration not limited** (*Ref. Cummings, 6th ed., page 2567; 2551*)
2. **(b) Direction fixed** (*Ref. Anirban Biswas, 5th ed., Vol 2; page 98*)
3. **(c) Cochlear disease** (*Ref. Cummings, 6th ed., page 2531*)
   - Nystagmus and vertigo per se are not the manifestations of cochlear diseases. Cochlear diseases lead to hearing loss. However as mentioned in Table 3.1 in the text in vestibular pathologies additionally there may be tinnitus and deafness when there occurs involvement of cochlea.
   - In Cerebellar disease the nystagmus is pendular.
   - In Vestibular disease the nystagmus is jerky.
   - In the Arnold-Chiari malformation a part of the brainstem and the cerebellum are herniated into the cervical vertebral canal. The Arnold-Chiari malformation is typically associated with vertical downbeat nystagmus.
4. **(a) Medulla** (*Ref. Cummings, 6th ed., page 2531*)
5. **(b) Left side** (*Ref. Anirban Biswas, 5th ed., Vol 2; 287*)
6. **(d) Torsional vertical nystagmus** (*Ref. Cummings, 6th ed., page 2531; Scott Brown, 8th ed., Vol 2; page 833*)
7. **(c) Vertebrobasilar insufficiency** (*Ref. Cummings, 6th ed., page 2531*)
   - Vertebrobasilar insufficiency is a central vestibular condition.
   - The two vertebral arteries on each side are branches of the subclavian arteries. They enter the skull through the foramen magnum and join at the pontomedullary junction to form the basilar artery which divides into two posterior cerebral arteries at the upper pons.
   - The vertebrobasilar arterial system perfuses the medulla, cerebellum, pons, midbrain, thalamus, and occipital cortex.
   - Therefore vertebrobasilar insufficiency leads to involvement of the central vestibular system.
8. **(b) and (d) Fistula test, Cold caloric test** (*Ref. Scott Brown, 8th ed., Vol 2; page 795*)
   - Acoustic reflex is a part of impedance audiometry which is a test of hearing.
9. **(a), (c), (e) Galvanic stimulation test, Fistula test, Cold caloric test** (*Ref. Scott Brown, 8th ed., Vol 2; page 795*)
   - Acoustic reflex and Impedance audiometry are tests of hearing.
10. **(b) Lateral semicircular canal** (*Ref. Cummings, 6th ed., page 2537*)
11. **(b) 30°** (*Ref. Cummings, 6th ed., page 2537*)
12. **(a) 30° and 44°** (*Ref. Cummings, 6th ed., page 2538*)
13. **(c) Both slow and fast components** (*Ref. Cummings, 6th ed., page 2510*)
14. **(a) Towards the opposite side** (*Ref. Cummings, 6th ed., page 2510*)

- In bi-thermal caloric test the normal response is *C O W S*, i.e. with Cold water nystagmus is towards the Opposite side and with Warm water it is towards the Same side.
- If both meatus are irrigated simultaneously with cold water the normal response is an up-beating nystagmus with torsion.

15. **(a) Nystagmus to the right side** (*Ref. Scott Brown, 8th ed., Vol 2; page 796*)
   - If the same is done with warm water the nystagmus will be towards the same side, i.e. left side.
   - Direction changing nystagmus is seen in central lesions.
   - Positional nystagmus is seen in BPPV.
16. **(d) None (all are true)** (*Ref. Scott Brown, 8th ed., Vol 2; page 796*)
17. **(a) Vertical upbeat with slow component downwards** (*Ref. Scott Brown, 6th ed., Vol 2; page 2/21/20*)
   - If both meatuses are irrigated simultaneously with cold water, under normal circumstances the effect within both horizontal semicircular canals is equal and self cancelling; this eventually causes an up beating vertical nystagmus.
   - Vertical upbeat means the fast component is upwards, hence the slow component will be downwards.
18. **(a) Cold air caloric test** (*Ref. Dhingra, 6th ed., page page 43*)
19. **(a) Lateral semicircular canal** (*Ref. Shambaugh, 6th ed., page 466*)
20. **(c) Hypermobile footplate of stapes** (*Ref. Cummings, 6th ed., page 2562*)
21. **(a) Congenital syphilis** (*Ref. Cummings, 6th ed., page 2562*)
22. **(b) Erosion of lateral semicircular canal** (*Ref. Shambaugh, 6th ed., page 181*)
23. **(a) Dead ear** (*Ref. Shambaugh, 6th ed., page 181*)
   - If there is a fistula on the medial wall but inner ear is dead (not responding to pressure changes), then in spite of presence of fistula, fistula test will be negative. This is false negative fistula test.
   - If the footplate of stapes is hypermobile, it results in false positive fistula test.
   - Fenestration operation is an iatrogenic cause of positive fistula test.
24. **(d) Posterior semicircular canal** (*Ref. Cummings, 6th ed., page 2550*)
25. **(a) Vestibular function** (*Ref. Cummings, 6th ed., page 2551*)
   - DIX-Hallpike manoeuvre is a manoeuvre to rule out BPPV (benign paroxysmal positional vertigo) in any patient presenting with vertigo.
26. **(d) Canalith repositioning procedure** (*Ref. Cummings, 6th ed., page 2552*)
   - Canalith repositioning procedure or the Epley's manoeuvre is the treatment for benign positional

Section I **Ear**

vertigo. In this manoeuvre the patient's head is moved into different positions in a sequence that will move the debris from the posterior semicircular canal back into the utricle.

- When the **vestibular organs are damaged** with disease or injury, the brain can no longer rely on them for accurate information about equilibrium and motion.

  Vestibular exercises promote CNS compensation for these permanent or **fixed** deficits.

- In Benign positional vertigo vestibular exercises are not required, as the cause of BPPV gets treated by Canalith repositioning procedure or the Epley's manoeuvre.

- Vestibular sedatives and antihistamines may be used to control the severe symptoms, though they are not of much benefit and repositioning or Epley's manoeuvre is the treatment of choice in BPPV.

27. **(d) Epley's manoeuvre or the repositioning mano-euvre** (*Ref. Cummings, 6th ed., page 2552*)

28. **(a) Positional vertigo** (*Ref. Cummings, 6th ed., page 2552*)

29. **(c) Inferior Vestibular Nerve** (*Ref. Scott Brown, 8th ed., Vol 2; page 829*)

30. **(a) Fistula test positive without fistula** (*Ref. Shambaugh, 6th ed., page 181*)

31. **(a) Towards the opposite side** (*Ref. Scott Brown, 8th ed., Vol 2; page 796*)

32. **(a) Diagnose benign paroxysmal positional vertigo** (*Ref. Scott Brown, 8th ed., Vol 2; page 833*)

33. **(d) Multiple sclerosis** (*Ref. Scott Brown, 8th ed., Vol 2; page 833*)

34. **(a) Assess vestibular function** (*Ref. Scott Brown, 8th ed., Vol 2; page 800*)

35. **(b) Spinning of world around sensation** (*Ref. Scott Brown, 8th ed., Vol 2; page 774*)

- Cerebellar pathologies present with ataxia and dysarthria

- Central causes of vertigo lead to deficits of cranial nerves III to XII which are closely associated with the brainstem.

36. **(b) Testing vestibulo-ocular reflex by injecting cold water** (*Ref. Scott Brown, 8th ed., Vol 2; page 795*)

- Vestibulo-ocular reflex or caloric test is a test to evaluate the vestibular system and hence the brainstem functioning. One of the utility of this test is to confirm brain death.

- Syringing is never done in a patient of CSOM.

- Politzerisation is for endotracheal tube function.

37. **(a) Hearing loss is often present** (*Ref. Cummings, 6th ed., page 2551*)

38. **(c) BPPV** (*Ref. Scott Brown, 8th ed., Vol 2; page 835*)

39. **(d) Stimulates Posterior Semicircular Canal** (*Ref. Scott Brown, 8th ed., Vol 2; page 796*)

- It stimulates horizontal/lateral semicircular canal

40. **(c) Injury to SCC and Vestibulo-ocular tract** (*Ref. Anirban Biswas, 5th ed., Vol 2; page 446*)

41. **(a) Fast component is to left** (*Ref. Cummings, 6th ed., page 2510*)

Diseases of External Ear

DISEASE OF PINNA

Hematoma

MC cause of hematoma of the pinna is blunt trauma. When this extravasated blood clots and gets organised, the swelling takes the contour of the pinna appearing like a cauliflower, hence known as **cauliflower ear**. Since it is commonly seen in boxers and wrestlers it is also called **Boxer's ear** or **wrestler's ear**.

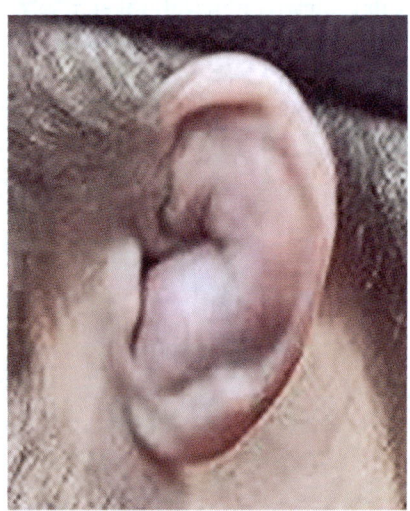

Management

Aspiration followed by pressure dressing according to the contour of pinna. If the aspiration fails, then incision and drainage (I and D) is done followed by contour dressing and prophylactic antibiotics.

Perichondritis

- It is an infection of the perichondrium of the pinna cartilage.
- MC cause of perichondritis of the pinna is trauma either iatrogenic (surgical incisions, ear piercing) or non-iatrogenic (lacerations, hematoma).
- MC organism causing perichondritis is *Pseudomonas aeruginosa*.
- The pinna appears red, hot, painful and stiff.

- Management: Antipseudomonal antibiotics, if abscess has formed then (I and D).

DISEASES OF EXTERNAL AUDITORY CANAL (EAC)/ OTITIS EXTERNA

Infections of the EAC (external auditory canal) are known as Otitis externa. These can be bacterial, fungal or viral. 90% of the cases of otitis externa are bacterial. Pseudomonas is overall the MC bacteria involved followed by Staph. The various Otitis externa are:

Bacterial Otitis Externa

Furuncle

Staphylococcal infection of the hair follicle is known as furuncle.

Hence a furuncle of EAC is localised to the outer 8 mm, i.e. the cartilaginous part, *see* chapter on anatomy.

Clinical Features

The patient presents with severe pain which increases on movements of pinna and jaw (while speaking or chewing).

The pinna is pushed outwards and forwards.

The retro-auricular groove is obliterated if the furuncle is on the posterior meatal wall. This is because the retro-auricular groove is formed by the cartilaginous part of EAC and a furuncle on its posterior wall causing oedema leads to obliteration of the retro-auricular groove.

On examination of the EAC there is edema and we might be able to see the furuncle or if it has ruptured then a frankly purulent (without mucus) discharge. Mucopurulent discharge comes only from the middle ear because EAC is lined by stratified squamous epithelium which has no mucus glands.

On pressing the tragus patient complains of pain. This is known as **tragal sign**.

Treatment

Treatment is by antistaphylococcal antibiotics. A 10% ichthammol glycerine pack can be put in the EAC to reduce oedema (due to hygroscopic action of glycerine) and pain.

I and D will be required if abscess has formed. Any patient with recurrent furunculosis should be investigated for diabetes mellitus.

Diffuse Otitis Externa

This is also known as **Tropical ear/telephonist ear/ swimmer's ear** as it is seen most commonly in tropical area, i.e. in hot and humid climate.

Excessive sweating or water of the swimming pool leads to a change in the acidic medium (pH 4–5) of meatal skin to alkaline, favouring growth of pathogens and subsequently with any scratching of EAC, there occurs abrasion followed by bacterial invasion.

The most common organism causing diffuse otitis externa is *Pseudomonas aeruginosa*. Other important organism is *Staph. aureus*.

Presentation

The patient here is immunocompetent (*see* below the malignant Otitis externa due to Pseudomonas in immunocompromised patients) and presents with pain(increase on manipulation of pinna), burning sensation, discharge and fullness. O/E there is erythema and oedema along the whole length of EAC.

Management

It is managed by antibiotics, ear toileting and by putting a medicated pack in the EAC.

Malignant Otitis Externa/Necrotising Otitis Externa

This is not a malignancy but an infective and locally invasive condition of the EAC caused by *Pseudomonas aeruginosa*. The term malignant signifies that it is a very aggressive and life threatening condition. It is seen in immunocompromised patients (diabetics, HIV positive and patients on steroids or immunosuppressive drugs). Most commonly these are elderly.

Presentation

The infection begins as an external otitis that spreads to the skull base through fissures of Santorini or bony cartilaginous junction of EAC, tympanomastoid and petrotympanic fissures. It then progresses into an osteomyelitis of the temporal bone. Malignant otitis externa is therefore also called **skull base osteomyelitis**.

Patient presents with severe excruciating pain in the ear, ear discharge and conductive hearing loss.

EAC shows oedema, erythema, granulations and discharge. The skin, subcutaneous tissue, and cartilage all get necrosed. Because of extensive necrosis it is confused with malignancy.

The patient can have nerve paralysis. The facial nerve **(VII)** is affected **most commonly**, usually at the stylomastoid foramen. As the disease progresses, cranial nerves IX, X, and XI can be affected at the jugular foramen, followed by XII in the hypoglossal canal. Cranial nerves V and VI can be affected if the disease extends to the petrous apex.

Diagnosis

- Microbial culture of the ear secretions.
- Due to extensive necrosis a biopsy of the external auditory canal is often required to be done to exclude carcinoma.
- For early **diagnosis Tc^{99}** scan is used. Tc^{99} is taken up by the osteoclasts and osteoblasts and therefore the scan picks up bony erosion even before structural changes appear on CT scan. However, Tc^{99} scan is not useful to document resolution of infection as bone remodelling (with the help of combined activity of osteoclasts and osteoblasts) continues even after the infection is over. For **resolution** of infection **Gallium citrate (Ga) 67 scan** and Indium (In) 111–labeled leukocyte scan is used as it is taken up by inflammatory cells.
- MRI and CT scanning are useful in detecting the extent of the disease, CT scan is sensitive for looking bone erosion but MRI is more sensitive for detecting intracranial complications.

Treatment

It is managed by antipseudomonal antibiotics (e.g. Ciprofloxacin, Ceftazidime, Piperacillin, Ticarcillin, Meropenem, aminoglycosides, etc.) for 3–6 weeks.

This being an invasive condition, the Erythrocyte sedimentation rate (ESR) is greatly increased at presentation. Although ESR is non-specific, but it being an affordable and easily available investigation, is used to follow treatment response and recurrence. In this regard evaluation of treatment response with a Gallium citrate (Ga) 67 scan is more accurate.

Debridement of necrotic material is done.

Fungal Otitis Externa

Fungal otitis externa is also known as "Otomycosis".

Otomycosis

It is seen in hot & humid climate. MC organism causing otomycosis is **Aspergillus (MC–niger),** followed by **candida**. Aspergillus infections have the appearance of

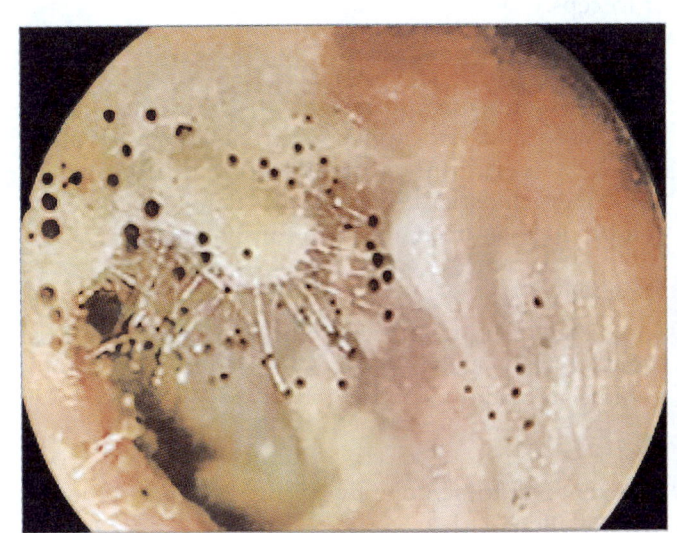

moist white plugs dotted with black debris (wet newspaper appearance) as shown below. Candida infections appear like a cotton like debris.

Patients present with itching, pain and ear blockade/discharge.

Management is by ear toileting and antifungal ear drops.

Otitis Externa Haemorrhagica/Bullous Myringitis/ Myringitis Bullosa

This is caused most commonly by bacteria (MC *Strept. pneumoniae*). Other important causes are Influenza virus and *Mycoplasma pneumoniae*.

It presents with otalgia and ear discharge. Here hemorrhagic bullae are formed on the TM and deep meatus (hence the name).

Management is by systemic antibiotics and antibiotic ear drops.

Viral Otitis externa

Herpes Zoster Oticus

Infection by herpes zoster virus is characterised by vesicles on TM, EAC skin, pinna and even skin around the pinna over the dermatome of the nerve involved (*see* nerve supply of external ear in the chapter on anatomy).

Herpes zoster oticus with facial palsy is known as **Ramsay Hunt syndrome**. Herpes zoster reactivation in the geniculate ganglion leads to Ramsay Hunt syndrome, *see* Chapter 11 on facial nerve.

Aural Myiasis

It is the infestation of the ear with the larvae (maggots) of flies.

It is seen commonly in tropical areas, in people with discharging ears with poor hygiene. The foul smelling discharge coming from the ear attracts flies which lay eggs. The eggs then hatch into larvae called maggots.

The patient presents with pain in the ear, bleeding and itching. There can be perforation of the TM.

It is managed by killing the maggots by chloroform water followed by removal of the maggots by syringing or forceps.

Wax

Wax is usually a mixture of secretions of ceruminous and sebaceous glands and desquamated epidermal cells of the EAC. The ceruminous glands are modified sweat (apocrine) glands, located in the cartilaginous part of EAC and produce cerumen, the main constituent of wax.

Presentation

The patient can present with blocked ear, hearing loss, earache, itching in the ear, reflex cough (via vagus nerve), tinnitus and giddiness.

Management

Wax removal to be done by syringing or instrumental manipulation.

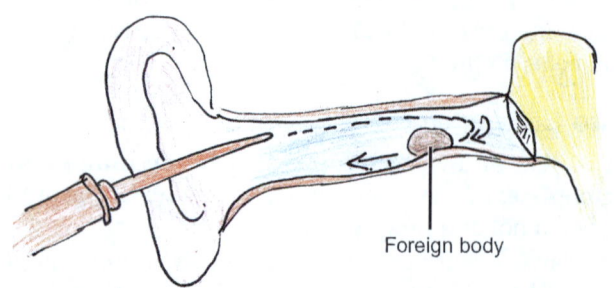

Fig. 4.1: Jet of water pushing the wax/foreign body out in syringing

Foreign Bodies (FB) in the External Auditory Canal (EAC)

Foreign bodies in the EAC are seen most commonly in children and may be organic (e.g. beans, live insects, etc.) or inorganic (e.g. cotton, paper, beads, button batteries, etc.).

Clinical Features

- Asymptomatic
- Pain
- Otitis externa

Management

The method of removal of FB depends on the nature of the foreign body.

- Inorganic round non graspable FB (e.g. beads, pellets, erasers) should be removed by syringing.
- Graspable non-living objects (e.g. cotton. Paper, dead insects) should be removed with a pair of crocodile forceps.
- Living insects should be first killed by putting oil into the meatus and then removal by syringing or forceps.
- Organic objects (e.g. beans) which absorb water and swell, should not be syringed. They should be removed with ear hook.
- Button batteries should not be syringed as they may leak on exposure of water.
- Firmly impacted FB medial to isthmus of EAC are removed surgically or by instrumentation.

Syringing: After pulling the pinna upward and backwards, water at body temperature is delivered through a syringe along the posterosuperior wall of EAC. The pressure of water builds up in the meatal recess and pushes the wax out.

Complications of syringing:

a. Vertigo (if water is too hot or too cold, i.e. not at body temperature, due to caloric stimulation)
b. Rupture of TM (if done too forcefully)
c. Reactivation of quiescent otitis media (if perforation is already present)

Contraindications of syringing:

- Acute inflammatory conditions of the external or middle ear.

- Perforation of the tympanic membrane
- Presence of a grommet
- History of ear surgery

Keratosis Obturans

Normally the epithelium from the surface of TM migrates into posterior meatal wall and gets extruded. Faulty epithelial migration pattern or obstruction of this migration can lead to collection of a dense plug of pearly white mass of desquamated epithelial cells (keratin) in the EAC. It is usually seen in people where the underlying epithelium is hyperplastic with an increased rate of desquamation and loss of normal migration.

Presentation

It is usually seen in young and can be B/L. The keratin plug can completely occlude the auditory canal (in a laminar onion skin arrangement) leading to conductive hearing loss. Ongoing keratin plug accumulation can cause widening of the EAC (this occurs due to build of pressure and not due to bony erosion) and thereby even facial nerve palsy. Frequently, these patients present with severe pain resulting from an aggressive secondary otitis externa.

Keratosis obturans should be differentiated from primary auditory canal cholesteatoma, *see* below.

It is managed by local debridement of the keratin plug.

Primary Cholesteatoma of the EAC

Primary auditory canal cholesteatoma is characterized by invasion of squamous tissue from the external auditory canal into a localized area of bone erosion.

Injury to the EAC following any infection or trauma can lead to the stratified squamous epithelium of the EAC invade inside the defect and get sequestered. This sequestered stratified squamous epithelium ultimately leads to formation of cholesteatoma. This was previously considered as a part of keratosis obturans but is now considered a separate clinical entity.

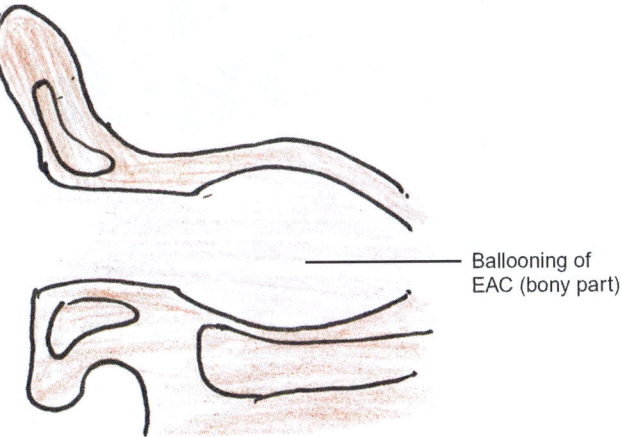

Fig. 4.2: Keratosis Obturans leading to dilatation of EAC

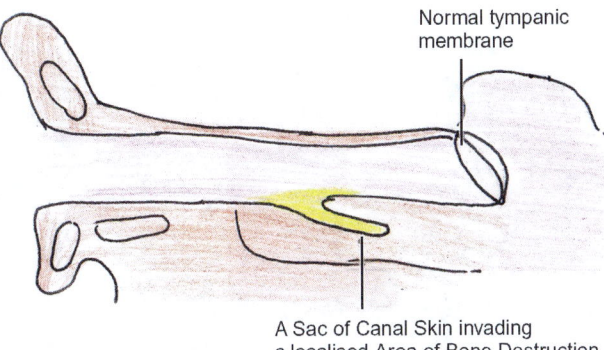

Fig. 4.3: Primary Cholesteatoma of EAC

Presentation

Patient presents with dull aching pain and foul smelling ear discharge (due to bone erosion) which appears to come from localised area of the external auditory canal with the rest of external auditory canal and tympanic membrane appearing normal. The hearing remains normal.

This should be differentiated from carcinoma and malignant Otitis externa by a detailed examination under the microscope of the EAC along with the biopsy.

Treatment is removal of the cholesteatoma and the necrotic bone and closure of the bony defect.

DISEASES OF TM

Traumatic Rupture

A traumatic perforation of the TM heals by itself in 6–12 weeks. If the edges of perforation are inverted towards the middle ear they have to be everted out.

A perforation of the TM heals only by two layers, the outer epithelial and the inner endothelial layer (the fibrous layer remains missing here).

Retraction of TM

Any condition leading to obstruction of Eustachian tube will lead to retraction of TM. The signs of a retracted TM are:

1. Loss of cone of light or distortion of cone of light leading to a dull, lustreless TM
2. Foreshortened handle of malleus resulting in non-prominent Umbo
3. Prominent lateral process of malleus
4. Sickling of anterior and posterior malleolar folds

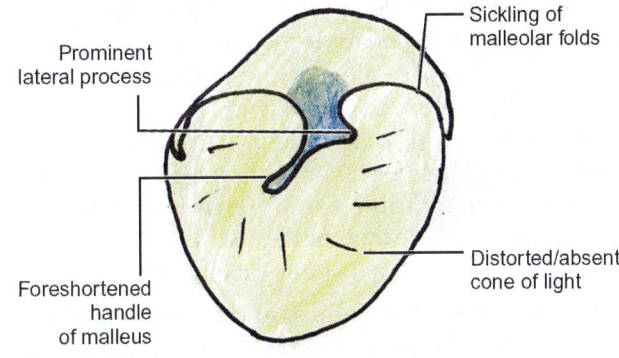

Fig. 4.4: Retracted tympanic membrane

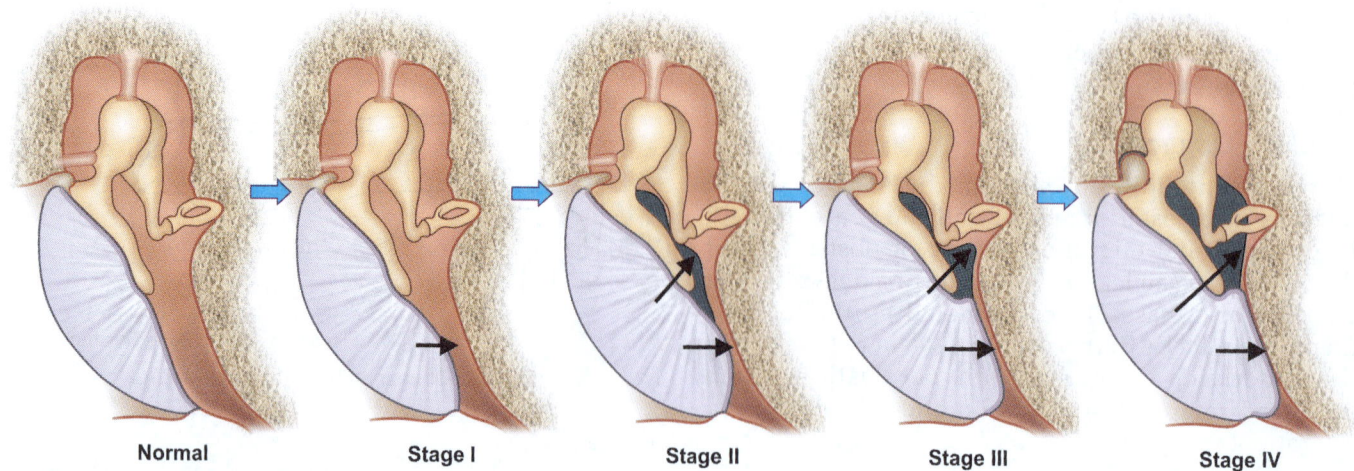

| Normal | Stage I | Stage II | Stage III | Stage IV |

Fig. 4.5: Blue arrows showing stages of retraction of pars flacida, Black arrows showing stages of retraction of pars tensa

There are four stages of tympanic membrane (Pars tensa part) retraction as described by **Sade:**

 i. *Stage 1:* TM is retracted but not in contact with incus

 ii. *Stage 2:* Retracted TM is in contact with incus

 iii. *Stage 3:* TM lies on the promontory. The middle ear space is obliterated but middle ear mucosa is intact. This is known as middle ear **atelectasis**.

 iv. *Stage 4:* TM is adherent to the promontory with no middle ear space remaining. This is known as **adhesive otitis media**.

Pars flaccida retractions have been classified by Tos as follows:

 i. *Stage 1:* Pars flaccida is retracted but not adherent to malleus

 ii. *Stage 2:* The Retraction is adherent to malleus and full extent of retraction may be seen.

 iii. *Stage 3:* Part of retraction is out of view and there may be partial erosion of the outer attic wall (scutum)

 iv. *Stage 4:* There is definite erosion of the scutum with full extent of retraction not seen.

TYMPANOSCLEROSIS

Tympanosclerosis is a condition in which hyaline and calcified deposits accumulate within the fibrous layer of the tympanic membrane and the submucosa of middle ear. Isolated involvement of tympanic membrane may occur and is known as myringosclerosis.

Factors which could result in the formation of tympanosclerosis are the following:

- Long term serous otitis media (glue ear) and CSOM: Chronic irritation or inflammation leads to connective tissue degeneration resulting in hyalinisation & dystrophic calcification of the TM.
- Insertion of a tympanostomy tube (grommet).

Tympanosclerotic plaques appear as chalky white plaque within the tympanic membrane and submucosa of middle ear.

In most patients, these plaques are clinically insignificant and cause a little or no hearing impairment.

Tympanosclerosis extending into the middle ear and leading to ossicular fixation can lead to conductive hearing loss.

EXAMINATION OF THE EAR

Examination of the ear, nose or throat in the ENT OPD is done with the head mirror attached to a head band. The head mirror reflects light from a light source known as the Bull's eye lamp (*see* Chapter on instruments in the end) to the part being examined. This head mirror is a concave mirror with a hole in the centre which allows binocular vision.

The **diameter of the head mirror** is 3.5 inch/9 cm /90 mm and the **diameter of the central hole** is 2 cm/ 20 mm. The **focal length** is approximately 25 cm/250 mm.

Examination of the ear can also be done with an Otoscope and a microscope (**EUM:** Examination under microscope) which has a **focal length** of 200–250 mm.

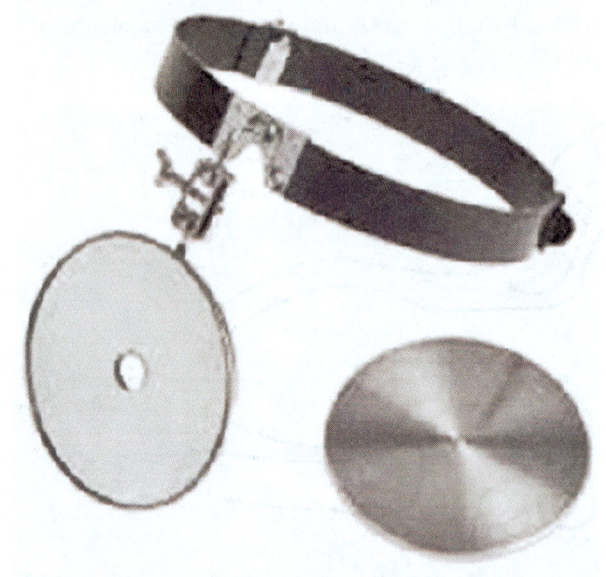

Pneumatic Otoscopy

Pneumatic otoscopy is an important diagnostic tool which is used in the ENT OPD and is done with a Siegel's pneumatic speculum. The Siegel's speculum has a convex lens with a magnification of 2.5 times connected to an aural speculum. A bulb with a rubber tube is provided to insufflate air via the aural speculum. When the speculum is attached and fitted snugly into the patient's external auditory canal, an air-tight chamber is produced.

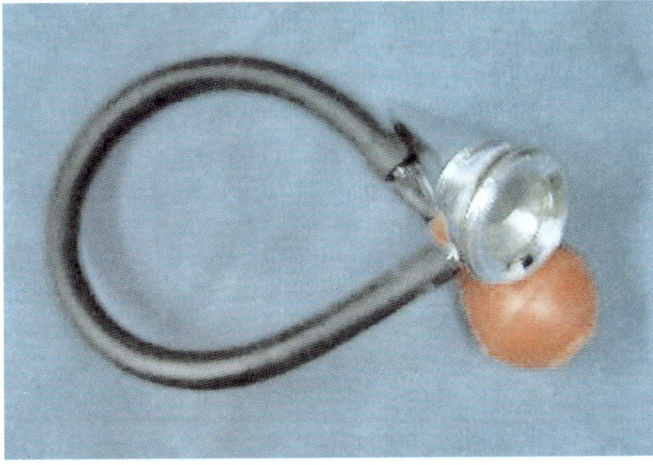

The advantages of this aural Siegel's speculum are:

1. It provides a magnified view of the ear drum
2. The pressure of the external canal can be varied by pressing the bulb, hence it can be used to assess the mobility of TM
3. By changing the pressure of EAC it can be used to elicit the fistula test (*see* Chapter on vestibular system), Gelle's test (*see* Chapter on audiology) and Brown's sign (*see* Chapter on Glomus)
4. Since it provides adequate suction effect, it can be used to suck out middle ear secretions in patients with CSOM.
5. Powdered antibiotic can be applied into the middle ear by using this speculum. Ear is first filled with the powdered antibiotic and a snugly fitting Siegel's speculum is applied to the external canal. Pressure in the external canal is varied by pressing and releasing the rubber bulb, this displaces the antibiotic into the middle ear cavity.

 "Points to Ponder/Points for Quick revision"

- **Hematoma of Pinna:** Boxer's/wrestler's/cauliflower ear due to blunt trauma.
- **Perichondritis of pinna cartilage:** MC Pseudomonas and follows laceration/ear piercing.
- **Diseases of EAC:**
  1. **Otitis externa;** Majority bacterial
     i. **Furuncle:** outer 8 mm in the cartilaginous part where hairs are present, MC-Staph., "tragal sign"
     ii. **Diffuse otitis externa:** Swimmer's ear-MC *Pseudomonas aeruginosa*
     iii. **Malignant otitis externa:**
        - Immunocompromised host
        - Pseudomonas
        - Invasive, extensive necrosis
        - Skull base osteomyelitis
        - Cranial N palsies: VII MC
     iv. **Otitis externa hemorrhagica/bullous myringitis:** hemorrhagic bullae; MC *Strept. pneumoniae*, also-Influenza and mycoplasma.
     v. **Otomycosis:** MC Aspergillus-"wet newspaper appearance". Candida → cotton wool debris.
     vi. **Ramsay Hunt syndrome:** Herpes Zoster Oticus + VII N palsy.
  2. **Myiasis:** Maggots of house fly. Treatment-killing by chloroform and removal.
  3. **Wax:** Cerumen + desquamated epithelial cells + sebaceous secretions. Syringing/instrumentation.
  4. **Keratosis Obturans:** Pearly white keratin plug in the EAC → CHL. Treatment-debridement.
  5. **Primary Cholesteatoma of the EAC:** Invasion of squamous cells which line the EAC into the underlying bone. Foul ear discharge, no hearing loss.
- **Diseases of TM:**
  i. **Traumatic rupture:** Healing in 2 layers in 6–12 weeks.
  ii. **Retraction of TM:** 2° to ET blocked; Sade's and Tos stages.
  iii. **Tympanosclerosis:** Calcification of the fibrous layer of TM 2° to chronic otitis media.

PREVIOUSLY ASKED QUESTIONS

1. **Cauliflower ear is:** *(Manipal 2006, 2009)*
   a. Keloid of pinna
   b. Hematoma of pinna in boxers
   c. Squamous cell carcinoma of pinna
   d. Anaplastic cell carcinoma of pinna

2. **Cauliflower ear is due to:** *(Kerala 99, Exam 2016)*
   a. Haematoma   b. Carcinoma
   c. Fungal infection   d. Herpes

3. **Chondritis of aural cartilage is most commonly due to:** *(NIMHANS 2006, Exam 2016)*
   a. Staphylococcus   b. Pseudomonas
   c. Candida   d. Streptococcus

4. **Fungus causing otomycosis is most commonly:** *(Delhi 96, Exam 2013)*
   a. *Aspergillus niger*   b. Candida
   c. Mucor   d. Penicillin

5. **Fungus causing otomycosis is most commonly:** *(Exam 2013)*
   a. Yeast
   b. Candida
   c. Mucor
   d. Penicillin

6. **Otomycosis is caused by:** *(PGI Dec 98, Exam 2012)*
   a. Candida   b. Aspergillus
   c. Both   d. None

7. **Diffuse otitis externa is also known as:** *(Exam 2003, Exam 2017)*
   a. Glue ear   b. Malignant otitis externa
   c. Swimmer's ear   d. ASOM

8. **Common causes of otitis externa:** *(PGI 2008, Exam 2013)*
   a. Aspergillus   b. Mucor
   c. Candida   d. Pseudomonas
   e. Klebsiella

9. **Malignant Otitis externa is caused by:** *(AP 96, Comed 2007, Exam 2013)*
   a. *S. aureus*   b. *S. albus*
   c. *P. aeruginosa*   d. *E. coli*

10. **Malignant Otitis externa is seen in:** *(MAHE 2005, Exam 2016)*
    a. Wax impaction
    b. Hypertension
    c. Diabetes
    d. All of the above

11. **Malignant Otitis externa is:** *(PGI Dec 99, Exam 2014)*
    a. Malignancy of external ear
    b. Caused by *H. influenzae*
    c. Blackish mass of aspergillus
    d. Pseudomonas infection in diabetic patient

12. **True statement about malignant Otitis externa is:** *(AIIMS 96, Exam 2017)*
    a. Not painful
    b. Common in diabetics and old age
    c. Caused by streptococcus
    d. All of the above

13. **Which of the following is not a typical feature of malignant Otitis externa:** *(AIIMS May 2006, Exam 2012)*
    a. Caused by *Pseudomonas aeruginosa*
    b. Patients are usually old
    c. Mitotic figures are high
    d. Patient is immunocompromised

14. **Malignant Otitis externa is characterised by:** *(PGI Dec 2003/June 2006, Exam 2010)*
    a. Caused by *Pseudomonas aeruginosa*
    b. Malignancy of external auditory canal
    c. Granulation tissue is seen in the floor of external auditory canal
    d. Radiotherapy can be given
    e. Gallium scan helpful for monitoring treatment

15. **Facial nerve palsy is seen in:** *(JIPMER 2003, Exam 2017)*
    a. Seborrhoeic Otitis externa
    b. Otomycosis
    c. Malignant Otitis externa
    d. Eczematous Otitis externa

16. **Regarding necrotizing otitis externa all are true except:** *(Exam 2013)*
    a. Caused by pseudomonas
    b. Surgery never done
    c. Facial nerve involved
    d. Common in diabetics

17. **An old diabetic male presented with rapidly spreading infection of the EAC with involvement of the bone and presence of granulation tissue. The drug of choice for this condition is:** *(AIIMS May 2006, AIIMS May 2014)*
    a. Ciprofloxacin
    b. Penicillin
    c. Second generation cephalosporin
    d. Clarithromycin

18. **A 60-year-old diabetic patient presents with extremely painful lesion in the external ear and otorrhoea. There is evidence of granulation type tissue in the external ear and bony erosion with facial nerve palsy is noted. The most likely diagnosis is:** *(Bihar 2004, AI 2012)*
    a. Malignant otitis externa
    b. Nasopharyngeal carcinoma
    c. Chronic suppurative otitis media
    d. Acute suppurative otitis media

19. An elderly diabetic male presents with severe pain in the ear. On examination he is found to have granulations in external ear (*see* picture given below) conductive deafness and facial palsy. He was found to be having increased uptake of Tc^{99}m. The most probable diagnosis is:

    (*Practice question by Author*)

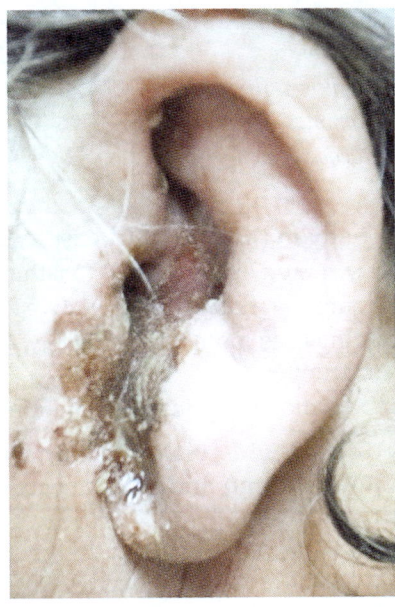

    a. Malignancy with middle ear infection
    b. Nasopharyngeal carcinoma with ET blockade
    c. Malignant otitis externa
    d. CSOM

20. Otitis externa Haemorrhagica is caused by:

    (*AIIMS 98, Exam 2017*)
    a. Influenza   b. Proteus
    c. Staph   d. Pseudomonas

21. Myringitis bullosa is caused by: (*AI 99, Exam 2017*)
    a. Protozoa   b. Fungus
    c. Bacteria   d. None

22. Direction of water jet while doing syringing of ear should be: (*MH 2002, Exam 2017*)
    a. Anteroinferior   b. Posterosuperior
    c. Anterosuperior   d. Posteroinferior

23. Dysfunction of tympanic membrane is characterized by all except: (*AP 2000, Exam 2016*)
    a. Normal 'cone of light'
    b. Retracted TM
    c. Non-prominent umbo
    d. Prominent malleolar folds

24. Features of moderately retracted tympanic membrane are all except: (*MH 2005, Exam 2016*)
    a. Handle of malleus appearance foreshortened
    b. Cone of light is absent or interrupted
    c. Lateral process of malleus becomes more prominent
    d. Shiny pearly grey tympanic membrane

25. Which of the following is false about tympanic membrane: (*Delhi 2008*)
    a. Cone of light is antero-inferior
    b. Shrapnell's membrane is also known as pars flaccida
    c. Healed perforation has 3 layers
    d. TM attachment to tip of malleus handle is called umbo

26. Chalky white tympanic membrane is seen in:

    (*RJ 2001, Exam 2016*)
    a. ASOM   b. Otosclerosis
    c. Tympanosclerosis   d. Cholesteatoma

27. Keratosis obturans is: (*TN 2007, Exam 2014*)
    a. Foreign body in external auditory canal
    b. Desquamated epithelial cells
    c. Cholesterol crystals surrounded by calcium
    d. Wax in external auditory canal

28. A 60-year-old male presented with left ear discharge for the past 7 years with dull ear ache. On examination intact TM on both the sides, with discharge coming from the posterior canal wall on the left side. Hearing is normal. Diagnosis is:

    (*AIIMS May 2013*)
    a. Keratosis obturans
    b. CSOM
    c. Complications of external otitis
    d. Carcinoma of external auditory canal

29. The focal length of the mirror used in head mirror: (*Exam 2014*)
    a. 85 mm   b. 150 mm
    c. 250 mm   d. 400 mm

30. Diameter of head mirror in ENT is:

    (*Bihar 2005, Exam 2016*)
    a. 15 cm   b. 22 cm
    c. 9 cm   d. 26 cm

31. Use of Siegel's speculum during examination of the ear provides all except: (*AI 2005, Exam 2016*)
    a. Magnification
    b. Assessment of the movement of TM
    c. Removal of foreign body from the ear
    d. As applicator for the powdered antibiotic of ear

32. The most common organism causing skull base osteomyelitis is: (*NIMHANS 2014*)
    a. Pneumococcus   b. *H. Influenzae*
    c. Aspergillus   d. Pseudomonas

33. External ear not washed with water in presence of: (*PGI 2013*)
    a. Ead   b. Wax
    c. Animate object   d. Vegetable matter
    e. Lead battery

Ear

Section I

34. **Which of the following is false regarding malignant otitis externa?** (*AIIMS 2014*)
    a. ESR is useful in the monitoring of response to antibiotics
    b. Sensory hearing loss is common presentation
    c. Common in diabetics
    d. Granulation tissue in external ear canal

35. **Child with battery as foreign body in nose. Which of the following is an important concern?**
    (*Exam 2014*)
    a. Refer to specialist and plan for elective removal
    b. Local release of chemical from battery and destruction of tissue
    c. Tetanus
    d. Anosmia

36. **Impaction of wax is treated by:** (*Exam 2016*)
    a. Syringing
    b. Softening followed by syringing
    c. Instrumentation
    d. Suction

37. **All of the following are risk factors for malignant otitis externa except:** (*Exam 2016*)
    a. Diabetes   b. Immunodeficiency
    c. Parotitis   d. Chemotherapy

38. **Most common cause of otitis externa is:**
    (*Exam 2016*)
    a. Fungal infection   b. Bacterial infection
    c. Seborrhoeic disease d. Herpes zoster

39. **The given appearance of pinna is suggestive of:**
    (*Practice question by Author*)

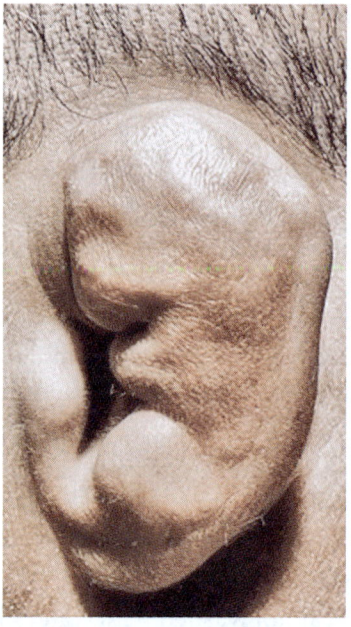

    a. Pseudomonas infection
    b. Aspergillus infection
    c. Post-traumatic
    d. Tuberculosis

40. **Retraction of TM lies on the promontory with intact middle ear mucosa. What is Sade's grade?**
    (*Exam 2016*)
    a. 1   b. 2
    c. 3   d. 4

41. **A 65-year-old diabetic presents with necrosis of the external auditory canal with foul smelling discharge. The probable organism associated with the conditions is:** (*Exam 2016*)
    a. *Hemophilus influenzae*
    b. *Pseudomonas aeruginosa*
    c. *Streptococcus pyogens*
    d. *E. coli*

42. **Foreign body in the ear not true is:** (*Exam 2016*)
    a. Most common site is medial to isthmus
    b. Syringing is not done for vegetative foreign body
    c. Syringing uses room temperature water directed at ear drum
    d. Can be removed by instrumentation

43. **Retraction of TM with TM adherent to the promontory with no middle ear space remaining. It is called:** (*Exam 2016*)
    a. Stage 1 Sade
    b. Stage 2 Sade
    c. Atelectasis
    d. Adhesive otitis media

44. **Which of the following is false regarding malignant otitis externa?** (*Exam 2016*)
    a. ESR is useful in the monitoring of response to antibiotics
    b. Sensorineural hearing loss is common presentation
    c. Common in diabetics
    d. Granulation tissue in external ear canal

45. **Malignant Otitis Externa is a:** (*Exam 2016*)
    a. Malignant condition
    b. Pre-malignant condition
    c. Infective condition
    d. Autoimmune condition

46. **Least life threatening condition in a diabetic patient is:** (*Exam 2016*)
    a. Emphysematous cholecystitis
    b. Emphysematous pyelonephritis
    c. Malignant otitis externa
    d. Mucor-mycosis
    e. Emphysematous appendicitis

47. **True about skull base osteomyelitis are all except:**
    (*WB PG 2015*)
    a. Frequent aural toileting is required
    b. High uptake on bone scan
    c. Causes pain in ear
    d. Most common organism is *Staph. aureus* and *Proteus mirabilis*

48. MC cranial nerve palsy in malignant otitis externa is: (*Exam 2016*)
   a. V
   b. VI
   c. VII
   d. VIII

49. Patient presents with pain and discharge in the ear. On examination the ear shows the following. He should be managed by:

   (*Practice question by Author*)

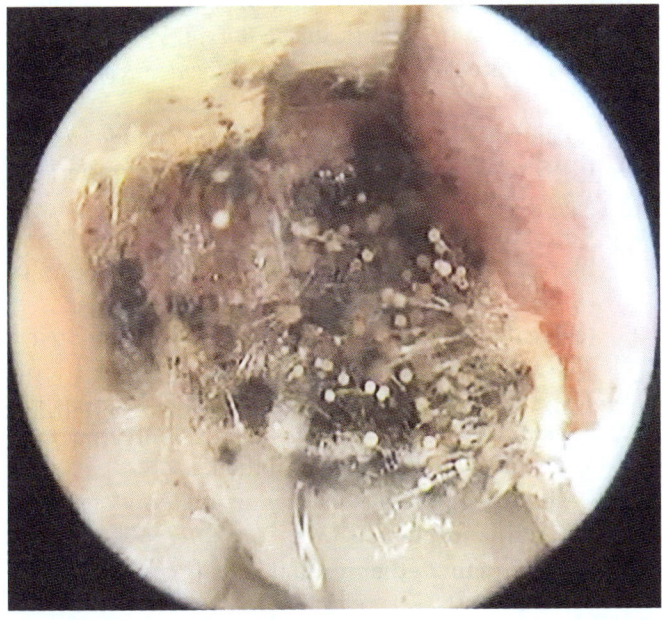

   a. Ciprofloxacin ear drops
   b. Clotrimazole ear drops
   c. Wax softening ear drops
   d. Steroid ear drops

50. Correct about the shown procedure:

   (*Practice question by Author*)

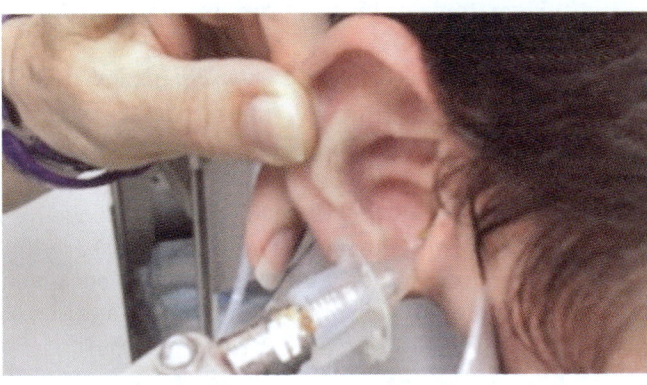

   a. Ear pulled up and backwards, syringe jet posterosuperiorly
   b. Ear pulled down and backwards, syringe jet anterosuperiorly
   c. Ear pulled down and forwards, syringe jet anteroinferiorly
   d. Ear pulled up and forwards, syringe jet anterosuperiorly

51. Aural Myiasis means: (*Exam 2016*)
   a. Otomycosis
   b. Maggots of the ear
   c. Swimmers ear
   d. Perichondritis of pinna

52. When irrigation of the ear canal is done to remove wax or foreign body, fluid used should be:

   (*Exam 2017*)
   a. 30°
   b. 44°
   c. 37°
   d. 15°

Section I | Ear

ANSWERS AND EXPLANATIONS

1. **(b) Hematoma of pinna in boxers** (*Ref. Scott Brown, 8th ed., Vol 2; 1102*)
2. **(a) Haematoma** (*Ref. Scott Brown, 8th ed., Vol 2; 1102*)
3. **(b) Pseudomonas** (*Ref. Scott Brown, 8th ed., Vol 2; 959*)
4. **(a) *Aspergillus niger*** (*Ref. Scott Brown, 8th ed., Vol 1; 206*)
5. **(b) Candida** (*Ref. Scott Brown, 8th ed., Vol 2; 956*)
   - MC organism causing otomycosis is *Aspergillus* followed by Candida. Since *Aspergillus* is not given in the choice, the next most common is Candida.
6. **(c) Both** (*Ref. Scott Brown, 8th ed., Vol 2; 956*)
7. **(c) Swimmer's ear** (*Ref. Cummings, 6th ed., 2116*)
8. **(a), (c), (d) Aspergillus, Candida, Pseudomonas** (*Ref. Cummings, 6th ed., 2116*)
   - Infections of the EAC (external auditory canal) are known as Otitis externa. These can be bacterial, fungal or viral, please refer the text.
9. **(c) *P. aeruginosa*** (*Ref. Scott Brown, 8th ed., Vol 2; 1421*)
10. **(c) Diabetes** (*Ref. Scott Brown, 8th ed., Vol 2; 1420*)
11. **(d) Pseudomonas infection in diabetic patient** (*Ref. Cummings, 6th ed., 2118*)
12. **(b) Common in diabetics and old age** (*Ref. Cummings, 6th ed., 2118*)
    - Malignant Otitis externa is extremely painful. It is caused by Pseudomonas.
13. **(c) Mitotic figures are high** (*Ref. Scott Brown, 8th ed., Vol 2; 1420*)
    - High mitotic figures are suggestive of a malignant condition. Malignant Otitis externa is not a malignancy but an infective and locally invasive condition.
14. **(a), (c) and (e)** (*Ref. Cummings, 6th ed., 2119*)
15. **(c) Malignant Otitis externa** (*Ref. Scott Brown, 8th ed., Vol 2; 1420*)
    - Malignant Otitis externa can lead to granulations and bony erosion leading to facial nerve palsy.
      The other options do not cause bony erosion and facial nerve palsy.
16. **(b) Surgery never done** (*Ref. Scott Brown, 8th ed., Vol 2; 1422*)
17. **(a) Ciprofloxacin** (*Ref. Scott Brown, 8th ed., Vol 2; 1422*)
    - Old diabetic with rapidly spreading infection and granulations, the diagnosis is malignant Otitis externa. The cause is pseudomonas.
    - Antipseudomonal antibiotics (e.g. Ciprofloxacin, Ceftazidime, Piperacillin/Ticarcillin, Meropenem, etc.) for 3–6 weeks are given and debridement of necrotic material is done.
18. **(a) Malignant otitis externa** (*Ref. Cummings, 6th ed., 2118*)
19. **(c) Malignant otitis externa** (*Ref. Scott Brown, 8th ed., Vol 2; 1422*)
    - This is a clear cut case of malignant Otitis externa. For early diagnosis Tc^{99} scan is used. Tc^{99} is taken up by the osteoclasts and osteoblasts and indicates the bony erosion during the malignant Otitis externa.
    - Malignancy of the EAC usually follows long standing ear discharge which has not been mentioned in the above question. A biopsy will be diagnostic of malignancy and Tc^{99} scan is not required here.
    - Nasopharyngeal carcinoma with ET blockade presents with upper deep cervical lymphadenopathy with U/L serous otitis media.
20. **(a) Influenza** (*Ref. Scott Brown, 8th ed., Vol 2; 936*)
21. **(c) Bacteria** (*Ref. Scott Brown, 8th ed., Vol 2; 936*)
22. **(b) Posterosuperior** (*Ref. Scott Brown, 8th ed., Vol 2; 235*)
23. **(a) Normal 'cone of light'** (*Ref. Dhingra, 6th ed., 55*)
24. **(d) Shiny pearly grey tympanic membrane** (*Ref. Dhingra, 6th ed., 55*)
    - Retracted tympanic membrane appears dull and lustreless due to absent or interrupted cone of light.
25. **(c) Healed perforation has 3 layers** (*Ref. Scott Brown, 8th ed., Vol 2; 529*)
    - The TM membrane which heals by itself does not have the fibrous layer. It has 2 layers only, the outer epithelial and the inner endothelial.
      Rest are true, see the chapter on anatomy of ear
26. **(c) Tympanosclerosis** (*Ref. Cummings, 6th ed., 2151*)
27. **(b) Desquamated epithelial cells** (*Ref. Scott Brown, 8th ed., Vol 2; 942*)
28. **(a) Keratosis obturans** (*Ref. Scott Brown, 8th ed., Vol 2; 942*)
    - Since the TM is intact so it cannot be CSOM
    - Otitis externa is an acute condition
    - Carcinoma of EAC of such a long duration will not remain localised
29. **(c) 250 mm** (*Ref. Dhingra, 6th ed., 374*)
30. **(c) 9 cm** (*Ref. Dhingra, 6th ed., 374*)
    - The diameter of the mirror is 3.5 inch/9 cm/90 mm
31. **(c) Removal of foreign body from the ear** (*Ref. Dhingra, 6th ed., 374*)
    - Removal of foreign body of ear is done by syringing or instrumentation.
32. **(d) Pseudomonas** (*Ref. Cummings, 6th ed., 2118*)
33. **(d), (e), Vegetable matter, Lead battery** (*Ref. Scott Brown, 8th ed., Vol 2; 386*)
34. **(b) Sensory hearing loss is common presentation** (*Ref. Cummings, 6th ed., 2118*)
35. **(b) Local release of chemical from battery and destruction of tissue** (*Ref. Scott Brown, 8th ed., Vol 2; 386*)
36. **(b) Softening followed by syringing** (*Ref. Scott Brown, 8th ed., Vol 2; 921*)
37. **(c) Parotitis** (*Ref. Scott Brown, 8th ed., Vol 2; 1421*)
38. **(b) Bacterial infection** (*Ref. Cummings, 6th ed., 2116*)
39. **(c) Post-traumatic** (*Ref. Scott Brown, 8th ed., Vol 2; 1102*)
    - This is the picture of hematoma of pinna showing the typical cauliflower appearance

40. **(c) 3** (*Ref. Shambaugh, 6th ed., 395*)

41. **(b)** *Pseudomonas aeruginosa* (*Ref. Scott Brown, 8th ed., Vol 2; 1420*)

42. **(c) Syringing uses room temperature water directed at ear drum** (*Ref. Scott Brown, 8th ed., Vol 2; 386*)

- Syringing uses body temperature water (37°C) and not room temperature.
- There is a chance of vegetative F B to get swollen up and therefore get stuck up. Therefore syringing is avoided here.

43. **(d) Adhesive otitis media** (*Ref. Shambaugh, 6th ed., 395*)

44. **(b) Sensorineural hearing loss is common presentation** (*Ref. Cummings, 6th ed., 2118*)
Invasion of inner ear to result into SN hearing loss is unusual and if it all occurs, will be a very late feature.

45. **(c) Infective condition** (*Ref. Scott Brown, 8th ed., Vol 2; 1419*)

46. **(c) Malignant otitis externa** (*Ref. Scott Brown, 8th ed., Vol 2; 1419*)

Though all are life threatening complications in a diabetic patient but since Malignant otitis externa can be picked up early (it being an external condition and therefore early management here), it is the least life threatening among the rest of the choices.

Emphysematous infections in a diabetic are caused by fermentation of glucose by bacterial and fungal pathogens. Also due to immunocompromised state in D/M, these infections of the internal organs may lead to perforation leading to high mortality. Mucormycosis being angio-invasive therefore spreads rapidly from nose to orbits to CNS and thus fatal. Malignant otitis externa may also lead to death, but for the reason mentioned, it is the least likely cause.

47. **(d) Most common organism is** *Staph. aureus* **and** *Proteus mirabilis* (*Ref. Cummings, 6th ed., 2119*)

48. **(c) VII** (*Ref. Scott Brown, 8th ed., Vol 2; 1420*)

49. **(b) Clotrimazole ear drops** (*Ref. Scott Brown, 8th ed., Vol 2; 956*)

50. **(a) Ear pulled up and backwards, syringe jet posterosuperiorly** (*Ref. Dhingra, 6th ed., 53*)

51. **(b) Maggots of the ear** (*Ref. Dhingra, 6th ed., 161*)

52. **(c) 37°** (*Ref. Dhingra, 6th ed., 53*)

Section I | Ear

Acute Infections of Middle Ear

Infection of the middle ear is known as Otitis media. It can be acute or chronic and accordingly known as acute Otitis media or chronic Otitis media.

ACUTE INFECTIONS OF MIDDLE EAR

Acute Otitis Media (AOM) or Acute Suppurative Otitis Media (ASOM)

Since the only connection of the middle ear to the rest of the body is through the Eustachian tube which opens in the nasopharynx, any infection of the nasopharynx (adenoiditis) and its vicinity, i.e. oropharynx (pharyngitis, tonsillitis, etc.) or nose (sinusitis) can ultimately reach the middle ear through the Eustachian tube leading to acute otitis media.

Therefore, the MC route of AOM is through Eustachian tube and also any ET dysfunction, i.e. interference with its physiological opening will predispose to ASOM. The less common routes are through traumatic perforation of the TM and hematogenous.

AOM can be viral or bacterial. The MC bacteria causing AOM is *Streptococcus pneumoniae* followed by *Haemophilus influenzae*. It is for these Pyogenic, i.e. pus-forming bacterial pathogens, the acute otitis media is also called as acute suppurative otitis media.

Pathogenesis

There are four stages in the course of AOM or ASOM:

1. **Stage of tubal occlusion:** The infection from the pharynx first infects the Eustachian tube (which opens 1 cm behind inferior turbinate in the nasopharynx). This leads to oedema and obstruction of Eustachian tube leading to a negative pressure in the middle ear and TM retraction (*see* features of retracted TM in Chapter 4). Patient here presents with blocked feeling of the ear and earache.

2. **Stage of hyperaemia or stage of pre-suppuration:** From the Eustachian tube the infection now reaches the middle ear. Infection in the middle ear causes inflammation and hyperaemia of middle ear mucosa leading to exudation of fluid.

   Here the patient presents with severe pain in the ear and on examination the TM appears very **red and**

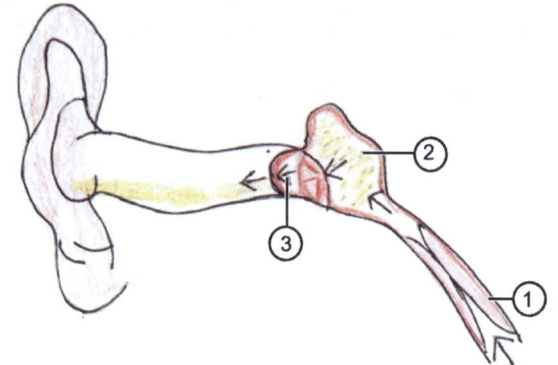

Fig. 5.1: Schematic diagram showing the initial three stages of ASOM

congested. Since the vessels on the TM run radially, this hyperaemic appearance is also known as **Cart wheel** appearance of TM.

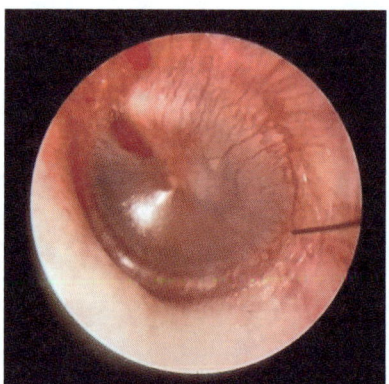

3. **Stage of suppuration:** Here the exudate in the middle ear along with WBC/pus cells forms the suppurate. As the suppurated fluid increases, the TM starts to bulge to the point of rupture. The patient here presents with severe pain and fever.

   On examination the TM is red and bulging. If the pressure increases further, the TM ruptures. The most common site of rupture following ASOM is in the **antero-inferior quadrant.**

   This antero-inferior perforation that occurs following rupture of the TM allows the pus to come out. This pus coming out from the middle ear being large and in a lot of pressure gives an appearance known as **"pulsatile otorrhoea or light house sign"**.

Patient here presents with the complaint of mucopurulent (which may be blood tinged also) discharge from the ears.

4. **Stage of resolution:** Resolution can occur in early stages also if the antibiotics are started early. With the release of pus, the pain and fever come down.

Or

Stage of complication: If virulence of the organism is high or the immunity of the patient is low then the patient might go into the stage of complication which results due to the further spread of infection. This spread occurs due to anatomical connections, congenital or surgical dehiscence or via hematogenous route. It can be intratemporal like acute mastoiditis, labyrinthitis, facial nerve palsy and petrositis or intracranial like extradural abscess, meningitis, brain abscess and lateral sinus thrombophlebitis, *see* Chapter 9.

Management

The treatment if started early will prevent the suppuration/rupture of TM.

a. Antibiotics against *Streptococcus pneumoniae* and *H. influenzae*

b. Nasal decongestants (drops) and oral decongestants to relieve Eustachian tube oedema

c. Analgesics, antipyretics and antihistaminics. And if required,

d. *Myringotomy:* As its name myring (TM) tomy (opening), this is a procedure of making an incision (opening) on the TM. **The indications of myringotomy in a patient of ASOM are as follows:**

1. **Red bulging TM with intense pain:** Slight bulge of TM may regress with antibiotics alone. Since myringotomy is an invasive procedure, it is done only when the TM is full and bulging and there is impending rupture because if the TM ruptures by itself, it will cause a greater damage to TM.

2. **Persistent effusion (>12 weeks):** Here the pain has subsided but effusion is still there causing deafness. This is because of inadequate dose or duration of antibiotics or due to the formation of biofilms and is now classified as serous otitis media (SOM). Please refer the chapter on Secretory Otitis Media.

3. **ASOM with facial nerve palsy:** Facial nerve is the only cranial nerve which runs in a bony canal in most of its course. This canal extends from its entry from IAM to its exit at the stylomastoid foramen and is known as fallopian canal. This fallopian canal is congenitally dehiscent in 50% cases. The most common site of dehiscence is the horizontal part just above the oval window. Increased pressure in the middle ear in a patient of AOM can get transmitted through the dehiscence to facial nerve leading to facial nerve palsy. In such a patient management of facial palsy will be by relieving the pressure on facial nerve by myringotomy along with the usual management of ASOM.

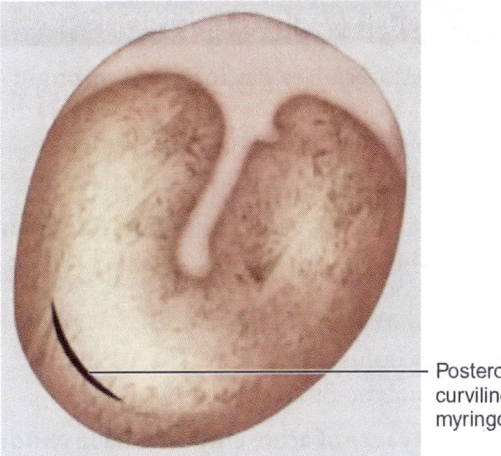

Postero-inferior curvilinear myringotomy

Fig. 5.2: Site and Shape of Myringotomy in ASOM

In ASOM myringotomy is done in the postero-inferior quadrant by a curvilinear J shaped incision (see details of myringotomy in chapter on serous otitis media).

Prognosis of ASOM: It usually resolves completely without sequelae.

ACUTE NECROTISING OTITIS MEDIA (ANOM)

When the organism is much more virulent and the immunity of the patient is low then the patient develops ANOM. Beta-hemolytic Streptococcus is the most common causative organism here.

The cardinal feature of ANOM is that it leads to a marginal or total perforation (i.e. the annulus of TM also gets destroyed). This **marginal perforation** can lead to **secondary cholesteatoma**, see chapter on CSOM, also *see* Chapter 9 for various intra-temporal and intra-cranial complications following ANOM.

🤔 **"Points to Ponder/Points for Quick revision"**

- MC route of Acute Otitis Media (AOM) is via Eustachian tube (ET)
- MC organism causing AOM-*Streptococcus pneumoniae*
- 4 stages of AOM:
  i. *Stage I*: ET occlusion → TM retraction
  ii. *Stage II*: Hyperaemia in middle ear → red and congested TM (cart wheel appearance)
  iii. *Stage III*: Suppuration in middle ear → bulging TM; if TM ruptures → pulsatile otorrhoea ("Light house sign")
  iv. *Stage IV*: Mostly resolution (with medical management); if highly virulent organisms or low host immunity → intra-temporal or intracranial complications
- Treatment:
- Antibiotics (systemic as well as local), decongestants, antihistaminics and antipyretics
- Myringotomy (J shaped incision in the postero-inferior quadrant of the TM) if:
  i. Full and bulging TM which can rupture soon any time
  ii. ASOM with facial nerve palsy
- Acute necrotising otitis media (ANOM): Beta hemolytic streptococcus → marginal/total perforation (i.e. involving annulus) → secondary cholesteatoma → squamosal chronic otitis media (COM).

Section I   Ear

PREVIOUSLY ASKED QUESTIONS

1. **Throat infection causes Ear infection through:**
   (PGI 2008)
   a. Blood spread   b. Eustachian tube
   c. Nasocranial spread d. Simultaneous infection

2. **Commonest causative organism for ASOM in a 2-year-old child is:** *(AIIMS Dec 99, 91, Exam 2016)*
   a. Pneumococcus
   b. *H. influenzae*
   c. Staphylococcus
   d. Beta-hemolytic Streptococcus

3. **Commonest cause of acute Otitis media in children is:** *(AIIMS June 2000, Delhi 2006, UP 2003, Exam 2017)*
   a. *H. influenzae*
   b. *Streptococcus pneumoniae*
   c. *Staph. aureus*
   d. Pseudomonas

4. **Cart Wheel sign is seen in:**   *(MP 2008)*
   a. ASOM   b. Glomus
   c. OME   d. CSOM

5. **Most common perforation site in tympanic membrane in ASOM:**   *(Exam 2013, 2016)*
   a. Antero-inferior   b. Postero-inferior
   c. Antero-superior   d. Postero-superior

6. **Light house sign characterizes:** *(RJ 2000, Exam 2016)*
   a. ASOM   b. CSOM
   c. Meniere's disease d. Cholesteatoma

7. **Pulsatile otorrhoea is seen in:** *(AP 97, Exam 2017)*
   a. Glomus tumour   b. CSF otorrhoea
   c. ASOM   d. Fistula

8. **Light house sign is seen in ASOM in which stage:**
   (Exam 2013, 2016)
   a. Stage of suppuration b. Stage of hyperaemia
   c. Stage of resolution d. Stage of pre-suppuration

9. **Myringotomy is:**   *(Exam 2013)*
   a. Surgical opening in Eustachian tube
   b. Surgical opening in tympanic membrane
   c. Surgical opening in semicircular canal
   d. None

10. **Myringotomy is indicated in:**   *(PGI 98, 2018)*
    a. Coalescent mastoiditis
    b. Cholesteatoma
    c. ASOM
    d. External otitis media

11. **For ASOM Myringotomy is done in which quadrant:**
    (AI 95, Exam 2016)
    a. Antero-inferior   b. Antero-superior
    c. Postero-superior   d. Postero-inferior

12. **A 3-year-old child presents with fever and ear ache. On examination there is congested with slight bulging tympanic membrane. The treatment of choice is:**   *(AI 2005, 2010)*
    a. Myringotomy with antibiotics
    b. Myringotomy with grommet insertion
    c. Oral antibiotics and decongestants
    d. Anti-allergic and decongestants only

13. **A 7-year-old child presenting with acute Otitis media, does not respond to amoxicillin-clavulanic acid. Examination reveals full and bulging tympanic membrane, the treatment of choice is:** *(AI 2004, 2009)*
    a. Systemic steroids   b. Ciprofloxacin
    c. Myringotomy   d. Cortical mastoidectomy

14. **Acute suppurative Otitis media (ASOM) is treated using all except:**   *(AIIMS 2000, 2012)*
    a. Erythromycin   b. Penicillin
    c. Streptomycin   d. Cephalosporin

15. **True statement about ASOM is:**   *(Exam 2016)*
    a. Most frequently it resolves without sequelae
    b. Commonly follows painful parotitis
    c. Radical mastoidectomy is required for treatment
    d. Most common organism is Pseudomonas

16. **Incision on tympanic membrane is called:**
    (Exam 2016)
    a. Myringoplasty   b. Tympanoplasty
    c. Myringotomy   d. Fenestration operation

IMAGE BASED PRACTICE QUESTIONS BY THE AUTHOR

17. **A 3-year-old child presents with fever and ear ache. Endoscopic appearance of the tympanic membrane is shown below. The treatment of choice is:**

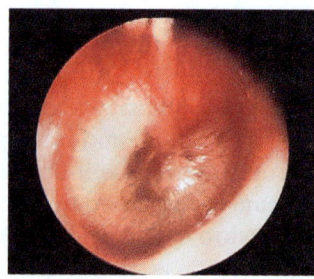

    a. Myringotomy with grommet insertion
    b. Oral antibiotics
    c. Anti-allergic and decongestants only
    d. Cortical mastoidectomy

18. **The following type of incision on the TM is given in which condition:**

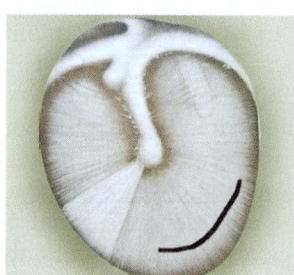

    a. ASOM   b. Safe CSOM
    c. SOM   d. Unsafe CSOM

ANSWERS AND EXPLANATIONS

1. **(b) Eustachian tube** (*Ref. Scott Brown, 8th ed., Vol 2; 140*)

2. **(a) Pneumococcus** (*Ref. Scott Brown, 8th ed., Vol 2; 139*)
   - The MC organism causing AOM is *Streptococcus pneumoniae* (pneumococcus) followed by *Haemophilus influenzae*.
   - In the ear Staphylococcus is the most common causative organism in furuncle of the EAC
   - Beta-hemolytic Streptococcus is the causative organism in ANOM and acute mastoiditis.

3. **(b) *Streptococcus pneumoniae*** (*Ref. Scott Brown, 8th ed., Vol 2; 139*)
   - Irrespective of the age of the patient suffering from AOM, the MC organism is *Streptococcus pneumoniae* followed by *Haemophilus influenzae*.
   - In the ear Pseudomonas causes perichondritis, diffuse Otitis externa and malignant Otitis externa and it is also the main organism in unsafe CSOM.

4. **(a) ASOM** (*Ref. Hazarika, 3rd ed., 149*)
   - In Glomus "rising sun sign" or "red reflex" is seen.
   - In Otitis media with effusion (OME) TM appears dull, retracted and sometimes bluish.
   - In CSOM the TM will be perforated (please refer the respective chapters)

5. **(a) Antero-inferior** (*Ref. Shambaugh, 6th ed., 437; Scott Brown, 8th ed., Vol 2; 147*).
   However this answer is controversial as according to Shambaugh it is most commonly anteroinferior but Scott Brown says it is the posterior half of pars tensa.

6. **(a) ASOM** (*Ref. Hazarika, 3rd ed., 150*)

7. **(c) ASOM** (*Ref. Hazarika, 3rd ed., 150*)

8. **(a) Stage of suppuration** (*Ref. Shambaugh, 6th ed., 426; Hazarika, 3rd ed., 150*)

9. **(b) Surgical opening in tympanic membrane** (*Ref. Scott Brown, 8th ed., Vol 2; 974*)

10. **(c) ASOM** (*Ref. Scott Brown, 8th ed., Vol 2; 143*)
    - Myringotomy is indicated in ASOM. Another indication of doing Myringotomy is in serous Otitis media (SOM). Here in SOM Myringotomy along with grommet insertion is done.

11. **(d) Postero-inferior** (*Ref. Hazarika, 3rd ed., 202*)
    - In ASOM myringotomy is done in the postero-inferior quadrant by a curvilinear J-shaped incision.
    - In serous Otitis media myringotomy along with grommet insertion is done in the antero-inferior quadrant by a radial incision (refer to chapter on serous Otitis media for the reason for these preferred sites of incision in the said two conditions).

12. **(c) Oral antibiotics and decongestants** (*Ref. Scott Brown, 8th ed., Vol 2; 142*)
    - The slight bulge of TM may regress with antibiotics alone. Myringotomy being an invasive procedure is done only when the TM is full and bulging.
    - Myringotomy with grommet insertion is the treatment modality in serous Otitis media

13. **(c) Myringotomy (please see the explanation to the above question)** (*Ref. Scott Brown, 8th ed., Vol 2; 143*)
    - Ciprofloxacin is given in pseudomonal and other Gram-negative infections.
    - Cortical mastoidectomy is done in acute mastoiditis
    - In ASOM steroids are not used

14. **(c) Streptomycin** (*Ref. Scott Brown, 8th ed., Vol 2; 142*)
    - Streptomycin—an aminoglycoside is used in anti-tubercular treatment.
    - The MC organism causing ASOM is *Streptococcus pneumoniae* followed by *Haemophilus influenzae*. So beta-lactum, macrolides and fluro-quinolones active against these bacteria, are the antibiotics of choice.

15. **(a) Most frequently it resolves without sequelae** (*Ref. Scott Brown, 8th ed., Vol 2; 141*)
    - ASOM usually resolves completely without complications.
    - ASOM commonly follows infection in the naso or oro-pharynx via Eustachian tube.
    - Most common organism causing ASOM is *Streptococcus pneumoniae*.
    - Myringotomy may be required to be done in ASOM.

16. **(c) Myringotomy** (*Ref. Dhingra, 6th ed., 63*)

17. **(b) Oral antibiotics** (*Ref. Cummings, 6th ed., 3020*)
    - Grommet insertion is not done in ASOM. It is put in SOM

18. **(a) ASOM** (*Ref. Hazarika, 3rd ed., 202*)

Serous Otitis Media, Functions of Eustachian Tube, Otitic Barotrauma

SEROUS OTITIS MEDIA (SOM)/SECRETORY OTITIS MEDIA/OTITIS MEDIA WITH EFFUSION/GLUE EAR

Serous otitis media is the collection of sterile fluid in the middle ear.

Causes of Serous Otitis Media

1. **Decreased drainage** through the Eustachian tube due to its obstruction or dysfunction. Here the Eustachian tube obstruction is non-infective, as an infective obstruction will lead to ASOM, *see* Chapter on ASOM.

   The Eustachian tube dysfunction/obstruction causes inadequate gas exchange into the middle ear space. This leads to the development of increasingly negative middle ear pressures, resulting in the formation of a transudate that fails to clear. The causes of Eustachian tube obstruction/dysfunction leading to serous otitis media can be the following:

   a. Any **non-infective nasopharyngeal mass** may cause Eustachian tube obstruction, which in a child is most commonly hypertrophied adenoids. Therefore, the most common cause of SOM in children is **hypertrophied adenoids**. Adenoids being midline, leads to obstruction of both the Eustachian tubes leading to B/L SOM.

      Adenoids disappear by 20 years of age, therefore, in adults **benign and malignant tumours of the nasopharynx**, e.g. nasopharyngeal carcinoma, can lead to Eustachian tube obstruction. This being one-sided causes **unilateral SOM**.

   b. **Interference with physiological opening:** Eustachian tube dysfunction, i.e. interference with physiological opening of Eustachian tube can occur due to

      i. **Conditions like palatal palsy and cleft palate** (here there occurs defective function of tensor veli palatini muscle which normally acts to open the Eustachian tube).

      ii. **Enlarged tonsils** mechanically obstructing movements of soft palate, thereby interfering with the Eustachian tube opening.

      iii. In **otitic barotraumas** (*see* at the end of this Chapter) the Eustachian tube gets locked by forcing of the soft tissues of the pharyngeal end of the tube into the lumen of the tube and oedema of the tube, leading to SOM.

2. **Increased production** as in allergic conditions.

3. **Persistent Effusion of ASOM:** SOM can also occur subsequent to inadequate treatment of ASOM and/or formation of biofilms.

   The colonies of bacteria at times produce a matrix of polysaccharides known as **biofilms**. These biofilms allow passage of nutrients and fluid and produce a favourable environment where the bacteria can persist in tissues and are shielded from eradication by host defence mechanisms and long-term antibiotic therapy. Their persistence results in proliferation of mucosal lining and excessive secretion of mucous, leading to SOM.

   Here the culture of this fluid from the middle ear is negative as the biofilm aggregated bacteria are not free floating in the fluid but are sequestered on the surface of the lining mucosa. Biofilms have been demonstrated in many cases of SOM.

Clinical Features

The following can be the clinical presentation of SOM:

a. Mostly children present with inability or delayed development of speech (due to reduced hearing) and learning difficulties.

b. Patients can also present with the complaint of decreased hearing. SOM is the MC cause of reduced hearing or deafness in children. SOM leads to **B/L painless, fluctuating** (due to changing fluid levels) **conductive hearing loss** in children. The underlying cause in children is most commonly hypertrophied adenoids which being a midline structure leads to B/L SOM in children. In adults the presentation is hearing loss which is either U/L (following nasopharyngeal carcinoma) or B/L (following allergy).

c. If SOM develops due to inadequate treatment or formation of biofilms following ASOM, then the

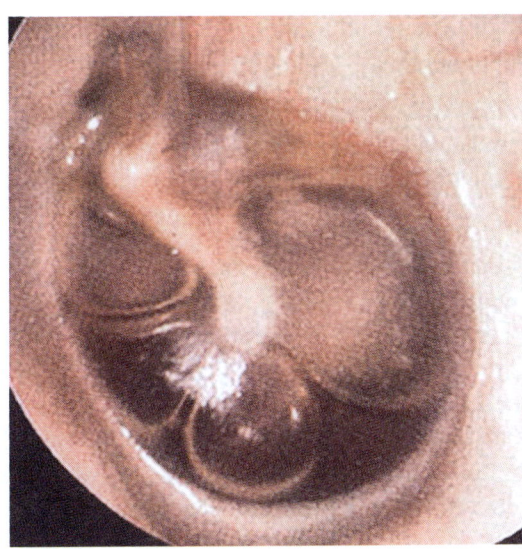

Fig. 6.1: Air bubbles and fluid level in SOM

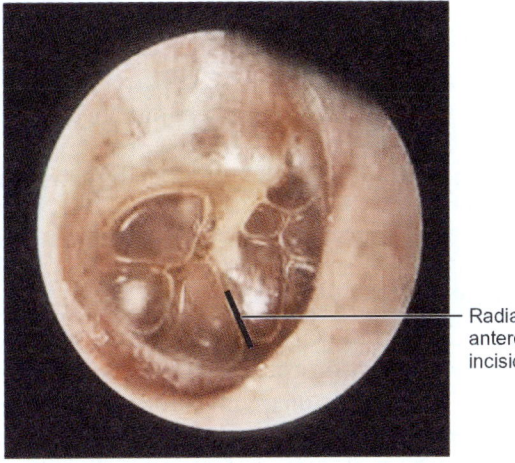

Radial, antero-inferior incision

Fig. 6.2: Site and shape of myringotomy in SOM

classical presentation is resolution of pain and fever due to ASOM but development of fluctuating deafness and a sensation of fullness in the ears.

Examination

On examination the TM appears **dull and retracted** because of the negative pressure in the middle ear due to Eustachian tube blockade. Sometimes **fluid level and air bubbles** may be seen through the TM.

If the fluid stays for a very long time in prolonged obstruction of the Eustachian tube, the fluid thickens due to precipitation of cholesterol in the effusion. This leads to the formation of cholesterol granulomas and gives the TM a bluish appearance. This thick effusion appearing like glue gives SOM its other nomenclature, the glue ear.

Prolonged SOM can lead to formations of retraction pockets in the attic as well as in the pars tensa. Later adhesions form between the retracted tympanic membrane and walls of middle ear leading to adhesive otitis media and can also lead to erosion of ossicles. These retraction pockets act as precursors to primary cholesteatoma formation.

Audiometry

The **hearing tests** suggest conductive pathology, *see* Chapter on audiology.

- **Rinne** → negative
- **Weber** → towards the affected ear
- **Schwabach's** → lengthened
- **Audiogram** → conductive hearing loss of 20–35 dB
- **Impedance** → B type curve **(diagnostic)**

Management

Medical Management

If the underlying cause of SOM is reversible, then the 1st line management is medical which consists of the following:

a. Antiallergics
b. Decongestants

c. If biofilms are involved in the persistent effusion cases subsequent to ASOM, then supposedly higher doses of antibiotics, than we usually use, are needed to treat these individuals.
d. Manoeuvres of auto inflation of Eustachian tube, like Valsalva, Toynbee, etc.

Surgical Management

If SOM **does not resolve after 3 months** of medical management and is associated with hearing loss > 25 dB in both the ears, then the best management of SOM is **surgical** removal of the middle ear fluid with correction of Eustachian tube blockade. Simultaneously a temporary replacement of Eustachian tube is also provided by grommet, see below. This is because the Eustachian tube function might not come back to normal immediately even after the obstructive cause has been treated.

Fluid in the middle ear is drained by giving an incision on the TM, i.e. myringotomy. Here the myringotomy is done by giving a **radial incision** in the **antero-inferior quadrant**. Along with the myringotomy, grommet is also inserted. Over a period of time the grommet gets extruded on its own and the incision site perforation heals by itself.

Grommet is a ventilation tube or tympanostomy tube for ventilating and draining the middle ear, i.e. the same function as that of Eustachian tube.

Hence to summarise the management of persistent (more than 3 months) SOM is **Myringotomy with Grommet** along with **treatment of causative factor (Adenoidectomy/ tonsillectomy,** etc.)

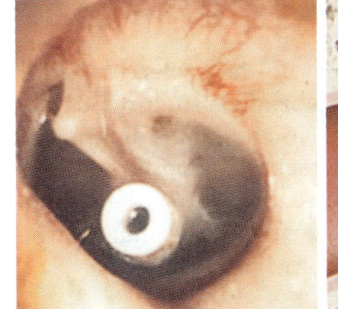
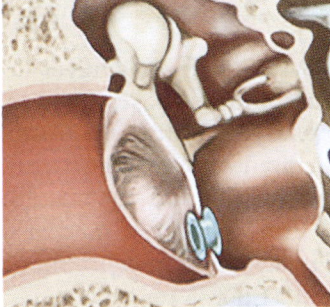

Fig. 6.3: Grommet *in situ*

Ear

Section I

According to the duration for which the grommet stays (after such a time it gets extruded spontaneously), grommet have been divided into:

1. *Short term:* Stay <6 months. These are Shepard and Donaldson grommets.
2. *Midterm:* 6 months–2 years, e.g. Shah, Amstrong grommet, etc.
3. *Long term:* Goldie T tube, Per Lee tube

Myringotomy in SOM *vs* ASOM

1. **In contrast to SOM the Grommet is not put in ASOM** as the Eustachian tube obstruction in ASOM is infective and will resolve quickly on giving antibiotics. It is put in SOM where the Eustachian tube function might not come back to normal immediately even after the ET obstructing cause has been treated.

   Myringotomy in SOM is by radial incision, whereas in ASOM it is by curvilinear incision. This is because the fibres of TM run radially. If we give a radial incision, it will not stay open on itself unless and until we put a grommet to keep the ends apart. Later on when the grommet gets extruded, there will be faster healing of TM.

   So in SOM where we put grommet we give a radial incision, whereas in ASOM where we do not have to put a grommet the incision is against the direction of fibres of TM, i.e. curvilinear or J-shaped so that the opening will stay open on itself and allow the drainage of infected secretions.

2. **In ASOM Myringotomy is done in postero-inferior quadrant because:**
   i. It is easily accessible (the posterior part of TM being more lateral)
   ii. No chance of damage to ossicular chain
   iii. No chance of damage to Chorda tympani nerve

   Whereas in **SOM, Myringotomy is done in antero-inferior quadrant (with grommet insertion) because:**
   i. To simulate Eustachian tube which also lies in the antero-inferior aspect of middle ear cavity.
   ii. It is a relatively avascular area, making the surgery bloodless
   iii. No important structure is present in this area making the surgery safe.

Myringotomy	SOM	ASOM
Grommet insertion	Yes	No
Incision	Radial	Curvilinear
Incision site on TM	Antero-inferior	Postero-inferior

Myringotomy is never done in the **postero-superior quadrant** as most of the important structures of the mesotympanum are present in the postero-superior quadrant and since the narrowest part of middle ear is the mesotympanum only, any of these structures can be injured:

From lateral to medial the **structures** that can be **damaged by a P**ostero-**S**uperior **M**yringotomy are:
1. **C**horda tympani
2. **F**acial nerve,

3. **I**ncudostapedial joint,
4. **O**val window.

Mnemonic: **P**reventive and **S**ocial **M**edicine (**PSM**) is about **C**hildren, **F**emale and **I**mmunization **O**verall.

FUNCTIONS OF EUSTACHIAN TUBE

The Eustachian tube connects the middle ear cavity with the nasopharynx.

The physiologic functions of the Eustachian tube are as follows:

a. **Ventilation or pressure regulation of the middle ear:** Normally the Eustachian tube is closed at rest.

   The Eustachian tube opens upon swallowing or yawning by contraction of the tensor veli palatini muscle. Defective **tensor veli palatini** muscle function in cleft palate results in Eustachian tube dysfunction

   Repeated opening of the Eustachian tube actively maintains middle ear pressure between +50 mm and –50 mm H_2O. Eustachian tube obstruction will lead to –ve pressure in the middle ear and thus retraction of TM and decreased mobility of ossicles and formation of transudate.

   This ventilatory function of the Eustachian tube is less efficient in children than in adults. In addition to this, repeated upper respiratory tract infections and enlarged adenoids in children further contribute to the increased incidence of middle ear disease in them as compared to adults.

b. **Protection of the middle ear from nasopharyngeal secretions and sound pressures:** The Eustachian tube is closed at rest. This prevents retrograde reflux of nasopharyngeal secretions into the middle ear. Also sudden loud sounds (say shouting by the person himself) are dampened before reaching the middle ear through the nasopharynx.

   However, forceful nose blowing creates high nasopharyngeal pressure and may force nasopharyngeal secretions into the middle ear.

   Patulous Eustachian tube is an abnormal condition in which the tube is abnormally patent. The patient often complains about echoing when he or she talks (**autophony**). This can occur due to rapid weight loss leading to decreased size of the Ostmann's pad of fat. This pad of fat is located in the inferolateral aspect of the Eustachian tube and is thought to be an important contributing factor in closing the tube.

c. **Clearance or drainage of middle ear secretions into the nasopharynx:** The Eustachian tube is responsible for drainage of middle ear secretions into the nasopharynx.

The Eustachian tube dysfunction/obstruction causes inadequate drainage of middle ear secretions leading to collection of secretions in the middle ear space.

TESTS OF EUSTACHIAN TUBE (ET) FUNCTION

Normal ET function is very important for the normal functioning of the middle ear. The middle ear will be able to do the impedance matching only if the middle ear pressure matches the ambient atmospheric pressure (read Chapter 2). Also the result of treatment of chronic otitis media and SOM depends on the functioning of the ET. The function of Eustachian tube can be tested by the following:

1. **Tympanometry:** Unlike the other tests mentioned below, which give an idea of the anatomical patency of the ET, tympanometry also assesses its physiological functioning. Hence this is the most reliable test for assessing the Eustachian tube function, also see chapter on audiology.

   High negative middle ear pressure (>90 daPa or mm H_2O) indicates Eustachian tube dysfunction.

   Tympanometry also helps to assess the Eustachian tube function in tympanic membrane perforation. The ear canal is sealed with a probe and a positive or negative pressure of +200 or –200 mm of H_2O is created. The patient is now asked to swallow five times in 20 seconds. If the Eustachian tube is functioning normally, the pressure gets equilibrated to atmospheric pressure following the swallows.

2. **Pneumatic Otoscopy:** Normal tympanic membrane mobility on pneumatic Otoscopy (siegelization) indicates good patency of the Eustachian tube.

3. **Nasopharyngoscopy:** The patency of the Eustachian tube can be tested by direct visualization of its nasopharyngeal opening, using a fiberoptic endoscope.

4. **Eustachian tube catheterization:** Catheterization of the Eustachian tube with a curved metal cannula via the transnasal approach has been used to assess tubal function. It can be done blindly or with the help of a nasopharyngoscope.

   The catheter is passed along the floor of the nose until it touches the posterior wall of the nasopharynx. The catheter is then rotated 90° medially and pulled forward until it impinges on the posterior free part of the nasal septum. The catheter is then rotated 180° laterally, so that its tip will now lie at the nasopharyngeal opening of the Eustachian tube. A Politzer bag is attached to the outer end of the catheter. Air is pushed into the catheter by means of the Politzer bag. Normal blowing sounds mean a patent Eustachian tube and absence of sounds indicates obstruction.

5. **Valsalva and Politzer tests:** In the Valsalva test, the Eustachian tube and middle ear are inflated by a forced expiration with the mouth closed and the nose pinched by the thumb and forefinger. When the tympanic membrane is intact, patent Eustachian tube leads to the overpressure in the middle ear which can be observed by Otoscopy as a bulging of tympanic membrane. When the tympanic membrane is perforated, the sound of the air escaping from the middle ear can be heard with a stethoscope.

   The Politzer test is similar to the Valsalva test, but instead of positive nasopharyngeal pressure being generated by the patient himself during Valsalva manoeuvre, the nasopharynx is passively inflated here. This is achieved by compressing one nostril into which the end of a rubber tube attached to an air bag has been inserted while simultaneously compressing the opposite nostril also by finger pressure.

6. **Toynbee test:** On closed nose swallowing, negative middle ear pressure develops in healthy persons. This negative pressure can be detected on pneumatic otoscopy or tympanometry.

7. **Frenzel Manoeuvre:** This manoeuvre is performed by scuba divers, free divers and by passengers on an aircraft as they descend. The manoeuvre is used to equalize pressure in the middle ear, like Valsalva.

   The Frenzel Manoeuvre is accomplished by pinching the nose and closing the back of the throat as if straining to lift a weight while making the sound of the letter "K". This forces the back of the tongue upward, compressing air against the openings of the Eustachian tubes, thereby equalising pressure in the middle ear.

8. **Sonotubometry:** It is based on the principle that on holding a source of sound in front of the nostrils of a test subject, the sound could be heard more loudly when the test subject swallows as the Eustachian tube opens during swallowing and conducts more sound into the middle ear. In sonotubometry the sound is measured by a microphone in the EAC while the patient keeps swallowing.

Otitic Barotrauma/Barotraumatic Otitis Media/ Aero-otitis Media

Repeated opening of the Eustachian tube actively maintains middle ear pressure between +50 mm and –50 mm H_2O.

During ascent, the atmospheric pressure lowers as compared to the middle ear. This leads to expansion of air in the middle ear and bulging of tympanic membrane. This can lead to a little pain in the ear. When the pressure difference exceeds 15 mm of H_2O, the Eustachian tube passively opens because of increased middle ear pressure and air moves from the high pressure area, i.e. middle ear to the low pressure area, i.e. nasopharynx (Boyle's law). This equalises pressure on both the sides.

During aircraft **descent** or scuba diving descent, the atmospheric pressure increases as compared to the middle ear. This leads to contraction of air in the middle ear and negative middle ear pressure. To equilibrate this pressure the Eustachian tube will have to be now actively opened. This can be done by yawning, swallowing, chewing or by doing valsalva or Frenzel manoeuvre.

Section I Ear

But when the atmospheric pressure gradient becomes >90 mm H$_2$O, i.e. when the external atmospheric pressure becomes higher than the middle ear **pressure by 90 mm of H$_2$O**, the Eustachian tube gets locked by forcing of the soft tissues of the pharyngeal end of the tube into the lumen of the tube. This may occur during fast descent of aircraft or scuba diving, travelling by air during upper respiratory infection and sleeping during descent. The equilibration of middle ear pressure through the Eustachian tube is not possible now. It is now not possible to actively open the Eustachian tube. So in this case the middle ear pressure is negative as compared to the EAC and inner ear. The increased pressure in the EAC pushes the TM inwards leading to retraction of TM or even may perforate it. The retracted TM may cause the foot plate of stapes to move in and the round window membrane to bulge out into the middle ear space. Since the inner ear pressure is already high compared to the middle ear, this can lead to rupture of round window membrane. Valsalva manoeuvre further aggravates the condition by increasing the CSF and inner ear pressure thereby further increasing the chances of rupture of round window membrane.

Also there is stagnation of secretions and hyperaemia leading to transudation and haemorrhages in the middle ear. All these cause ear fullness, otalgia and deafness.

Management

Initially management is conservative. Opening of Eustachian tube can be helped by taking antihistamines or decongestants (pseudoephedrine). Politzerization and Catheterization can be done to actively insufflate air into the middle ear. If the above methods fail and transudate persists, myringotomy can be done.

"Points to Ponder/Points for Quick revision"

- SOM: Collection of sterile fluid in the middle ear.
- 2° to non-infective ET obstruction:
  a. Hypertrophied adenoids in children → B/L SOM, Nasopharyngeal tumour in adults → U/L SOM
  b. Enlarged tonsils
  c. Otitic barotrauma
- 2° to interference with ET opening, e.g. in palatal palsy and cleft palate
- 2° to increased production in allergies
- 2° to biofilms formation in inadequately treated ASOM
- CFs: B/L fluctuating painless CHL in children (SOM is the MC underlying cause) → delayed development of speech. U/L CHL in adults with nasopharyngeal Ca.
- Dull, retracted, bluish TM (glue ear, due to precipitation of cholesterol) with fluid level and air bubbles
- Long standing SOM → Adhesive otitis media
- If no resolution even after 3 months of medical treatment → Myringotomy (radial incision, antero-inferior quadrant) with grommet insertion (for functional recovery of ET) along with treatment of underlying cause, e.g. adenoidectomy, tonsillectomy, etc.
- ET: Maintains middle ear pressure, protect it from nasopharyngeal secretions, drains its secretions.
- Loss of Ostmann's pad of fat → patulous opened ET → Autophony.
- Tympanometry-most reliable test of ET functioning (tests physiological functioning as well as its anatomical patency).
- Pneumatic Otoscopy, Nasopharyngoscopy, ET catheterisation, Valsalva and Politzer tests, Toynbee test and Frenzel manoeuvre are the tests for checking ET patency.
- Otitic barotrauma: Rapid (pressure gradient >90 mm H$_2$O) aircraft or Scuba diving descent → locked ET (Valsalva now cannot open it) → Severely retracted TM or even perforation of TM and round window, haemorrhage. Treatment-mainly Conservative.

PREVIOUSLY ASKED QUESTIONS

1. **Glue ear:** *(Exam 2003, 2017)*
   a. Is painful
   b. Is painless
   c. Radical mastoidectomy is required
   d. Na F is useful

2. **A boy with ASOM underwent treatment for the same. Now presents with subsidence of pain but persistence of deafness. O/E TM appears dull, diagnosis is:** *(Kolkata 2003, 2017)*
   a. Ototoxicity
   b. Secretory otitis media
   c. Adhesive otitis media
   d. Tympanosclerosis

3. **Blue ear drum is seen in:** *(Exam 2013)*
   a. Serous otitis media
   b. CSOM
   c. Perforation
   d. None

4. **U/L non-suppurative Otitis media in adults is due to:** *(UP 2003, 2017)*
   a. Allergic rhinitis
   b. URTI
   c. Trauma
   d. Malignancy

5. **All are false in a case of secretory otitis media except:** *(MAHE 2005, 2016)*
   a. Red TM
   b. B-shaped tympanogram
   c. Marginal perforation most common
   d. Rinne test +ve

6. **A 55-year-old man presented with U/L conductive hearing loss, fullness sensation in ear, no discharge, TM Normal, Tympanometry shows B type graph. What is the Next Step of management:** *(AIIMS 2012, 2013)*
   a. Myringotomy with grommet
   b. Evaluation for Nasopharyngeal Mass
   c. Antibiotics
   d. Observation

7. **Cause of unilateral secretory Otitis media in an adult is:** *(PGI Dec 99, UP 2004, Exam 2013)*
   a. CSOM
   b. Nasopharyngeal carcinoma
   c. Mastoiditis
   d. Foreign body of external ear

8. **Secretory Otitis media (SOM) is diagnosed by:** *(PGI June 98, 2013)*
   a. Impedance audiometry
   b. Pure tone audiometry
   c. X-ray
   d. Otoscopy

9. **In serous Otitis media which one of the following statements is true:** *(AIIMS 2004)*
   a. Sensorineural deafness occurs as a complication in 80% of the cases
   b. Intracranial spread of the infection complicates the clinical courses
   c. Tympanostomy tubes are usually required for treatment
   d. Gram-positive organisms are grown routinely in culture in the aspirate

10. **Following statements are true about otitis media with effusion in a child:** *(PGI Dec 2003, 2009)*
    a. Immediate myringotomy is done
    b. Type B tympanogram
    c. The effusion of middle ear is sterile
    d. Most common cause of deafness in children in daycare patients

11. **Treatment of choice for glue ear is:** *(AIIMS May 2007)*
    a. Myringotomy with cold knife
    b. Myringotomy with diode laser
    c. Myringotomy with ventilation tube insertion
    d. Conservative treatment with analgesics and antibiotics

12. **Grommet insertion with myringotomy is done at:** *(CUPGEE 2002, Kolkata 2002, RJ 2001, Exam 2013)*
    a. Antero-inferior quadrant
    b. Postero-inferior quadrant
    c. Antero-superior quadrant
    d. Postero-superior quadrant

13. **Grommet tube is used in:** *(TN 2002, 2017)*
    a. Chronic otitis media
    b. Necrotising otitis media
    c. Serous otitis media
    d. All of the above

14. **Procedure for serous otitis media is:** *(AP 2002, 2017)*
    a. Tympanoplasty
    b. Mastoidectomy
    c. Myringotomy
    d. Stapedotomy

15. **To do myringotomy in ASOM, the incision is given in posteroinferior region, this is the preferred region for all the following reasons except:** *(AI 2007, 2017)*
    a. It is easily accessible
    b. Damage to ossicular chain does not occur
    c. Damage to chorda tympani is avoided
    d. It is the least vascular region

16. **Cause for grommet insertion:** *(TN 2008, Exam 2013)*
    a. Secretory otitis media
    b. Otosclerosis
    c. CSOM
    d. Cholesteatoma

Section I Ear

17. A child has Adenoidectomy done but he has effusion in middle ear. What is done next:
                                                        (*Exam 2014*)
    a. Grommet insertion
    b. Mastoidectomy
    c. Tympanoplasty
    d. None

18. A 6-yr-old child presents with recurrent URTI with mouth breathing and failure to grow with high arched palate and impaired hearing. His tympanogram finding is given below. He should be managed by:
                                    (*Practice question by Author*)

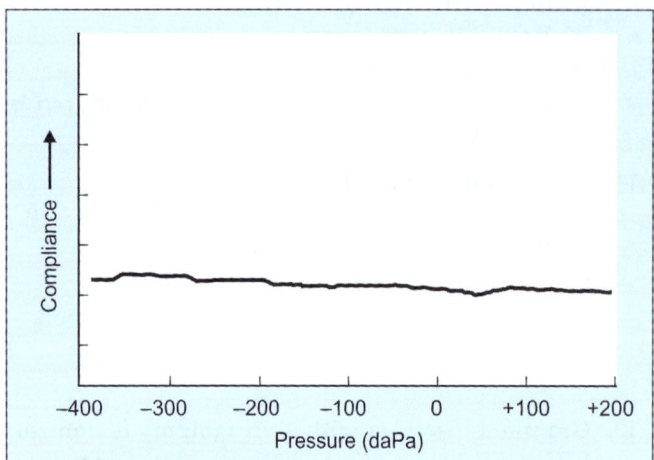

    a. Myringotomy
    b. Grommet insertion
    c. Myringotomy with grommet insertion
    d. Adenoidectomy with grommet insertion

19. A child presenting with recurrent respiratory tract infection, mouth breathing and decreased hearing. Treatment is: (*PGI 2008*)
    a. Tonsillectomy   b. Adenoidectomy
    c. Grommet insertion   d. Myringotomy
    e. Myringoplasty

20. Autophony is seen in which condition of Eustachian tube: (*Exam 2010*)
    a. Blocked Eustachian tube
    b. Eustachian tube dysgenesis
    c. Patulous Eustachian tube
    d. Retraction of Eustachian tube

21. All are tests to check Eustachian tube patency except: (*AIIMS 98, 2015*)
    a. Valsalva manoeuvre
    b. Fistula test
    c. Frenzel manoeuvre
    d. Toynbee's manoeuvre

22. Eustachian tube gets blocked if pressure difference is more than: (*Exam 2012*)
    a. 15 mm of H_2O b. 30 mm H_2O
    c. 50 mm H_2O d. 90 mm H_2O

23. At what atmosphere pressure gradient barotraumatic otitis media occurs: (*JIPMER 2002, Delhi 2008, 2016*)
    a. 80 mm of H_2O
    b. 90 mm of H_2O
    c. 100 mm of H_2O
    d. 120 mm of H_2O

24. Otitic barotrauma results due to:
                                    (*PGI June 97, Exam 2013*)
    a. Ascent in air
    b. Descent in air
    c. Linear acceleration
    d. Sudden acceleration

25. A child presents with barotrauma pain without middle ear inflammation. Treatment:
                                    (*Jharkhand 2003, Exam 2017*)
    a. Antibiotics
    b. Myringotomy
    c. Supportive
    d. Grommet

26 After what duration of medical management in SOM, is myringotomy done: (*Exam 2013*)
    a. 1 month   b. 3 months
    c. 6 months   d. 1 year

27. All of the following are tests for patency of the Eustachian tube except: (*Exam 2013*)
    a. Valsalva test
    b. Caloric test
    c. Tympanometry
    d. Politzer test

28. Ventilation tube is put in the ear in cases of:
                                                        (*Exam 2016*)
    a. Otosclerosis
    b. Labyrinthitis
    c. Serous otitis media
    d. CSOM

29. During flying in an aeroplane, barotrauma occurs with: (*Exam 2016*)
    a. Ascent   b. Descent
    c. Both   d. None

30. Glue ear is also known as: (*Exam 2016*)
    a. Serous otitis media
    b. Chronic suppurative Otitis media
    c. Acute mastoiditis
    d. Acute suppurative otitis media

31. A 7-year-old child presents with bilateral hearing difficulty for three months. Impedance audiometry shows type B Curve. There is bilateral conductive hearing deficit. There is no sign of infection. Next step is: (*Exam 2016*)
    a. Wait and watch
    b. Antibiotics
    c. Myringotomy and grommet
    d. Canal wall down procedure

32. **In the given condition which one of the following statements is true:** (*Practice question by Author*)

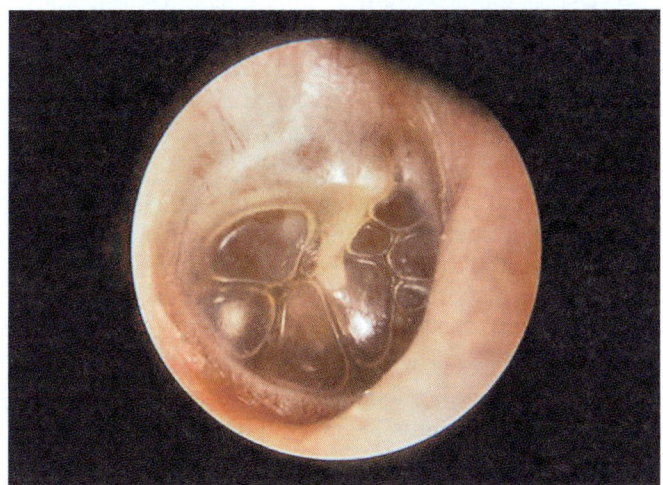

a. Sensorineural deafness occurs as a complication in 80% of the cases
b. Intracranial spread of the infection complicates the clinical courses
c. Tympanostomy tubes are usually required for treatment
d. Gram-negative organisms are grown routinely in culture in the aspirate

33. **Eustachian tube function is best assessed by:** (*AIIMS 2015*)
a. Politzerisation   b. Tympanometry
c. VEMP   d. Rhinomanometry

34. **In a child with serous otitis media, hearing loss is typically:** (*JIPMER 2015*)
a. 10–20 dB   b. 20–40 dB
c. 40–60 dB   d. 60–80 dB

35. **The most reliable method of detecting otitis media with effusion is** (*Kerala PGMEE 2015*)
a. Pure tone audiometry
b. Otoscopic examination
c. X-ray mastoids
d. Tympanometry

36. **True about grommet insertion:** (*PGI May 2015*)
a. Small plastic tube aerating middle ear
b. Maximum duration of grommet insertion is 5 months

c. Healing occurs spontaneously after extrusion
d. It is placed anteriorly on tympanic membrane
e. Surgery is always needed to remove it

37. **The treatment of choice of glue ear is:** (*JIPMER 2015*)
a. Myringoplasty
b. Decongestants and antiallergics
c. Steroid drops
d. Low power hearing aid

IMAGE BASED PRACTICE QUESTIONS BY THE AUTHOR

38. **The following type of incision on the TM is given in which condition:**

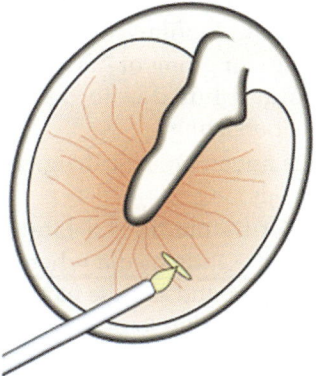

a. ASOM   b. Safe CSOM
c. SOM   d. Unsafe CSOM

39. **The following are used in:**

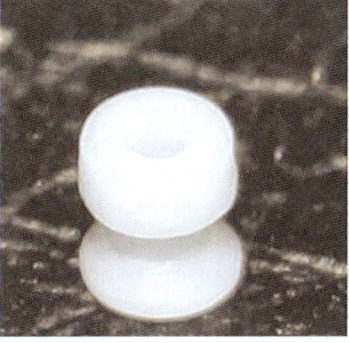 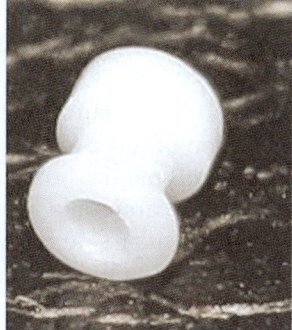

a. ASOM
b. CSOM
c. SOM
d. All of the above

Section I ‖ **Ear**

ANSWERS AND EXPLANATIONS

1. **(b) Is painless** (*Ref. Scott Brown, 8th ed., Vol 2; 115*)
   - Unlike ASOM Glue ear being a non-infective condition (or the biofilm aggregated bacteria being sequestered), is therefore painless.
   - Radical mastoidectomy is done in unsafe CSOM. In Glue ear if medical management does not help then the best management is Myringotomy with Grommet insertion along with Adenoidectomy/tonsillectomy.
   - Na F is given in active Otosclerosis.

2. **(b) Secretory otitis media** (*Ref. Cummings, 6th ed., 2139*)
   - This is a case of SOM developing over ASOM probably due to Biofilms formation, (please see the text) so some symptoms of ASOM, i.e. pain and fever have subsided but due to persistence of fluid deafness is persisting.
   - Penicillin is not an ototoxic drug, *see* Chapter 12 for ototoxic drugs.
   - Adhesive Otitis media is a late complication of chronic serous Otitis media where adhesions form between the TM and middle ear structures leading to conductive hearing loss.
   - Tympanosclerosis is also a late complication of chronic serous Otitis media. It can also follow CSOM. Here there is hyalinisation and calcification of tympanic membrane seen as thickened white patches on the TM. In most patients, these plaques are clinically insignificant and cause a little or no hearing impairment.

3. **(a) Serous otitis media** (*Ref. Cummings, 6th ed., 3020*)

4. **(d) Malignancy** (*Ref. Scott Brown, 8th ed., Vol 2; 973*)
   - Any adult presenting with U/L non-suppurative Otitis media should be investigated for nasopharyngeal carcinoma which might be obstructing that particular side Eustachian tube.
   - If serous Otitis media occurs because of overproduction of middle ear fluid due to allergy, it will be bilateral.
   - URTI may lead to ASOM.
   - Trauma does not lead to Serous Otitis media.

5. **(b) B-shaped tympanogram** (*Ref. Shambaugh, 6th ed., 427*)
   - In SOM Tympanic membrane is dull and retracted and may appear bluish. Perforation is not seen here and Rinne test is –ve.

6. **(b) Evaluation for Nasopharyngeal Mass** (*Ref. Cummings, 6th ed., 2035*)
   - This man is suffering from U/L SOM. Any adult presenting with U/L SOM should be investigated for nasopharyngeal carcinoma. If this is ruled out, then initially conservative management in the form of antihistaminics and decongestants and later if no relief Myringotomy with grommet insertion is done.

7. **(b) Nasopharyngeal carcinoma** (*Ref. Cummings, 6th ed., 2035*)
   - CSOM and Mastoiditis do not lead to Serous Otitis media.
   - Foreign body of external ear will not lead to fluid collection in middle ear.

8. **(a) and (d) Impedance audiometry, otoscopy** (*Ref. Cummings, 6th ed., 3020*)
   - A patient presenting with painless blocked feeling of ear in a sub-acute fashion and on otoscopy TM appearing dull and retracted and showing fluid levels or air bubbles, a diagnosis of SOM is considered. The diagnostic investigation is impedance audiometry which shows B type curve.
   - Pure tone audiometry shows conductive hearing loss of approximately 20–35 dB which can also be seen in complete obstruction of EAC or in TM perforation, *see* Chapter 2.
   - X-ray of the mastoid may show clouding which can also be seen in ASOM and mastoiditis.

9. **(c) Tympanostomy tubes are usually required for treatment** (*Ref. Cummings, 6th ed., 3031*)
   - SOM leads to conductive deafness of approximately 20–35 dB.
   - SOM does not lead to intracranial complications.
   - If medical management does not help, then the best management of SOM is surgical, i.e. Myringotomy (to remove the collected fluid) with tympanostomy tube (or Grommet or ventilation tube) insertion (to provide ventilation to middle ear for the time being till Eustachian tube opens up) along with treatment of causative factor (Adenoidectomy/tonsillectomy).
   - SOM being non-infective or the biofilm aggregated bacteria being sequestered, there are no organisms in the fluid.

10. **(b), (c) and (d)** (*Ref. Scott Brown, 8th ed., Vol 2; 121*)
    - The initial management of otitis media with effusion consists of Antiallergics and Decongestants. Myringotomy is done in patients not responding to medical management after a duration of 3 months and an associated hearing loss of > 25 dB in both the ears.

11. **(c) Myringotomy with ventilation tube insertion** (*Ref. Scott Brown, 8th ed., Vol 2; 125*)

12. **(a) Antero-inferior quadrant** (*Ref. Scott Brown, 8th ed., Vol 2; 126*)

13. **(c) Serous otitis media** (*Ref. Scott Brown, 8th ed., Vol 2; 126*)

14. **(c) Myringotomy** (*Ref. Scott Brown, 8th ed., Vol 2; 125*)
    - Tympanoplasty constitutes surgical repair of the TM, i.e. myringoplasty along with replacement of ossicles, i.e. ossiculoplasty and is the procedure for CSOM.

15. **(d) It is the least vascular region** (*Ref. Scott Brown, 8th ed., Vol 2; 126*)

16. **(a) Secretory otitis media** (*Ref. Scott Brown, 8th ed., Vol 2; 125*)

17. **(a) Grommet insertion** (*Ref. Scott Brown, 8th ed., Vol 2; 125*)
    - Since Eustachian tube function takes time to come back to normal Myringotomy with grommet should have been done along with adenoidectomy in the mentioned child.

18. **(d) Adenoidectomy with grommet insertion** (*Ref. Scott Brown, 8th ed., Vol 2; 125*)
    - This child is suffering from adenotonsillar hypertrophy which is causing recurrent URTI, mouth breathing, failure to grow and high-arched palate, refer the chapter on adenoids.
    - Hypertrophied adenoids may have led to Eustachian tube blockade with a resultant SOM which explains impaired hearing.
    - So the treatment is adenoidectomy with grommet insertion. It is understood that the grommet has to be put by radial Myringotomy in the antero-inferior quadrant.

19. **(a), (b), (c) and (d)** (*Ref. Scott Brown, 8th ed., Vol 2; 126*)
    - This child is probably suffering from adenotonsillar hypertrophy which is causing recurrent respiratory tract infections and mouth breathing.
    - Hypertrophied adenoids/tonsils might have led to Eustachian tube blockade with a resultant SOM which explains decreased hearing.
    - So the treatment is Myringotomy with grommet insertion along with Adeno-tonsillectomy in the same sitting.
    - Myringoplasty is the surgical repair of TM and is done in CSOM.

20. **(c) Patulous Eustachian tube** (*Ref. Scott Brown, 8th ed., Vol 2; 1041*)
21. **(b) Fistula test** (*Ref. Cummings, 6th ed., 2036*)
    Fistula test is a test of vestibular function, *see* Chapter 3.
22. **(d) 90 mm H$_2$O** (*Ref. Scott Brown, 8th ed., Vol 2; 1119*)
23. **(b) 90 mm of H$_2$O** (*Ref. Scott Brown, 8th ed., Vol 2; 1119*)
24. **(b) Descent in air** (*Ref. Scott Brown, 8th ed., Vol 2; 1121*)
25. **(c) Supportive** (*Ref. Scott Brown, 8th ed., Vol 2; 1123*)
26. **(b) 3 months** (*Ref. Scott Brown, 8th ed., Vol 2; 130*)
27. **(b) Caloric test** (*Ref. Cummings, 6th ed., 2036*)
28. **(c) Serous otitis media** (*Ref. Scott Brown, 8th ed., Vol 2; 125*)
29. **(b) Descent** (*Ref. Scott Brown, 8th ed., Vol 2; 1121*)
30. **(a) Serous otitis media** (*Ref. Scott Brown, 8th ed., Vol 2; 115*)
31. **(c) Myringotomy and grommet** (*Ref. Scott Brown, 8th ed., Vol 2; 125*)
32. **(c) Tympanostomy tubes are usually required for treatment** (*Ref. Scott Brown, 8th ed., Vol 2; 125*)
33. **(b) Tympanometry** (*Ref. Cummings, 6th ed., 2036*)
34. **(b) 20–40 dB** (*Ref. Scott Brown, 8th ed., Vol 2; 122*)
35. **(d) Tympanometry** (*Ref. Scott Brown, 8th ed., Vol 2; 120*)
36. **(a), (c) and (d) Small plastic tube aerating middle ear. Healing occurs spontaneously after extrusion. It is placed anteriorly on tympanic membrane** (*Ref. Scott Brown, 8th ed., Vol 2; 126*)
37. **(b) Decongestants and antiallergics** (*Ref. Scott Brown, 8th ed., Vol 2; 126*)
38. **(c) SOM** (*Ref. Scott Brown, 8th ed., Vol 2; 126*)
39. **(c) SOM** (*Ref. Scott Brown, 8th ed., Vol 2; 126*)

Tubotympanic or Chronic Mucosal Otitis Media

Chronic infection of the middle ear and mastoid is known as chronic suppurative Otitis media or nowadays preferably as chronic otitis media (COM).

Pathophysiology

The characteristic of CSOM is a **permanent perforation** in TM.

When a TM perforation heals by itself, it heals in two layers only, the outer epithelial layer of one end of perforation meets the epithelial layer of other end and the inner endothelial layer of one end of perforation meets the endothelial layer of the other end leading to healing of the perforation. This is what usually happens following traumatic perforation or perforation during ASOM.

However, if the epithelial layer grows towards the inside and meets the endothelial layer all along the margins of perforation, i.e. epithelisation of the margin occurs then the perforation does not heal and becomes permanent. This will now lead to CSOM.

If a perforation heals by itself it usually heals by 6–12 weeks so if the perforation persists after 12 weeks it is considered permanent and now the condition leads to CSOM.

Any perforation either following ASOM or trauma, if becomes permanent will ultimately lead to CSOM.

CSOM (as its name) is caused by **mixed aerobic and anaerobic bacteria**. MC aerobic being **Pseudomonas** others include *Staph. aureus*, Proteus, *E. coli*, etc. Among anaerobes are mainly bacteroides.

Types of CSOM

CSOM can be of two types:
1. **Tubotympanic or safe CSOM/mucosal COM (safe chronic suppurative otitis media is now preferably called as mucosal chronic otitis media)**
2. **Atticoantral or unsafe CSOM** (*see* next Chapter)

Tubotympanic CSOM

It is also known as safe or benign disease or mucosal disease. It is associated with **a permanent perforation anywhere in the pars tensa which is not marginal,** *see* photo below. This perforation exposes the middle ear to

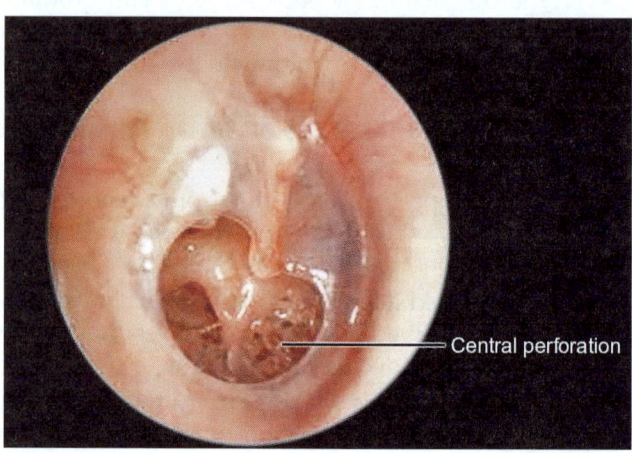

Central perforation

repeated infections from the external ear leading to ear discharge. Also any infection of the naso or oropharynx, which reaches the middle ear through the Eustachian tube, will lead to discharge (mucoid or mucopurulent) from the middle ear (called active mucosal COM). Since here the part of the ear developing from tubo-tympanic recess (from 1st and 2nd pouch), i.e. Eustachian tube and tympanic cavity gets affected, it is known as tubo-tympanic. In between the infection episodes when the ear is dry and the middle ear and mastoid are not inflamed it is known as inactive mucosal COM.

Clinical Features

The patient here presents with:
  i. **Painless mucoid or mucopurulent, ear discharge** with non-offensive odour.
 ii. **Conductive hearing loss (CHL)** (of 10–40 dB depending upon the size and the site of perforation). In long standing disease ossicles might also get necrosed because of repeated episodes of infection, leading to increase in hearing loss. The **MC ossicle** to get **necrosed** is **long process of incus** because of its precarious blood supply. It is important to remember that in safe CSOM/mucosal COM, there is no erosion of bony walls of middle ear. Erosion of bones is seen in unsafe CSOM characterised by cholesteatoma, *see* next Chapter.

Management

Medical Management

A permanent perforation does not heal by medical management. It has to be repaired surgically. But the pre-requisite for surgical repair is that the ear should be dry and free of infection. For this ear toileting is done and local and systemic antibiotics are given.

SURGICAL REPAIR

Myringoplasty

Once the ear is **dry for 6 weeks** (i.e. the disease is in inactive mucosal form now) without antibiotics, surgical repair is taken up.

Surgical repair of TM is known as myringoplasty. This is done with an operating microscope with a focal length of 200–250 mm. Here the perforation is repaired by a graft which is most commonly taken from the fascia overlying the temporalis muscle of the patient, hence called the **temporalis fascia autograft**. The graft can also be taken from the tragal perichondrium, tragal or conchal cartilage or fat.

There are 2 primary grafting techniques **employed while performing myringoplasty:**

1. **Overlay technique** (lateral grafting)
2. **Underlay technique** (medial grafting)

These terms refer to the **position of the graft in relation to the fibrous annulus (and not to the malleus for** in both a portion of the graft is tucked medial to the malleus handle, read below). The basic procedure for both is to excise the rim of perforation so that there is raw surface from which new tissue will grow. The graft acts as a scaffold for the growth of the new squamous epithelial layer on the EAC side of TM and growth of mucosal layer on the middle ear side of TM. The graft itself becomes the middle fibrous layer.

Overlay technique: After excising the rim of perforation, the squamous epithelial layer of the tympanic membrane remnant is completely raised, keeping the fibrous layer along with the annulus and endothelial layer of tympanic membrane in place. The fascia graft is then placed **(over), i.e. lateral to the** fibrous middle layer of tympanic membrane and its annulus. During this overlay placement a part of the fascia graft over the perforation is insinuated through the perforation and made to lie under the handle of malleus. This is done to prevent lateralisation of the fascia graft. The previously raised tympanic membrane epithelium is then replaced lateral to the graft.

Disadvantage of overlay technique: Despite the insinuation of graft there is still a risk of lateralization of the graft and resultant blunting of anterior meatal recess.

Underlay technique: After excising the rim of perforation, the entire TM along with its annulus is raised. The fascia graft is then placed (under) medial to the tympanic membrane and its annulus, and a part of the graft is passed under the malleus.

Disadvantage of underlay technique: Overall underlay technique is better than overlay technique. Underlay technique is associated with rare chances of reduction in middle ear space which may lead to medialisation or adhesions between the graft and medial wall of middle ear, thereby causing atelectasis of middle ear cavity.

Ossiculoplasty

While doing myringoplasty if any ossicle is found to be necrosed, then it is replaced, i.e. ossiculoplasty is done. This replacement is done either with tragal or conchal cartilage or resculptured autograft ossicles or prosthetic implants, e.g. TORP/PORP (*see* below).

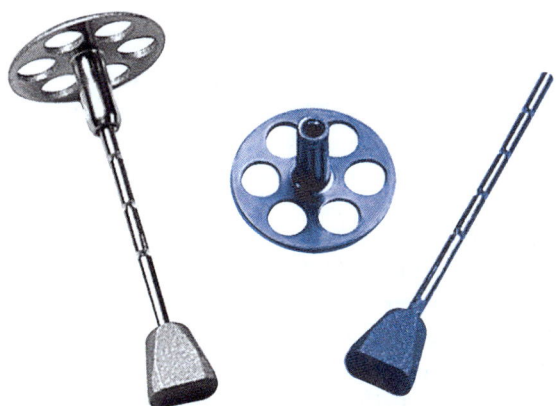

Fig. 7.1: TORP and PORP Prosthesis

The prosthetic implants used during the ossiculoplasty are:

1. **TORP:** Total ossicular replacement prosthesis. This is used when all the ossicles are missing or only the malleus handle is present. It is kept in **between the tympanic membrane/malleus handle and stapes footplate**.

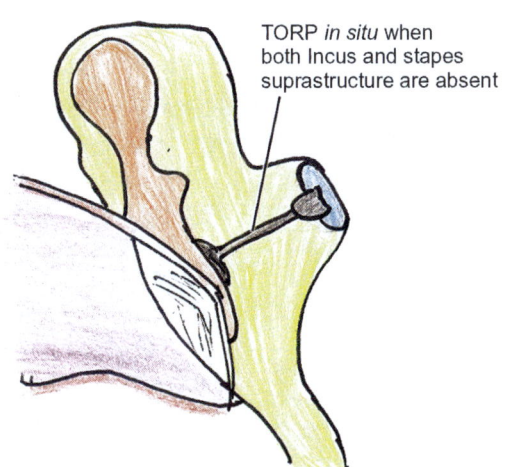

TORP *in situ* when both Incus and stapes suprastructure are absent

Fig. 7.2: TORP

2. **PORP:** Partial ossicular replacement prosthesis. This is used when the malleus and incus are absent or when only incus is absent. It is kept in **between the tympanic membrane and stapes head**.

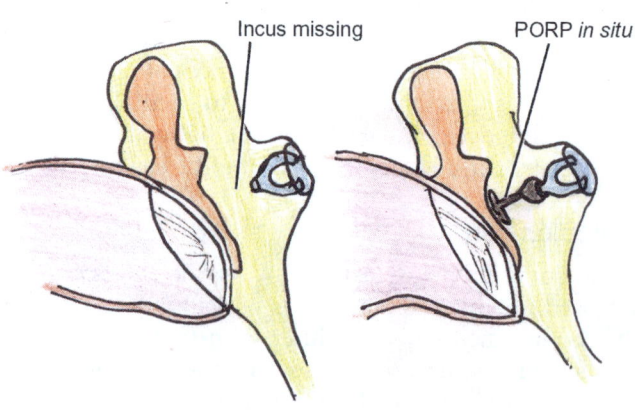

Fig. 7.3: PORP

The use of TORP or PORP or any other prosthesis depends on which ossicles are eroded.

Austin classified the ossicular erosions into four types. Since the most common ossicle to get eroded as mentioned above is incus, this classification is **based on the presence or absence of malleus handle (M) and stapes suprastructure (S)** (i.e. head, neck, anterior and posterior crura of stapes), **assuming the incus to be absent in all cases** since it is the first ossicle to be eroded.

a. *Type A:* **M+S+**; Both malleus handle and stapes suprastructure are present here and only the incus is absent. Therefore, reconstruction is by PORP.

b. *Type B:* **M+S−**; Here malleus handle is present, incus and stapes suprastructure are absent. Therefore, reconstruction is by TORP.

c. *Type C:* **M−S+**; Both malleus handle and incus are absent here and only the stapes suprastructure is present. Therefore, reconstruction is by PORP.

d. *Type D:* **M−S−**; All the ossicles are missing. Therefore, reconstruction is by TORP.

Tympanoplasty

Surgical repair of the TM (myringoplasty) with ossiculoplasty is together known as tympanoplasty.

Wullstein Divided Tympanoplasty into 5 Types

Type I: It is done when tympanic membrane is perforated but the ossicles are intact. Here we put the temporalis fascia graft over 1st ossicle (so type 1), i.e. malleus. It is known as type I tympanoplasty. This is the same as **myringoplasty**.

Type II: It is done for tympanic membrane perforation with erosion of malleus only. Here we put the temporalis fascia graft anywhere over the 2nd ossicle (so type 2), i.e. incus, or the remnant of malleus.

Type III: It is done for tympanic membrane perforation with erosion of malleus and incus. Since the most common ossicle to be necrosed is the incus, this is the most commonly done tympanoplasty. Here we put the temporalis fascia graft anywhere over the 3rd ossicle (so type 3), i.e. stapes (either head or footplate of stapes) after keeping an autograft or PORP/TORP (type C/type D Austin ossicular erosion). Therefore, Type III tympanoplasty is also known as **myringostapediopexy**.

Another term to describe type III tympanoplasty is **"Columella tympanoplasty"** (this is because in the middle ear of birds there is only one ossicle which is named columella and here also the middle ear is left with only one ossicle).

Type IV: All the three ossicles are absent here. The graft (Temporalis fascia) is placed in between the oval window

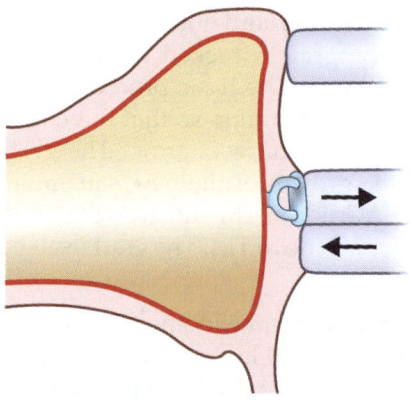

Fig. 7.5: Type 3 Myringo-stapediopexy

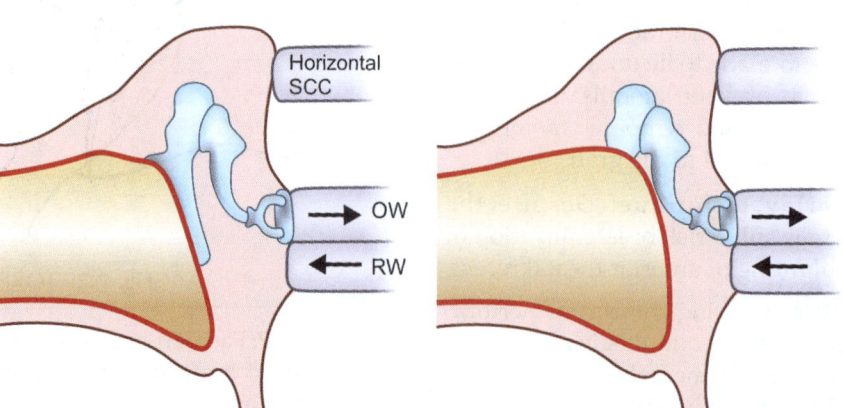

Fig. 7.4: Type 1 Myringoplasty; Type 2 Myringo-incudopexy

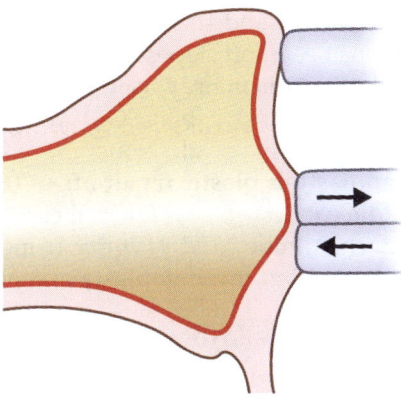

Fig. 7.6: Type 4 Cavum minor

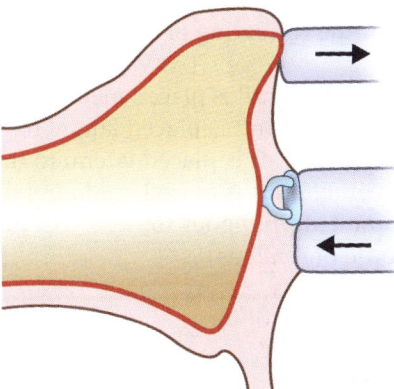

Fig. 7.7: Type 5 Fenestration

above and round window below. The Temporalis fascia graft which now forms the tympanic membrane covers the round window and Eustachian tube. The Stapes foot plate overlying the oval window is kept outside the middle ear cavity, exposed to the exterior so that sound waves hit the oval window directly. The round window being covered the **phase difference is maintained** (so type 4) as the sound does not reach both the windows at the same

time. Here the middle ear becomes small. This small middle ear cavity is known as cavum minor.

Type V: When the footplate of stapes is completely fixed, leading to fixity of oval window also which now can no longer vibrate to sound waves, a fenestra (an opening) is made on the bulge of lateral semicircular canal just above the oval window. This is known as **fenestration operation**. However, it is no more done now. Fenestration operation is an iatrogenic cause of positive fistula test, *see* chapter on vestibular system.

 "Points to Ponder/Points for Quick revision"

- Tubotympanic/Safe CSOM—now called Tubotympanic/mucosal COM.
- Permanent perforation (non-marginal) ± ossicular necrosis (MC—incus, Austin classification—M ± S±).
- Active or inactive mucosal COM—terms used depending upon whether infection is presently there or not.
- CFs—Mucoid/mucopurulent, painless, non-offensive discharge and CHL
- Definitive treatment of surgery:
  i. Myringoplasty—if only perforation is there, ear dry for >6 weeks, autologous temporalis fascia graft, underlay preferred
  ii. Ossiculoplasty—if ossicles are additionally necrosed, ossicular replacement prosthesis used either total or partial (TORP/PORP)
  iii. Tympanoplasty—Myringoplasty + Ossiculoplasty (types I–V by Wullstein)
     – Type 1—Myringoplasty
     – Type II—Graft placed over IInd ossicle, i.e. incus
     – Type III—MC (Myringostapediopexy/columella tympanoplasty)
     – Type IV—Stapes foot plate overlying oval window is kept outside the middle ear cavity
     – Type V—Fenestration operation.

PREVIOUSLY ASKED QUESTIONS

1. **True about safe CSOM:** *(PGI Dec 2000, 2011)*
   a. Aetiology is multiple bacteria
   b. Oral antibiotics are not effective
   c. Ear drops have no role
   d. Otic hydrocephalus is a complication
   e. Ossicular erosion is not seen

2. **Treatment of choice in central safe perforation is:** *(AI 94, Exam 2014)*
   a. Modified mastoidectomy
   b. Tympanoplasty
   c. Myringoplasty
   d. Conservative management

3. **Ossicle most commonly involved in CSOM:** *(Kolkata 2004, Exam 2016)*
   a. Stapes
   b. Long process of incus
   c. Head malleus
   d. Handle of malleus

4. **In tubo-tympanic CSOM commonest operation done is:** *(AI 97, Exam 2016)*
   a. Modified radical mastoidectomy
   b. Radical mastoidectomy
   c. Simple mastoidectomy
   d. Tympanoplasty

5. **Surgery on ear drum is done using:** *(Kerala 91, Exam 2011)*
   a. Operative microscope
   b. Laser
   c. Direct vision
   d. Blindly

6. **The focal length of the lens used in microscopic ear surgeries is:** *(JIPMER 2002, AIIMS 2005, 2014)*
   a. 300 mm
   b. 150 mm
   c. 250 mm
   d. 400 mm

7. **What is tympanoplasty?** *(Exam 2013)*
   a. Eradication of middle ear disease with reconstruction of tympanic membrane and ossicles
   b. Eradication of disease from internal ear
   c. Eradication of middle ear disease with repair of tympanic membrane only
   d. Eradication of middle ear disease with repair of ossicles only

8. **Columella effect is seen in:** *(TN 2005, Exam 2017)*
   a. Tympanoplasty
   b. Septoplasty
   c. Tracheostomy
   d. None of the above

9. **Columella tympanoplasty is:** *(Exam 2016)*
   a. Type I
   b. Type II
   c. Type III
   d. Type IV

10. **Myringoplasty is done using:** *(RJ 2003, Exam 2017)*
    a. Temporalis fascia
    b. Dura mater
    c. Periosteum
    d. Mucous membrane

11. **Material used in Tympanoplasty:** *(PGI 98, 2003, 2013)*
    a. Temporalis fascia
    b. Cartilage
    c. Muscle
    d. Mucous membrane

12. **Austin's classification for ossicular chain defects depends on:** *(DPG 2009)*
    a. Malleus head and stapes footplate
    b. Malleus handle and stapes suprastructure
    c. Malleus head and stapes suprastructure
    d. Malleus head and stapes head

13. **Tympanoplasty is mainly used for:** *(Exam 2013)*
    a. Otosclerosis
    b. CSOM
    c. ASOM
    d. None

14. **Myringoplasty is plastic repair of:** *(Exam 2011)*
    a. Middle ear
    b. Internal ear
    c. Eustachian tube
    d. Tympanic membrane

15. **All are true about myringoplasty except:** *(Delhi 2008)*
    a. It is done by overlay and under lay techniques
    b. Temporalis fascia graft is the most commonly used graft
    c. Reconstruction of the TM is done
    d. If required malleus is also reconstructed

16. **Which of the following is true regarding myringo-plasty:** *(AI 2013)*
    a. In underlay graft is placed medial to the annulus
    b. In underlay graft is placed lateral to the malleus
    c. In overlay graft is placed lateral to the malleus
    d. In overlay graft is placed medial to the annulus

17. **Least blood supply goes to:** *(Exam 2016)*
    a. Handle of malleus
    b. Body of incus
    c. Long process of incus
    d. Stapes

18. **In tympanic membrane perforation, graft is taken from temporalis muscle fascia. What type of graft is this?** *(Exam 2016)*
    a. Autograft
    b. Allograft
    c. Xenograft
    d. Isograft

19. **All of the following are features of Tubotympanic CSOM except:** *(Exam 2016)*
    a. Profuse painless discharge
    b. Hearing loss
    c. Marginal Perforation
    d. Central perforation

20. **Wullstein type III tympanoplasty is:** *(Exam 2016)*
    a. Myringoplasty
    b. Myringo-ossiculoplasty
    c. Myringostapediopexy
    d. Fenestration operation

21. **A 35-years old patient with 6 months of non-foul smelling ear discharge and hearing loss. The TM appearance is given below. Treatment includes all except:** *(Practice question by Author)*

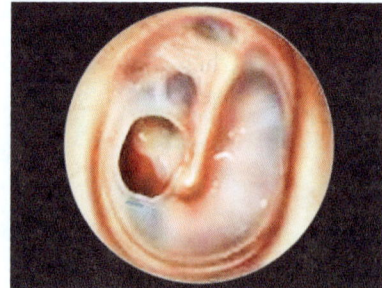

   a. Topical antibiotics
   b. Systemic antibiotics
   c. Mastoidectomy
   d. Tympanoplasty

ANSWERS AND EXPLANATIONS

1. **(a) Aetiology is multiple bacteria** (*Ref. Scott Brown, 8th ed., Vol 2; 1001*)
   - CSOM is caused by mixed aerobic and anaerobic organisms. MC aerobic organism being Pseudomonas, others include Proteus, *E. coli* and *Staph. aureus*. Bacteroids are the anaerobic bacteria here.
   - Oral antibiotics and antibiotic ear drops are given to control the infection and once the ear is dry for 6 weeks without antibiotics surgical repair is taken up.
   - Otic hydrocephalus is a complication of unsafe CSOM, *see* next Chapter.
   - Resorption of bony ossicles in safe CSOM is due to repeated infections with resultant local inflammatory cytokines and local acidosis mainly in the area of low blood supply (most commonly long process of incus and incudo-stapedial joint).

2. **(b) Tympanoplasty** (*Ref. Scott Brown, 8th ed., Vol 2; 997*)
   - Surgical repair of TM is known as myringoplasty. If while doing the surgery any ossicle is found to be necrosed, then ossiculoplasty is also done.
   - This repair of the TM (myringoplasty) with ossiculoplasty is together known as tympanoplasty.
   - Since here the ossicular status has not been mentioned the preferable answer is tympanoplasty because myringoplasty is type 1 tympanoplasty.
   - Modified mastoidectomy is done in unsafe CSOM.
   - Conservative management is the strategy in acute perforations following trauma and ASOM.

3. **(b) Long process of incus** (*Ref. Scott Brown, 8th ed., Vol 2; 997*)
   - Ossicle most commonly involved in CSOM is long process of incus because of its poor blood supply.

4. **(d) Tympanoplasty** (*Ref. Scott Brown, 8th ed., Vol 2; 997*)
   - Management of tubo-tympanic CSOM is tympanoplasty
   - Radical and modified radical mastoidectomy are done for unsafe CSOM.
   - Simple mastoidectomy or Schwartze operation is done for acute and coalescent mastoiditis.

5. **(a) Operative microscope** (*Ref. Shambaugh, 6th ed., 508; Scott Brown, 8th ed., Vol 2; 1021*)

6. **(c) 250 mm** (*Ref. Dhingra, 6th ed., 374*)
   - Also remember that the focal length of the lens used in microscopic laryngeal surgeries is 400 mm.

7. **(a) Eradication of middle ear disease with reconstruction of tympanic membrane and ossicles** (*Ref. Shambaugh, 6th ed., 465*)

8. **(a) Tympanoplasty** (*Ref. Shambaugh, 6th ed., 491*)

9. **(c) Type III** (*Ref. Shambaugh, 6th ed., 491*) (mnemonic- Collumela, letter **C** is the **III**rd alphabet). This is the MC type of tympanoplasty done.

10. **(a) Temporalis fascia** (*Ref. Scott Brown, 8th ed., Vol 2; 1025*)

11. **(a), (b) Temporalis fascia, Cartilage** (*Ref. Scott Brown, 8th ed., Vol 2; 997*)

12. **(b) Malleus handle and stapes suprastructure** (*Ref. Scott Brown, 8th ed., Vol 2; 1030*)

13. **(b) CSOM** (*Ref. Cummings, 6th ed., 2177*)
    - Active otosclerosis is managed by Na F, whereas mature otosclerosis is managed by stapedotomy.
    - ASOM responds to antibiotics, antihistaminics, decongestants and analgesics.

14. **(d) Tympanic membrane** (*Ref. Scott Brown, 8th ed., Vol 2; 1021*)

15. **(d) If required malleus is also reconstructed** (*Ref. Shambaugh, 6th ed., 491*)

16. **(a) In underlay graft is placed medial to the annulus** (*Ref. Scott Brown, 8th ed., Vol 2; 1026*)
    - In both underlay and overlay, a portion of the graft is placed medial to the malleus.
    - In underlay, graft is placed medial to the annulus, whereas in overlay graft is placed lateral to the annulus.

17. **(c) Long process of incus** (*Ref. Scott Brown, 8th ed., Vol 2; 1023*)

18. **(a) Autograft** (i.e. from the same individual) (*Ref. Scott Brown, 8th ed., Vol 2; 1025*)
    - Allograft or homograft is a graft from another human being, i.e. from the same species.
    - Xenograft is a graft from a different species, e.g. animals
    - Isograft is a graft from an identical/monozygotic twin.

19. **(c) Marginal Perforation** (it is a feature of atticoantral CSOM) (*Ref. Scott Brown, 8th ed., Vol 2; 989*)

20. **(c) Myringostapediopexy** (*Ref. Shambaugh, 6th ed., 491*)

21. **(c) Mastoidectomy** (*Ref. Scott Brown, 8th ed., Vol 2; 1022*)
    - Non-foul smelling discharge of 6 months duration suggests that the above is a case of safe CSOM. Hence management is ear toileting, local and systemic antibiotics and once the ear is dry for 6 weeks without antibiotics, surgical repair by tympanoplasty.

Chapter
8

Atticoantral or Squamous Chronic Otitis Media

PATHOPHYSIOLOGY

Atticoantral CSOM also known as **unsafe or dangerous CSOM** is now preferably called as squamous chronic otitis media. It can lead to serious complications. These complications occur because of the **bone eroding property of cholesteatoma,** a pathology associated with unsafe CSOM.

Cholesteatoma is neither cholesterol crystals nor a tumour (oma) but is the presence of **keratinizing stratified squamous epithelium** (hence called squamosal disease) **in any part of temporal bone where it is usually not present**, e.g. middle ear, mastoid, petrous apex (these are normally lined by mucosa).

In its basal layer cholesteatoma has got **enzymes** like collagenases and acid phosphatases which cause the bony erosion, helping the middle ear infection to reach the surrounding areas leading to the various complications (*see* below).

Types of Cholesteatoma

Refer to Table 8.2, at the end of this chapter Cholesteatoma has been divided into:
1. Congenital Cholesteatoma
2. Acquired Cholesteatoma; this is further of two types:
   a. Primary
   b. Secondary

Congenital Cholesteatoma

It develops from congenital cell, rests present in any part of temporal bone which are destined to form some other epithelium but develop into stratified squamous epithelium. Congenital cholesteatoma is most commonly present in **antero-superior quadrant** of middle ear.

Levenson gave the following criteria for the diagnosis of congenital cholesteatoma:
   a. A white mass medial to an intact tympanic membrane.
   b. Normal pars flaccida and tensa
   c. No history of otorrhoea or perforations
   d. No prior otologic procedures

   e. Past history of Acute Otitis media is not an exclusion criteria, i.e. even if there is a history of ASOM in the past, congenital cholesteatoma is still a possibility. This is because even if a child has had ASOM leading to perforation, it usually heals, and congenital cell rests might have been present from before.

PRIMARY CHOLESTEATOMA

It is called primary since it does not occur secondary to a perforation on the TM. There are various theories for the formation of primary cholesteatoma:

a. **Wittmaack's/invagination theory of retraction pocket:** This is the most accepted theory.

The obstruction of Eustachian tube leads to negative pressure in the middle ear and retraction of TM. If this obstruction becomes very prolonged, persistent negative pressure leads to formation of retraction pocket in the TM(inactive squamous COM). Since the pars flaccida is less fibrous and the most mobile part of TM, the most common site of formation of retraction pocket is in the pars flaccida. The pars flaccida retraction pocket retracts into the attic (i.e. epitympanum) in its Prussak's space (*see* Chapter 1).

Keratin debris accumulates in this retraction pocket. Repeated infection by mixed organisms of this keratin

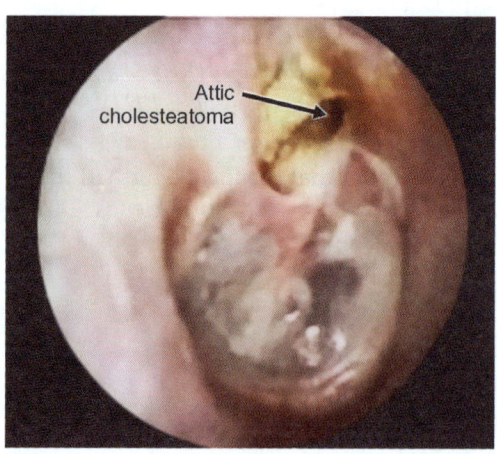

Attic cholesteatoma

Fig. 8.1

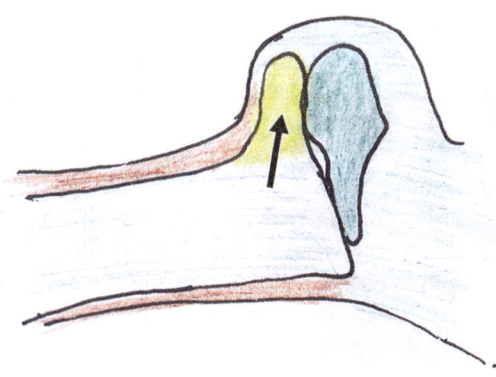

Fig. 8.2: Retraction pocket

in a more or less closed space leads to an increase in macrophages, lymphocytes and monocytes. These in turn release TNF and interleukins which stimulates osteoclasts. The activated osteoclasts release enzymes (acid phosphatases, collagenases and acid proteases) which lead to erosion and perforation into the attic or simply called attic perforation (active squamous COM).

The MC route of primary cholesteatoma is through retraction pocket and the MC site of retraction pocket formation is pars flaccida/attic/**Prussak's space.** The retraction pocket may also form in the posterosuperior part of Pars tensa of TM.

Hence **any retraction pocket, perforation or granulations of the pars flaccida has to be considered as unsafe** and treated accordingly.

b. **SADE'S theory of Squamous metaplasia:** Because of the repeated infection of the middle ear through Eustachian tube, the normal ciliated columnar epithelium of the middle ear undergoes metaplasia (which is the replacement of one **differentiated cell type** with another mature differentiated cell type) and changes to stratified squamous epithelium. This is known as SADE's theory of squamous metaplasia.

c. **RUEDI's theory of Basal cell hyperplasia:** Following repeated infection (of deep meatus and TM), the basal epithelial cells of the outer layer of TM proliferate and invade the subepithelial tissue. Repeated infections lead to disruptions in the basal lamina. The proliferating keratinocytes invade through the basal lamina.

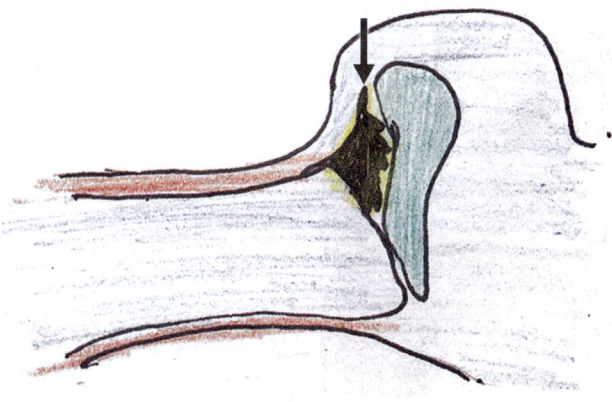

Fig. 8.3: Basal cell hyperplasia

SECONDARY CHOLESTEATOMA

Secondary cholesteatoma occurs **secondary to a marginal or total perforation** on the TM. Perforation of a part of pars tensa with destruction of tympanic annulus is called marginal perforation. Total perforation is perforation of whole of the pars tensa along with its annulus.

This marginal or total perforation **follows ANOM,** *see* chapter on ASOM.

Habermann's theory of migration through marginal perforation: The MC route of secondary cholesteatoma is migration of keratinising stratified squamous epithelium of the external auditory canal through marginal perforation of TM into the middle ear.

The most common site of marginal perforation through which **migration occurs is postero-superior marginal perforation.**

CLINICAL FEATURES OF UNSAFE CSOM

Discharge

Patient presents here with **scant, painless and foul smelling discharge** (because of osteitis and bone erosion by cholesteatoma and infection with anaerobic bacteria).

Hearing Loss

The deafness can be conductive or mixed (eroding cholesteatoma causing ossicular necrosis and involvement of the inner ear leading to conductive deafness and SN deafness respectively).

The patient can also present with any of the **complications of CSOM** (*see* next chapter on complications of CSOM).

On Examination

Cholesteatoma can be seen along with marginal perforation, total perforation, attic or posterosuperior retraction pocket, attic perforation or attic granulations.

MANAGEMENT

The main management of unsafe CSOM is **mastoid exploration** (mastoidectomy) with removal of disease from the mastoid, followed by removal of disease from the middle ear. Discharge in unsafe CSOM is mainly because of bony erosion so medical management with local and systemic antibiotics is indicated only in superimposed acute infection or in infection causing extra or intracranial complications assisted by erosion due to cholesteatoma, *see* next chapter.

The main aim of the surgery is to give the patient a **safe, dry and hearing ear** by eradicating the disease and reconstructing the hearing mechanism. When surgery is required for intracranial complications that follow unsafe CSOM the intracranial complications are managed first. The surgery for unsafe CSOM can be:

1. Intact canal wall Mastoidectomy
2. Canal wall down Mastoidectomy

Here canal wall refers to the posterior wall of the middle ear which is the common wall between middle

Section I | **Ear**

ear and mastoid. As per the name in Canal wall down mastoidectomy, this common wall is removed. In Intact Canal wall mastoidectomy, just a small opening is made in this common wall, read below.

Mastoid Exploration/Mastoidectomy

The initial mastoid exploration till the mastoid antrum is reached is the same for all surgeries of the mastoid.

This is done with an operating microscope with a focal length of 250 mm. Post-auricular incision (known as wilde's incision) is given. Macewen's triangle is exposed. Mastoid exploration is done by drilling, at the Macewen's triangle, *see* chapter on anatomy.

The drilling is started with cutting drill burs which are sharp and drill away the mastoid air cells. In areas which are close to the important structures, e.g. facial nerve etc, diamond burrs are used which cut the bone very slowly. Adequate irrigation is done while drilling to wash away bone dust generated by the drill to improve visualization. Irrigation also decreases the risk of injury from the heat produced by drilling.

Haemostasis is achieved with bipolar cautery, bone wax or using a diamond burr (as it produces lots of bone dust which seals of the bleeding vessel).

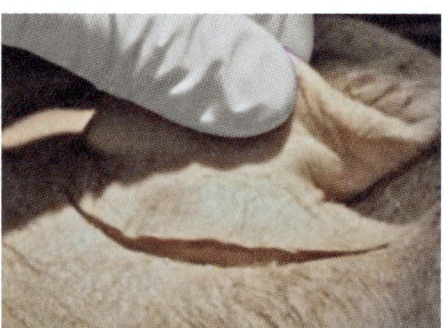

Fig. 8.4: Post-aural incision (Wilde's)

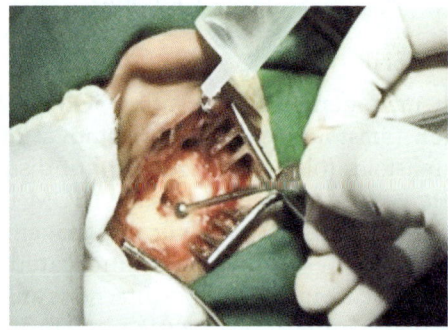

Fig. 8.5: Mastoid exploration of the right ear started by drilling at Macewen's triangle

INTACT CANAL WALL PROCEDURE

Posterior Tympanotomy Approach

All the mastoid air cells are exenterated (exenteration means removing all the contents of a cavity). On reaching the mastoid antrum (which lies around 1.5 cm deep to the Macewen's triangle) the disease of the antrum is removed. If it is found that the disease in the antrum is minimal, considering the disease in the middle ear to be also

minimal, to remove the disease from the middle ear through the mastoid, a small **opening is made in the facial recess area** on the posterior wall of tympanic or middle ear cavity (lying lateral to the bulge of vertical part of fallopian canal, *see* chapter on anatomy). This is known as posterior tympanotomy approach (i.e. opening the tympanic cavity through the posterior wall). The **sinus tympani** area lying medial to the bulge of vertical part of fallopian canal (i.e. mastoid part of facial nerve), is the **hidden area** of the middle ear and the most common site of residual cholesteatoma. It can be visualised through the posterior tympanotomy approach and disease can be removed from here.

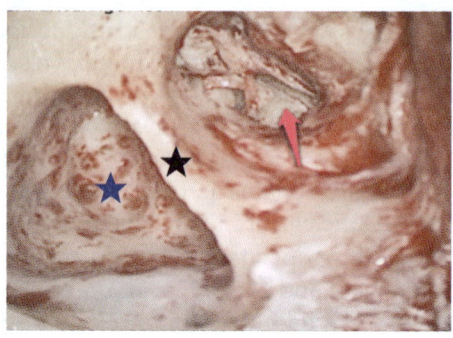

Fig. 8.6: Operative picture of right ear showing intact canal wall procedure. Pink arrow shows middle ear cavity. Black star shows the posterior wall of EAC (which has been left intact) and blue star shows the operated mastoid cavity

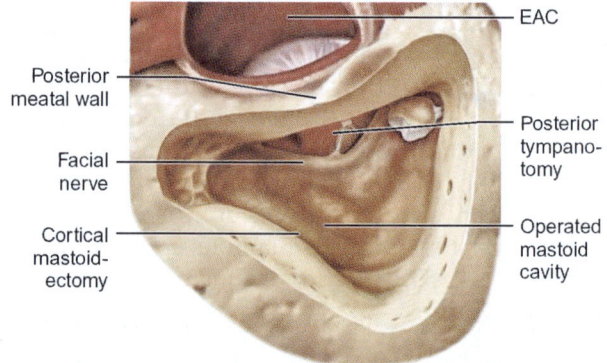

Fig. 8.7: Operative picture of left ear showing an opening made in the facial recess area (posterior tympanotomy). The posterior meatal/canal wall is intact

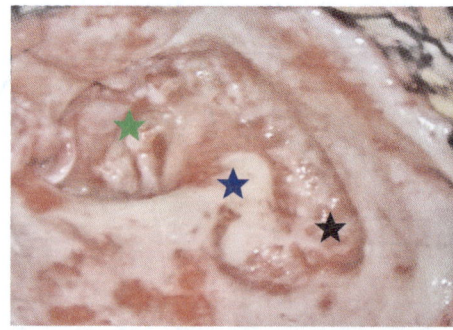

Fig. 8.8: Operative picture of left ear showing the posterior canal wall removed and mastoid and middle ear becoming a common cavity. Black star shows the operated mastoid cavity. Blue star shows the lowered posterior canal wall (facial ridge) and green star shows the operated middle ear cavity

In intact canal wall procedure the disease of middle ear is also removed by permeatal route, i.e. through the EAC side and possible reconstruction by tympanoplasty is also done. Since here in intact canal wall we approach the middle ear by both postaural and transmeatal route, it is also known as **combined approach tympanoplasty**.

The chances of **residual and recurrent** cholesteatoma is high in intact canal wall procedure.

CANAL WALL DOWN PROCEDURE

It can be either:
a. Radical Mastoidectomy
b. Modified Radical Mastoidectomy (MRM)

Mastoid exploration and Lowering the posterior canal wall: In a patient of unsafe CSOM, the mastoid exploration is started as mentioned above. On reaching the mastoid antrum, the disease of the antrum is removed. If it is found that the disease in the antrum is very extensive, considering the disease in the middle ear to be also extensive, to remove the disease from the middle ear the posterior canal wall, i.e. **the posterior wall of the middle ear (common wall between mastoid and middle ear), along with the posterior wall of EAC is drilled down up till the level of descending part of facial nerve** and now the disease of the middle ear is also removed. This removing of the posterior canal wall lateral to the mastoid segment of facial nerve, is known as lowering of facial ridge. **Lowering** of **facial ridge** should be done carefully keeping in mind the important landmarks of mastoid segment of facial nerve (please *see* chapter on facial nerve) as the most common site of injury to facial nerve during mastoid surgeries is this mastoid segment, specifically the second genu area.

So here after exenterating all the mastoid air cells we convert mastoid and middle ear into a common cavity by removing the common posterior wall between them. This procedure has disadvantage of a big mastoid cavity leading to cavity problems like retention of debris, wax, etc. which may get infected leading to discharge.

Meatoplasty

This big mastoid cavity should be exposed properly for proper drainage. For this purpose we widen the external acoustic meatus by removing a piece of conchal cartilage. This procedure is known as meatoplasty and is mandatory for all canal wall down procedures.

Cavity Obliteration

To prevent the complications of a big cavity, e.g. accumulation of cerumen, debris and difficulty with fitting in a hearing aid, cavity obliteration and canal wall reconstruction can be carried out in cases of unsafe CSOM **without complications** at the time of surgery.

The two important canal wall down procedures are **radical mastoidectomy** and **modified radical mastoidectomy**. The above mentioned procedures of exenterating

all mastoid air cells, removing the posterior canal wall and doing a meatoplasty are same for both.

RADICAL MASTOIDECTOMY

As its name this surgery is radical, in the sense that all (healthy as well as unhealthy) remnants of TM, middle ear mucosa and all the ossicles except for footplate is removed and along with this the **Eustachian tube is closed** to reduce the risk of a chronic otorrhoea resulting from acute infections of the pharynx. During lowering of posterior canal wall the **Chorda tympani** nerve has to be **sacrificed**.

MODIFIED RADICAL MASTOIDECTOMY

In MRM all the healthy remnants of TM, healthy mucosa of middle ear and healthy ossicles are preserved for a **next stage reconstruction** or if possible reconstruction at the time of primary surgery. The reconstruction of ossicles along with TM is called tympanoplasty. So tympanoplasty is a part of MRM. Here in MRM the Eustachian tube is not closed because normal Eustachian tube is required for a functional middle ear, however during lowering of posterior canal wall the Chorda tympani nerve has to be sacrificed.

The aim of the surgery for unsafe CSOM is to give the patient a hearing ear along with a safe and dry ear. Since reconstruction of hearing (i.e. tympanoplasty) is done in Modified radical Mastoidectomy, **MRM is preferred over radical mastoidectomy in the treatment of unsafe CSOM with or without complications**.

Though MRM in general is the preferred treatment of unsafe CSOM, **Radical mastoidectomy** is **indicated** in the following:

i. Unsafe CSOM with dead ear (no good hearing left).
ii. Unresectable cholesteatoma extending onto the Eustachian tube or to petrous apex.
iii. Promontory cochlear fistula due to cholesteatoma.
iv. When cholesteatoma cannot be removed and must be cleaned or inspected periodically.
  • Radical Mastoidectomy is also done during resection of temporal bone neoplasm.

TUBERCULAR OTITIS MEDIA

• It occurs most commonly following pulmonary tuberculosis.
• Patient presents with **painless** foul smelling (because of bony erosion) ear discharge with **severe hearing loss** (because of ossicular necrosis)
• On examination: **Multiple perforations** on the TM which may coalesce to form a single large perforation and **pale granulations** are seen.
• Most common complication of TB Otitis media is **facial palsy**. The others being mastoiditis, labyrinthitis, postauricular fistula, osteomyelitis, etc.
• Treatment: Medical management with anti-tubercular drugs (ATT).

Section I   **Ear**

To summarise:

Table 8.1: Tubotympanic *vs* Atticoantral CSOM

Type of CSOM	Tubo-tympanic	Attico-antral
Also called	Safe/benign/mucosal CSOM	Unsafe/dangerous/squamosal CSOM
Main pathology	Permanent perforation of TM leads to repeated infections, no cholesteatoma.	Cholesteatoma present
TM perforation	Non-marginal, sub-total	Marginal or total
Ear discharge	Non-offensive	Very foul smelling
Deafness	Conductive	Conductive or Mixed
Ossicular necrosis	Due to repeated and prolonged infections	Due to erosion by cholesteatoma
Extent of disease	Limited to middle ear	Go beyond middle ear to involve inner ear and cranium
Complications	No	Present due to eroding cholesteatoma
Surgical treatment	Myringoplasty or Tympanoplasty	Intact canal wall surgery, Canal wall down surgery (MRM)

Table 8.2: Various theories of cholesteatoma formation

Cholesteatoma	Criterion/theory	Develops from	Follows
Congenital	Levenson's	Congenital cell rests	—
Primary	Wittmaack's/Invagination	Retraction pocket in pars flaccida	Prolonged Eustachian tube obstruction
	Sade's	Squamous metaplasia	Repeated middle ear infection through Eustachian tube
	Ruedi's	Basal cell hyperplasia	Repeated infections of deep meatus and TM
Secondary	Habermann's	Migration of EAC epithelium via marginal/total perforation	ANOM

 "Points to Ponder/Points for Quick revision"

- Atticoantral/unsafe CSOM—now called Atticoantral/ Squamous chronic otitis media.
- Pathology: Enzymatic bone erosion by Keratinizing stratified squamous epithelium called "CHOLESTEATOMA"
- Pathogenesis:
  1. Congenital Cholesteatoma–Levenson criteria
  2. Primary Cholesteatoma
     i. Wittmaack's retraction pocket formation and invagination (MC–in pars flaccida) secondary to ET obstruction.
     ii. Sade's–middle ear mucosa developing squamous metaplasia due to repeated infections.
     iii. Ruedi's–repeated otitis externa involving deep meatus and TM → basal cell hyperplasia of the epithelial layer of TM → invasion of the basal lamina.
  3. Secondary Cholesteatoma–2° to total/marginal perforation, i.e. involving the tympanic annulus (Habermann's migration).
- Active or inactive squamous COM – terms used depending upon whether cholesteatoma is causing on going erosion or is relatively dormant.
- CFs-Permanent marginal perforation, painless offensive ear discharge, mixed hearing loss ± complications.
- Treatment–Surgery; with the aim of giving safe, dry and hearing ear to the patient.
  i. Intact canal wall Mastoidectomy:
     – Less extensive procedure–done for minimal disease.
     – Opening is made in the common posterior wall between the mastoid and middle ear to enter the facial recess.
     – Sinus tympani–the hidden area–can be explored.
     – Tympanoplasty, i.e. Myringoplasty + Ossiculoplasty– is done subsequently.
     – Recurrence issue.
  ii. Canal wall down Mastoidectomy:
     – Extensive procedure–done when disease is extensive.
     – The common posterior wall between the mastoid and external auditory canal along with middle ear is removed (hence the name)–Chorda tympani nerve sacrificed.
     – Two types:
        a. Radical Mastoidectomy (RM)
           ▪ Healthy as well as unhealthy TM and ossicles (except foot plate) is removed
           ▪ ET–closed
           ▪ Done–if no hearing left or unresectable choles-teatoma
        b. Modified Radical Mastoidectomy (MRM)
           ▪ As per the Aim—Preferred over RM
           ▪ Only the unhealthy tissues removed along with cholesteatoma
           ▪ ET–patent
           ▪ Tympanoplasty done subsequently
- Tubercular otitis media–often 2° to pulmonary TB, multiple perforations over TM, granulations, facial nerve palsy, ATT.

PREVIOUSLY ASKED QUESTIONS

1. **What is true in case of perforation of pars flaccida:**
   (AIIMS May 93, 2001, Exam 2017)
   a. CSOM is a rare cause
   b. Associated with cholesteatoma
   c. Usually due to trauma
   d. All of the above

2. **Perforation of a part of tympanic membrane with destruction of tympanic annulus is called:**
   (Bihar 2004, Exam 2017)
   a. Attic
   b. Marginal
   c. Subtotal
   d. Total

3. **Cholesteatoma occurs in:**
   (AIIMS May 94, 2002, Exam 2017)
   a. CSOM with central perforation
   b. Masked mastoiditis
   c. Coalescent mastoiditis
   d. Acute necrotising Otitis media

4. **Levenson's criteria for diagnosing congenital cholesteatoma includes:** *(PGI Nov 2010)*
   a. Whitish mass behind intact TM
   b. Normal pars tensa and pars flaccida
   c. Recurrent attacks of otorrhoea
   d. Prior otitis media is not an exclusion criteria
   e. Prior history of ear surgery

5. **Most accepted theory for the formation of secondary cholesteatoma:** *(AI 2004, Exam 2017)*
   a. Congenital
   b. Squamous metaplasia
   c. Migration of squamous epithelium
   d. Retraction pocket

6. **The postero-superior retraction pocket, if allowed to progress, will lead to:** *(AI 2003, Exam 2017)*
   a. Sensorineural hearing loss
   b. Secondary cholesteatoma
   c. Tympanosclerosis
   d. Tertiary cholesteatoma

7. **Cholesteatoma is usually present at:**
   (Delhi 2001, Exam 2017)
   a. Anteroinferior quadrant of TM
   b. Posteroinferior quadrant of TM
   c. Attic region
   d. Central part

8. **Cholesteatoma is commonly caused by:**
   (AI 94, Exam 2011)
   a. Attic perforation
   b. Tubo-tympanic disease
   c. Central perforation of tympanic membrane
   d. Meniere's disease

9. **Cholesteatoma commonly associated with:**
   (PGI 2008)
   a. Atticoantral CSOM b. Tubotympanic CSOM
   c. Tympanosclerosis   d. Foreign body in ear
   e. Keratosis obturans

10. **Scanty, foul smelling painless discharge from the ear is characteristic feature of which of the following lesions:**
    (AIIMS Nov 2000/2004, Exam 2013)
    a. ASOM   b. Cholesteatoma
    c. Central perforation d. Otitis externa

11. **Cholesteatoma (atticoantral) true about:**
    (PGI June 2006, Exam 2014)
    a. Scanty, malodorous discharge
    b. Otalgia
    c. Central perforation
    d. Ossicular necrosis
    e. Convulsions

12. **True about cholesteatoma is/are:**
    (PGI Dec 2002/2004, Exam 2015)
    a. It is a benign tumour
    b. Metastasises to lymph node
    c. Contains cholesterol
    d. Erodes the bone
    e. Malignant potential

13. **Which is true of cholesteatoma:**
    (AI 2004, Exam 2017)
    a. Physiological   b. Erodes bone
    c. Benign neoplasm   d. Contains cholesterol

14. **All of the following are the features of the disease shown in the picture except:** *(Exam 2016)*

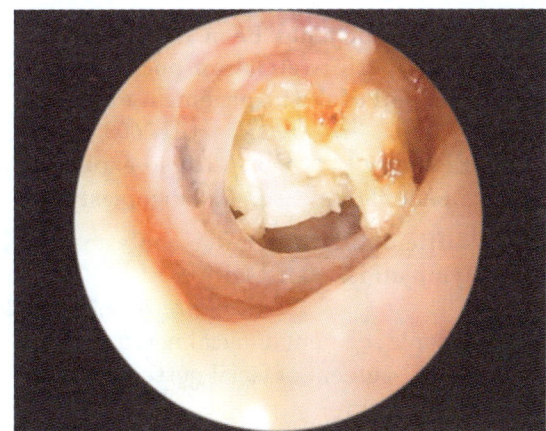

   a. Filled with keratinised stratified squamous epithelium
   b. Deafness
   c. Erodes bone
   d. Lymphatic permeation

15. **Cholesteatoma is seen in:** *(RJ 2006, Exam 2017)*
    a. ASOM   b. CSOM
    c. Secretory Otitis media d. Otosclerosis

16. **Primary treatment of middle ear cholesteatoma is:** *(AI 2000, Exam 2017)*
    a. Surgery   b. Medical treatment and surgery
    c. Radiotherapy   d. Chemotherapy

17. **The treatment of choice for atticoantral variety of CSOM is:** *(AIIMS Nov 2002, Exam 2017)*
    a. Mastoidectomy
    b. Medical management
    c. Underlay myringoplasty
    d. Insertion of ventilation tube

18. **Treatment of choice for perforation in pars flaccida of the tympanic membrane with cholesteatoma is:** *(AI 96, Exam 2012)*
    a. Myringoplasty
    b. Modified radical mastoidectomy
    c. Antibiotics
    d. Radical mastoidectomy

19. **All of the following techniques are used to control bleeding from bone during mastoid surgery except:** *(Exam 2010, AIIMS 2004)*
    a. Cutting drill over the bleeding area
    b. Diamond drill over the bleeding area
    c. Bipolar cautery over the bleeding area
    d. Bone wax

20. **A child presents with foul smelling ear discharge. On further exploration a small perforation is found in the pars flaccida of the tympanic membrane. Most appropriate next step in the management would be:** *(AIIMS 2007, Exam 2017)*
    a. Topical antibiotics and decongestants for 4 weeks
    b. I/V antibiotics and follow up after a month
    c. Tympanoplasty
    d. Tympanomastoid exploration

21. **A 5-year-old boy has been diagnosed to have posterior superior retraction pocket. All would constitute part of the management except:** *(AI 2003, Exam 2017)*
    a. Audiometry   b. Mastoid exploration
    c. Tympanoplasty   d. Myringoplasty

22. **Most difficult site to remove cholesteatoma, i.e. sinus tympani is related with:** *(Kolkata 2001, Exam 2017)*
    a. Tympanic segment of facial nerve
    b. Mastoid segment of facial nerve
    c. Epitympanum
    d. Hypotympanum

23. **A 30-year-old male is having Attic Cholesteatoma of left ear with lateral sinus thrombophlebitis. Which of the following will be the operation of choice:** *(AI 2006)*
    a. Intact canal wall mastoidectomy
    b. Simple mastoidectomy with tympanoplasty
    c. Canal wall down mastoidectomy
    d. Mastoidectomy with cavity obliteration

24. **Medical treatment is not effective in which type of suppurative Otitis media:** *(UP 2007)*
    a. Tuberculous Otitis media
    b. Secretory Otitis media
    c. Acute suppurative Otitis media
    d. Chronic suppurative Otitis media

25. **Modified radical mastoidectomy is indicated in all except:** *(Exam 2001, Exam 2017)*
    a. Safe CSOM
    b. Atticoantral disease
    c. Unsafe CSOM with facial palsy
    d. Unsafe CSOM with intracranial complications

26. **Radical mastoidectomy is done for:** *(Exam 2000, Exam 2017)*
    a. ASOM
    b. Safe CSOM
    c. Atticoantral cholesteatoma
    d. Acute mastoiditis

27. **All of the following steps are done in radical mastoidectomy except:** *(AI 97, Exam 2015)*
    a. Lowering of facial ridge
    b. Removal of middle ear mucosa and muscles
    c. Removal of all ossicles except stapes footplate
    d. Maintenance of patency of Eustachian tube

28. **Radical mastoidectomy includes all except:** *(AIIMS 2000, Exam 2012)*
    a. Closure of the auditory tube
    b. Ossicles removed
    c. Cochlea removed
    d. Exteriorization of mastoid

29. **Communication between middle ear and Eustachian tube is obliterated in which surgery:** *(Delhi 2005, Exam 2017)*
    a. Tympanoplasty
    b. Schwartz operation
    c. Modified radical mastoidectomy
    d. Radical mastoidectomy

30. **Nerve which can get damaged in radical mastoidectomy is:** *(MH 2000, Exam 2017)*
    a. Facial   b. Cochlear
    c. Vestibular   d. All

31. **Tubercular otitis media is characterized by all except:** *(AP 2004, PGI Dec 99, Exam 2017)*
    a. Multiple perforations
    b. Pale granulations
    c. Pain
    d. Foul smelling ear discharge

32. **Which of the following is characteristic of TB otitis media?** *(AIIMS May 95, 2004, Exam 2017)*
    a. Marginal perforation
    b. Attic perforation
    c. Central perforation
    d. Multiple perforation

33. Schuller's view and Law's view is for:
    (Rj 2003, Exam 2017)
    a. Sphenoid sinus
    b. Mastoid air cells
    c. Foramen ovale and spinosum
    d. Carotid canal

34. Stenver's view is used for: *(AI 99, Exam 2017)*
    a. Temporal bone
    b. Nasopharyngeal carcinoma
    c. Paranasal sinuses
    d. Larynx

35. What is the treatment of choice of atticoantral CSOM?   *(Exam 2016)*
    a. Antibiotics
    b. Tympanoplasty
    c. Myringoplasty
    d. Modified radial mastoidectomy

36. All of the following are removed in radical mastoidectomy except: *(Exam 2016)*
    a. Chorda tympani
    b. Incus
    c. Posterior meatal wall
    d. Stapes footplate

37. All of the following are theories for acquired cholesteatoma except: *(Exam 2016)*
    a. Squamous metaplasia
    b. Basal cell hyperplasia
    c. Retraction pocket
    d. Pressure of keratin

38. In radical mastoidectomy it is necessary to preserve: *(Exam 2016)*
    a. Tympanic membrane and its remnants
    b. Stapes footplate
    c. Facial bridge and ridge
    d. Function of the Eustachian tube

39. Which one of the following is the most likely diagnosis of the picture depicted below?
    (APPG 2015)

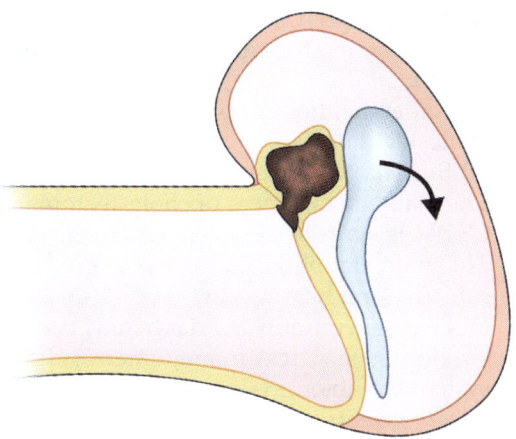

a. CSOM with attic perforation and cholesteatoma
b. Herpes zoster oticus
c. CSOM with tubo-tympanic perforation
d. ASOM with bulging eardrum

40. A 30-year-old male presents with foul smelling ear discharge. On examination the tympanic membrane appeared as the picture given below. Most appropriate next step in the management would be:
    (AIIMS 2007, Exam 2017)

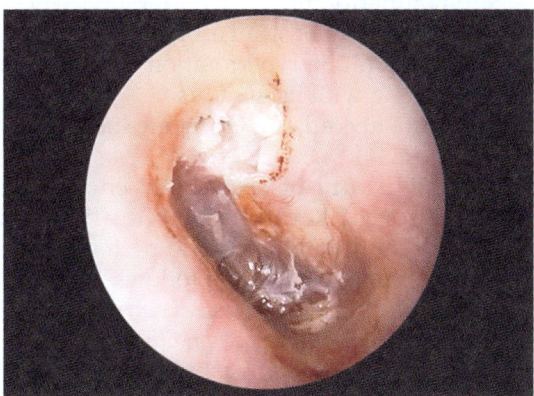

a. Topical antibiotics and decongestants for 4 weeks
b. Modified radical mastoidectomy
c. Schwartze operation
d. Myringoplasty

41. Child with adenoids hypertrophy and blockage of Eustachian tube has future risk for: *(Exam 2016)*
    a. Primary acquired cholesteatoma
    b. Secondary acquired cholesteatoma
    c. Congenital cholesteatoma
    d. Tertiary cholesteatoma

42. Below is an endoscopic picture of a patient who presented with foul smelling ear discharge. Most probable diagnosis is: *(Exam 2019)*

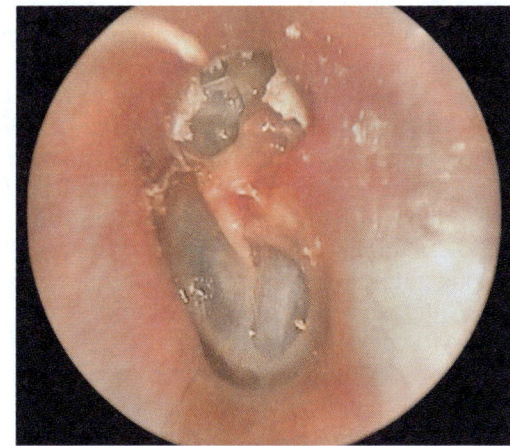

a. Congenital cholesteatoma
b. Primary cholesteatoma
c. Secondary cholesteatoma
d. Tubotympanic CSOM

ANSWERS AND EXPLANATIONS

1. **(b) Associated with cholesteatoma** (*Ref. Scott Brown, 8th ed. Vol 2; 989*)
   - Any perforation of pars flaccida is unsafe CSOM because it is associated with cholesteatoma.
2. **(b) Marginal** (*Ref. Scott Brown, 8th ed. Vol 2; 989*)
   - Perforation of a part of pars tensa with destruction of tympanic annulus is called marginal perforation.
   - Attic perforation is perforation of the pars flaccida.
   - Subtotal perforation is a perforation when a small margin of pars tensa all around is still there.
   - Total perforation is perforation of whole of the pars tensa along with its annulus.
3. **(d) Acute necrotising Otitis media** (*Ref. Cummings, 6th ed., 2146*)
   - The MC route of secondary cholesteatoma is migration of keratinising stratified squamous epithelium through marginal perforation of TM.
   - This marginal perforation follows ANOM.
   - Rest of the choices are not associated with cholesteatoma.
4. **(a), (b), (d)** (*Ref. Shambaugh, 6th ed. 429*)
5. **(c) Migration of squamous epithelium** (*Ref. Cummings, 6th ed., 2146*)
   - The MC route of secondary cholesteatoma is migration of keratinising stratified squamous epithelium through marginal perforation of TM (Habermann's theory).
   - Congenital cholesteatoma is due to the presence of congenital cell rests which later on form stratified squamous epithelium in any part of temporal bone.
   - Squamous metaplasia and retraction pocket are theories for primary cholesteatoma.
6. **(a) Sensorineural hearing loss** (*Ref. Cummings, 6th ed., 2143*)
   - A postero-superior retraction pocket, if allowed to progress, will lead to primary cholesteatoma which in turn can lead to sensorineural hearing loss.
   - Secondary cholesteatoma is migration of keratinising stratified squamous epithelium through marginal perforation of TM.
   - Tympanosclerosis is hyalinisation and calcification of the fibrous layer of tympanic membrane. There is no condition called tertiary cholesteatoma.
7. **(c) Attic region** (*Ref. Cummings, 6th ed., 2143*)
   - Most common site of primary cholesteatoma is attic.
   - The most common site of marginal perforation through which migration occurs leading to secondary cholesteatoma is postero-superior marginal.
   - Congenital cholesteatoma is most commonly present in Anterosuperior quadrant of middle ear.
8. **(a) Attic perforation** (*Ref. Cummings, 6th ed., 2143*)
   - Central perforation of the TM leads to safe CSOM, i.e. Tubo-tympanic disease and is not associated with cholesteatoma.
   - Meniere's disease is endolymphatic hydrops.
9. **(a) Atticoantral CSOM** (*Ref. Scott Brown, 8th ed. Vol 2; 989*)
   - Tympanosclerosis is hyalinisation and calcification of the fibrous layer of tympanic membrane. It is not associated with cholesteatoma. Foreign body in ear does not lead to cholesteatoma formation.
   - Keratosis obturans is the collection of desquamated keratin debris in the external auditory canal. This keratin debris comes from the external auditory canal stratified squamous epithelium.
10. **(b) Cholesteatoma** (*Ref. Cummings, 6th ed., 2141*)
    - In cholesteatoma the ear discharge is due to bone erosion, hence it is scanty and foul smelling. It is painless.
    - In central perforation, i.e. safe CSOM the ear discharge is painless, on and off and is mucopurulent, non-foul smelling and moderate in amount.
    - In ASOM following rupture of TM, there is relief of pain and the ear discharge is profuse, mucopurulent and non-foul smelling.
    - In Otitis externa, e.g. furuncle, the ear discharge is only purulent and characteristically lacks the mucoid component which indicates that it is not coming from the middle ear. It is associated with pain.
11. **(a), (d) and (e)** (*Ref. Cummings, 6th ed., 2141*)
    - Unsafe CSOM (atticoantral) presents with scant foul smelling discharge (because of osteitis and bone erosion) and deafness.
    - The patient can also present with any of the complications of CSOM. Convulsions can be due to temporal lobe abscess, *see* next Chapter.
    - Ossicular necrosis is seen in both unsafe and safe CSOM. In unsafe CSOM it is mainly due to eroding cholesteatoma and in safe CSOM ossicular necrosis is due to repeated infections. The MC ossicle to get necrosed is long process of incus because of its precarious blood supply.
    - Central perforation is a feature of tubo-tympanic safe CSOM.
    - Otalgia is a feature of ASOM not CSOM.
12. **(d) Erodes the bone** (*Ref. Cummings, 6th ed., 2148*)
    - Cholesteatoma word is misnomer. It does not contain cholesterol. It is not a malignant tumour and therefore does not metastasise. It is also not a benign tumour; however, its bone eroding property justifies the suffix 'oma'.
13. **(b) Erodes bone** (*Ref. Shambaugh, 6th ed. 453*)
14. **(d) Lymphatic permeation** (*Ref. Cummings, 6th ed., 2143*)
    - Cholesteatoma spreads by eroding bone and not by lymphatics.
15. **(b) CSOM** (*Ref. Cummings, 6th ed., 2141*)
    - Cholesteatoma formation is characteristic of unsafe CSOM.
    - The other mentioned options are not associated with cholesteatoma.
16. **(a) Surgery** (*Ref. Cummings, 6th ed., 2145*)
    - The main management of cholesteatoma, i.e. unsafe CSOM is surgery.
    - The main aim of the surgery is to give the patient a safe, dry and hearing ear.
    - Discharge in unsafe CSOM is mainly because of bony erosion so medical management with local and systemic antibiotics is indicated only in superimposed acute infection or infection causing extra or intracranial complications assisted by erosion due to cholesteatoma, *see* next chapter.

17. **(a) Mastoidectomy** (*Ref. Cummings, 6th ed., 2145*)
- The main management of unsafe CSOM is mastoid exploration by mastoidectomy which can be intact canal wall or canal wall down procedure (please refer the text for details of these procedures).
- Initial medical management of atticoantral CSOM with local and systemic antibiotics is indicated only in superimposed acute infection or complication.
- Underlay myringoplasty is done in tubo-tympanic CSOM.
- Ventilation tube or grommet is inserted in serous Otitis media.

18. **(b) Modified radical mastoidectomy** (*Ref. Cummings, 6th ed., 2145*)
- Since reconstruction of hearing is not done in radical mastoidectomy, so MRM is preferred over radical mastoidectomy in the treatment of unsafe CSOM to give the patient a hearing ear besides making the ear safe and dry, please refer the text.

19. **(a) Cutting drill over the bleeding area**, please see the text (*Ref. Shambaugh, 6th ed., 511*)

20. **(d) Tympanomastoid exploration** (*Ref. Cummings, 6th ed., 2145*)
- Foul smelling discharge and perforation in the pars flaccida of the tympanic membrane indicates that it is an unsafe CSOM patient. So the management is Tympanomastoid exploration.
- Tympanoplasty is done as a part of Modified radical mastoidectomy in unsafe CSOM and per se is not the primary management. It is the primary management of tubo-tympanic disease or safe CSOM.

21. **(d) Myringoplasty** (*Ref. Cummings, 6th ed., 2145*)
- Any retraction pocket of the pars flaccida or postero-superior part of TM has to be considered as unsafe CSOM and has to be treated by mastoid exploration with tympanoplasty (MRM).
- Audiometry is done pre- and post-operatively to assess the improvement in hearing.
- Myringoplasty alone is done in safe CSOM.

22. **(b) Mastoid segment of facial nerve** (*Ref. Cummings, 6th ed., 2193*)
- The sinus tympani area is the hidden area of the middle ear and is the most common site of residual cholesteatoma. It lies medial to the bulge of the vertical part of fallopian canal, i.e. mastoid segment of facial nerve. It being a hidden area, it is the most difficult site to remove cholesteatoma.
- It can be visualised through the posterior tympanotomy approach. Please *see* the text.

23. **(c) Canal wall down mastoidectomy** (*Ref. Cummings, 6th ed., 2175*)
- Intact canal wall mastoidectomy is done in unsafe CSOM with limited and minimal disease.
- Simple mastoidectomy is done for acute and coalescent mastoiditis, *see* next Chapter.
- Cavity obliteration and canal wall reconstruction is carried out in cases of unsafe CSOM without complications.

24. **(d) Chronic suppurative Otitis media** (*Ref. Cummings, 6th ed., 2145*)

- In secretory Otitis media initially the treatment is medical for 3 months and if not responding treatment is surgical, i.e. myringotomy with grommet insertion. Also it is not a suppurative Otitis media.
- Of the remaining 3 options of suppurative Otitis media CSOM being characterised by permanent perforation requires surgical treatment. Tympanoplasty is for safe CSOM and MRM for unsafe CSOM.
- Tubercular Otitis media responds to ATT and antibiotics are the treatment modality in ASOM.

25. **(a) Safe CSOM** (*Ref. Cummings, 6th ed., 2148*)
- In Safe CSOM tympanoplasty is done.

26. **(c) Atticoantral cholesteatoma** (*Ref. Cummings, 6th ed., 2190*)
- These days MRM is preferred over radical mastoidectomy in the management of unsafe CSOM with or without complications except for a few areas, please *see* the text.

27. **(d) Maintenance of patency of Eustachian tube** (*Ref. Shambaugh, 6th ed. 516*)

28. **(c) Cochlea removed** (*Ref. Shambaugh, 6th ed. 516*)

29. **(d) Radical mastoidectomy** (*Ref. Cummings, 6th ed., 2190*)

30. **(a) Facial** (*Ref. Shambaugh, 6th ed. 518*)

31. **(c) Pain** (*Ref. Cummings, 6th ed., 2303*)
- Tubercular otitis media is a painless condition. Rest are true, refer the text

32. **(d) Multiple perforation** (*Ref. Cummings, 6th ed., 2304*)

33. **(b) Mastoid air cells** (*Ref. Cummings, 6th ed., 105*)
- Schuller's view and Law's view are lateral oblique views of mastoid to see the extent of pneumatisation and destruction, and the dural and sinus plate.
- X-ray of the ear was formerly the standard method of diagnosing diseases of mastoid but now HRCT scan shows a much clearer picture of the mastoid and other structures and thus is of greater utility in assessing the various conditions of the ear and their complications. Therefore the use of standard X-rays has now declined.

34. **(a) Temporal bone** (*Ref. Cummings, 6th ed., 105*)
- Stenver's view is to see the whole of the petrous pyramid (internal acoustic meatus, labyrinth, cochlea, mastoid antrum). Nowadays HRCT is done to assess temporal bone pathologies.

35. **(d) Modified radial mastoidectomy** (*Ref. Cummings, 6th ed., 2145*)

36. **(d) Stapes footplate** (*Ref. Cummings, 6th ed., 2190*)

37. **(d) Pressure of keratin** (*Ref. Cummings, 6th ed., 2144*)

38. **(b) Stapes footplate** (*Ref. Cummings, 6th ed., 2190*)

39. **(a) CSOM with attic perforation and cholesteatoma** (*Ref. Cummings, 6th ed., 2143*)

40. **(b) Modified radical mastoidectomy** (*Ref. Cummings, 6th ed., 2145*)

41. **(a) Primary acquired cholesteatoma** (*Ref. Cummings, 6th ed., 2143*)

42. **(b) Primary cholesteatoma** (*Ref. Cummings, 6th ed., 2145*)
- The picture shows attic retraction pocket with whitish cholesteatoma flakes.

Ear

Section I

Complications of Suppurative Otitis Media

Unsafe CSOM and ASOM/ANOM can lead to intratemporal and intracranial complications by spreading through the following pathways:

i. **Preformed pathways:**

  a. *Natural openings:* Through **oval** and **round window** into the **inner ear** and from inner ear through **internal acoustic meatus** and **cochlear aqueduct** to the cranium.

  b. *Congenital dehiscence:* Over fallopian canal to the facial nerve or on the floor of middle ear over jugular bulb.

  c. *Surgical or traumatic:* Mastoid exploration leading to exposure of dura superiorly and sigmoid/lateral sinus posteriorly, Fenestration operation and previous skull fractures.

ii. **Bone erosion:** In unsafe CSOM cholesteatoma causes bony erosion.

iii. **Venous thrombophlebitis:** The bacteria propagate in and around the venous channels that lead from the mastoid into the adjacent brain parenchyma.

While in unsafe CSOM, the complications occur mainly due to bone erosion, in ASOM the complications develop by venous thrombophlebitis or by direct extension along preformed pathways.

The complications of ASOM/ANOM and unsafe CSOM can be extracranial (i.e. limited to intratemporal areas) and intracranial.

EXTRACRANIAL (INTRATEMPORAL) COMPLICATIONS

The **extracranial or intratemporal** complications are the following:

i. Posterior to the middle ear is the mastoid so the patient can have **mastoiditis**.

ii. Medial to middle ear is the inner ear (labyrinth). So the patient can have **labyrinthitis**.

iii. In the middle ear is the nerve of temporal bone, the facial nerve, so the patient can have **facial nerve palsy**

iv. When the infection goes up to the petrous apex, patient has **petrositis**.

1. Acute Mastoiditis

This is the most common intratemporal complication. The most common organism causing acute mastoiditis is *Streptococcus pneumoniae* followed by β haemolytic streptococcus.

Pathophysiology

In a patient of ASOM infection from the pharynx comes to the middle ear via Eustachian tube. If the patient's immunity is less or there is infection with a highly virulent organism then the infection spreads from middle ear through the aditus to involve the mucosal lining of mastoid. This is known as mastoiditis.

Here again in the mastoid air cells, like ASOM, infection leads to hyperaemia, exudation and suppuration. Thus all the mastoid air cells get filled with pus.

Because of increased surface area from which the pus is being produced (air cells), the production of pus is more than that can be drained through TM perforation, or via Eustachian tube. Also the thickened, swollen mucosa of the antrum and aditus impairs drainage of pus leading to accumulation of pus under tension in all the air cells.

The hyperaemia of mucosal lining leads to venous stasis leading to local acidosis and dissolution of calcium from the bone leading to hyperaemic decalcification and hence destruction of bony septa of mastoid leading to coalescence of air cells and ultimately the whole of mastoid gets filled with pus. Here it is known as **coalescent mastoiditis**.

The destruction of the bony septa of the air cells can also lead to the conversion of the mastoid air cells into a common cavity. This pus can rupture into adjoining areas leading to respective abscesses, *see* below.

Clinical Features

Since it usually follows ASOM, a patient of acute mastoiditis presents with a history of persistence of pain, fever, deafness and ear discharge even after 3 weeks of the episode of ASOM.

On examination:

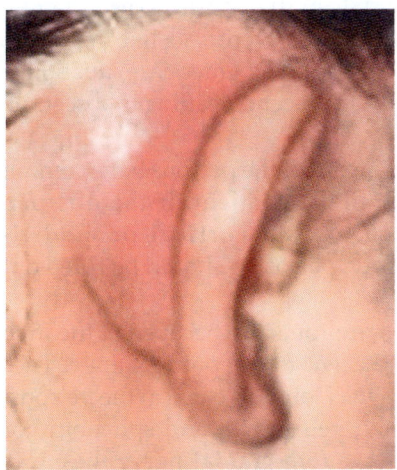

Pinna → The swelling over the mastoid pushes the pinna downwards, forwards and laterally.

Postauricular area → Because of abscess and infection in the mastoid air cells the periosteum overlying the mastoid gets inflamed and becomes oedematous. This oedema over the mastoid makes the mastoid appear very smooth as if we have ironed it. So it is known as **ironed out appearance** of mastoid, see the clinical picture above.

There is also **tenderness over the mastoid** mainly in the middle and tip. This is the most common sign of mastoiditis.

Retroauricular groove → Because of oedema over the mastoid the retroauricular groove appears deepened. Since it is not actually deepened, it is known as **apparent deepening.**
External auditory canal → There is mucopurulent discharge in the EAC (as it is coming through the perforation on the TM, from middle ear where mucus glands are present).

Reservoir sign → The moment we clean the EAC of the discharge it again refills with discharge. This is because of the reservoir of pus in the middle ear and mastoid. This is known as reservoir sign.

Light house sign → The pus coming through the antero-inferior perforation on the TM (*see* Chapter 5) from the mastoid and middle ear being large and in a lot of pressure gives an appearance known as **"pulsatile otorrhoea or light house sign".**

Sagging of postero-superior meatal wall → When the EAC is cleaned of the discharge we see sagging of the posterosuperior meatal wall. Since the posterior wall is the common wall between middle ear, deep EAC and mastoid, abscess in the mastoid will lead to periosteitis and periosteal oedema of this common wall. This through the EAC appears as sagging of postero-superior deep meatal wall.

When the abscess of the mastoid erodes this common wall and ruptures anteriorly towards the EAC, then this sagging increases and it is known as **Luc abscess.** (*Mnemonic:* **LUC** in **EAC**)

When the abscess ruptures laterally eroding the mastoid cortex over the Macewen's triangle, it is known as **postauricular abscess or subperiosteal abscess.** The **most common abscess** following mastoiditis is postauricular abscess or subperiosteal abscess.

When the abscess ruptures superiorly (mainly seen with involvement of zygomatic air cells) over the posterior root of zygoma, it is known as **zygomatic abscess**.

When the abscess ruptures inferiorly there can be two abscesses in relation to the two muscles that attach to the **tip of mastoid** (sternocleidomastoid and digastric).

a. If the abscess tracks down along the sterno-cleidomastoid it is known as **Bezold abscess.** It can also reach the parapharyngeal space leading to parapharyngeal abscess.

b. If the abscess tracks down along the **posterior belly of digastric**, it is known as **Citelli's abscess.** (*Mnemonic:* **C D:** **C**itelli-**D**igastric)

Investigation

X-ray mastoid and **CT scan** shows clouding of air cells because of the collection of exudates in them. Later on mastoid pneumatisation is lost and a single mastoid cavity may be seen.

Management

Pus anywhere has to be drained. So here also the management will be antibiotics and I and D.

In late cases or in cases not responding to antibiotics for 48 hrs, to drain the pus from mastoid air cells the air cells will have to be opened for which we have to drill the mastoid. Drilling is started over the Macewen's triangle.

As we go on drilling, the air cells go on opening and the pus comes out of them. When we have reached the deepest air cell, i.e. the antrum, we have converted the whole of mastoid into a single cavity. This operation is known as **cortical mastoidectomy, simple mastoidectomy or Schwartze operation.**

Masked mastoiditis: When a patient of mastoiditis is given antibiotics but in inadequate dose and duration, the symptoms of pain, fever subside but the collection in the mastoid and middle ear is still there leading to hearing loss and mild chronic auricular and post auricular pain and tenderness. This is known as masked or latent mastoiditis.

Management

It is managed by antibiotics and cortical mastoidectomy.

2. Labyrinthitis

It can be of 3 types:

a. **Circumscribed labyrinthitis:** Here there is exposure of a localised part of membranous labyrinth due to erosion of the overlying bone which might also proceed to fistula formation. The MC site of erosion and fistula formation is at the **bulge of lateral semicircular canal.**

The exposed part of membranous labyrinth becomes exposed to pressure changes leading to positive fistula test, *see* Chapter on vestibular system.

Patient presents with vertigo and partial SN hearing loss.
Management: Mastoid exploration with closure of fistula.

Section I || Ear

b. **Diffuse serous labyrinthitis:** This is diffuse sterile inflammatory response to the toxins from middle ear infection (entering into the inner ear fluid through the bone erosions by cholesteatoma, round window membrane or oval window annulus). There is no bacterial invasion or pus formation in the labyrinth.

Clinical features: Patient here presents with vertigo and **partial SN hearing loss.**

In diffuse serous labyrinthitis the nystagmus is towards the same side of lesion as it is an irritative lesion of the labyrinth, see chapter on vestibular system.

Management: Management is by antibiotics to control the middle ear infection, labyrinthine sedatives to control vertigo and mastoid exploration (if unsafe CSOM is the underlying cause). The hearing loss is reversible if the treatment is started early.

c. **Diffuse suppurative/Purulent labyrinthitis:** It follows serous labyrinthitis when direct spread of infection occurs into the inner ear. This leads to **complete destruction** of membranous labyrinth leading to necrosis, fibrosis and even ossification (labyrinthitis ossificans).

Clinical features: As it is a destructive lesion it leads to **total loss of hearing** and equilibrium leading to very severe vertigo and nystagmus towards the normal side, i.e. opposite side of lesion, as it is a destructive lesion.

The vertigo subsides in 2–3 weeks due to central compensation and compensation from the normal side.

Nystagmus may be absent. In this situation the diagnosis of serous or purulent labyrinthitis will be retrospective. If the vestibular and auditory functions are partially or completely retained it is assumed that the infection was serous.

Management: Antibiotics, labyrinthine sedatives and mastoid exploration in unsafe CSOM.

3. Facial Nerve Palsy

Facial nerve is the only cranial nerve that runs in a bony canal in most of its course. This canal is called fallopian canal. This canal can be dehiscent congenitally in 50% individuals. The MC site of this dehiscence is the horizontal segment just above the oval window. So if a child with congenital dehiscence of fallopian canal develops acute Otitis media, the increased pressure of the middle ear will get transmitted through the dehiscence to the facial nerve leading to facial palsy.

So in this patient of **ASOM with facial palsy** the management will be antibiotics to treat ASOM and a myringotomy to relieve the pressure on the facial nerve.

In **unsafe CSOM the facial palsy** occurs because of erosion of fallopian canal by cholesteatoma. This can be managed by immediate mastoid exploration and facial nerve decompression.

4. Petrositis

Petrous part of temporal bone is a pneumatised bone in approximately 30% people with air cells extending from the mastoid/middle ear uptill the petrous apex.

When the infection goes from the mastoid/middle ear up to the air cells in the petrous part of temporal bone, it is known as petrositis. Here also, like mastoiditis, infection of the air cells leads to hyperaemia, exudation, suppuration and ultimately coalescence leading to abscess at the petrous apex.

Since the air cells of the petrous bone communicate with the mastoid, in any patient, if there is **persistent ear discharge following cortical or modified radical mastoidectomy,** petrositis should be ruled out by CT and MRI.

Here the symptoms are because of the involvement of the nerves adjacent to the petrous apex. The **6th cranial nerve** runs in the Dorello's canal at the petrous apex (canal in between the petrous tip and sphenoid bone) and the trigeminal nerve (**5th cranial nerve**) lies in the Meckel's cave which is a concavity on the anterior slant of petrous part of temporal bone near the petrous apex in which the V nerve ganglion (gasserian ganglion) rests.

So there is palsy of the 6th nerve leading to lateral rectus palsy causing diplopia and retro-orbital and deep facial pain due to involvement of ophthalmic division of 5th cranial nerve.

The 6th nerve palsy, 5th nerve involvement (ophthalmic division) and the persistent ear discharge in petrositis is called **Gradenigo triad or syndrome**.

Mnemonic: G   γ   a   d e n i g   o
              6   V   **a**nd   **d**ischarge **o**phthalmic
              division

Treatment: It is managed by antibiotics and mastoid exploration along with curettage of the fistulous track to drain abscess from the petrous apex.

INTRACRANIAL COMPLICATIONS OF CSOM

1. Meningitis

This is the **MC intracranial complication** of unsafe CSOM and ASOM.

The MC organism causing otogenic meningitis is Streptococcus pneumoniae, followed by *H. influenzae*.

Though the incidence of meningitis has gone down because of availability of vaccinations (against Hib and Pneumococcal) and antibiotics, but still the most common intracranial complication of CSOM is Meningitis.

Clinical features: Patient presents with fever and features suggestive of increased intracranial tension (headache, vomiting, drowsiness) and meningeal irritation (neck rigidity and irritability).

The two signs seen here are:

1. **Kernig's sign:** Pain on extending the leg with thigh flexed on abdomen.
2. **Brudzinski's sign:** Flexion of hip and knee occurs on flexion of neck.

Diagnosis: Lumbar puncture

Management: Antibiotics followed by mastoid exploration once the general condition improves.

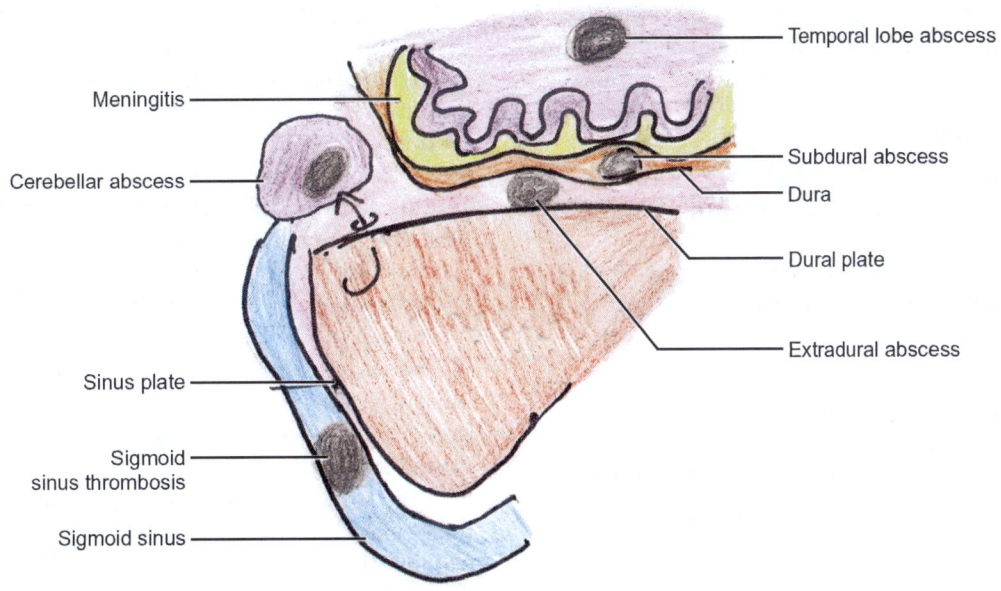

Fig. 9.1: Intracranial Complications of Atticoantral CSOM

2. Brain Abscess

The **most common** otogenic brain abscess is **temporal lobe abscess** followed by cerebellar abscess. Temporal lobe abscess is the second most common intracranial complication of unsafe CSOM.

The **organisms** isolated in brain abscess are both aerobic (Gram-negative—Pseudomonas, Proteus, *E.coli*; Gram-positive—Streptococcus and Staphylococcus) and anaerobic (Peptostreptococcus and *Bacteroides fragilis*).

H. influenzae which was previously the most common cause of otogenic meningitis is rarely found in otogenic brain abscess.

Clinical Features

Temporal lobe abscess

A patient of temporal lobe abscess, along with the other features of brain abscess, i.e. features of increased intracranial pressure due to space occupying lesion (headache, vomiting) and features of infection (fever), presents with the following localising features:

  i. **Nominal aphasia** (inability to name the common things)
 ii. **Homonymous supra quadrantanopia:** As the name, corresponding upper quadrants of each field (right or left), i.e. the upper half of ipsilateral nasal and the upper half of contralateral temporal have been lost. (*Mnemonic:* Pie in the sky appearance) This is due to involvement of the ventral band of optic radiation which passes through the temporal lobe in its course from the lateral geniculate body to the occipital lobe.
iii. Contralateral hemiparesis and
 iv. Seizures

Cerebellar abscess

It will additionally present with the following:
1. Ataxia
2. Dysmetria
3. Dysdiadochokinesia and other cerebellar manifestations.

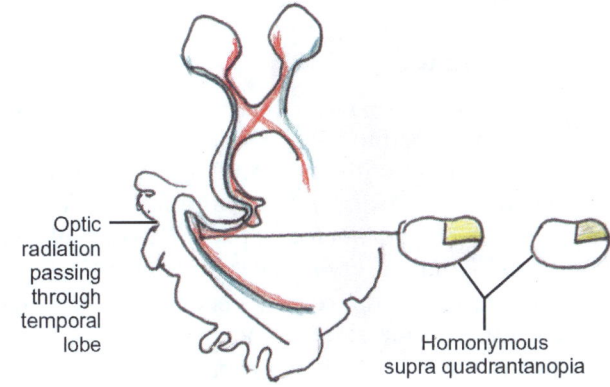

Fig. 9.2: Homonymous Supra Quadrantanopia

Diagnosis: MRI/CT (MRI is better than CT) shows '**ring sign'** (abscess surrounded by a zone of oedema).

Management: Abscess drainage followed by mastoid exploration once the patient's condition improves.

3. Extradural (Epidural/Peridural Abscess)

Any infection of the mastoid whether it be acute (e.g. mastoiditis following acute Otitis media) or chronic (unsafe CSOM) can erode the bone forming the roof of mastoid (tegmen antri) that separates the mastoid from middle cranial fossa or the posterior wall of mastoid (sinus plate) separating the mastoid from sigmoid/lateral sinus leading to an extradural abscess. This abscess lies in between the dura and skull bone.

This is known as **silent complication** as here most of the times, the patient does not present with any features of brain abscess and it is an accidental finding seen during mastoid exploration.

Management: Since the abscess is related to the roof or posterior wall of mastoid, it can be drained only once the disease of mastoid is removed and these walls exposed.

Section I ‖ Ear

So here the abscess drainage is done at the same time as mastoid exploration (MRM, RM or cortical mastoidectomy). Postoperatively antibiotics are given.

4. Subdural Abscess

This is the rarest complication of Otitis Media.

Here there is collection of pus in between the dura and arachnoid.

Patient presents with features of brain abscess, i.e. fever, headache, vomiting and focal neurological signs.

Investigation: MRI

Management: Abscess drainage and antibiotics followed by mastoid exploration once the patient is stabilised.

5. Lateral Sinus or Sigmoid Sinus Thrombophlebitis

The posterior wall of the mastoid antrum is formed by bone covering the lateral sinus or sigmoid sinus.

Disease of the antrum can erode this bone and form a perisinus abscess which can then lead to intrasinus inflammation, damage to intima of the blood vessel initiating hyper coagulation, and thrombus formation. Subsequently the thrombus gets infected and enlarges occluding the sinus.

Clinical features: Whenever the infected thrombus is released as embolus into the systemic circulation, patient has a peak of fever with chills and rigors returning to baseline, when he feels well till another embolus is released leading to another febrile peak. This type of fever is known as "**hectic fever or picket fence fever**".

Due to interruption of cortical venous drainage there may be features of increased intracranial tension.

When the thrombophlebitis propagates superiorly, it extends to the tributary of the sigmoid sinus draining the mastoid; the mastoid emissary vein. The thrombosis of this vein leads to impaired drainage of the mastoid leading to oedema over the mastoid. This is known as '**Griesinger's sign**'.

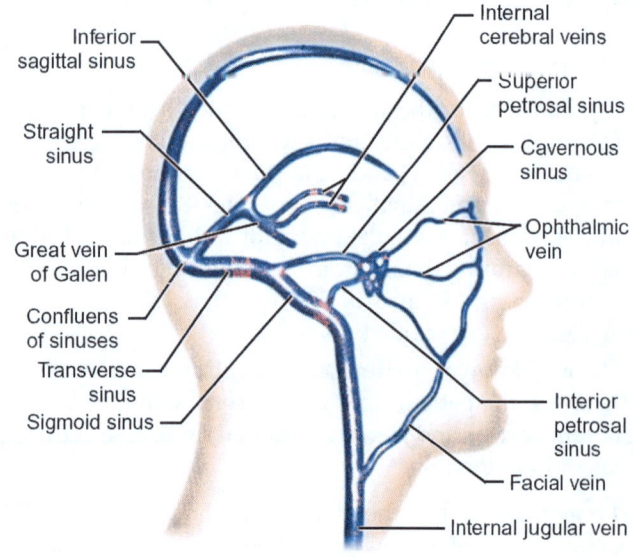

Fig. 9.3

When the thrombophlebitis propagates inferiorly, it involves the internal jugular vein which is the inferior extension of sigmoid sinus. The jugular vein becomes cord like and very tender. The patient presents with **tenderness on the neck over the jugular vein area**. In a patient with thrombosis and obstruction of one jugular vein, the normal side jugular vein takes over the function. In such a patient with only one functioning jugular vein, pressure over this normal side jugular vein will increase the CSF pressure, whereas pressure on the obstructed jugular vein will cause no change in CSF pressure.

The above test to look for increase in CSF pressure (as measured on lumbar puncture) by alternately pressing jugular vein of both sides is known as "**Tobey Ayer test**" (**Queckenstedt's test**).

If the same increase in CSF pressure is seen as retinal vein engorgement or papilloedema on fundus examination, it is known as "**Crowe-Beck sign.**" Pressure on jugular vein leading to retinal vein engorgement means that side is normal and no retinal engorgement on pressing the jugular vein suggest obstruction of jugular vein.

Diagnosis: Contrast enhanced MRI (better) or CECT (show the typical "**delta sign**" or **empty triangle sign Δ**) (the thrombus does not take up the contrast, the walls appear enhanced giving the above picture).

Treatment: Treatment is by I/V antibiotics with mastoid exploration (MRM).

Since the sigmoid sinus can be exposed only after opening up the mastoid antrum as it forms its posterior wall, a preliminary modified radical mastoidectomy (canal wall down surgery, please *see* chapter on CSOM) will have to be done to remove the disease from the mastoid and the middle ear following which the bone covering the dura of the sinus is removed and the perisinus or intrasinus thrombophlebitic abscess is drained.

6. Otitic Hydrocephalus

This usually follows lateral sinus thrombosis, when an embolus obstructs the transverse sinus and other dural venous sinuses. Due to obstruction and impairment of the venous outflow there is increase in intracranial pressure leading to hydrocephalus (benign intracranial HTN/ pseudotumour cerebri).

Clinical features: The patient presents with features of increased CSF pressure, i.e. headache, vomiting, blurring of vision (due to papilloedema).

Investigation: HRCT

Treatment: The management involves reducing the CSF pressure; medically (diuretics) or surgically by a VP (ventriculo-peritoneal) shunt.

7. Encephalocele (Brain Hernia/Brain Fungus)

Erosion leading to defects of tegmen tympani or tegmen mastoideum can lead to encephalocele or even CSF leakage. These defects can be repaired through middle ear and mastoid or middle cranial fossa approach after removing the disease.

"Points to Ponder/Points for Quick revision"

- The complications occur in Atticoantral/squamosal chronic otitis media (COM) (unsafe CSOM) mainly due to bone erosion by the cholesteatoma.
- The complications may also be seen at times in Acute otitis media (AOM) and Acute necrotising otitis media (ANOM) due to the high virulence or low immunity through venous thrombophlebitis or by direct extension along preformed pathways (natural openings or congenital/surgical/traumatic dehiscences).
  A. Extracranial complications (intratemporal):
  i. Acute Mastoiditis (MC):
     - MC–*Strept. pneumoniae* (the causative organism of AOM)
     - Infection comes through the aditus
     - Hyperemia, exudation and suppuration of mastoid air cells → pus under tension → damage to the bony septa between air cells → coalescent mastoiditis and other abscesses
     - Postauricular abscess (MC), LUC abscess in the deep postero-superior EAC, Bezold abscess (along sternocleidomastoid) and Citelli's abscess (along digastric)
     - CFs: Persistence of symptoms after AOM, tenderness over mastoid (MC sign), ironed out appearance, apparent deepening of retro-auricular groove, reservoir and light house sign
     - Antibiotics ± Cortical/Simple mastoidectomy (Schwartze operation)
  ii. Labyrinthitis:
     - CFs: Vertigo and SN hearing loss
     - 3 types:
       a. Circumscribed:
          - Due to localised erosion with ± fistula formation (MC–bulge of lateral SCC)
          - + fistula test
       b. Diffuse serous:
          - Sterile inflammation
          - Nystagmus towards the lesion
       c. Diffuse purulent:
          - Infection → Complete destruction of the labyrinth
          - Nystagmus towards normal
          - Treatment: Antibiotics, labyrinthine sedatives ± mastoid exploration (if cholesteatoma)

  iii. Facial N palsy:
     - Though facial N is in a bony canal (fallopian canal), but it being commonly congenitally dehiscent, therefore may get involved in ASOM (t/t antibiotics + myringotomy to relieve the pressure)
     - Cholesteatoma erodes the fallopian canal in squamosal COM (t/t–mastoid exploration)
  iv. Petrositis:
     - Air cells in the petrous bone in communication with the mastoid air cells
     - Therefore Mastoiditis → petrositis → abscess formation at the petrous apex → Gradenigo triad or syndrome
     - Gradenigo triad: 6th N palsy → LR palsy → diplopia + involvement V_1 → retro-orbital and deep facial pain + persistent ear discharge
  B. Intracranial complications:
  i. Meningitis (MC):
     - MC–Strept. pneumoniae
     - CFs–fever, headache, vomiting, alteration of consciousness. Neck rigidity, Brudzinski's and Kernig's sign
  ii. Brain abscess:
     - MC–Temporal lobe
     - Mixed organisms
     - CFs–fever, headache, vomiting, nominal aphasia, homonymous supra quadrantanopia, hemiparesis, seizures
     - MRI–ring sign
  iii. Epidural abscess: silent
  iv. Subdural abscess: rarest
  v. Lateral sinus/Sigmoid sinus thrombophlebitis:
     - Erosion of the posterior wall of mastoid → sigmoid sinus intima damage → thrombus formation
     - CFs:
       a. Infected emboli into the systemic circulation → Picket fence fever
       b. Emboli obstructing other dural venous sinuses → impairment of venous outflow → ↑ intracranial pressure and hydrocephalus
       c. Propagation of thrombus—Mastoid emissary vein; Griesinger's sign; Internal jugular vein; tenderness, Tobey Ayer test (Queckenstedt's test), Crowe-Beck sign
     - MRI/CECT–delta sign or empty triangle sign
  vi. Encephalocele (Brain hernia/brain fungus)

PREVIOUSLY ASKED QUESTIONS

1. **Middle ear infections are known to spread to the adjacent areas via all of the following routes, except:** *(AI 2012)*
   a. Direct Bony Invasion
   b. Oval/Round Window
   c. Venous thrombophlebitis
   d. Lymphatic spread

2. **Most common complication of acute Otitis media in children:** *(SRMC 2002, Exam 2017)*
   a. Deafness
   b. Mastoiditis
   c. Cholesteatoma
   d. Facial nerve palsy

3. **Extracranial complications of CSOM:** *(PGI Dec 2002, Exam 2015)*
   a. Epidural abscess
   b. Facial nerve palsy
   c. Hearing loss
   d. Labyrinthitis
   e. Sigmoid sinus thrombosis

4. **Extracranial complications of CSOM:** *(PGI June 2001, Exam 2014)*
   a. Labyrinthitis
   b. Otitic hydrocephalus
   c. Bezold abscess
   d. Facial nerve palsy
   e. Lateral sinus thrombophlebitis

5. **Most common extracranial complication of ASOM is:** *(UP 2001, Exam 2013)*
   a. Facial nerve paralysis
   b. Lateral sinus thrombosis
   c. Mastoiditis
   d. Brain abscess

6. **Acute mastoiditis is characterised by all except:** *(AP 97, Exam 2010)*
   a. Deafness
   b. Outward and downward deviation of the pinna
   c. Vertigo
   d. Clouding of air cells

7. **Essential radiological feature of acute mastoiditis is:** *(UP 2003, Exam 2017)*
   a. Temporal bone pneumatisation
   b. Clouding of air cells of mastoid
   c. Rarefaction of petrous bone
   d. Thickening of temporal bone

8. **Mastoid tip is involved in:** *(UP 2006, Exam 2017)*
   a. Bezold abscess
   b. Luc abscess
   c. Subperiosteal abscess
   d. Parapharyngeal abscess

9. **Bezold abscess is located in:** *(AIIMS 92/Exam 2007)*
   a. Submandibular region
   b. Sternocleidomastoid muscle
   c. Digastric triangle
   d. Infratemporal region

10. **Mastoid reservoir sign is positive in:** *(AI 2001, Exam 2017)*
    a. CSOM   b. Petrositis
    c. Serous Otitis media d. Coalescent mastoiditis

11. **Schwartz operation is also called:** *(UP 2000, Exam 2017)*
    a. Cortical mastoidectomy
    b. Modified radical mastoidectomy
    c. Radical mastoidectomy
    d. Fenestration operation

12. **Schwartz operation is done in:** *(MP 2004, Exam 2017)*
    a. CSOM   b. Serous otitis media
    c. Otosclerosis   d. Acute mastoiditis

13. **Simple mastoidectomy is done in:** *(MP2000, AIIMS 93, Exam 2017)*
    a. Acute mastoiditis
    b. Cholesteatoma
    c. Safe CSOM
    d. Localized chronic otitis media

14. **Cortical mastoidectomy is indicated in:** *(AI 2000, Exam 2017)*
    a. Cholesteatoma without complication
    b. Coalescent mastoiditis
    c. CSOM with brain abscess
    d. Perforation in Pars flaccida

15. **Most common nerve to be damaged in CSOM is:** *(Exam 2013)*
    a. III   b. VII
    c. IV   d. VI

16. **Treatment of cholesteatoma with facial paresis in a child is:** *(AIIMS 93, 2000, Exam 2017)*
    a. Antibiotics to dry ear and then mastoidectomy
    b. Immediate mastoidectomy
    c. Observation
    d. Only antibiotic ear drops

17. **Treatment of choice for CSOM with vertigo and facial nerve palsy is:** *(AI 96, 2003, Exam 2016)*
    a. Antibiotics and labyrinthine sedatives
    b. Myringoplasty
    c. Immediate mastoid exploration
    d. Labyrinthectomy

18. **Cholesteatoma perforates:** *(PGI 2000, Exam 2016)*
    a. Lateral semicircular canal
    b. Superior semicircular canal
    c. Promontory
    d. Oval window
    e. Posterior semicircular canal

19. Cranial nerves related to the apex of petrous temporal bone: *(PGI 2005, Exam 2013)*
    a. V
    b. VI
    c. VII
    d. VIII
    e. IX

20. The diagnosis in a patient with 6th nerve palsy, retro-orbital pain and persistent ear discharge is: *(AI 2004, Exam 2017)*
    a. Gradenigo syndrome
    b. Sjögren's syndrome
    c. Frey's syndrome
    d. Rendu-Osler-Weber disease

21. A patient presents with diplopia, pain side of head, fever and ear discharge. The most probable diagnosis is: *(Exam 2014)*
    a. CSOM
    b. Meningitis
    c. Lateral sinus thrombosis
    d. Petrositis

22. All are true for Gradenigo syndrome except: *(AI 2005, Exam 2017)*
    a. It is associated with jugular vein tenderness
    b. It is caused by an abscess in the petrous apex
    c. It leads to involvement of the cranial nerves V and VI
    d. It is characterised by retro-orbital pain

23. Gradenigo syndrome involves the following cranial nerves: *(AI 2004, Exam 2017)*
    a. IV, VII
    b. V, VI
    c. VI, IX
    d. VII, VIII

24. Gradenigo triad is characterised by all except: *(MH 2004, Exam 2017)*
    a. Retro-orbital pain
    b. Profuse discharge from the ear
    c. VII nerve palsy
    d. Diplopia

25. Components of Gradenigo triad: *(PGI 2008)*
    a. Abscess petrous apex
    b. Retro-orbital pain
    c. Cranial nerve VI involved
    d. Ear discharge
    e. Conductive deafness

26. Ramu presented with persistent ear discharge and hearing loss. Modified radical mastoidectomy was done to him. Patient comes back with persistent ear discharge and retro-orbital pain. What is your diagnosis: *(AIIMS May 2007)*
    a. Diffuse serous labyrinthitis
    b. Purulent labyrinthitis
    c. Petrositis
    d. Latent mastoiditis

27. A patient with h/o right ear discharge undergoes mastoidectomy but now he presents with vertigo and deafness. Diagnosis is: *(AIIMS 2013)*
    a. Labyrinthitis
    b. Thrombophlebitis
    c. Temporal lobe abscess
    d. Mastoiditis

28. A case of CSOM presenting with vertigo can have any of the following except: *(AI 99, Exam 2009)*
    a. Extradural abscess
    b. Cerebellar abscess
    c. Fistula of semicircular canal
    d. Labyrinthitis

29. A patient of CSOM has cholesteatoma and presents with vertigo. Treatment of choice would be: *(AI 98, Exam 2011)*
    a. Myringotomy
    b. Myringoplasty
    c. Immediate mastoid exploration
    d. Labyrinthectomy

30. The most common complication of chronic suppurative Otitis media is: *(Kerala 96, UPSC 2005, Exam 2013)*
    a. Meningitis
    b. Intracerebral abscess
    c. Cholesteatoma
    d. Conductive deafness

31. Commonest intracranial complication of CSOM is: *(DPG 2009, Comed 2008)*
    a. Sub-periosteal abscess
    b. Mastoiditis
    c. Brain abscess
    d. Meningitis

32. Most potential route for transmission of labyrinthitis leading to meningitis: *(AI 2009)*
    a. Cochlear aqueduct
    b. Endolymphatic sac
    c. Vestibular aqueduct
    d. Hyrtle fissure

33. Patient presents with high fever, neck rigidity, signs of raised ICT and a past history of chronic otitis media likely diagnosis is: *(DPG 2009)*
    a. Brain abscess
    b. Pyogenic meningitis
    c. Acute subarachnoid haemorrhage
    d. Lateral sinus thrombosis

34. A 6-month-old infant was treated for *H. influenzae* meningitis. Most important investigation to be done before discharging the patient is: *(JIPMER 2008, Exam 2014)*
    a. MRI
    b. Brainstem evoked response audiometry
    c. Growth screening test
    d. Psychotherapy

Section I || Ear

35. **Commonest cause of otogenic meningitis is:**
(*AI 2000, Exam 2017*)
a. *Streptococcus pneumoniae*
b. *H. influenza*
c. Pseudomonas
d. *E. coli*

36. **True about otogenic brain abscess is:**
(*AI 2004, Exam 2017*)
a. *H. influenzae* is most common causative organism
b. CSOM with lateral sinus thrombosis in turn can cause brain abscess
c. Most common intracranial complication of CSOM
d. Temporal lobe abscess is associated with personality changes

37. **Lateral sinus thrombosis is associated with all except:** (*AP 2008*)
a. Griesinger's sign
b. Gradenigo triad
c. Crowe-Beck sign
d. Tobey-Ayer test

38. **Tobey Ayer test is positive in:** (*Exam 2013*)
a. Lateral sinus thrombosis
b. Petrositis
c. Cerebral abscess
d. Subarachnoid haemorrhage

39. **Griesinger's sign is seen in:**
(*TN 2003, DPG 2008, Exam 2013*)
a. Lateral sinus thrombosis
b. Meningitis
c. Brain abscess
d. Cerebellar abscess

40. **A 30-year-old male is having attic cholesteatoma of left ear with lateral sinus thrombophlebitis. Which of the following will be the operation of choice:**
(*AI 2006, Exam 2017*)
a. Intact canal wall mastoidectomy
b. Simple mastoidectomy with tympanoplasty
c. Canal wall down mastoidectomy
d. Mastoidectomy with cavity obliteration

41. **Which sign is seen due to thrombosis of mastoid emissary veins?** (*Exam 2016*)
a. Battle sign   b. Griesinger's sign
c. Irwin Moore sign   d. Hennebert's sign

42. **Edema over the mastoid is seen in:** (*Exam 2016*)
a. Bell's Palsy
b. Lateral sinus thrombophlebitis
c. CSOM
d. Labyrinthitis

43. **Picket fence fever is a feature of:** (*Exam 2016*)
a. Acute mastoiditis
b. Lateral sinus thrombophlebitis

c. Temporal lobe abscess
d. Atticoantral CSOM

44. **Tobey Ayer's test is done for:** (*Exam 2016*)
a. Acute mastoiditis   b. BPPV
c. Glomus jugulare   d. Jugular vein thrombosis

45. **Griesinger's sign is:** (*Exam 2016*)
a. Mastoid bone edema
b. Jugular vein tenderness
c. Tenderness over mastoid
d. Sagging of posterosuperior meatal wall

46. **Given is the CECT of a patient of foul smelling ear discharge with convulsions. He should be managed by:** (*Exam 2015*)

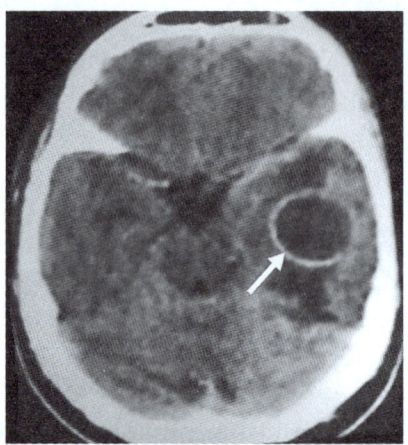

a. Abscess drainage followed by MRM
b. MRM followed by abscess drainage
c. Myringoplasty
d. Only MRM

47. **Which of the following is not related to the complication of cholesteatoma:** (*Exam 2016*)
a. Tobey-Ayer test
b. Crowe-Beck sign
c. Griesinger sign
d. Hitzelberger sign

48. **A patient presents with deep retro orbital pain, pain in eye movement, compensatory head tilt and ear discharge. His diagnosis is:** (*WB PG 2015*)
a. Gradenigo syndrome
b. Temporal lobe abscess
c. Malignant otitis externa
d. Vestibular Schwannoma

49. **The delta sign is seen in:** (*APPG 2015*)
a. Lateral sinus thrombosis
b. Petrositis
c. Meningitis
d. Brain abscess

50. **A 5-year-old child presents with continuing pain and discharge from right ear since one month after an episode of ASOM. The appearance of the ear is**

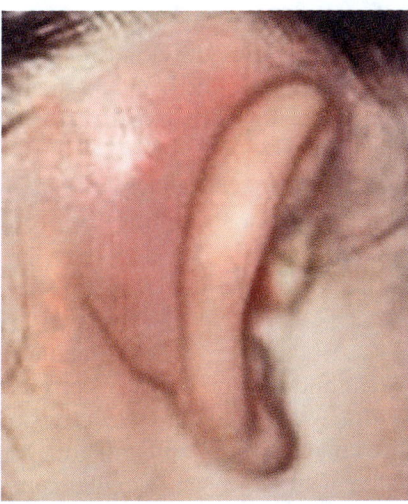

given in the picture below. Examination of the EAC shows reservoir sign and sagging of posterosuperior meatal wall. He should be managed by:

(Practice question by Author)

a. Schwartze operation
b. Modified radical mastoidectomy
c. Radical mastoidectomy
d. Myringoplasty

51. **Which of the following is not the component of Gradenigo triad:** *(Exam 2016)*
    a. Involvement of the V and VI nerve
    b. Persistent otorrhoea
    c. Palatal palsy
    d. Retro-orbital pain

52. **Treatment of Brain fungus in mastoid cavity is:** *(Karnataka 2005, Exam 2017)*
    a. Amphotericin therapy
    b. Miconazole powder application
    c. Surgical repair
    d. Syringing

53. **False regarding Gradenigo syndrome is:** *(Exam 2016)*
    a. Retro-orbital pain
    b. Persistence of ear discharge
    c. Facial palsy
    d. Petrositis

Section I | **Ear**

ANSWERS AND EXPLANATIONS

1. **(d) Lymphatic spread** (*Ref. Shambaugh, 6th ed., 453*)
2. **(b) Mastoiditis** (*Ref. Cummings, 6th ed., 2157; Scott Brown, 8th ed., Vol 2; 972*)
   - This is the most common complication following ASOM.
   - Facial nerve palsy is an uncommon complication of ASOM
   - Deafness (along with Pain and ear discharge) is the presenting feature of ASOM
   - Cholesteatoma is not associated with ASOM.
3. **(b) and (d) Facial nerve palsy, labyrinthitis** (*Ref. Cummings, 6th ed., 2157*)
   - Hearing loss is the presentation of CSOM.
   - Epidural abscess and sigmoid (lateral) sinus thrombosis are intracranial complications, please see the text.
4. **(a), (c) and (d) Labyrinthitis, Bezold abscess, facial nerve palsy** (*Ref. Cummings, 6th ed., 2157*)
5. **(c) Mastoiditis** (*Ref. Cummings, 6th ed., 2157*)
6. **(c) Vertigo** (*Ref. Cummings, 6th ed., 2160*)
7. **(b) Clouding of air cells of mastoid** (*Ref. Cummings, 6th ed., 2161*)
   - X-ray mastoid and CT scan shows clouding of air cells because of the collection of exudates in them. Later on mastoid pneumatisation is lost and a single mastoid cavity may be seen.
8. **(a) Bezold abscess, please refer the text** (*Ref. Cummings, 6th ed., 2163*)
9. **(b) Sternocleidomastoid muscle** (*Ref. Cummings, 6th ed., 2164*)
10. **(d) Coalescent mastoiditis,** (*Ref. Dhingra, 6th ed. 78*) **please refer the text**
11. **(a) Cortical mastoidectomy** (*Ref. Shambaugh, 6th ed., 501*)
12. **(d) Acute mastoiditis** (*Ref. Shambaugh, 6th ed., 501*)
13. **(a) Acute mastoiditis** (*Ref. Shambaugh, 6th ed., 509*)
14. **(b) Coalescent mastoiditis** (*Ref. Cummings, 6th ed. 2161*)
15. **(b) VII** (*Ref. Shambaugh, 6th ed., 512*)
    - Most common nerve to be damaged in CSOM is the facial nerve as it passes through the middle ear.
    - Rest of the nerves mentioned are not related to the ear.
16. **(b) Immediate mastoidectomy** (*Ref. Cummings, 6th ed., 2169*)
    - In a patient of unsafe CSOM the cholesteatoma may erode the fallopian canal and cause facial nerve paresis. So here immediate mastoidectomy is done to remove the disease. There is no role of antibiotics.
17. **(c) Immediate mastoid exploration** (*Ref. Shambaugh, 6th ed., 448*)
    - This is an unsafe CSOM. Here cholesteatoma eroding fallopian canal and causing fistula formation on the medial wall of middle ear (lateral semicircular canal, promontory, oval window) is causing facial nerve palsy and vertigo respectively. So the management is immediate mastoid exploration to remove cholesteatoma.
18. **(a), (c) and (d)** (*Ref. Cummings, 6th ed., 2167*)
    - Cholesteatoma most commonly erodes Lateral semicircular canal.
    - It can also erode the oval window and promontory.
    - All these structures are on the medial wall of the middle ear and erosion of these leads to a fistula on the medial wall leading to vertigo on external pressure changes and positive fistula test.
    - The bulge of superior semi-circular canal is present on the anterior slant of the petrous part of temporal bone and not on the medial wall. Hence a middle ear cholesteatoma does not erode it.
19. **(a), (b) V, VI** (*Ref. Cummings, 6th ed., 2165*)
20. **(a) Gradenigo syndrome** (*Ref. Scott Brown, 8th ed., Vol 2; 1318*)
21. **(d) Petrositis** (*Ref. Scott Brown, 8th ed., Vol 2; 1318*)
    The given patient has developed petrositis which explains fever, ear discharge, diplopia (due to involvement of VI nerve) and pain side of head (in the distribution of the ophthalmic division of trigeminal).
    The rest of the choices are clearly not the considerations, see the text for their presentation.
22. **(a) It is associated with jugular vein tenderness** (*Ref. Scott Brown, 8th ed., Vol 2; 1318*)
23. **(b) V, VI** (*Ref. Cummings, 6th ed. 2165*)
24. **(c) VII nerve palsy** (*Ref. Cummings, 6th ed. 2165*)
25. **(b), (c) and (d)** (*Ref. Scott Brown, 8th ed., Vol 2; 1318*)
    - The Gradenigo triad is caused by petrositis (or abscess of petrous apex) and constitutes:
      i. VI nerve involvement leading to diplopia
      ii. V nerve involvement (ophthalmic division) leading to retro-orbital pain
      iii. Ear discharge
    - Conductive deafness is also seen in petrositis (or abscess petrous apex) as petrositis follows otitis media but it is not a part of the triad.
26. **(c) Petrositis** (*Ref. Cummings, 6th ed., 2165*)
    - Since the air cells of the petrous bone communicate with the mastoid, in any patient, if there is persistent ear discharge following cortical or modified radical mastoidectomy, petrositis should be ruled out by CT and MRI. Also retroorbital pain is suggestive of petrositis (due to involvement of ophthalmic division of trigeminal).
    - Labyrinthitis per se does not lead to ear discharge once the middle ear and mastoid disease has been cleared by surgery. Moreover, in labyrinthitis there will be vertigo along with hearing loss. So this is not the complication in the given case.

- Latent mastoiditis or masked mastoiditis can be a consequence of inadequate medical management; but there is no question of it arising after modified radical mastoidectomy.

27. **(a) Labyrinthitis** (*Ref. Cummings, 6th ed., 2169*)
- Following mastoidectomy deafness along with vertigo is suggestive of labyrinthitis.

28. **(a) Extradural abscess** (*Ref. Shambaugh, 6th ed., 447*)
- Extradural abscess is most often a silent complication and is detected accidently during mastoid exploration.

29. **(c) Immediate mastoid exploration** (*Ref. Cummings, 6th ed., 2169*)
- This is an unsafe CSOM with labyrinthitis. So the management is immediate mastoid exploration to remove cholesteatoma.

30. **(a) Meningitis** (*Ref. Cummings, 6th ed., 2157*)
- The most common intracranial complication of chronic suppurative Otitis media is meningitis followed by intracerebral abscess (temporal lobe abscess)
- Cholesteatoma promotes the above complications in unsafe CSOM.
- Conductive deafness is one of the presenting features of CSOM.

31. **(d) Meningitis** (*Ref. Cummings, 6th ed., 2157*)
- The most common intracranial complication of chronic suppurative Otitis media is meningitis followed by brain abscess (temporal lobe abscess).
- Mastoiditis is the most common extracranial complication.
- Subperiosteal or postauricular abscess is the most common abscess following mastoiditis.

32. **(a) Cochlear aqueduct** (*Ref. Cummings, 6th ed., 2169; Scott Brown, 8th ed., Vol 2; 1012*)
- Most potential route for transmission of labyrinthitis leading to meningitis or vice versa is through cochlear aqueduct. From the inner ear the infection can spread to the cranium via.
  - i. Cochlear aqueduct (which connects the CSF to the scala tympani and is the site of entry of CSF leading to the formation of perilymph)
  - ii. Internal acoustic meatus.
- Endolymphatic sac is a part of membranous labyrinth. It is a closed sac, present extradurally and responsible for absorption of endolymph.
- Vestibular aqueduct is the part of bony labyrinth which surrounds the endolymphatic duct.
  Hyrtle fissure is the tympanomeningeal hiatus present at 16–18 week stage during fetal life. It connects round window to the posterior cranial fossa. It fuses and disappears by 26 weeks.

33. **(b) Pyogenic meningitis** (*Ref. Scott Brown, 8th ed., Vol 2; 1012*)
- Focal neurological deficits being not mentioned so brain abscess is not the right choice. Also meningismus causing neck rigidity is generally not present in brain abscess.

- Acute subarachnoid haemorrhage is due to rupture of intracranial aneurysm or head trauma. It presents with sudden loss of consciousness. It may also present with sudden onset very severe headache described as worst ever headache.
- Lateral sinus thrombosis presents with fever, tenderness over jugular vein and oedema over the mastoid.

34. **(b) Brainstem evoked response audiometry** (*Ref. Cummings, 6th ed., 2076*)
  Meningitis can lead to labyrinthitis and thereby deafness which an infant will not report and if diagnosed early, cochlear implantation will have good results, so BERA needs to be done.

35. **(a) *Streptococcus pneumoniae*** (*Ref. Cummings, 6th ed., 2171*)
  MC cause of otogenic meningitis was *H. influenzae* but after the introduction of Hib vaccine in the universal immunisation programme, it is *Streptococcus pneumoniae* now.

36. **(b) CSOM with lateral sinus thrombosis in turn can cause brain abscess** (*Ref. Cummings, 6th ed., 2172*) (please refer to the spreading pathways for complications of CSOM in the beginning of the chapter)
- *H. influenzae* which was previously the most common cause of otogenic meningitis is rarely found in otogenic brain abscess, refer the text for organisms causing brain abscess.
- Most common intracranial complication of CSOM is meningitis.
- Personality changes are associated with Frontal lobe abscess.

37. **(b) Gradenigo triad** (*Ref. Cummings, 6th ed., 2165*)
- Gradenigo triad is seen in association with abscess of petrous apex or petrositis. Rest all are seen in lateral sinus thrombosis.

38. **(a) Lateral sinus thrombosis** (*Ref. Shambaugh, 6th ed., 459*)

39. **(a) Lateral sinus thrombosis** (*Ref. Shambaugh, 6th ed., 459*)

40. **(c) Canal wall down mastoidectomy** (*Ref. Cummings, 6th ed., 2175*)
- Intact canal wall down mastoidectomy is done when there is limited disease in the mastoid.
- Simple mastoidectomy also known as cortical mastoidectomy is done for acute and coalescent mastoiditis.
- Following any canal wall down procedure the big mastoid cavity can be obliterated to prevent cavity related problems but if the unsafe CSOM is associated with complications this is postponed to a next stage.

41. **(b) Griesinger's sign** (*Ref. Shambaugh, 6th ed., 459*)
- Battle's sign represents ecchymosis around the mastoid process from head trauma that has caused a temporal bone fracture.

Section I

Ear

- Irwin Moore sign: On pressure of anterior pillar there is expression of cheesy material from the tonsil. It is a feature of chronic tonsillitis.
- Hennebert's sign is False positive fistula test.

42. (b) Lateral sinus thrombophlebitis (*Ref. Shambaugh, 6th ed., 459*)

43. (b) Lateral sinus thrombophlebitis (*Ref. Cummings, 6th ed., 2175*)

44. (d) Jugular vein thrombosis (*Ref. Shambaugh, 6th ed., 459*)

45. (a) Mastoid bone edema (*Ref. Shambaugh, 6th ed., 459*)

46. (a) Abscess drainage followed by MRM (*Ref. Cummings, 6th ed., 2172*)

The ring enhancing lesion that is being seen here is temporal lobe abscess following unsafe CSOM. Intracranial complication has to be managed first.

47. (d) Hitzelberger sign (*Ref. Shambaugh, 6th ed., 647*)

48. (a) Gradenigo syndrome (*Ref. Cummings, 6th ed., 2165*)

Diplopia is causing compensatory head tilt in the said patient.

49. (a) Upper part of neck (*Ref. Cummings, 6th ed., 2164*) (along the sternocleidomastoid muscle)

50. (a) Schwartze operation (*Ref. Cummings, 6th ed., 2160*)

51. (c) Palatal palsy (*Ref. Scott Brown, 8th ed., Vol 2; 1318*)

52. (c) Surgical repair (*Ref. Cummings, 6th ed., 2169*)

53. (c) Facial palsy (*Ref. Scott Brown, 8th ed., Vol 2; 1318*)

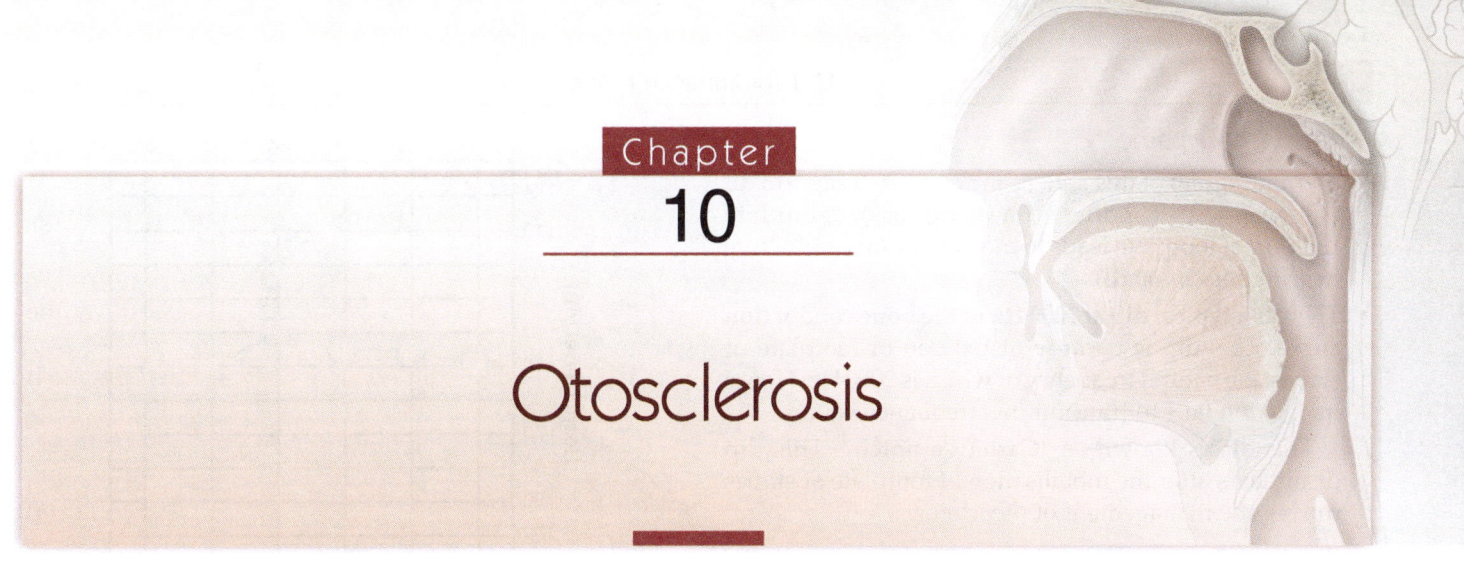

Otosclerosis

PATHOPHYSIOLOGY

There are a few areas in the bony labyrinth where immature cartilaginous cell rests are present throughout life. Their significance is that they retain their capacity to divide. One of these important areas is fissula ante fenestrum. As its name it lies anterior to the fenestra of oval window.

Whenever fissula ante fenestrum gets triggered by viral infection (possible association with **measles virus** has been postulated), autoimmunity, mutation, etc. it starts dividing. Since it lies anterior to the oval window, the overgrowth comes on the oval window on which is present the footplate of stapes, so it comes over the footplate and fixes it. Here to be fixed first is the area of the anterior crura of stapes.

This condition is known as Otosclerosis.

The most common site of origin of otosclerosis is **fissula ante fenestrum**.

Because of repeated division, modelling and remodelling, the normal enchondral bone is replaced by wavy spongy bone/immature bone, hence otosclerosis is also known as **otospongiosis**. This area when seen histologically shows a lot of **osteoclasts**, osteoblasts, new blood vessels and new bone formation. The new blood vessels are surrounded by a layer of new bone which stains blue on H and E stain hence known as blue mantle of Manasse (discovered by Manasse, mantle meaning envelope).

Clinical Features

Otosclerosis usually presents in the third decade, i.e. **20–30 years** of age, seen more commonly in **females** with a ratio of 2:1. It is aggravated by any hormonal change, be it pregnancy or menopause.

It is inherited as autosomal dominant and a positive family history is therefore usually present. It is seen more commonly in **white people**.

In 70–85% of patients it is a bilateral condition. Patient presents with **B/L progressive conductive hearing loss**.

In fact Otosclerosis is the **most common cause of B/L progressive conductive hearing loss in adults**.

This patient gives the typical history of hearing better in noisy surroundings, which is known as **Paracusis Willisii phenomenon**. This is because the speaker raises his voice in noisy surroundings which now crosses the hearing threshold of the patient.

The patient of otosclerosis has low tone speech (read under the topic Weber's in Chapter 2).

At times sensorineural hearing loss occurs in otosclerosis. The site of active division lies anterior to oval window on the medial wall of middle ear. If the overgrowth occurs towards the inner ear side or if during active division on this common wall the toxins are released into the inner ear fluid, there occursdamage and hyalinisation of the spiral ligament leading to cochlear otosclerosis and SN hearing loss.

Therefore in otosclerosis there can be mixed hearing loss.

Less commonly tinnitus can also occur in otosclerosis, particularly in cochlear otosclerosis and active otosclerosis (when active division is occurring).

Sometimes otosclerosis is associated with Osteogenesis Imperfecta and blue sclera, when it constitutes **van der Hoeve syndrome**.

On Examination

90% patients of otosclerosis have mature otosclerosis, here the tympanic membrane appears normal, i.e. **pearly white**.

10% cases of otosclerosis are active. In these the active division is taking place on the medial wall of middle ear leading to increased vascularity. This appears pinkish through the intact tympanic membrane leading to **flamingo pink** appearance of TM also known as **Schwartze sign**.

Audiometric Tests

Tuning fork tests indicate conductive pathology unless and until cochlear involvement is present, also *see* chapter on audiology:

Tuning fork test	Finding
Rinne's	**Negative**
Weber's	**Lateralised to the worst ear.**
ABC	**Same as examiner**
Schwabach	**Lengthened**
Gelle's	**Negative** (i.e. change in the pressure of EAC does not produce any change in hearing as ossicular chain is already fixed)

Pure Tone Audiometry

- The **audiogram** of this patient shows an A-B gap >15 dB (suggestive of conductive hearing loss). **Complete fixation** of footplate leads to the **maximum conductive hearing loss of 60 dB**.

- There is a **typical dip at 2000 Hz in the bone conduction curve**. This dip is because of fixation of footplate of stapes, the natural frequency of which is 2000 Hz. Hence its fixation fails to transmit this frequency sound.

    This dip is known as **"Carhart's notch"**. This dip disappears after the mobilisation of footplate of stapes during the management of otosclerosis.

    Figure 10.1 upper curve showing **Carhart's notch: BC** threshold of approximately 5 dB, 10 dB and 15 dB at 500, 1000, 2000 Hz respectively. *Mnemonic*: **C BC, C**arhart's show dip in **B**one **C**onduction.

Note:

This Carhart's notch disappears after mobilisation of foot plate of stapes.

- A **Cookie bite curve,** i.e. a dip in mid-frequency region in both BC and AC is seen in cochlear otosclerosis. *Mnemonic*: Cookie Bite should be shared so seen in both AC and BC.

Impedance Audiometry

Tympanometry → shows **As type** curve (normal middle ear pressure with reduced compliance). This is diagnostic of otosclerosis as the most common ossicular fixation is fixation of footplate of stapes.

Stapedial reflex is **absent** in complete fixation of footplate of stapes. This is due to inability of the stapes to move.

Management

Active Cases

a. **Sodium fluoride (Na F):** In active cases, i.e. when Schwartze sign is present, medical management with sodium fluoride (Na F) is done. Na F accelerates the maturation of the focus by **increasing osteoblastic** and **decreasing osteoclastic activity**. It also **inhibits the proteolytic enzymes** that release cytotoxic chemicals to cochlea.

    Fluoride therapy is contraindicated in chronic nephritis, rheumatoid arthritis, pregnancy, lactation, allergy to fluoride, etc. Another complication with fluoride is that it can lead to skeletal fluorosis.

b. Bisphosphonates have also been used as they inhibit bone resorption.

Mature Otosclerosis Cases

a. **Surgery:** In mature otosclerosis when the footplate is fixed and active division has stopped the treatment consists of **mobilisation of footplate of stapes**.

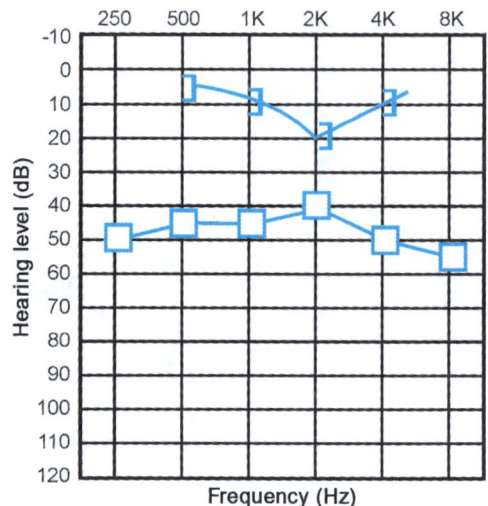

Fig. 10.1: Carhart's Notch in Bone Conduction Curve

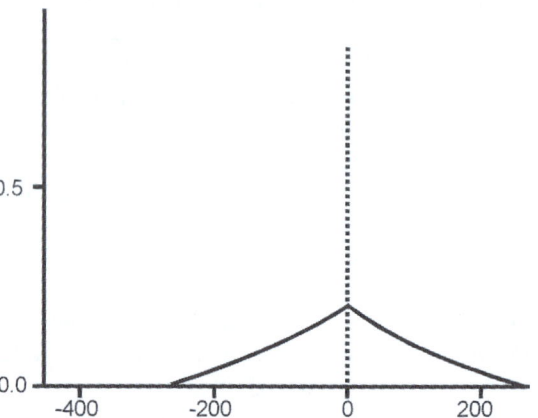

Fig. 10.2: Tympanogram showing as type curve (reduced compliance normal pressure). X axis showing pressure in mm H_2O and Y axis showing compliance in ml.

Indications of surgery

Surgery is done only when the patient's hearing threshold is 30 dB or more and an A-B gap of 25 dB or more is present.

This surgery involves the footplate of stapes, hence any complication might lead to fistula on the medial wall leading to leakage of perilymph and labyrinthitis. Therefore, always the **worst ear is operated upon 1st** so that if any complication occurs, the better ear is still left behind.

If no complication occur in the worst ear, for one year following surgery, the better ear can be operated upon.

This surgery is preferably done under local anaesthesia so that hearing can be tested immediately and if while operation the patient complains of vertigo, the surgeon can become cautious not to cause further injury to the vestibule of inner ear.

The surgical procedures done here are as follows:

1. *Stapedectomy:* Here the whole of the stapes is removed and the oval window is then covered with a fascia graft and prosthesis is placed over the graft with the other end of prosthesis attached to the long

process of incus. The chance of perilymph fistula , SN hearing loss and vertigo is higher in stapedectomy as compared to stapedotomy. Stapedotomy is hence not preferred nowadays.

2. *Stapedotomy:* This is a more conservative and better procedure where the incudostapedial joint is separated, the stapedial tendon is cut and the suprastructure of stapes (head, neck, anterior and posterior crura) is removed leaving the fixed footplate behind. An opening/fenestra is made either with instrument, electric microdrill or LASER (CO_2, Argon, KTP-532) in the fixed footplate. On this opening one end of the prosthesis is placed with the other end attached to the long process of incus. The **most common prosthesis** used here is **Teflon piston**. The other pistons that can be used are platinum, titanium, stainless steel, etc.

Figure 10.3 showing piston *in situ* following stapedotomy: Piston placed on the opening on the footplate with the suprastructure of stapes removed.

Note:

Following stapedotomy the compliance increases and the tympanogram shows A_d type curve.

Postoperative complications:

i. Conductive hearing loss: This can occur due to the following reasons:
   a. Displacement of the piston which can occur immediately or later.
   b. Incus erosion: Due to pressure on the long process by the piston loop.
   c. Bony regrowth over the fenestra.
ii. Perilymph fistula: This can lead to vertigo and persistent or fluctuating hearing loss which can be SN, mixed or conductive.
iii. Facial nerve palsy.

Contraindications of surgery:

Stapedotomy/stapedectomy is **contraindicated in an only hearing ear**.

The other important contraindications are active otosclerosis, pregnancy and professionals, e.g. pilots and divers (in whom there occurs sudden change of middle ear pressure which may lead to perilymph fistula).

Previously surgeons used to think that since footplate is fixed, making an opening, i.e. fenestra on the lateral semicircular canal will solve the purpose. This is known as **fenestration operation**. It is no longer done nowadays. It is an iatrogenic cause of positive fistula test.

b. **Hearing aid:** In patients not willing or unfit for surgery, hearing aid is the alternative treatment.

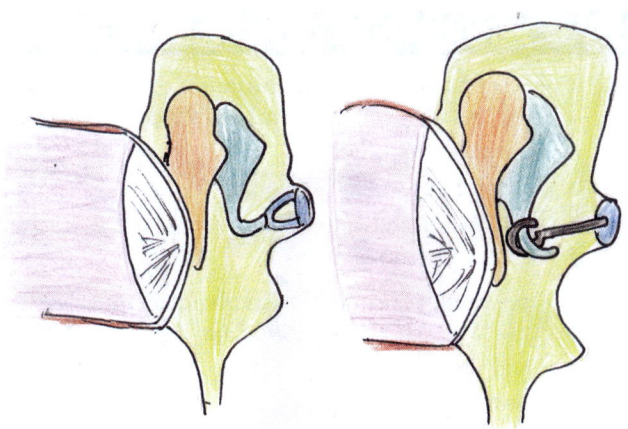

Fig. 10.3: Footplate of Stapes which is completely fixed is replaced by a Teflon Piston after making an opening in the footplate

c. **Cochlear implantation:** In patients with far advanced otosclerosis in both the ears, with significant SN involvement, who progress to profound hearing loss with significant deterioration in speech discrimination despite hearing aids, may be candidates for cochlear implant.

"Points to Ponder/Points for Quick revision"

- Immature cartilaginous cell rests in the bony labyrinth (MC at "fissula ante fenestrum") start growing (triggered by virus infections, e.g. measles, autoimmune insults, etc.) → fixation of the footplate → otosclerosis (also known as Otospongiosis/blue mantles)
- AD, Whites, 20–30 years, F > M, aggravated by pregnancy
- CFs: B/L progressive conductive hearing loss (CHL) (MC underlying cause), sometimes mixed hearing loss, i.e. SN—if cochlear involvement, better hearing in noisy surroundings (Paracusis Willisii phenomenon). Low tone voice
- Vander Hoeve syndrome—otosclerosis, osteogenesis imperfecta and blue sclera
- Majority—Normal pearly grey TM, in active otosclerosis-flamingo pink appearance of TM (Schwartze sign)
- Tuning fork tests
- Audiogram—Carhart's notch (dip at 2000 Hz in the BC curve); Cookie bite curve (seen with cochlear involvement, dip in both AC and BC)
- Tympanometry—A_s type curve, stapedial reflex absent
- Treatment—Active otosclerosis-Na F; Mature otosclerosis-Stapedotomy, hearing aid
- Stapedotomy (better than stapedectomy):
  - Stapedial tendon and stapes supra-structure removed, Teflon piston is placed between incus and the opening made in the foot plate.
  - Complications—CHL, perilymph fistula(far less incidence than stapedectomy), facial N palsy.
  - Contraindications—single hearing ear, active otosclerosis and pregnancy.

Section I   Ear

PREVIOUSLY ASKED QUESTIONS

1. **Most common site for the initiation of otosclerosis:** *(Karnataka 2006, Exam 2017)*
   a. Footplate of stapes
   b. Margins of stapes
   c. Fissula ante-fenestrum
   d. Fissula post-fenestrum

2. **The part most commonly involved in otosclerosis is:** *(PGI June 99, Comed 2007, UP 2008)*
   a. Oval window
   b. Round window
   c. Tympanic membrane
   d. Malleus

3. **Common age for otosclerosis is:** *(UP 2006, Exam 2016)*
   a. 5–10 yrs
   b. 10–15 yrs
   c. 20–30 yrs
   d. 30–45 yrs

4. **Otospongiosis is inherited as:** *(AI 95, Exam 2016)*
   a. Autosomal dominant
   b. Autosomal recessive
   c. X-linked dominant
   d. X-linked recessive

5. **True about otosclerosis:** *(PGI June 2003, 2014)*
   a. Family history is usually present
   b. Males are affected twice than females
   c. More common in Negro's and Africans
   d. Deafness occurs in 20–30 yrs
   e. Pregnancy has bearing on it

6. **A 30-year-old woman with family history of hearing loss from mother's side developed hearing problem during pregnancy. Hearing loss is B/L, slowly progressive. Pure tone audiometry shows an apparent bone conduction hearing loss at 2000 Hz. What is the most likely diagnosis:** *(AIIMS May 2006)*
   a. Otosclerosis
   b. Acoustic neuroma
   c. Otitis media with effusion
   d. Sigmoid sinus thrombosis

7. **Otospongiosis causes:** *(AI 96, Exam 2015)*
   a. U/L conductive deafness
   b. B/L conductive deafness
   c. U/L sensorineural deafness
   d. B/L sensorineural deafness

8. **A 30-year-old woman presents with progressive conductive deafness bilaterally. The most common cause is:** *(Exam 2013, AIIMS NOV 2009, AIIMS 93)*
   a. Tympanosclerosis
   b. Otospongiosis
   c. Meniere's disease
   d. B/L otitis media

9. **Paracusis Willisii is feature of:** *(MH CET 2016, Exam 2013, MHPG/MCET 2002/MH 2005)*
   a. Tympanosclerosis
   b. Otosclerosis
   c. Meniere's disease
   d. Presbycusis

10. **A patient hears better in noise. The diagnosis is:** *(Karnataka 95, Exam 2013)*
    a. Hyperacusis
    b. Diplacusis
    c. Presbycusis
    d. Paracusis

11. **In otosclerosis tinnitus is due to:** *(Bihar 2005, Exam 2017)*
    a. Cochlear otosclerosis
    b. Increased vascularity in lesion
    c. Conductive deafness
    d. All

12. **In majority of cases with otosclerosis the tympanic membrane is:** *(Kerala 94, Exam 2014)*
    a. Normal
    b. Flamingo pink
    c. Blue
    d. Yellow

13. **Pink tympanic membrane is seen in:** *(AIIMS 2010)*
    a. Otosclerosis
    b. Glomus
    c. Acute otitis media
    d. Serous otitis media

14. **Schwartze sign seen in:** *(MAHE 2005, PGI 98, Exam 2016)*
    a. Glomus jugulare
    b. Otosclerosis
    c. Meniere's disease
    d. Acoustic neuroma

15. **Feature in otosclerosis includes:** *(AP 2003, Exam 2017)*
    a. Sounds not heard in noisy environment
    b. Normal tympanic membrane
    c. More common in males
    d. Malleus is most commonly affected

16. **True statements about otosclerosis:** *(PGI June 2005, 2015)*
    a. Unilateral
    b. Carhart's notch seen
    c. Fluctuating hearing loss
    d. Progressive deafness
    e. Males are commonly affected

17. **Characteristic feature of otosclerosis are all except:** *(AIIMS June 97, 2004)*
    a. Conductive deafness
    b. Positive Rinne test
    c. Paracusis Willisii
    d. Pearly white ear drum

18. **Not true regarding hearing loss in otosclerosis:** *(Maharashtra 2010, Exam 2018)*
    a. Common in female of age around 30 years
    b. Vertigo present
    c. Paracusis Willisii
    d. Schwartze sign

19. **Gelle's test is for:** *(Bihar 2006, Exam 2017)*
   a. Otosclerosis
   b. NHL
   c. Sensorineural deafness
   d. None

20. **A lady has B/L hearing loss since 4 years which worsened during pregnancy. Type of impedance audiometry graph will be:** *(AIIMS May 2007)*
   a. Ad
   b. As
   c. B
   d. C

21. **In otosclerosis the tympanogram is:**
   (Exam 2013, Exam 2016)
   a. Low compliance
   b. High compliance
   c. Normal compliance
   d. None of the above

22. **In otosclerosis Carhart's notch dips at:**
   (TN 2004, Exam 2017)
   a. 1000 Hz in AC
   b. 1000 Hz in BC
   c. 2000 Hz in AC
   d. 2000 Hz in BC

23. **Carhart's notch in audiogram is deepest at the frequency of:** *(AI/TN 2003, Exam 2017)*
   a. 0.5 kHz
   b. 2 kHz
   c. 4 kHz
   d. 8 kHz

24. **A pure tone audiogram with a dip at 2000 Hz is characteristic of:** *(Exam 2013, Exam 2016)*
   a. Presbycusis
   b. Ototoxicity
   c. Otosclerosis
   d. Noise induced hearing loss

25. **Otosclerosis treatment includes all except:**
   (AI 2011, 2010)
   a. Sodium fluoride
   b. Hearing Aids
   c. Stapedectomy
   d. Radical mastoidectomy

26. **Carhart's notch in audiometry is seen in:**
   (MAHE 2005, Exam 2017)
   a. Meniere's
   b. Labyrinthitis
   c. Acoustic neuroma
   d. Otosclerosis

27. **All are true about otosclerosis except:**
   (PGI June 2006, 2016)
   a. Increased incidence in females
   b. Conductive deafness
   c. Irreversible loss of hearing
   d. Carhartz notch at 2000 Hz
   e. Family history positive

28. **Medication which may prevent rapid progression of cochlear Otosclerosis is:**
   (Karnataka 94, Exam 2016)
   a. Steroids
   b. Antibiotics
   c. Fluorides
   d. Vitamins

29. **All of the following statements about sodium fluoride in otosclerosis are true, except:**
   (AIIMS 2011)
   a. Acts by inhibiting proteolytic enzymes in cochlea
   b. Acts by inhibiting osteoblastic activity
   c. Is contraindicated in chronic nephritis
   d. Is indicated in patients with a positive Schwartze sign

30. **A 31-year-old female patient complains of B/L impairment of hearing for the past 5 years. Audiogram shows a B/L conductive deafness. Impedance audiometry is given below. All constitute part of treatment except:** *(Practice question by Author)*

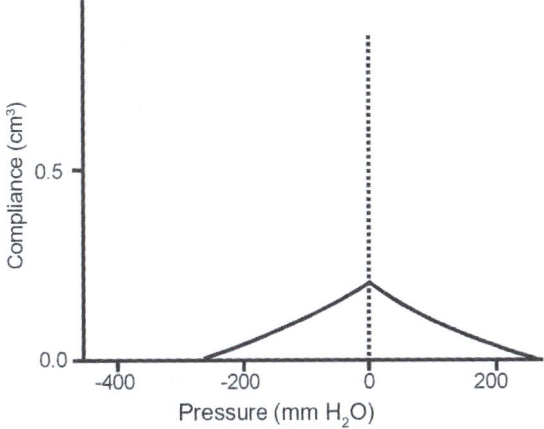

   a. Hearing aid
   b. Stapedectomy
   c. Sodium fluoride
   d. Gentamicin

31. **Following operation is the most preferred in case of otosclerosis:** *(Exam 2016)*
   a. Stapedectomy
   b. Fenestration
   c. Stapedotomy
   d. Sacculotomy

32. **In otosclerosis during stapes surgery prosthesis used is:** *(UP 2006)*
   a. Teflon piston
   b. Grommet
   c. Total ossicular replacement
   d. All

33. **Stapedotomy includes removal of all except:**
   (AIIMS May 2014)
   a. Anterior crura of stapes
   b. Posterior crura of stapes
   c. Stapedius tendon
   d. Lenticular process of Incus

34. **What is the role of sodium fluoride in otosclerosis:**
   (Exam 2017)
   a. It restores the electrolyte equilibrium
   b. It hastens recovery of the overstimulated Cochlea
   c. It quickens the maturity of the active focus and reduces osteoclastic resorption
   d. It repolarises the cochlear cells

Section I · Ear

35. Otosclerosis most commonly affects which race:
    (Exam 2016)

    a. White race   b. Negros
    c. Japanese   d. Chinese

36. A 25-year-old female patient presented with history of bilateral hearing loss and tinnitus which worsened during pregnancy. She can hear better in noisy environment. She speaks in a low volume monotonous voice. Examination showed intract ear drums bilaterally and Rinne test negative bilaterally. Pure tone audiometry is given below. What is the most probable diagnosis:
    (Practice question by Author, Exam 2018)

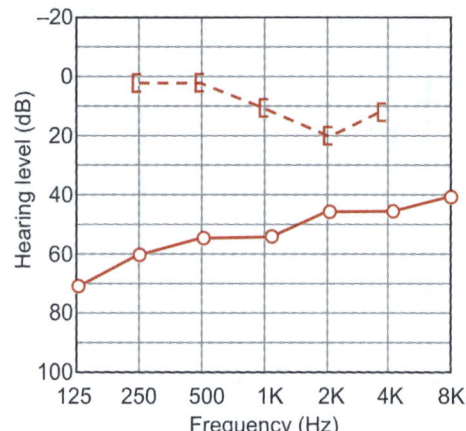

   a. Meniere's disease
   b. Secretory otitis media
   c. Bilateral acoustic neuroma
   d. Otosclerosis

37. In the above patient, dip in bone conduction at 2 kHz is called: *(COMEDK 2013)*
    a. Moore's sign
    b. Carhart's notch
    c. Schwartz's sign
    d. Thumb sign

38. The treatment of this patient is: *(COMEDK 2013)*
    a. Endolymphatic sac decompression
    b. Myringotomy and grommet insertion
    c. Stapedotomy and piston insertion
    d. Retrosigmoid approach and excision

39. The finding of impedance audiometry in a long standing case of otosclerosis is: *(Exam 2017)*
    a. A_s graph alone
    b. B graph with loss of stapedial reflex
    c. A_s graph with increased stapedial reflex
    d. A_s graph with loss of stapedial reflex

40. Post stapes surgery produces which curve in impedance audiometry: *(Exam 2017)*
    a. A   b. B
    c. C   d. A_d

ANSWERS AND EXPLANATIONS

1. **(c) Fissula ante-fenestrum** (*Ref. Cummings, 6th ed., 2212*)
- Though otosclerosis ultimately results in the fixation of the footplate and margins of stapes which is lying over the oval window, it actually gets initiated most commonly in the **immature cartilaginous area of the bony labyrinth** which lies anterior to the fenestra of oval window and hence called fissula ante fenestrum.
- Fissula post-fenestrum area of the bony labyrinth is also cartilaginous but otosclerosis is uncommon here.

2. **(a) Oval window** (*Ref. Cummings, 6th ed., 2211*)
- Since the most common site of origin of otosclerosis is fissula ante fenestrum, the overgrowth from here comes over the footplate of stapes lying over the oval window. So the part most commonly involved in otosclerosis is oval window.

3. **(c) 20–30 yrs** (*Ref. Cummings, 6th ed., 2211*)

4. **(a) Autosomal dominant** (*Ref. Cummings, 6th ed., 2211*)

5. **(a), (d) and (e) are correct** (*Ref. Cummings, 6th ed., 2211*)

6. **(a) Otosclerosis** (*Ref. Cummings, 6th ed., 2211*)
30-yr-old woman with family history of hearing loss, presenting with B/L hearing loss during pregnancy, pure tone audiometry showing an apparent bone conduction hearing loss at 2000 Hz, i.e. Carhartz notch is diagnostic of otosclerosis.
- Acoustic neuroma is seen in the age group of 40–70 yrs and presents with U/L SN hearing loss and tinnitus.
- Otitis media with effusion or glue ear is seen most commonly in children and presents with B/L conductive hearing loss. Tympanic membrane here is dull retracted with fluid level and air bubbles seen behind.
- Sigmoid sinus thrombosis is a complication of unsafe CSOM and presents with hectic fever, jugular vein area tenderness, oedema of the mastoid and features of unsafe CSOM, i.e. ear discharge, cholesteatoma, and hearing loss.

7. **(b) B/L conductive deafness** (*Ref. Cummings, 6th ed., 2213*)
- Otospongiosis causing fixation of foot plate of stapes is a conductive pathology.
- Uncommonly when there occurs cochlear otosclerosis (please refer to the text) it leads to, B/L SN hearing loss along with conductive, i.e. mixed hearing loss.

8. **(b) Otospongiosis** (*Ref. Cummings, 6th ed., 2211*)
- Otosclerosis is the most common cause of B/L progressive conductive hearing loss in adults.
- Meniere's disease presents with U/L SN hearing loss, vertigo and tinnitus.
- With the kind of presentation mentioned the remaining two options of conductive hearing loss are less common than otosclerosis.

9. **(b) Otosclerosis** (*Ref. Cummings, 6th ed., 2213*)
- The patient of otosclerosis gives the typical history of hearing better in noisy surrounding which is known as Paracusis Willisii.
- Hyalinisation and calcification of the fibrous layer of TM is known as tympanosclerosis. Here a very mild conductive hearing loss is present.
- Meniere's disease being a U/L condition leads to distortion of sound which is known as diplacusis, i.e. both the cochleas sense the same sound as different.
- Presbycusis is the age related B/L SN hearing loss.

10. **(d) Paracusis** (*Ref. Cummings, 6th ed., 2213*)
See the explanation to the above question
- Hyperacusis is because of absence of stapedial reflex seen in facial nerve palsy. Here normal sounds appear abnormally loud.

11. **(d) All** (*Ref. Scott Brown, 8th ed., Vol 2; 755*)
Tinnitus in otosclerosis is not common; if present it is due to:
   i. Active otosclerosis because of increased vascularity
   ii. Cochlear otosclerosis
- Any hearing loss condition, be it conductive or SN can as such lead to tinnitus. So all are possible mechanisms.

12. **(a) Normal** (*Ref. Shambaugh, 6th ed., 531*)
- In 90% patients of otosclerosis the tympanic membrane appears normal, i.e. pearly white.
- In 10% cases which are active tympanic membrane is flamingo pink.
- Blue TM is a feature of glue ear because of cholesterol granuloma.
- Yellow TM is not seen in any condition

13. **(a) Otosclerosis** (*Ref. Cummings, 6th ed., 2213*)
- In active otosclerosis the TM appears pink known as flamingo (a bird) pink, though 90% cases are mature otosclerosis where TM is pearly white.
- In Glomus the vascular mass abutting on TM gives it a red reflex.
- In acute otitis media the increased vascularity on the TM makes it appear red.
- In serous otitis media or glue ear the TM is blue.

14. **(b) Otosclerosis** (*Ref. Cummings, 6th ed., 2213*)
- 10% cases of otosclerosis are active. In these the active division is taking place on the medial wall of middle ear leading to increased vascularity. This appears pinkish through the intact tympanic membrane leading to flamingo pink appearance of TM also known as Schwartze sign.
- In Glomus jugulare the vascular tumour coming from the floor of the middle ear gives a rising sun appearance on the TM. This is also known as red reflex.
- In Meniere's and Acoustic neuroma the TM appears no3rmal, i.e. pearly white.

15. **(b) Normal tympanic membrane** (*Ref. Cummings 6th ed., 2213*)

- Sounds are rather better heard in noisy environment, the Paracusis Willisii phenomenon.
- Otosclerosis is seen more commonly in females.
- The ossicle affected is Stapes.

16. **(b) and (d)** (*Ref. Scott Brown, 8th ed., Vol 2 page 1068*)
- In 70–85% of patients otosclerosis is a bilateral condition.
- The audiogram of a patient of otosclerosis shows an A-B gap >15 dB and typical dip at 2000 Hz in the bone conduction curve. This dip is known as "Carhart's notch".
- Fluctuating conductive hearing loss is seen in serous Otitis media, whereas fluctuating SN hearing loss is seen in Meniere's disease.
- Due to progressive fixation of the footplate of stapes, there is progressive conductive hearing loss in otosclerosis.

17. **(b) Positive Rinne test** (*Ref. Cummings, 6th ed., 2213*)
- Since otosclerosis majorly leads to conductive deafness so Rinne test is negative.

18. **(b) Vertigo present** (*Ref. Cummings, 6th ed., 2213*)
- Vertigo is not a feature of otosclerosis

19. **(a) Otosclerosis** (*Ref. Dhingra, 6th ed., 22*)
- Gelle's is negative in otosclerosis, i.e. change in the pressure of EAC does not produce any change in hearing as Ossicular chain is already fixed.

  Please refer to Gelle's test in audiometry chapter.

20. **(b) As** (*Ref. Cummings, 6th ed., 2213*)

  Lady with B/L hearing loss with history of worsening during pregnancy is suggestive of otosclerosis.
- Impedance audiometry shows As type curve (normal middle ear pressure with reduced compliance). This is diagnostic of otosclerosis.
- Ad type curve is seen in ossicular discontinuity.
- B type curve is seen in serous Otitis media.
- C curve is seen in early stages of Eustachian tube obstruction.

21. **(a) Low compliance** (*Ref. Scott Brown, 8th ed., Vol 2 1071*)
- The As type of curve in otosclerosis is low compliance and normal pressure type.
- High compliance, normal pressure type of curve is Ad, seen in ossicular discontinuity.
- Normal compliance, normal pressure is A type, i.e. normal curve.

22. **(d) 2000 Hz in BC** (*Ref. Shambaugh, 6th ed., 532*)

  In otosclerosis the dip at 2000 Hz is seen in bone conduction curve which is known as Carhart's notch.
  Mnemonic: Carhart's in **B**one **C**onduction, **CBC**.

23. **(b) 2 kHz or 2000 Hz** (*Ref. Scott Brown, 8th ed., Vol 2 1070*)
- In otosclerosis there is an increase in BC threshold of approx. 5 dB, 10 dB and 15 dB at 500, 1000, 2000 Hz respectively. So the deepest dip is at 2 kHz which is known as Carhart's notch.
- At 4 or 8 kHz, there is no hearing loss in otosclerosis.

24. **(c) Otosclerosis** (*Ref. Shambaugh, 6th ed., 532*)

25. **(d) Radical mastoidectomy** (*Ref. Cummings, 6th ed., 2213*)
26. **(d) Otosclerosis** (*Ref. Scott Brown, 8th ed., Vol 2 page 1070*)
27. **(c) Irreversible loss of hearing** (*Ref. Cummings, 6th ed., 1071*)
- Since the hearing loss in otosclerosis is due to fixation of footplate of stapes so the mobilisation of stapes by stapedotomy reverses the hearing loss.
- Largely there occurs conductive deafness but when there is involvement of cochlea, i.e. cochlear otosclerosis SN deafness is also seen.

  Rest options have been discussed previously.

28. **(c) Fluorides** (*Ref. Cummings, 6th ed., 2218*)
- In active otosclerosis cases, i.e. when Schwartz sign is present medical management with sodium fluoride (Na F) decreases the progression by accelerating the maturation and inhibiting proteolytic enzymes. Please *see* text.
- As per the pathogenesis of otosclerosis steroids, antibiotics and vitamins have no role in the management of otosclerosis.

29. **(b) Acts by inhibiting osteoblastic activity** (*Ref. Cummings, 6th ed., 2218*)

30. **(d) Gentamicin** (*Ref. Cummings, 6th ed., 2213*)

  The given tympanogram shows As type of curve and as per the description the diagnosis is clearly otosclerosis.

  Gentamicin is a vestibulotoxic drug given in Meniere's to relieve vertigo. It has no role in otosclerosis.

31. **(c) Stapedotomy** (*Ref. Cummings, 6th ed., 2213*)
- In mature otosclerosis when the footplate is fixed and active division has stopped the treatment consists of mobilisation of footplate of stapes. This can be done either by Stapedectomy or Stapedotomy. Fenestration operation is no longer done now.
- Previously Sacculotomy used to be done in Meniere's to decompress the endolymph. It is no longer done now.

32. **(a) Teflon piston** (*Ref. Cummings, 6th ed., 2215*)
- Grommet insertion is required in serous Otitis media.
- Total ossicular replacement prosthesis (TORP) is used when it is required to reconstruct whole of the ossicular chain, for example, in unsafe CSOM when there occurs complete necrosis of all the three ossicles.

33. **(d) Lenticular process of Incus** (*Ref. Cummings, 6th ed., 2213*)

  Please refer to the text.

34. **(c) It quickens the maturity of the active focus and reduces osteoclastic resorption** (*Ref. Scott Brown, 8th ed., Vol 2 1074*)

35. **(a) White races** (*Ref. Cummings, 6th ed., 2211*)
36. **(d) Otosclerosis** (*Ref. Cummings, 6th ed., 2213*)
37. **(b) Carhart's notch** (*Ref. Scott Brown, 8th ed., Vol 2 1070*)
38. **(c) Stapedotomy and piston insertion** (*Ref. Scott Brown, 8th ed., Vol 2 1086*)
39. **(d) A$_s$ graph with loss of stapedial reflex** (*Ref. Anirban Biswas 5th ed., 118*)
40. **(d) A$_d$** (*Ref. Anirban Biswas, 5th ed., 90*)

Facial Nerve and its Disorders

Facial, the 7th cranial nerve is a mixed nerve, i.e. with both sensory and motor components.

The sensory part of facial nerve is known as **nervus intermedius or nerve of Wrisberg**.

SUPRANUCLEAR PALSY

The facial motor nucleus lying in the anterior pons, is divided into dorsal and ventral parts. The **dorsal part** contains lower motor neurons supplying the muscles of the **upper face** whereas the **ventral part** carries lower motor neurons to the **lower part** of the face.

The dorsal part receives bilateral upper motor neuron input (i.e. from both sides of the brain) while the ventral part receives only contralateral input (i.e. from the opposite side of the brain).

Thus, **lesions of** one-sided corticobulbar tract or **supranuclear pathway** (i.e. lesions anywhere between the cerebral cortex and facial motor nucleus in the pons) destroy input to the contralateral ventral division but input to the contralateral dorsal division is retained (due to its dual supply).

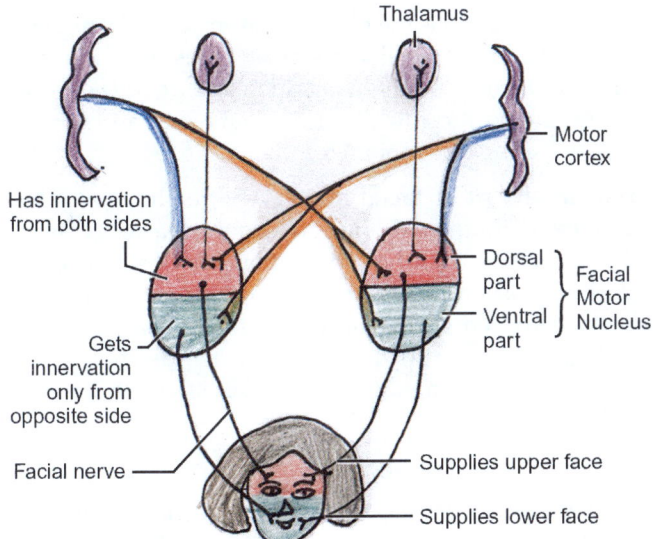

Fig. 11.1: Innervation and supply of motor nucleus of facial nerve

As a result, central facial palsy is characterized by **hemiparalysis or hemiparesis of the muscles of lower half of one side of the face. The forehead is spared here**.

COURSE OF FACIAL NERVE

The course of facial nerve from its nucleus till the facial muscles is divided into three parts:

1. **Intracranial:** The facial nerve after originating from its nucleus in the pons, hooks around the nucleus of 6th cranial nerve. As a result brainstem lesions involving the seventh nerve also usually involve the sixth nerve leading to ipsilateral complete facial palsy along with ipsilateral lateral rectus palsy. These along with contralateral hemiplegia constitutes Millard-Gubler syndrome.

   The facial nerve finally emerges from the brainstem and courses across the cerebellopontine angle to reach the internal acoustic meatus. From its origin in the nuclei till its entry into the internal acoustic meatus (IAM), is the **intracranial part** of facial nerve.

2. **Intratemporal (longest):** From the IAM till the stylomastoid foramen is the **intratemporal part** of facial nerve. Most of the facial nerve is intratemporal and is described below.

3. **Extracranial:** From where it exits the stylomastoid foramen constitutes the extracranial part of facial nerve, *see* below.

Intratemporal Part of Facial Nerve

Facial nerve is the only cranial nerve which runs in most of its course through a bony canal (known as **fallopian canal**). The fallopian canal extends from the entry of the facial nerve in the inner ear from the internal acoustic meatus, till its exit from the stylomastoid foramen.

This canal is dehiscent congenitally in 50% cases. **The most common site of congenital dehiscence of fallopian canal is in the horizontal part**, just above the oval window (please read below).

In its intratemporal part, the facial nerve is divided into various segments:

1. **Meatal segment:** In the IAM facial nerve occupies the antero-superior part separated posteriorly from

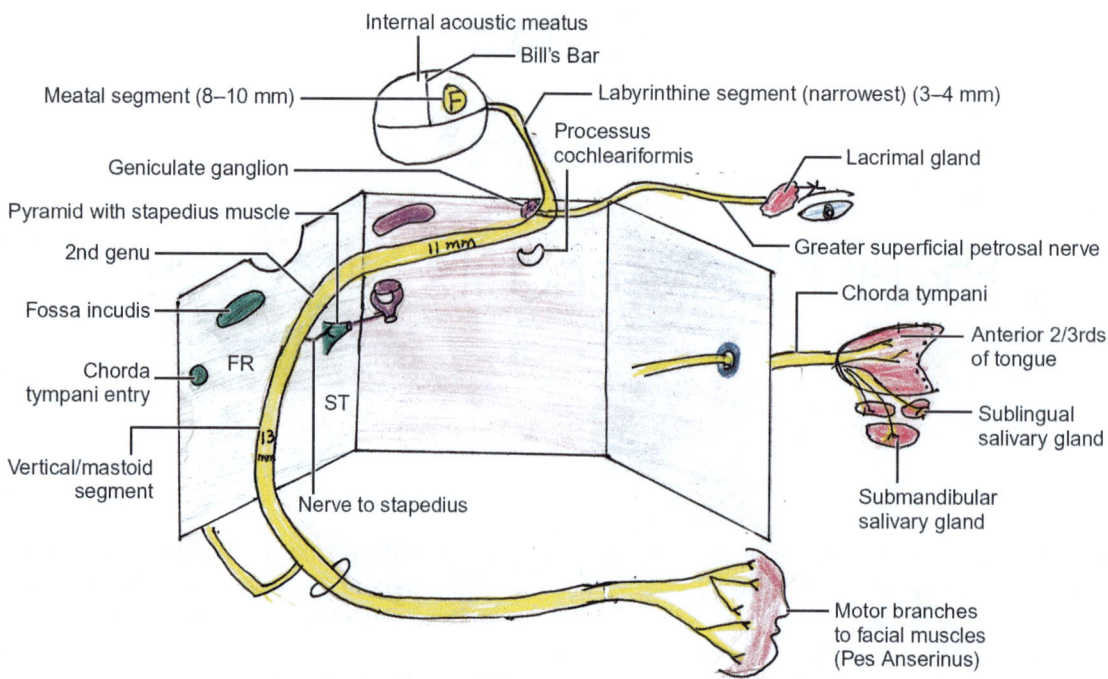

Fig. 11.2: The Course and Branches of Facial Nerve

superior vestibular nerve by a bar of bone known as **'Bills Bar'**, see diagram above. This segment is known as the meatal segment of facial nerve and measures approximately 8–10 mm.

2. **Labyrinthine segment:** From the IAM the facial nerve enters the inner ear. This is known as the labyrinthine segment measuring 3–4 mm. This is the shortest segment of facial nerve and also the **narrowest segment** of the fallopian canal with a diameter of only 0.68 mm.

So in this part, the facial nerve is most prone to compression following edema leading to ischemia and palsy (e.g. Bell's palsy).

The labyrinthine segment ends at the first genu which is the first turn of facial nerve as it enters the middle ear.

3. **Tympanic segment or Horizontal segment:** The facial nerve after passing through the inner ear enters the middle ear on its medial wall which is the common wall between the inner ear and middle ear. Where it enters the middle ear it takes a turn known as first genu (genu means knee like) and then runs a horizontal course on the medial wall. At the first genu is present the geniculate ganglion. This segment of facial nerve on the medial wall of middle ear is known as horizontal or tympanic segment of facial nerve. It is approximately 11 mm. *See* diagram above.

The **landmarks** of this tympanic segment are

a. **Processus cochleariformis:** The first genu of facial nerve lies antero-superior to the Processes cochleariformis.

b. **Cog:** A ridge of bone extends inferiorly from the tegmen tympani (roof) just anterior to the processus cochleariformis. It is known as cog, it also acts as a landmark of the first genu of facial.

c. **Posteriorly** the facial nerve lies in between bulge of lateral semicircular canal above and oval window below.

4. **Mastoid or Vertical segment:** At the junction of the medial and posterior wall of middle ear the facial nerve takes another turn known as second genu and then runs vertically down on the posterior wall, till it exits from the stylomastoid foramen. This part of facial nerve is known as the vertical or the mastoid segment of the facial nerve. Its length is 13 mm.

The landmarks of this segment are:

a. **Pyramid:** The nerve lies lateral and posterior to the pyramid.

b. **Fossa Incudis which is produced by the short process of incus:** The nerve lies medial and inferior to it.

The second genu is the **most common site of iatrogenic (surgical) injury** to facial nerve during mastoid surgeries. Lateral to vertical or the mastoid segment of the facial nerve on the posterior wall is the facial recess and medial to it is the sinus tympani area.

Extracranial part of facial nerve: After exiting from the stylomastoid foramen (lying between the mastoid tip and styloid process) starts the extracranial part of facial nerve. Here the facial nerve passes into the parotid gland dividing into the two, temporofacial and cervicofacial branches which then divide to form pes anserinus (temporal, zygomatic, buccal, mandibular and cervical). *See* diagram above.

Branches of Facial Nerve in the Temporal Bone

In the temporal bone, facial nerve gives various branches:

i. The first branch is the **greater superficial petrosal** nerve. It arises from the geniculate ganglion and goes

Segment	Length	Important landmarks	Blood supply	Remarks
Meatal (in IAM)	8–10 mm	Bill's bar	**Labyrinthine artery** (a branch of anterior inferior cerebellar artery)	**Bill's bar separates it from the superior vestibular nerve in IAM**
Labyrinthine (in inner ear)	3–4 mm	—	**Labyrinthine artery**	• Narrowest segment (0.68 mm) of fallopian canal • Most common segment involved in Bell's palsy
Horizontal/Tympanic (on medial wall of middle ear)	11 mm	**Processes cochleariformis, bulge of lateral semicircular canal and Oval window**	**Superior petrosal artery** (a branch of middle meningeal artery)	• Most common site of congenital dehiscence of fallopian canal • From this segment arises the greater superficial petrosal nerve (from geniculate ganglion)
Vertical/Mastoid (on posterior wall of middle ear)	13 mm	**Pyramid, Short process of incus**	**Stylomastoid artery** (a branch of postauricular artery which is a branch of external carotid)	• 2nd most common site of iatrogenic injury to facial nerve (most common being 2nd genu). • From this segment arises nerve to stapedius, Chorda tympani and sensory auricular branch, *see* below

to the sphenopalatine/pterygopalatine ganglion and gives secretomotor fibres to lacrimal, nasal and palatine glands. Its section will lead to **dry eye** which can be tested by **Schirmer test with the help of Whatman filter paper**.

ii. The second branch is the **nerve to stapedius.** It is given off at the pyramid. This is the first motor branch of facial. It supplies the stapedius muscle which attaches to the neck of stapes. It mediates the **stapedial reflex**. Section of this branch will lead to **hyperacusis** (normal sounds appearing abnormally loud).

iii. The third branch is given from the vertical segment, 4–6 mm before the exit of facial nerve from the stylomastoid foramen. This is the **chorda tympani**. After being given off from the facial it ascends up and enters the middle ear cavity through an opening on the posterior wall, just medial to the tympanic annulus (*see* Chapter on anatomy). Passing between the fibrous and mucosal layers of TM, it then runs in between malleus and incus and exits through the anterior wall of middle ear (through foramen of Huguier). It gives taste to the anterior 2/3rd of the tongue and parasympathetic secretomotor supply to the sublingual and submandibular salivary glands. Section of this nerve will lead to **loss of taste** of anterior 2/3rd and reduced salivary flow which can be tested by electrogustometry and **salivary flow** studies respectively.

iv. The **sensory auricular branch** is given in the vertical part and gives sensory supply to the pinna and external auditory canal.

Localisation of Site of Lesion/Topodiagnostic Tests

These branches are important to us as they help us to find the site of injury in a patient of facial nerve palsy.

• If in a patient following injury, the **Schirmer test is normal, but stapedial reflex is absent**, the lesion is after the geniculate ganglion but before the pyramid i.e. in the **horizontal part**.

• If the **stapedial reflex is normal but taste of the anterior 2/3rd of tongue is gone**, lesion is after pyramid and before chorda tympani origin, i.e. the **vertical or mastoid segment**.

• If the **taste of anterior 2/3rd of tongue is normal but corneal reflex**, see below, is absent the injury is after the origin of chorda tympani, i.e. at or beyond the stylomastoid foramen.

Corneal reflex: In this reflex a piece of cotton wool is touched on the cornea lateral to the pupil. Normally there occurs bilateral blink. The sensory nerve of this reflex arc is the ophthalmic division of trigeminal and motor is the facial (pes anserinus). In Vth nerve lesions there will be no response from either lid when the abnormal side is stimulated and a normal response from both lids when the normal side is stimulated. In VIIth nerve lesions there will be no response from the side of the facial paralysis no matter which side is stimulated and a blink on the normal side even when the abnormal side is touched.

• If **all Schirmer, stapedial reflex, taste anterior 2/3rd of tongue and corneal reflex is absent,** injury is proximal, i.e. before geniculate ganglion, i.e. in the **labyrinthine segment**.

These tests which help us to find out the site of the lesion of facial nerve palsy are known as **topodiagnostic tests**.

Section I **Ear**

- So the topodiagnostic tests of facial are the Schirmer test, stapedial reflex, taste anterior 2/3rd of tongue (Electrogustometry) and salivary flow studies.

Infranuclear Palsy

Injury anywhere in the **infranuclear course** of facial nerve will lead to paralysis of the complete **ipsilateral half of face** (upper as well as lower, please compare from supranuclear palsies written above), supplied by pes anserinus, manifested as obliteration of nasolabial fold, loss of facial movements and incomplete closure of the eye on the affected side. The face deviates to the opposite side because of the pull of the normal side facial muscles.

Electrophysiological Tests

Incomplete facial N paresis has a high chance of full recovery. In patients with complete paralysis or in paresis not improving with time, to find out the prognosis of facial nerve injury, the tests that are done are known as electrophysiological tests.

The two most significant electrophysiological tests are **Electroneuronography (ENOG)** and **Electromyography (EMG)**.

- These tests give us an idea of the severity of injury to the nerve which helps to indirectly decide the overall spontaneous recovery.
- Following any severe injury the Wallerian degeneration of the nerve takes 2–3 days to set in during which the conduction in the nerve continues. So these tests are falsely normal and are therefore not of any use during this period.

1. **ENOG:** Also known as Evoked Electroneuronography.

   In ENOG a supramaximal stimulus is given to the facial nerve trunk as it exits from the stylomastoid foramen and the response to this is recorded in the form of compound muscle action potential (CMAP) by using surface electrodes in the facial muscles. The response is compared with the normal side.

   If the CMAP is 10% of the normal side, it means that only 10% nerves are remaining, the rest 90% being lost to injury.

   Interpretation: If there is > 90% decrease in CMAP within the first 14 days of paralysis, the chances of spontaneous recovery of facial nerve function is negligible and surgical decompression might be considered.

2. **Electromyography (EMG):** Here the action potential in the facial muscles is recorded during rest and during voluntary contraction.

   EMG testing is performed in facial nerve palsies of > 3 weeks duration.

   A degenerating nerve produces fibrillation potential 2–3 weeks after injury whereas the regenerating nerve produces active motor unit potentials.

   Interpretation: If motor unit potentials are present it suggests that the nerve is regenerating and surgical intervention is not needed. If fibrillation potentials are present chances of spontaneous recovery is negligible and surgical decompression is indicated.

   No electric output (flat curve) on EMG suggests long term denervation and that the motor end plates are no longer viable and muscle has been replaced by fibrous tissue. Then facial reanimation is indicated.

Causes of Facial Nerve Palsy

a. **Intracranial part**

   Cerebellopontine angle mass:
   i. Facial nerve schwannoma
   ii. Acoustic neuroma
   iii. Meningioma
   iv. Congenital cholesteatoma (also called epidermoid)

b. **Intratemporal part**

   1. *Idiopathic (MC cause):*
      i. Bell's palsy (the MC idiopathic facial nerve palsy)
      ii. Melkersson Rosenthal syndrome
   2. *Secondary to infectious involvement of ear:*
      i. Malignant otitis externa
      ii. Ramsay Hunt syndrome
      iii. ASOM/ANOM
      iv. Unsafe CSOM
   3. *Traumatic:*
      i. Iatrogenic (second most common cause of facial nerve palsy)
      ii. Non-iatrogenic (temporal bone fractures)

c. **Extracranial part**
   i. Parotid tumours
   ii. Parotid surgery
   iii. Sarcoidosis (Heerfordt's syndrome)

BELL'S PALSY

This is the most common idiopathic cause of facial nerve (labyrinthine segment) palsy.

Largely the aetiology of Bell's palsy remains unclear. However, viral etiology is most widely accepted. **Herpes Simplex Virus (HSV) - type 1** is the most likely causative agent. Hence acyclovir/valacyclovir is also used in the management of Bell's palsy.

It is **acute onset, unilateral, rapidly progressing lower motor neuron facial palsy**. Here Facial palsy may be associated with other cranial nerve neuropathies (V, VIII, IX and X). Because of involvement of Vth nerve pain and numbness affecting midface can be present.

Presenting features: Since the site of involvement is the labyrinthine segment (narrowest segment of facial N), the clinical features are because of involvement of all the branches distal to it. Hence the patient presents with dry eye, hyperacusis, loss of taste from the anterior 2/3rd of the tongue and complete LMN palsy of ipsilateral half of the face including the forehead.

Poor Prognostic Signs

a. Complete palsy
b. Loss of both flows that facial nerve regulates, i.e. tearing and salivation.

A good prognostic sign is incomplete palsy.

It may be self limiting condition, but steroids given in the treatment have been found to prevent the progression of disease and hasten the recovery. Steroids also help in complete normal recovery preventing synkinesis, *see* below.

Therefore patients who are treated with steroids early in the course of the disease show good prognosis with **complete recovery in 70–80%** of cases.

Recurrence is uncommon and occurs in about 10% patients.

There is **increased susceptibility of Bell's palsy in diabetes, pregnancy and AIDS patients**.

Management

1. Oral steroids
2. Valacyclovir/Acyclovir—should be started within 72 hrs of palsy.
3. Vitamin B complex as a nerve nourisher.
4. Physiotherapy—this comprises of electrical stimulation of facial muscles and facial massage and exercises.
5. Eye care, in the form of lubrication and covering during sleep, is done to prevent drying and damage to cornea (exposure keratitis).

In patients not responding to medical management electrophysiological assessment should be done. If recovery is seen then the steroids are continued and the electrophysiological tests are repeated.

If recovery is not seen an immediate surgical decompression of mainly the labyrinthine segment is performed. This being the narrowest segment therefore the facial nerve is most prone to compression here, due to edema, following a possible viral infection (HSV-1).

MELKERSSON ROSENTHAL SYNDROME

It constitutes **recurrent** alternating facial palsy along with swelling of lips and fissuring of tongue. Main management here too is steroids.

RAMSAY HUNT SYNDROME

Herpes zoster of external ear with facial palsy is known as Ramsay Hunt syndrome. It is because of reactivation of latent Varicella Zoster virus (VZV) in the geniculate ganglion.

Patients usually complain of pain followed by vesicles over the ear canal, pinna and skin around the pinna and facial palsy. Extension of the infection to the 8th nerve will lead to hearing loss and vertigo. Other cranial nerves might also be involved (e.g. 5th, 9th and 10th).

Management is the same as Bell's palsy. Prognosis is poorer than Bell's palsy.

ASOM

In a patient of ASOM, if the fallopian canal is dehiscent (most commonly in the horizontal segment), the increased pressure is transmitted through the dehiscence leading to facial nerve palsy.

This can be managed by antibiotics and myringotomy.

UNSAFE CSOM

In unsafe CSOM due to erosion of fallopian canal by cholesteatoma facial nerve can get exposed and paralysed. Management is mastoid exploration (MRM) with decompression of the involved segment.

TRAUMATIC FACIAL NERVE PALSY

1. Iatrogenic

The **most common iatrogenic cause** of facial nerve palsy is **parotid surgery** followed by mastoid surgery. This is because in the parotid the facial nerve lies exposed dividing the parotid into a superficial and deep part whereas in the ear the facial N lies protected in the fallopian canal.

In mastoid surgeries the most common site of injury is the 2nd genu followed by mastoid segment.

Following any mastoid surgery if the patient presents with facial palsy immediately, i.e. once the effect of anaesthesia is gone, the patient should be taken up for re-exploration and facial nerve decompression or repair by end to end anastomosis or nerve grafting should be done.

The **grafting** of facial nerve is most commonly done with greater auricular nerve. This nerve supplies the greater part of pinna and lies very superficially in the neck. Longer graft, if required, is taken from sural nerve.

If the patient following surgery develops delayed onset facial palsy, the management is steroids and watchful waiting as this delayed palsy is because of nerve getting compressed due to surrounding oedema.

2. Non-iatrogenic Palsy

It occurs in fractures of temporal bone.

Temporal bone fractures are of two types according to their axis in reference to the long axis of petrous part of temporal bone. They are classified as either longitudinal (parallel to the axis) or transverse (perpendicular to the axis).

1. **Longitudinal fracture:** They are frequently caused by a lateral force over the mastoid or temporal squama, usually produced by temporal or parietal blows.

   In this fracture, the **fracture line runs parallel along the long axis of petrous part of temporal bone.** Here the fracture line runs from the roof of external auditory canal (EAC) through the tympanic membrane to the roof of middle ear but fortunately not involving the inner ear. This is the less severe and **more common fracture** constituting 80% of temporal bone fractures.

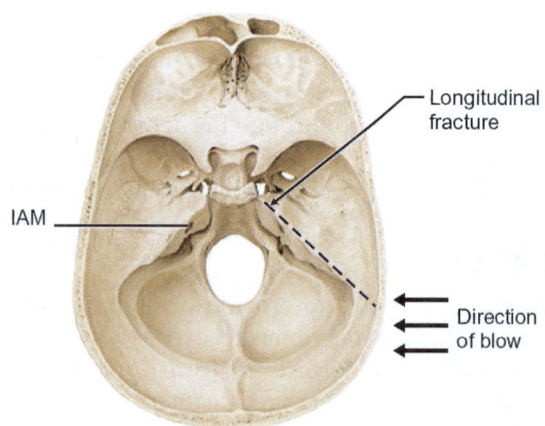

Fig. 11.3: Longitudinal Fracture

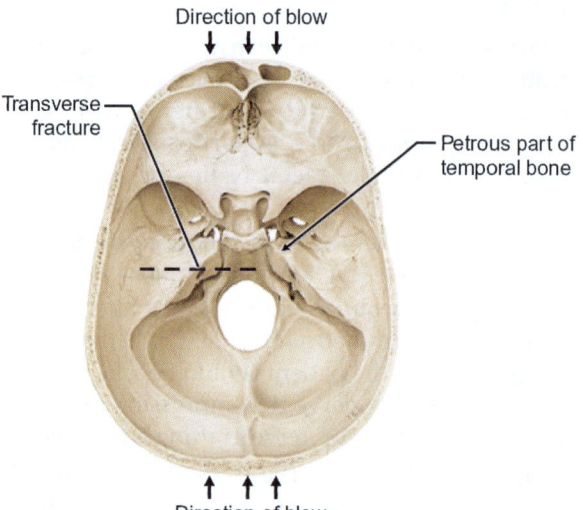

Fig. 11.4: Transverse Fracture

Clinical features: The longitudinal fracture leads to rupture of tympanic membrane. It also leads to the dislocation of ossicles lying in the epitympanum. So this fracture leads to conductive hearing loss. Since the roof of middle ear (tegmen tympani) separating the middle ear from middle cranial fossa is ruptured, the CSF may leak into the middle ear and come out through the ruptured tympanic membrane presenting as CSF otorrhoea.

The injury site of facial nerve is usually where it enters the middle ear from inner ear, i.e. the **first genu. Injury can also occur to the horizontal segment** of the facial nerve.

Facial nerve palsy is **seen only in 20%** of longitudinal fractures.

2. **Transverse fracture:** They are usually caused by a frontal but may also result from an occipital blow.

This is the more severe but less common fracture of temporal bone **constituting 20%** of temporal bone fractures.

Here the fracture line runs **perpendicular (transverse) to the petrous part of temporal bone** involving the internal acoustic meatus, roof of inner ear, and roof of middle ear. Patient here will have **sensorineural hearing loss and vertigo. The facial nerve palsy occurs more commonly here (in 50% cases).**

The CSF leaks into the inner ear and middle ear but it is not able to come from middle ear into the EAC because the TM is intact, so it comes through the Eustachian tube into the nasopharynx and then through the nose presenting as CSF rhinorrhoea (CSF otorhinorrhoea).

	Longitudinal fractures	Transverse fractures
Incidence	Approximately 80%	Approximately 20%
Mechanism	Temporal or parietal trauma	Frontal or occipital trauma
Tympanic membrane perforation	Common	Not present
Facial nerve damage	20%	50%
Hearing loss	Conductive	Severe sensorineural or mixed
Vertigo	Absent	Severe
CSF otorrhoea	Common	Not present
CSF rhinorrhoea	Absent	Present

Investigation

The best investigation for a petrous temporal bone fracture is **HRCT** of temporal bone to visualise the middle ear, inner ear structures and the facial nerve.

Management

It is like in iatrogenic palsy. In **sudden onset** complete palsy, which is the usual scenario, early exploration and decompression of facial nerve or nerve repair should be carried out.

Delayed onset palsy, which might be because of surrounding edema, should be treated with steroids and watchful waiting.

HEERFORDT'S SYNDROME

This is seen in association with sarcoidosis and is also known as **uveo-parotid fever**.

It is characterised by B/L parotid enlargement, facial palsy and uveitis.

ABERRANT REGENERATION OF FACIAL NERVE

Synkinesis and Crocodile Tears

Any injured facial nerve during regeneration can aberrantly interconnect with other facial branches leading to complications like synkinesis and crocodile tears.

Synkinesis

When patient uses one group of facial muscles, the other group also aberrantly contracts for example when the patient smiles, he winks also. This can be managed by intramuscular botulinum toxin injection.

Crocodile Tears

This is **unilateral gustatory lacrimation** and is also known as gustatolacrimal reflex or paroxysmal lacrimation. When the facial nerve gets injured **before the geniculate ganglion,** i.e.1st genu (e.g. in Bell's palsy), during regeneration the fibres which are destined to go to chorda tympani aberrantly interconnect with the greater superficial petrosal nerve. So now when the patient eats, along with salivation, he has tearing also.

Management

Surgical management consisting of sectioning the greater superficial petrosal nerve (vidian neurectomy) used to be done previously but now the treatment of choice of crocodile tears is **botulinum toxin A injection** into the affected lacrimal gland.

ABERRANT REGENERATION OF AURICULOTEMPORAL NERVE

Frey's Syndrome

Frey's syndrome is **gustatory sweating,** i.e. when the patient eats, he has sweating over the cheek skin over the parotid.

Frey's syndrome is because of injury and aberrant regeneration of **auriculotemporal nerve** (a branch of mandibular division of trigeminal) following parotid surgery.

The pathway of parotid gland secretion is as follows:

Inferior salivary nucleus → 9th nerve → Tympanic plexus (TP) → lesser superficial petrosal nerve → Otic ganglion → auriculotemporal nerve → Parasympathetic supply of parotid.

In section of auriculotemporal nerve during parotid surgery, the nerve aberrantly reconnects with the sympathetic sweat glands of the skin overlying the parotid. So now when the patient eats, along with the salivation from the parotid, there is sweating from the skin overlying the parotid.

Note:

Since the most common iatrogenic cause of facial nerve palsy is also parotid surgery so both Frey's syndrome and facial palsy can occur together, Frey's syndrome being due to injury to auriculotemporal nerve.

Diagnosis

In patients affected by gustatory sweating, a Minor's test (iodine-starch test) is performed for diagnosis. Iodine solution is applied to the affected area and it is let dry. Corn starch is then dusted on the area. Chewing some bread, for some minutes, leads to areas of sweating. This causes dried iodine turning aqueous, which then reacts with starch to cause blue colouration in the affected region. The Minor's test also help us localise the area where Botox has to be injected, read below.

Management

Systemic or topical applications of various anticholinergic agents (scopolamine, glycopyrrolate) have been unsuccessful.

- Recently, good results have been obtained with local injection of botulinum toxin (BTX). At present, BTX therapy is considered the gold standard for curative treatment of Frey. However, it needs to be injected periodically.
- In severe Frey's syndrome or in patients opting for permanent treatment, surgical management can be done, e.g. cervical sympathectomy or Tympanic neurectomy (i.e. disrupting parasympathetic fibres as they pass through the middle ear).

  Other surgical treatments include sternocleidomastoid transfer, dermis-fat, fascia grafts and various materials, as inter positional barriers. These techniques aim to create a physical barrier between the divided fibres of the auriculotemporal nerve and the sweat glands in the facial skin.

"Points to Ponder/Points for Quick revision"

- Supranuclear (UMN) facial palsy → paralysis of the lower half of contralateral face (forehead is spared).
- Millard—Gubler syndrome: A brain stem lesion → ipsilateral complete (LMN) facial + ipsilateral lateral rectus palsy + contralateral hemiplegia
- Of the 3 parts of facial nerve, i.e. intracranial, intra-temporal and extracranial; the intra-temporal part is the longest and lies in a bony canal (fallopian canal).
- Intra-temporal part of facial N course is divided into 4 segments: Meatal, Labyrinthine, Tympanic or horizontal and Mastoid or vertical (summarised in a table in the chapter).
- Branches of facial N in the temporal bone:
  i. Greater superficial petrosal: Secretomotor fibres to lacrimal and nasal glands. Damage → dry eyes and nose.
  ii. Nerve to stapedius: Mediates the stapedial reflex; damage → hyperacusis.
  iii. Chorda tympani: Taste sensations anterior 2/3 tongue and secretomotor to sublingual and submandibular salivary glands.
  iv. Sensory auricular branch to the pinna and EAC.
- Topodiagnostic tests; Along with the ipsilateral LMN palsy of the entire face (including forehead) if there is ipsilateral:
  a. Schirmer test abnormal, stapedial reflex absent, taste anterior 2/3 tongue gone, corneal reflex absent—injury in the labyrinthine segment.
  b. Schirmer test N, stapedial reflex absent, taste anterior 2/3 tongue gone, corneal reflex absent—injury to the horizontal part.
  c. Schirmer test N, stapedial reflex N, taste anterior 2/3 tongue gone, corneal reflex absent—injury to the vertical part.
  d. Schirmer test N, stapedial reflex N, taste anterior 2/3 tongue N, corneal reflex absent—injury at or after exiting stylomastoid foramen.
- Electrophysiological tests (falsely negative initially):
  i. ENOG: Assesses the severity of facial N injury—CMAP of >90% at 2 weeks—consideration for N decompression

ii. EMG: Performed after 3 weeks after facial N palsy (if no satisfactory recovery by this time):
   a. Motor unit potentials indicate N regeneration.
   b. Fibrillation potentials indicate poor chances of spontaneous recovery and bad prognosis—consideration for N decompression.
   c. Flat curve indicate long term denervation and loss of viability of motor end plates.

- Bell's palsy (MC cause of facial N paralysis). Next common cause is traumatic (following parotid and mastoid surgeries).
- Bell's palsy:
  – Acute onset, U/L, LMN facial palsy (MC–labyrinthine segment).
  – Idiopathic (though HSV 1 is thought to be the likely underlying cause).
  – Self-limiting (though steroids, if started early on, hasten the recovery, prevents further progression and synkinesis formation).
  – Complete recovery in 70–80%.
  – T/t: Oral steroids, Acyclovir/Valacyclovir (to be started with in 3 days), Vitamin B complex, Physiotherapy, eye care.
- Melkersson Rosenthal syndrome: recurrent alternating facial N palsy, swelling of the lips and tongue fissuring.
- Ramsay Hunt syndrome: Herpes zoster of external ear with facial palsy ± other cranial N palsies, management similar to Bell's palsy.
- Temporal bone fractures (summarised in a table in the chapter). T/t–sudden onset complete palsy → nerve decompression/nerve repair, delayed onset → steroids.
- Heerfordt's syndrome: B/L parotid enlargement, facial palsy and uveitis; Sarcoidosis.
- Aberrant regeneration of facial nerve:
  – Synkinesis (e.g. when patient smiles, he winks also).
  – Crocodile tears: U/L gustatory lacrimation. T/t– Botulinum toxin A.
- Frey's syndrome: U/L gustatory sweating (aberrant regeneration of auriculotemporal N). T/t–Botulinum toxin A.

PREVIOUSLY ASKED QUESTIONS

1. **Right upper motor neuron/supranuclear lesion of facial nerve causes:** (*Exam 2013, AIIMS 95*)
   a. Loss of taste sensation in right anterior part of tongue
   b. Loss of corneal reflex on right side
   c. Loss of wrinkling of forehead on left side
   d. Paralysis of lower facial muscles on left side

2. **Which part of the facial nerve is commonly exposed through natural dehiscence in the fallopian canal?** (*Exam 2013*)
   a. Horizontal part
   b. Upper half of the vertical part
   c. Lower half of the vertical part
   d. Labyrinthine part

3. **First branch of the facial nerve is:** (*UP 2004, Exam 2017*)
   a. Greater petrosal nerve
   b. Lesser petrosal nerve
   c. Chorda tympani nerve
   d. Nerve to the stapedius

4. **Dryness of mouth with normal Stapedial reflex in facial nerve injury—site of lesion is at:** (*UP 2008*)
   a. Chorda tympani nerve
   b. Cerebellopontine angle
   c. Geniculate ganglion
   d. Concussion of tympanic membrane

5. **Nerve involved in hyperacusis:** (*Exam 2013*)
   a. Facial nerve
   b. Glossopharyngeal
   c. Vagus
   d. Trigeminal

6. **Which test can detect facial nerve palsy occurring due to lesion at the outlet of stylomastoid:** (*AIIMS Nov 93, Exam 2015*)
   a. Deviation of angle of mouth towards opposite site
   b. Loss of taste sensation in anterior 2/3rd of tongue
   c. Loss of sensation over right cheek
   d. Deviation of tongue towards opposite side

7. **Dryness of eye is caused by injury to facial nerve at:** (*AI 96, Exam 2015*)
   a. Chorda tympani
   b. Vertical segment
   c. Tympanic segment
   d. Geniculate ganglion

8. **Lacrimation is affected when facial nerve injury is at:** (*AI 98, Exam 2014*)
   a. Geniculate ganglion
   b. Mastoid segment
   c. At Otic ganglion
   d. At Stylomastoid foramen

9. **Facial nerve injury at stylomastoid foramen can cause:** (*AIIMS June 99, Exam 2013*)
   a. Loss of corneal reflex at side of lesion
   b. Loss of taste sensation in anterior 2/3rd of ipsilateral half of tongue
   c. Loss of lacrimation at side of lesion
   d. Hyperacusis

10. **Which one of the following statements is correct in facial paralysis:** (*MP 2009*)
    a. The nasolabial fold is obliterated on same side
    b. The nasolabial fold is obliterated on opposite side
    c. The face deviates to the same side
    d. The eyes do not close completely on the opposite side

11. **Intratemporal lesion of chorda tympani nerve results in:** (*AIIMS Dec 94, May 2005, Exam 2017*)
    a. Loss of taste sensations from circumvallate papillae of tongue
    b. Loss of taste sensations from anterior 2/3rd of tongue
    c. Loss of taste sensations from posterior 1/3rd of tongue
    d. Loss of secretomotor fibres to the parotid

12. **A patient presents with hyperacusis, loss of lacrimation and loss of taste sensation in the anterior 2/3rd of the tongue. Injury extends up to which level of facial nerve:** (*AIIMS 2008*)
    a. Horizontal part
    b. Vertical part proximal to nerve to stapedius
    c. Vertical part beyond nerve to stapedius
    d. Proximal to geniculate ganglion

13. **Surgical landmarks for the identification of facial nerve in mastoid surgeries are all except:** (*DPG 2008*)
    a. Below the processus cochleariformis
    b. Above and posterior to oval window
    c. Medial to short process of incus
    d. Behind the pyramid

14. **Blood supply of facial nerve:** (*PGI 2005, 2006*)
    a. Ascending palatine artery
    b. Facial artery
    c. Labyrinthine artery
    d. Ascending pharyngeal artery
    e. Stylomastoid artery

15. **Aetiology of facial nerve paralysis include all of the following except:** (*Karnataka 2011*)
    a. Otosclerosis
    b. Bell's palsy
    c. Acoustic neuroma
    d. Modified Radical Mastoidectomy

16. **Facial nerve palsy is seen:** (*Exam 2013*)
    a. Sarcoidosis   b. VZV
    c. Acoustic neuroma   d. All

17. **Facial nerve palsy is seen in this condition:**
(*JIPMER 2003, Exam 2017*)
a. Seborrhoeic Otitis externa
b. Otomycosis
c. Malignant Otitis externa
d. Diffuse Otitis externa

18. **Most common cause of facial palsy:** (*Exam 2014*)
a. Post-operative
b. Trauma
c. Ramsay Hunt syndrome
d. Bell's palsy

19. **Most common cause of lower motor neuron facial palsy is:** (*MP 2004, Exam 2017*)
a. Cholesteatoma
b. Cerebellopontine angle tumours
c. Bell's palsy
d. Postoperative (after ear surgery)

20. **Bell's palsy is paralysis of:** (*Comed 2007*)
a. UMN Vth nerve b. UMN VIIth nerve
c. LMN Vth nerve d. LMN VIIth nerve

21. **Patient with Bell's palsy all true except:**
(*AIIMS 2013*)
a. Immediate surgical decompression
b. Acute onset unilateral palsy
c. Herpes simplex virus is a cause
d. Steroid is the choice of treatment

22. **All of the following are seen in Bell's palsy except:**
(*SGPGI 2005, Exam 2014*)
a. I/L facial palsy b. I/L loss of taste sensation
c. Hyperacusis d. I/L ptosis

23. **Hyperacusis in Bell's palsy is due to the paralysis of the following muscle:** (*AIIMS May 2006*)
a. Tensor tympani b. Levator palatini
c. Tensor veli palatini d. Stapedius

24. **Which of the following is not true of Bell's palsy:**
(*Delhi 2008*)
a. Acute onset
b. Always recurrent
c. Spontaneous remission
d. Increased predisposition in diabetes mellitus

25. **True about Bell's palsy is/are:** (*PGI 2000, 2013*)
a. Most common cause of facial palsy
b. Associated with diplopia
c. Crocodile tears and synkinesis may occur
d. No role of steroids
e. Can recur

26. **True about Bell's palsy:** (*Exam 2014*)
a. Spontaneous recovery
b. Steroid contraindicated
c. 25% recover completely
d. Antibiotics mainstay of treatment

27. **True about lower motor palsy of VIIth nerve:**
(*PGI Nov 2009*)
a. Other motor cranial nerves are also involved
b. Melkersson syndrome cause recurrent paralysis
c. Eye protection done
d. Prognosis can be predicted by serial electrical studies
e. Bell's palsy is commonest cause

28. **Which one of the following statements truly represents Bell's paralysis?**
(*AIIMS May 2005/AI 2004, Exam 2017*)
a. Facial nerve paralysis and contralateral Hemiparesis
b. Combined paralysis of the facial, trigeminal and abducens nerves
c. Idiopathic ipsilateral paralysis of the facial nerve
d. Facial nerve paralysis with uveitis and parotid enlargement

29. **Bell's palsy patient comes on day 3. Treatment given would be:** (*AIIMS Nov 2009*)
a. Intratympanic steroids
b. Oral steroids + vitamin B complex
c. Oral steroids + Acyclovir
d. Vasodilators + vitamin B complex

30. **Bell's palsy not responding to steroids. What will be the further line of management?**
(*MP 2000, Exam 2017*)
a. Increase the dose of steroid
b. Vasodilators and ACTH
c. Surgical decompression
d. Electrophysiological nerve testing
e. Physiotherapy

31. **Ramsay Hunt syndrome is caused by:**
(*AI 2004, Exam 2017*)
a. H. simplex b. H. zoster
c. Influenza d. HIV

32. **A man presents with vesicles over external acoustic meatus with ipsilateral facial palsy of LMN type. The cause is:** (*AP 2003, Exam 2017*)
a. Herpes zoster
b. Herpes simplex virus I
c. Both a and b
d. None of the above

33. **All are true about Ramsay Hunt syndrome except:**
(*UP 2000, Exam 2017*)
a. Involves VII nerve
b. May involve VIII nerve
c. Surgical treatment gives excellent prognosis
d. Causative agent is virus

34. **All of the following are true for Ramsay Hunt syndrome, except:** (*MH 2005, Exam 2017*)
a. It has viral aetiology
b. Involves VII nerve

c. May involve VIII nerve

d. Results of spontaneous recovery are excellent

35. Iatrogenic traumatic facial nerve palsy is most commonly caused during: *(Exam 2014)*

a. Myringoplasty

b. Stapedectomy

c. Mastoidectomy

d. Ossiculoplasty

36. Which fracture of the petrous bone will cause facial nerve palsy more commonly? *(AI 2007)*

a. Longitudinal fractures

b. Transverse fractures

c. Mastoid

d. Cribriform plate

37. Which is the correct statement regarding facial nerve palsy in temporal bone fractures? *(AI 2008, AIIMS May 2008)*

a. More common with transverse fractures

b. More common with longitudinal fractures

c. Facial palsy is usually of delayed onset

d. It is not associated with CSF leakage

38. CSF otorrhoea is caused by: *(AIIMS 2000, Karnataka 2009)*

a. Rupture of tympanic membrane

b. Fracture of cribriform plate

c. Fracture of parietal bone

d. Fracture of petrous temporal bone

39. The most common cause of cerebrospinal otorrhoea is: *(UP 97, Exam 2013)*

a. Rupture of tympanic membrane

b. Fracture of petrous ridge

c. Fracture of mastoid air cells

d. Fracture of parietal bone

40. Treatment of choice for temporal bone fracture with facial nerve palsy: *(AIIMS June 99, May 2003)*

a. Nerve decompression

b. Wait and watch

c. Sling operation

d. Repair the fracture

41. Treatment of choice in traumatic facial nerve injury is: *(AIIMS Dec 96, Exam 2013)*

a. Facial sling

b. Facial nerve repair

c. Conservative management

d. Systemic corticosteroids

42. A patient presents with facial nerve palsy following head trauma with fracture of the temporal bone. Best intervention here is: *(AI 2001, Exam 2017)*

a. Immediate decompression

b. Wait and watch

c. Facial sling

d. Steroids

43. Crocodile tears are due to: *(Delhi 2005, Exam 2017)*

a. Cross innervations of facial nerve fibres

b. Cross innervations of trigeminal nerve fibres

c. Improper regeneration of trigeminal nerve

d. Cross innervation of auriculotemporal nerve

44. Frey's syndrome is caused by: *(Exam 2013)*

a. Aberrant reinnervation of parasympathetic fibres of auriculotemporal nerve with sympathetic sweat glands

b. Aberrant reinnervation of parasympathetic fibres of auriculotemporal nerve with greater superficial petrosal nerve

c. Abnormal cross innervation of facial nerve with greater auricular nerve

d. Abnormal cross innervation of facial nerve with auriculotemporal nerve

45. For crocodile tears to occur, injury should be: *(DPG 2007, Exam 2018)*

a. Before greater superficial petrosal

b. Beyond greater superficial petrosal

c. At Chorda tympani

d. Beyond stylomastoid foramen

46. Most accepted management of crocodile tears is: *(JIPMER 2006, Exam 2017)*

a. Section of greater superficial petrosal

b. Removal of lacrimal gland

c. Inj. Botulinum toxin in lacrimal gland

d. Section of Chorda tympani

47. Best investigation for petrous temporal bone fracture is: *(AIIMS 2009)*

a. NCCT

b. CECT

c. HRCT

d. MRI

48. Secretomotor fibres of facial nerve does not supply: *(AIIMS May 2014)*

a. Lacrimal gland

b. Parotid gland

c. Submandibular glands

d. Nasal

49. Lacrimal gland is supplied by: *(Bihar PGMAT 2014)*

a. Otic ganglion

b. Ciliary ganglion

c. Sphenopalatine ganglion

d. Sympathetic chain ganglion

50. Level of Facial nerve. lesion with Intact lacrimation on Schirmer test and loss of taste in anterior 2/3rd of tongue is: *(Exam 2015)*

a. Horizontal segment

b. Labyrinthine segment

c. Internal auditory canal

d. Stylomastoid foramen

Section I | **Ear**

51. **Two months following parotid surgery patient presents with flushing and sweating of cheek while having his meals. Which of the following is false about this condition:** (*Exam 2019*)

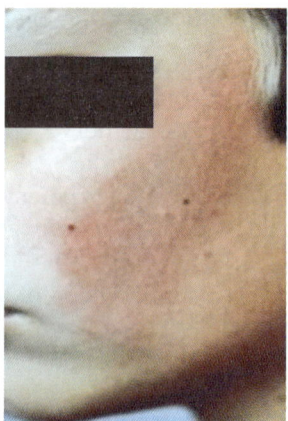

    a. Tympanic neurectomy is contraindicated
    b. Due to faulty regeneration of parasympathetic nerves
    c. Sternocleidomastoid flap is used in treatment
    d. Inj. Botulinum toxin is given

52. **What is the mainstay of treatment for Bell's palsy:** (*Exam 2016*)
    a. Prednisolone
    b. Facial nerve decompression
    c. Eye drops
    d. Electric stimulation

53. **Frey's syndrome occurs due to damage to which nerve during Parotid gland surgery:** (*Exam 2016, 2018, 2019*)
    a. Trigeminal nerve
    b. Lesser petrosal nerve
    c. Vidian nerve
    d. Auriculotemporal nerve

54. **Frey's syndrome is due to cross connection of auriculotemporal nerve with which nerve after parotid surgery:** (*Exam 2015*)
    a. Sympathetic cholinergic fibres
    b. Facial nerve
    c. Glossopharyngeal
    d. Greater superficial petrosal

55. **Frey syndrome includes:** (*Exam 2016*)
    a. Crocodile tears
    b. Anosmia
    c. Gustatory sweating
    d. None of the above

56. **Most appropriate treatment of facial nerve injury in lateral facial wound is:** (*MH CET 2016*)
    a. Secondary repair
    b. Primary repair
    c. Secondary repair with grafting
    d. Healing with secondary intention

57. **Facial nerve is related to which wall of middle ear during mastoid surgeries?** (*WB PG 2016*)
    a. Roof   b. Posterior wall
    c. Medial wall   d. Anterior wall

58. **The nerve that supplies skin over the angle of mandible, if involved in parotid injuries forms a part of anatomical basis for gustatory sweating:** (*NIMHANS 2015*)
    a. Auriculotemporal nerve
    b. Greater auricular nerve
    c. Zygomaticotemporal nerve
    d. Buccal nerve

59. **The given patient comes on day 3. Treatment given would be:** (*Practice question by Author*)

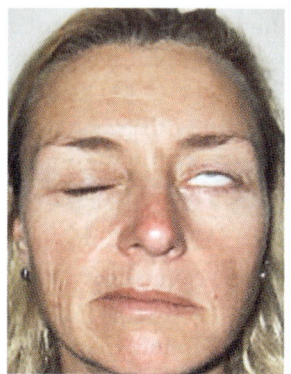

    a. Intratympanic steroids
    b. Oral steroids + vitamin B complex
    c. Oral steroids + Acyclovir
    d. Vasodilators + vitamin B complex

60. **A patient presents with LMN facial nerve palsy along with pain in the ear. The appearance of the ear is given below. Following is true about the disease:** (*Practice question by Author*)

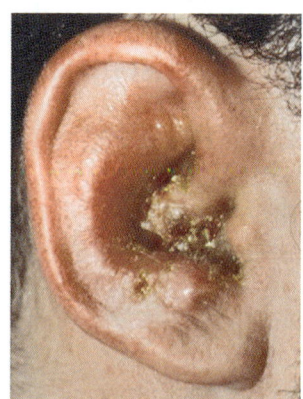

    a. Due to reactivation of Herpes simplex virus in the geniculate ganglion
    b. Due to reactivation of Herpes zoster virus in the geniculate ganglion
    c. Due to reactivation of Herpes simplex virus in the Otic ganglion
    d. Due to reactivation of Herpes zoster virus in the Otic ganglion

ANSWERS AND EXPLANATIONS

1. **(d) Paralysis of lower facial muscles on left side** (*Ref. Scott Brown, 6th ed., 1639*)

2. **(a) Horizontal part, refer the text** (*Ref. Scott Brown, 6th ed., 1386*)

3. **(a) Greater petrosal nerve** (*Ref. Scott Brown, 6th ed., 1385*)
   - The greater superficial petrosal nerve arises from the geniculate ganglion at the first genu. This is the first branch.
   - The 2nd branch is the nerve to the stapedius given at the pyramid.
   - The 3rd is the chorda tympani given 4–6 mm before the exit of facial nerve from stylomastoid foramen.
   - Lesser superficial petrosal nerve is not a branch of facial. It arises from tympanic plexus and supplies the Otic ganglion. Otic ganglion is for the parasympathetic supply to the parotid. Secretomotor fibres to the parotid arise from glossopharyngeal nerve, reach the otic ganglion through the lesser superficial petrosal nerve via the tympanic plexus and then reach the parotid through the auriculotemporal nerve arising from the otic ganglion.

4. **(a) Chorda tympani nerve** (*Ref. Scott Brown, 6th ed., 1934*)
   - Chorda tympani nerve gives taste to the anterior 2/3rd of the tongue and parasympathetic supply to the sublingual and submandibular salivary glands. Here in this question since the Stapedial reflex is normal so injury is beyond the nerve to stapedius, i.e. at or before Chorda tympani but after the pyramid and will lead to loss of taste from anterior 2/3rd of tongue and reduced salivary flow leading to some dryness of mouth.
   - Stapedial reflex will also be absent with facial nerve injury at CP angle and geniculate ganglion.

5. **(a) Facial nerve** (*Ref. Cummings, 6th ed., 2620*)

6. **(a) Deviation of angle of mouth towards opposite site.** (*Ref. Scott Brown, 6th ed., 1387*)
   - When there is lesion at the outlet of stylomastoid foramen the motor fibres which supply the facial muscles on the same side are affected leading to deviation of angle of mouth towards opposite side due to the pull of the normal side facial muscles.
   - The chorda tympani originates before the stylomastoid foramen so taste sensation in anterior 2/3rd of tongue is preserved here.
   - Sensation over cheek is by trigeminal nerve and the motor supply of tongue is by hypoglossal, both of which will not be affected in facial nerve palsy.

7. **(d) Geniculate ganglion** (*Ref. Cummings, 6th ed., 2606*)
   - Whenever there is injury before or at the origin of the greater superficial petrosal nerve (i.e. before or

at the Geniculate ganglion) which is responsible for lacrimation there will be dry eye on the same side.
   - Tympanic segment, Vertical segment and Chorda tympani all are beyond the geniculate ganglion.

8. **(a) Geniculate ganglion** (*Ref. Cummings, 6th ed., 2606*)
   - Mastoid segment and Stylomastoid foramen are beyond the geniculate ganglion.
   - Otic ganglion is for the parasympathetic supply to the parotid.

9. **(a) Loss of corneal reflex at side of lesion.** (*Ref. Cummings, 6th ed., 2606*)
   - When the injury is at the stylomastoid foramen, the extracranial motor part of facial is affected leading to loss of corneal reflex, see the text above.
   - The branches of facial before the stylomastoid foramen, i.e. greater superficial petrosal, nerve to stapedius and Chorda tympani will all be preserved therefore there won't be any loss of lacrimation, hyperacusis and loss of taste respectively

10. **(a) The nasolabial fold is obliterated on same side** (*Ref. Scott Brown, 6th ed., 1370*)
    - In facial nerve palsy, the motor supply of the facial muscles on the same side will be affected leading to obliteration of nasolabial fold, loss of facial movements and incomplete closure of the eye on the affected side.
    - The face deviates to the opposite side because of the pull of the normal side facial muscles.

11. **(b) Loss of taste sensations from anterior 2/3rd of tongue** (*Ref. Scott Brown, 6th ed., 1387*)
    - The innervation of most of the posterior 1/3rd of tongue and circumvallate papillae is by glossopharyngeal nerve.
    - Secretomotor fibres to the parotid arise from glossopharyngeal nerve; reach the otic ganglion through the lesser petrosal nerve and then reach the parotid through the auriculotemporal nerve.

12. **(d) Proximal to geniculate ganglion** (*Ref. Cummings, 6th ed., 2606*)
    - Since all the intratemporal branches of facial are involved, the injury should be before the 1st branch (i.e. greater superficial petrosal) which is given off at the geniculate ganglion.

13. **(a) Below the processus cochleariformis** (*Ref. Scott Brown, 6th ed., 1386, 1387*)
    - The first genu of facial nerve lies antero-superior to the Processes cochleariformis.

14. **(c) and (e) labyrinthine artery, stylomastoid artery,** (*Ref. Scott Brown, 6th ed., 1388*) please refer the text.

15. **(a) Otosclerosis** (*Ref. Scott Brown 6th ed., 1401*)

16. **(d) All** (*Ref. Scott Brown, 6th ed., 1401*)

17. **(c) Malignant Otitis externa** (*Ref. Cummings, 6th ed., 2618*)
    - Among the given options Malignant Otitis externa is locally invasive infective condition and leads to facial nerve palsy. It is seen in immunocompromised patients and is caused most commonly by pseudomonas.

Section I | Ear

18. **(d) Bell's palsy** (*Ref. Scott Brown, 6th ed., 1400*)
   - The MC cause of facial nerve palsy is idiopathic. The MC idiopathic facial nerve palsy is Bell's palsy.
   - The second most common cause of facial nerve palsy is iatrogenic. The most common iatrogenic cause of facial nerve palsy is parotid surgery followed by mastoid surgery.
   - Non iatrogenic trauma causing temporal bone fractures can lead to facial nerve palsy. Here transverse fractures leads to facial nerve palsy more commonly than the longitudinal fractures.
   - Ramsay Hunt syndrome is an infective cause of facial nerve palsy due to Herpes zoster.

19. **(c) Bell's palsy** (*Ref. Scott Brown, 6th ed., 1400*)

20. **(d) LMN VIIth nerve** (*Ref. Cummings, 6th ed., 2619*)
   - In LMN VIIth nerve palsy (Most common being Bell's palsy) the complete half of the ipsilateral side of face gets involved.
   - In UMN VIIth nerve palsy the lower half of the opposite side of face gets involved.

21. **(a) Immediate surgical decompression**, (*Ref. Cummings, 6th ed., 2621*) please refer to text.

22. **(d) I/L ptosis** (*Ref. Scott Brown, 6th ed., 1370*)
   - In Bell's palsy because of involvement of the facial nerve, the muscles of the ipsilateral face are paralysed which leads to incomplete closure of the eye but not ptosis.
   - Ptosis is seen in 3rd nerve palsy.

23. **(d) Stapedius** (*Ref. Cummings, 6th ed., 2620*)
   - Hyperacusis is normal sounds perceived as abnormally loud. This is due to loss of Stapedial reflex. In Bell's palsy this is due to paralysis of the facial nerve which supplies the stapedius.
   - Tensor tympani which also helps in protecting the ear from loud noise, is supplied by the mandibular nerve.
   - The other muscles in the options are not involved in hyperacusis.

24. **(b) Always recurrent** (*Ref. Scott Brown, 6th ed., 1400*)
   - Recurrence is uncommon. There may occur spontaneous remission but steroids are very important in the management, please see the text.

25. **(a), (c), (e)** (*Ref. Scott Brown, 6th ed., 1400*)

26. **(a) Spontaneous recovery** (please refer the text) (*Ref. Cummings, 6th ed., 2621*)

27. **(a), (b), (c), (d), (e)** (*Ref. Scott Brown, 6th ed., 1394, 1400*) all are true

28. **(c) Bell's palsy is idiopathic LMN palsy of facial nerve causing ipsilateral paralysis of face.** (*Ref. Scott Brown, 6th ed., 1400*)
   - Ipsilateral Facial nerve paralysis and contralateral Hemiparesis along with ipsilateral VI nerve palsy constitutes Millard Gubler syndrome. It is a form of "crossed hemiplegia," as the paralysis of muscles controlled by the facial nerve occurs on the same side as the lesion, while the hemiplegia of muscles below the neck occurs on the opposite side from the lesion

   - In Bell's palsy facial palsy may be associated with other cranial nerve neuropathies which are Vth, VIIIth, IXth and Xth.
   - Facial nerve paralysis with uveitis and parotid enlargement constitutes Heerfordt's syndrome.

29. **(c) Oral steroids + Acyclovir is the best answer.** (*Ref. Cummings, 6th ed., 2621*)
   - Antiviral has to be started within 3 days. Since the patient has presented on the 3rd day, acyclovir should also be started here along with the steroids.
   - If the patient comes after 3 days he should be given only the steroid and vitamin B.
   - Intratympanic steroids and vasodilators are not used for Bell's palsy. Please refer the text.

30. **(d) Electrophysiological nerve testing.** (*Ref. Cummings, 6th ed., 2622*)
   - If on electrophysiological tests the signs of regeneration are not present surgical decompression is indicated.
   Vasodilators and ACTH have no role.
   - Physiotherapy is started from the 1st day itself while treating Bell's palsy.
   - Steroids in Bell's palsy are given in the dosage of 1 mg/kg body weight and gradually tapered. If there is no response electrophysiological nerve testing is done.

31. **(b) H. zoster** (*Ref. Cummings, 6th ed., 2622*)
   - Herpes Zoster of external ear with facial palsy is known as Ramsay Hunt syndrome.
   - H. simplex is being reported to be associated with Bell's palsy.
   - Facial nerve palsy can also be caused by other viruses, for example HIV, influenza, polio, EBV, etc.

32. **(a) Herpes zoster** (*Ref. Cummings, 6th ed., 2622*)
   Ramsay Hunt syndrome is the underlying condition.
   - H. simplex is found to be associated with Bell's palsy in some patients but there are no vesicular eruptions in Bell's palsy.

33. **(c) Surgical treatment gives excellent prognosis** (*Ref. Scott Brown, 6th ed., 1403*)
   - Treatment is steroids and acyclovir like Bell's palsy. Rest are true please refer the text.

34. **(d) Results of spontaneous recovery are excellent** (*Ref. Cummings, 6th ed., 2622*)

35. **(c) Mastoidectomy** (*Ref. Scott Brown, 6th ed., 1405*)
   - The most common iatrogenic cause of facial nerve palsy is parotid surgery.
   - The next common iatrogenic cause of facial nerve palsy is mastoid exploration.
   - It may also occur following rest of the options.

36. **(b) Transverse fractures** (*Ref. Scott Brown, 6th ed., 1404*) please refer the text.

37. **(a) More common with transverse fractures** (*Ref. Scott Brown, 6th ed., 1404*)
   Facial nerve palsy is usually of immediate onset.
   Mnemonic: **T**ransverse fracture **T**raumatises the facial nerve whereas **L**ongitudinal fracture **L**eaves it usually.

38. **(d) Fracture of petrous temporal bone** (*Ref. Scott Brown, 6th ed., 1110*)

39. **(b) Fracture of petrous ridge** (*Ref. Scott Brown, 6th ed., 1110*)

40. **(a) Nerve decompression** (*Ref. Scott Brown, 6th ed., 1404*)
    - In sudden onset complete palsy following fracture (which is the common presentation) early exploration and decompression of facial nerve or nerve repair should be carried out.
    - Delayed onset palsy, which might be because of surrounding edema, should be treated with steroids and watchful waiting.

41. **(b) Facial nerve repair** (*Ref. Scott Brown, 6th ed., 1404*)
    - Since generally following trauma the facial nerve injury occurs as sudden onset. Facial decompression should be the best option.

42. **(a) Immediate decompression** (*Ref. Scott Brown, 6th ed., 1404*)

43. **(a) Cross innervations of facial nerve fibres.** (*Ref. Scott Brown, 6th ed., 1370*)

44. **(a) aberrant reinnervation of parasympathetic fibres of auriculotemporal nerve with sympathetic sweat glands** (*Ref. Cummings, 6th ed., 1257*)

45. **(a) Before greater superficial petrosal** (*Ref. Scott Brown, 6th ed., 1370*)

46. **(c) Injection Botulinum toxin in lacrimal gland** (*Ref. Scott Brown, 6th ed., 1408*)

47. **(c) HRCT** (*Ref. Scott Brown, 6th ed., 1399*)

48. **(b) Parotid gland** (*Ref. Cummings, 6th ed., 2606*)
    - lacrimal and nasal mucosal glands are supplied by greater superficial petrosal nerve. Submandibular and sublingual glands are supplied by Chorda tympani. Parotid is supplied by the otic ganglion through the Auriculotemporal nerve.

49. **(c) Sphenopalatine ganglion** (*Ref. Shambaugh, 6th ed., 621*)

50. **(a) Horizontal segment** (*Ref. Scott Brown, 6th ed., 1394*)

51. **(a) Tympanic neurectomy is contraindicated** (*Ref. Cummings, 6th ed., 1257*)

52. **(a) Prednisolone** (*Ref. Cummings, 6th ed., 2621*)

53. **(d) Auriculotemporal nerve** (*Ref. Cummings, 6th ed., 3107*)

54. **(a) Sympathetic cholinergic fibres** (*Ref. Cummings, 6th ed., 3107*)

55. **(c) Gustatory sweating** (*Ref. Cummings, 6th ed., 1257*)

56. **(b) Primary repair** (*Ref. Scott Brown, 6th ed., 1403*)
    - Any sudden onset palsy following injury (iatrogenic or non iatrogenic trauma), should be managed by immediate exploration and repair.

57. **(b) Posterior wall** (*Ref. Shambaugh, 6th ed., 621*)

58. **(b) Greater auricular nerve** (*Ref. Cummings, 6th ed., 1254*)
    - The nerve that supplies skin over the angle of mandible is Greater auricular Nerve. Sometimes during parotid surgeries, Greater auricular Nerve also gets injured along with the Auriculotemporal Nerve. In this situation with the aberrant regeneration of the Auriculotemporal Nerve, the parasympathetic fibres (of the auriculotemporal nerve) to salivary glands become aberrantly connected with the sympathetic cholinergic fibres to sweat glands of the skin overlying the parotid as well as overlying the angle of mandible (the territory of Greater auricular nerve).

59. **(c) Oral steroids + Acyclovir** (*Ref. Cummings, 6th ed., 2621*)

60. **(b) Due to reactivation of Herpes zoster virus in the geniculate ganglion** (*Ref. Cummings, 6th ed., 2622*)

Section I | Ear

Meniere's Disease and Disorders of Vestibular System

MENIERE'S DISEASE

Meniere's is also known as **endolymphatic hydrops**.

As the name endolymphatic hydrops, endolymph which is present in the membranous labyrinth, increases here leading to dilatation of the membranous labyrinth.

Meniere's is largely **idiopathic**. If it occurs secondary to infection, trauma, allergy, autoimmune or any other known cause it is known as **secondary Meniere's** disease.

Most of the cases are sporadic however a positive family history is found in 10–15% cases. The genetic predisposition might be caused by mutations on the short arm of **chromosome 6**.

It is frequently a **unilateral** condition with M:F ratio - 1:1

Etiopathogenesis

Endolymph is the constituent of whole of the membranous labyrinth so the features of Meniere's are because of involvement of whole of the membranous labyrinth.

The increase of endolymph in Meniere's is either due to its increased production (e.g. sodium and water retention) or reduced absorption (due to endolymphatic sac obstruction), *see* Chapter 1 on anatomy. The dilatation of the membranous labyrinth, in Meniere's, starts from the scala media since the production of endolymph occurs from here from the stria vascularis, *see* Fig. 12.1.

The dilatation starts from the apex of scala media and goes down to involve the rest of the cochlear turns and then finally involves the vestibular part of membranous labyrinth.

As the endolymph further increases in amount it leads to bulging of the Reissner's membrane (the roof of scala media) into the scala vestibuli above. When the pressure increases further the Reissner's membrane ruptures, *see* Fig. 12.2. This rupture leads to mixing of endolymph and perilymph. In the perilymph there is more of sodium and in endolymph we have more of potassium.

This chemical mixture transiently irritates and damages the vestibular and cochlear nerve endings. This irritation leads to a depolarization blockade and transient loss of function of vestibular and cochlear pathways.

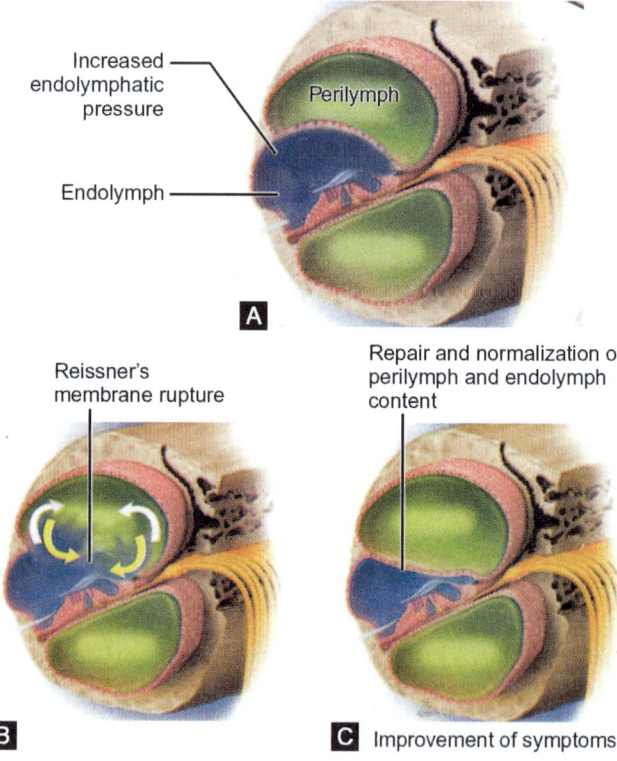

Increased endolymphatic pressure

Perilymph

Endolymph

A

Reissner's membrane rupture

Repair and normalization of perilymph and endolymph content

B   **C** Improvement of symptoms

Fig. 12.2: Rupture and healing of Reissner's membrane during an attack of Meniere

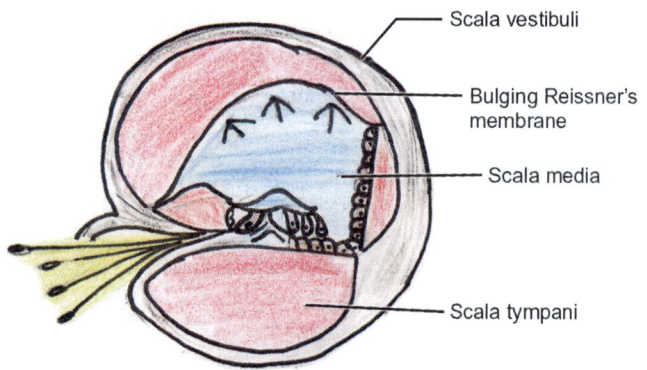

Scala vestibuli

Bulging Reissner's membrane

Scala media

Scala tympani

Fig. 12.1: Bulging Reissner's membrane in endolymphatic hydrops

Clinical Features

1. **Vertigo: The sudden change in the rate of vestibular nerve firing creates an acute vestibular imbalance (i.e. vertigo).** Vertigo is therefore the first symptom of Meniere's and it lasts for at least 20 minutes till a maximum of up to 24 hours. This sudden onset Vertigo of Meniere's is associated with **vagal symptoms** i.e. nausea, vomiting, abdominal cramps, diarrhoea and bradycardia. The attacks are usually preceded by an aura that is usually a sense of fullness in the ear. The vertigo is accompanied by nystagmus of peripheral origin, *see* Chapter 3.

2. **SN hearing loss and tinnitus:** The damage to the cochlear nerve endings and hair cells leads to the 2nd symptom of Meniere, i.e. SN hearing loss and tinnitus. Since the dilatation starts from the apex of scala media going down, so **low frequency** sounds are affected early here.

   Once the mixing has occurred the pressure on both sides equalises. With time the Reissner's membrane heals and the nerve endings also regenerate leading to normalisation of vertigo and hearing defect, till there is another attack of Meniere.

   This type of hearing loss is known as **fluctuating SN hearing loss**. Since Meniere is a unilateral condition, both the ears sense the same sound as different leading to distortion of sound known as Bin aural diplacusis.

   Gradually because of repeated rupture and damage, the cochlear hair cells and the nerve endings get permanently damaged and this leads to progressive hearing loss, which does not revert back to normal and becomes permanent.

   So the **presenting triad** of Meniere is episodic vertigo followed by deafness and tinnitus.

   In a variant of Meniere the deafness occurs before vertigo, this is known as **Lermoyez syndrome** (therefore, also called reverse Meniere).

   (*Mnemonic:* **Ler-m**oyez—Ist **L**istening problem then **M**otion sickness, i.e. vertigo).

   The dilatation reaching the other part of the membranous labyrinth, i.e. saccule and utricle causes two more symptoms in Meniere.

   1. **Drop crisis or Tumarkin's crisis:** Because of the dilatation of utricle and saccule there is distortion of the macular membrane (otolith) affecting the linear acceleration. Therefore when the patient walks he suddenly falls down, without any loss of consciousness. This is known as drop crisis or Tumarkin's crisis (or otolithic crisis).
   2. **Tullio phenomenon:** Because of their dilatation the utricle and saccule come to lie very near to the oval window so that whenever there is a very loud sound the footplate happens to touch and stimulate the saccule and utricle leading to vertigo. **Sound induced** vestibular symptoms such as vertigo, nystagmus, oscillopsia and postural imbalance is known as Tullio phenomenon. Other than Meniere, Tullio phenomenon can also be seen in Superior canal dehiscence and perilymph fistula, read below.

Investigations

Any patient presenting with vertigo, deafness, tinnitus and fullness in the ear should be investigated for Meniere.

The audiological tests in Meniere are suggestive of cochlear pathology, *see* also Chapter on audiology.

Rinne → positive
Weber → towards the normal ear
ABC → shortened
Schwabach shortened
Recruitment → **positive**. Because of recruitment patient does not tolerate loud sounds.
SISI → 70–100% (because of recruitment)

Mitz Recruitment test, i.e. stapedial reflex threshold is decreased: Stapedial reflex is present even at 60 dB or less (threshold is decreased), i.e. much before the normal threshold of 70–100 dB. This occurs because of recruitment leading to abnormal growth of loudness making a sound less than 70 dB loud enough, for stapedial reflex to be present.

Caloric test: There is a reduction in caloric response.

Electrocochleography → Here SP/AP > 30% is suggestive of Meniere. This is the most sensitive test for Meniere.

Glycerol test → Here glycerol is given orally. Since it is an osmotic diuretic it reduces the hydrops, improves the vertigo and hearing which is manifested in the Electrocochleography.

Glycerol test along with Electrocochleography is diagnostic of Meniere.
Tone decay → <30 dB

Speech Discrimination score → reduced (which is in proportion to hearing loss).

Audiogram → In early stages low frequencies are affected so it is **up sloping/rising** audiogram which in later stages becomes flat due to involvement of other frequencies, *see* the audiogram below.

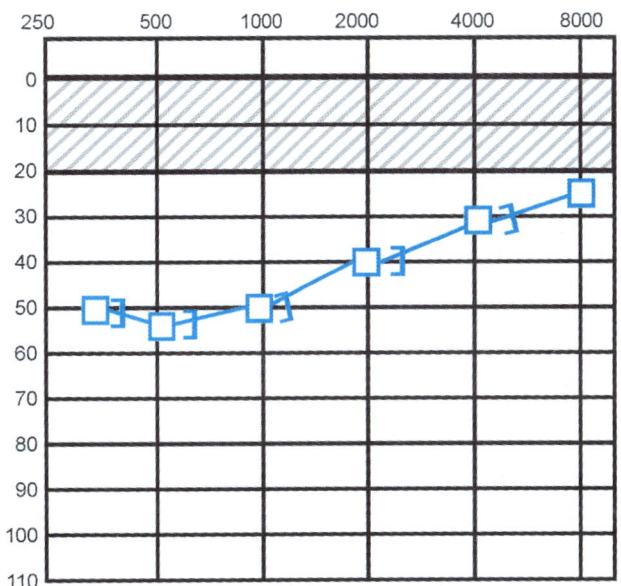

Fig 12.3: Audiogram showing low frequency hearing loss in left ear (up sloping type)

MRI with Gadolinium Contrast

Recently an upcoming diagnostic technique for Meniere's is intratympanic or intravenous injection of gadolinium based contrast followed by MRI to evaluate the perilymphatic and the endolymphatic space separately. In normal ears gadolinium loads only in the perilymphatic space without entering into the endolymph. In Meniere's because of rupture of Reisener's membrane there is mixing of perilymph and endolymph, hence gadolinium can be seen in both the spaces.

Management

1. **Salt restricted diet.** Any vasoconstrictors like nicotine (smoking), tea and coffee should be avoided.
2. Diuretics.
3. **Labyrinthine sedatives:** The main disturbing feature of Meniere is vertigo. So the medical management aims at relieving the vertigo. This can be done by labyrinthine sedatives, e.g. promethazine (phenargan), prochlorperazine (stemetil), cinnarizine (stugerone).
4. **Vasodilators:** These are used here since it has been postulated that vasoconstriction of labyrinthine artery precipitates the attack of Meniere. Moreover vasodilators also increase the reabsorption of endolymph.

   The MC vasodilator that is used is **Betahistine** (vertin), which is an oral histamine analogue. The other vasodilators that are used are **nicotinic acid (compare from nicotine)/niacin** (vitamin B3) and inhalation of Carbogen.
5. **Systemic and intratympanic steroids** have shown improvement in the symptoms of secondary Meniere where an autoimmune or allergic cause has been there.
6. **Meniett device:** It has been seen that application of external pressure to the middle ear decreases the symptoms of Meniere by redistribution of endolymph and facilitating the absorption of endolymph. This can be done by an external hand held air pressure generator device known as meniett device, through which pressure is delivered in complex pulses to the middle ear by a ventilation tube.

If the patient does not respond to the medical management, the surgical management options are the following:

1. **Endolymphatic sac decompression:** Endolymphatic sac is approached through the antrum by a cortical mastoidectomy. The endolymphatic sac lies below the **Donaldson line** (the line passing from the lateral semicircular canal, bisecting the posterior semicircular canal, *see* Fig. 1.20 in Chapter 1). In endolymphatic sac decompression surgery, the bone of the posterior fossa overlying the endolymphatic sac is removed thereby relieving pressure.
2. **Shunt operation:** A one way shunt is made between the membranous labyrinth and CSF so that the endolymph can drain but CSF cannot enter.
3. **Selective vestibular nerve destruction:** Initially when the hearing is preserved we go for selective vestibular nerve destruction to treat vertigo.

This can be done by LASER or surgical section of the vestibular nerve or by vestibulotoxic drugs, e.g. **Gentamicin** which is delivered to the inner ear via the **round window membrane** through a **microwick** (a small wick soaked with the drug) which is passed into the middle ear through a tympanostomy tube. This is known as chemical labyrinthectomy.

4. **Total labyrinthectomy:** This is done when the patient presents at a very late stage, i.e. with permanent hearing loss (here the inner ear which has two functions, the hearing and balance, hearing is of no good and vestibular part is creating imbalance therefore the whole of labyrinth is destroyed).

Note:

- Vestibular destruction therapy is effective in controlling vertigo associated with Meniere's disease.
- No therapy to date has been proven to be effective in the treatment of the permanent hearing loss in Meniere.

BENIGN PAROXYSMAL POSITIONAL VERTIGO (BPPV)

This is the most common cause of peripheral vertigo in clinical practice. Here the patient complains of **episodic vertigo lasting for seconds, in certain head positions**. Hearing is absolutely normal here (also *see* BPPV in the chapter on vestibular physiology).

Pathogenesis

BPPV occurs because of free floating debris which are detached otoconia from the utricular macula which reach the endolymph of most commonly the posterior semicircular canal (*Mnemonic:* BPPV—Posterior). This **occurs most commonly following head trauma**. Other causes are middle ear infection, viral labyrinthitis and prolonged bed rest.

This free floating debris moves in certain head positions, stimulating the cupula leading to vertigo. This vertigo disappears when the debris settles down in 10–20 seconds.

Diagnosis

It is diagnosed by doing '**DIX-HALLPIKE test**'which is a positional test, in which the nystagmus is watched for while changing the position of the head of the patient while sitting and lying down. The posterior canal BPPV elicits a vertical upbeating geotropical tortional nystagmus (i.e. fast phase upwards and outwards towards the ground).

Management

This involves repositioning the debris from posterior semicircular canal back into the utricle by placing the patient's head in a sequence of five positions. This manoeuvre is known as **"Epley's** manoeuvre" or canalith **repositioning** manoeuvre.

VESTIBULAR NEURONITIS

This condition is characterised by acute onset vertigo, associated with nausea and vomiting lasting for days to weeks. This, as the name, is most likely because of **viral infection** involving the **vestibular nerve**.

The cochlear part is not involved so the **hearing remains normal**. The **caloric test shows diminished response**.

It is a self limiting condition, the acute phase is managed by labyrinthine sedatives. Full recovery occurs within 6–12 weeks.

NOISE INDUCED HEARING LOSS (NIHL)

The various sound intensities in different voices perceived by normal ears are:

If tested at a distance of 1 metre, in a normal person:

Intensity of sound	Different voices
30 dB	Whisper
60 dB	Normal conversation
90 dB	Shouting
100–120 dB	Discomfort
120–130 dB (or more)	Pain

Easy to remember, a change by 30 dB in the sound changes the comfort level.

The normal **safe limit** of noise which a human ear can tolerate without damage is 85 dB for 8 hours a day, for 5 days a week (easy to remember people usually work 8 hours a day and 5 days in a week).

Any increase in loudness or duration of exposure can lead to noise induced hearing loss. NIHL was earlier known as Boiler maker's deafness.

It can be:

a. **Temporary threshold shift/Auditory fatigue:** Auditory fatigue is defined as a temporary loss of hearing after exposure to sound. This change of hearing recovers within 24 hrs.

b. **Permanent threshold shift:** Due to damage of organ of Corti, this hearing loss is permanent.

The inner ear is protected from loud noise by "acoustic/stapedial reflex", but there is a delay in onset of this reflex of approx. 100–200 ms.

Therefore, when an intense short impulse high intensity noise >140 dB (e.g. gun shot, bomb explosion, etc.) is subjected to the ear suddenly, it reaches the cochlea before acoustic reflex is activated leading to permanent hearing loss.

Diagnosis

Audiometry

Noise exposure initially causes high frequency hearing loss therefore initially the frequencies involved are > 8000 Hz to 20,000 Hz. These frequencies have to be tested by **high frequency audiometry** which tests frequencies from 8000 Hz to 20,000 Hz since a conventional pure tone audiogram tests frequencies of only up to 8000 Hz. Early detection of loss of high frequencies with the help of high frequency audiometry will prevent the involvement of

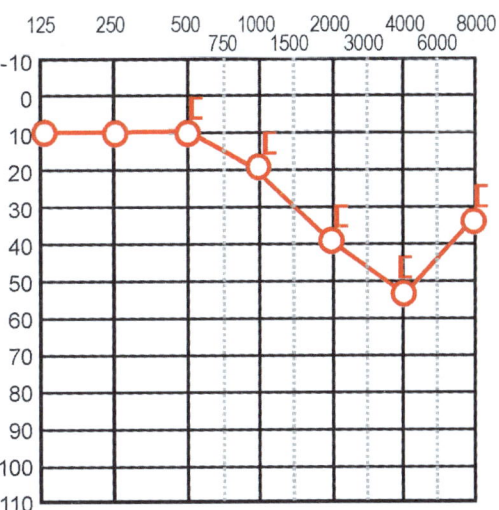

Fig. 12.4: Audiogram showing Acoustic dip at 4000 Hz in right ear

lower frequencies especially speech frequencies. However, the earliest change seen in the conventional pure tone audiogram is a **dip at 4000 Hz** which is known as 'acoustic dip.'

Oto Acoustic Emissions (OAE)

The outer hair cells are more prone to damage by noise trauma. Since the otoacoustic emissions (OAE) are produced by the outer hair cells, evoked OAE are very important diagnostic tool in detecting early noise induced hearing loss, like high frequency audiometry. Distortion product OAE are more useful in this regard.

Management

Noise induced hearing loss can be prevented. People working in noisy environment can use ear plugs which can provide protection of 30 dB. Ear muffs are more effective and give a protection of 40 dB.

Since NIHL is an irreversible and progressive disorder, therefore, early detection by high frequency audiometry and OAE is important to prevent the involvement of hearing loss in lower speech frequencies.

Hearing rehabilitation can be done by hearing aids.

PRESBYCUSIS

Presbycusis is known as age related hearing loss.

It is **slowly progressive, bilaterally symmetrical**, sensorineural hearing loss, usually starts after 50 years.

Changes associated with aging occur throughout the auditory system, from the hair cells of the cochlea, till the auditory cortex in the temporal lobe of the brain.

Six types of presbycusis are seen, *see* Table 12.1, the first three are cochlear the fourth type is retrocochlear (neural) and the last two are intermediate and mixed. The neural type is most common.

Treatment

Presbycusis is neither curable nor preventable. However properly fitted hearing aids may contribute to the rehabilitation of a patient with presbycusis.

Section I | **Ear**

Table 12.1			
Type of presbycusis	*Site of involvement*	*Type of audiogram*	*Speech Discrimination Score (SDS)*
Sensory	Hair cells in the organ of Corti	Down sloping (initially high frequency hearing loss)	Reduced in proportion to hearing loss
Mechanical/cochlear-conductive	Thickening and stiffening of the basilar membrane of cochlea	As above	As above
Metabolic/vascular	Atrophy of the Stria vascularis leading to decreased production of endolymph	Flat audiogram (involve all the frequencies)	Good
Neural (most common)	Atrophy of cochlear nerve	Down sloping	Severe decrease in speech discrimination which is out of proportion to hearing loss

Cochlear implants: Cochlear implants are indicated for people with bilateral severe hearing loss that is not significantly improved with hearing aid. Patients with cochlear changes only along with relatively normal cochlear nerve and central pathways are the candidates for cochlear implant.

OTOTOXICITY

Drug-induced damage to the structures of the auditory and balance system, i.e. the inner ear is known as ototoxicity.

Some drugs lead to permanent damage whereas others, cause temporary or reversible damage.

Irreversible or permanent damage occurs by formation of reactive oxygen species, by the offending drug, leading to primarily damage of outer hair cells (**note: NIHL, presbycusis and ototoxicity**, they all involve **outer hair cells**), whereas drugs causing **reversible** damage do so mainly by temporarily changing the metabolic milieu of perilymph/endolymph.

The following drugs lead to damage to the inner ear (cochlea/vestibule): (*Mnemonic:* **A C D**)

A:

1. Aminoglycosides: They vary greatly in their differential effects on the vestibular and cochlear systems.
   a. **Cochleotoxic aminoglycosides** are (*Mnemonic:* "**KAN**" (means ear in Hindi)—Kanamycin, Amikacin and Neomycin). Of these Neomycin is the most cochleotoxic (as well as nephrotoxic) aminoglycoside therefore it is not used (**neomycin—no**) systemically. Its use is restricted to topical antibiotic applications.
   b. **Predominantly vestibulotoxic aminoglycosides:** Of all ototoxic drugs, the aminoglycosides are the most vestibulotoxic. Among them Netilmicin, **Streptomycin, Gentamicin,** and Tobramycin are predominantly vestibulotoxic (*Mnemonic:* **NSG-T**—on seeing National Security Guards-Terrorists feel vertiginous). In very high doses they can affect the cochlear system also.

Therapeutic Toxicity

Intratympanic Gentamicin has become a major treatment modality for intractable Meniere's disease. It is more vestibulotoxic than cochleotoxic and therefore

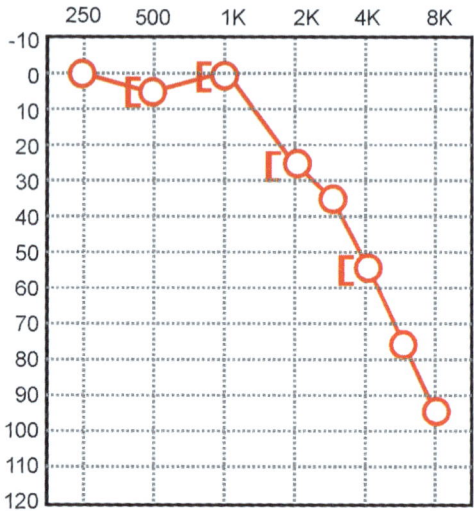

Fig. 12.5: Ototoxicity: High frequency (down sloping) hearing loss in right ear

ablates the vestibular function while preserving hearing. The idea is that unilateral vestibular loss allows compensation from the contralateral vestibular system, allowing for improved overall function.

2. **A**nalgesics (NSAIDs): Aspirin.
3. **A**ntimalarials: Quinine, Chloroquine

C:

1. **C**ytotoxic drugs: Cisplatin, Carboplatin
2. **C**helating agents: Desferrioxamine

D:

1. **D**iuretics: Loop—Furosemide, Ethacrynic acid

The ototoxic effects of loop diuretics seem to be associated with the **stria vascularis**. It blocks the **Na$^+$ K$^+$ 2Cl$^-$** channel in the stria vascularis tissue thereby changing the chemical milieu of endolymph. This leads to changes in the ionic gradients between the perilymph and endolymph. These changes cause edema of the epithelium of the stria vascularis.

Others:

Vancomycin is a commonly used antibiotic in methicillin-resistant *Staphylococcus aureus* (MRSA) infections. High doses attributed to renal failure can also lead to ototoxicity. Ototoxicity has also been reported with macrolides (Erythromycin, Azithromycin) and orgatnic solvents (e.g. toluene, ethyl benzene, etc).

As potentiation and **synergism** of ototoxic effects occur, co administration of these ototoxic agents is not recommended.

Clinical Features

Cochlear Symptoms

Cochlear toxicity is typically associated with **bilateral high-frequency sensorineural hearing loss and tinnitus**. The hearing loss usually begins in the high frequencies usually more than 4000 Hz. This is due to the involvement of outer hair cells in the organ of Corti, predominantly at the basal turn of the cochlea.

Early hearing loss may go unrecognized by the patient as the patient initially has high frequency **(>4000 Hz)** hearing loss. With progression, lower speech frequencies are affected and the patient may become profoundly deaf if the drug is continued.

Reversible/Temporary hearing loss	Irreversible/Permanent hearing loss
Aspirin	Aminoglycosides
Antimalarials	Cisplatin
Diuretics	

Vestibular Symptoms

Vestibular toxicity occurs due to damage to type 1 (more rapidly and severely) and type 2 hair cells and manifests as vertigo and nystagmus. Clinically, nystagmus may be present as an early sign.

Investigation

Baseline testing of hearing should be done. Monitoring should continue during therapy at regular intervals.

The outer hair cells are more prone to damage by ototoxicity. Since the **OAE** are produced by outer hair cells, the absence of OAE can be an early indication of ototoxicity. OAE is done along the bed side. Subsequently **high frequency audiometry** can confirm and also tell the degree of hearing loss.

Management

i. Prevention by withdrawing the drug, if possible, once toxicity is documented
ii. Hearing aids and cochlear implantation
iii. Vestibular rehabilitation

PERILYMPH FISTULA

The bony labyrinth contains the fluid known as perilymph. Perilymphatic or labyrinthine fistula is a condition in which an abnormal communication is present between the perilymphatic space of the inner ear and the middle ear.

Causes of perilymphatic fistula:

1. **Conditions causing Oval Window fistula** are the following:
   a. Stapedectomy surgery (for Otosclerosis)
   b. Rupture following Acoustic trauma
2. **Lateral semicircular canal fistula:**
   a. Fenestration operation: It is a surgical procedure previously done for otosclerosis where a fenestra is made in the lateral semicircular canal
3. **Conditions causing Round window fistula** are the following:
   a. Forced Valsalva manoeuvre or suppressed sneezing.
   b. The Hyrtl's fissure (this is the tympanomeningeal hiatus present at 16–18 week stage during foetal life. It connects round window to the posterior cranial fossa. It fuses and disappears by 26 weeks).

Common causes of fistula formation at the above three sites:
a. Erosion following Cholesteatoma
b. Rupture following barotrauma (e.g. SCUBA diving) or head injury

Clinical Features

In perilymph fistula whenever there occurs pressure changes, e.g. on valsalva, straining, weight lifting, etc. the perilymph leaks from the perilymphatic spaces of the bony labyrinth into the middle ear space. The loss of perilymph alters the balance between perilymph and endolymph within the membranous labyrinth. As a result the patient presents with **sudden persistent or fluctuating sensorineural hearing loss, tinnitus, vertigo, nystagmus, light headedness and disequilibrium. In contrast to Meniere's the vertigo here, is precipitated by pressure changes and is transient. There will also be a history of surgery, trauma, unsafe CSOM, etc. on examination. The fistula test is positive here,** *see* Chapter 3.

Treatment

Medical management includes bed rest, propped up position, use of stool softeners and avoidance of Valsalva manoeuvre, heavy lifting and straining.

The definitive treatment of perilymphatic fistula (PLF) is surgical exploration with grafting of the fistula.

SUPERIOR SEMICIRCULAR CANAL DEHISCENCE (SSCD)

The bulge of superior semicircular canal is present on the anterior slant of petrous part of temporal bone in the base of skull. This bulge of Superior semicircular canal on the floor of middle cranial fossa is known as arcuate eminence.

Superior semicircular canal dehiscence is a rare condition where the bone between the Superior semicircular canal and the middle cranial fossa is missing or thin, *see* Fig. 12.6.

This can be either congenital or acquired (following trauma).

Ear

Section I

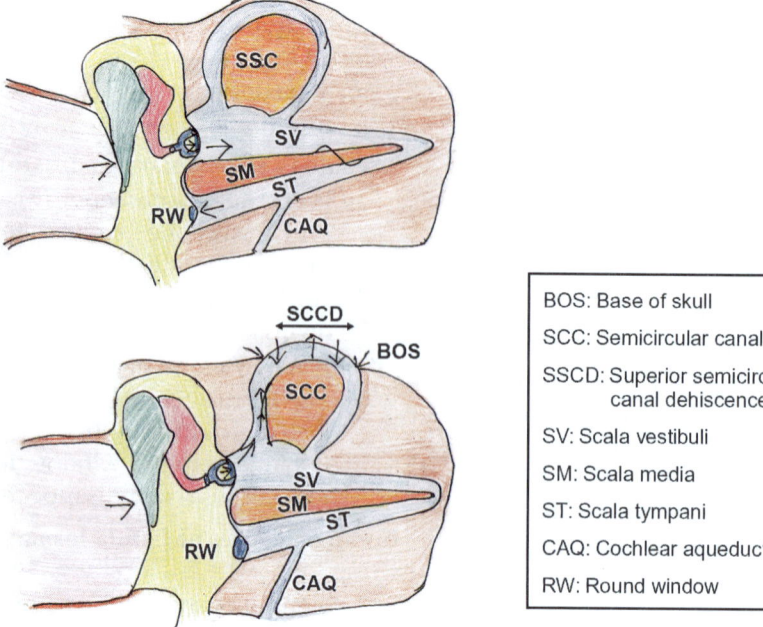

Fig. 12.6: Dissipation of sound energy and inner ear becoming susceptible to external and intracranial pressure changes in Superior Semicircular Canal Dehiscence

This leads to the formation of a **3rd mobile window** in the inner ear facing the middle cranial fossa (the other two being the round and oval window). The other conditions which can lead to 3rd window are dilated internal acoustic meatus and enlarged vestibular aqueduct (bony labyrinth surrounding the endolymphatic duct).

Clinical Features

This dehiscence leads to exposure of inner ear to changes in external pressure and intracranial pressure causing symptoms very similar to that of a round or oval window fistula.

Vestibular Symptoms

Under normal circumstances, pressure enters the inner ear through the stapes footplate in the oval window, passes through the cochlea and then exits through the round window. The presence of a dehiscence in the superior canal allows this canal to respond to sound and pressure stimuli.

Any loud noise (see **Tullio phenomenon** in Meniere's above), pressure on external auditory canal by tragal compression (see **Hennebert's sign** in the chapter on vestibular function), or raised pressure of middle ear like nose blowing, Valsalva or changes in intracranial pressure like jugular vein compression can stimulate the labyrinth leading to vertigo. This vertigo is accompanied by peripheral nystagmus.

Cochlear Symptoms

The 3rd mobile window leads to the acoustic energy getting dissipated leading to **conductive hearing loss** (**note**—otherwise in any condition of the inner ear the hearing loss is sensorineural, but here in SSCD it is Conductive).

The **stapedial reflex** is preserved here which helps in differentiating this conductive hearing loss in superior semicircular canal dehiscence from middle ear ossicular pathology where along with conductive hearing loss, the stapedial reflex is also absent. The BC threshold is decreased leading to increased sensitivity to bone conducted sounds and patients report hearing bone conduction sounds very loudly (ex. hearing their eye movements, footsteps or their pulse). There can also be autophonia (increased loudness of patient's own voice).

Diagnosis

Diagnosis is by HRCT.

Treatment

 i. Avoidance of provoking stimuli.
 ii. Surgical repair of the dehiscence.

SUDDEN SENSORINEURAL HEARING LOSS (SSNHL)

Sensorineural hearing loss of **greater than 30 dB over 3 contiguous** pure-tone frequencies occurring within **3 days period** is known as sudden sensorineural hearing loss. It is frightening to loose 30 dB hearing in three days and hence it is an otologic emergency. The prompt diagnosis is essential for starting prompt treatment as the prognosis is good only if the treatment is started immediately.

Causes

a. **Idiopathic:** Largely the aetiology of SSNHL remains idiopathic. However of the possible causes, clinical data and studies support viral origin. The various **viruses** implicated here are **Mumps (most common), Measles, Rubella, Varicella, Influenza, Herpes simplex type 1 and 2 and Cytomegalovirus** (easy to remember most of these are the viruses against which vaccines are available and additionally HSV and CMV).

The postulated pathophysiologies for idiopathic sudden sensory hearing loss are the following:

   i. Immune-mediated inner ear disease.

   ii. Labyrinthine vascular compromise.

b. **Trauma:** Temporal bone fracture, Acoustic trauma and Barotraumas leading to Intracochlear membrane ruptures and perilymph leak.

c. **Tumour:** Vestibular schwannoma (though most commonly it presents as slowly progressive SN hearing loss), *see* Chapter 14.

d. **Toxins:** Aminoglycosides, cisplatin, at times can present with SSNHL.

Management

The patient should be investigated for the probable causes.

1. *Corticosteroids:* Oral steroids should be started immediately. This along with intratympanic injection of dexamethasone is shown to effectively improve hearing in patients with severe or profound SSNHL.

2. *Antiviral agents:* Acyclovir and Amantadine presuming a viral aetiology.

3. Vasodilators

4. Hyperbaric oxygen

5. Carbogen (95% oxygen + 5% CO_2)

Tinnitus

Tinnitus is a ringing, roaring, hissing or clicking sound for more than 5 minutes perceived by the patient in the absence of any external stimuli.

It can be:

- Subjective; only the patient perceives it
- Objective; even the examiner can hear it unaided or using a stethoscope

Tinnitus in itself is not a disease but a symptom of many diseases. Any disease that leads to conductive or SN hearing loss can lead to tinnitus.

Pathophysiology

- *Pathological afferent excitation of the cochlear activity:* Since glutamate and calcium are the main excitatory neurotransmitter, over excitation leading to their overload can be toxic to nerves and can lead to tinnitus.

- *Decrease inhibition of cochlear activity:* Since GABA is the main inhibitory neurotransmitter, decreased inhibition can also lead to tinnitus.

Causes

Subjective	Objective
• CHL: Wax, TM perforation, AOM, SOM, COM, Otosclerosis, etc. • SNHL: NIHL, Meniere's, Acoustic neuroma, presbycusis, ototoxicity, SSNHL, etc. • Neurological disorders: Head injuries, # temporal bone, Multiple sclerosis, CNS tumours • Cardiovascular disorders (HTN, anemia) • Metabolic and endocrine disorders	• Vascular lesions: Glomus, carotid artery aneurysm, AV fistula (here the tinnitus is synchronous with pulse, hence called pulsatile tinnitus) • Palatal myoclonus • TM joint disorders

Management

- Treatment of underlying cause.
- *Tinnitus maskers:* These are wearable devices.
- *Tinnitus retraining therapy:* It is done by low level sound generators which provide constant low level sound which competes with the tinnitus sound and gradually lead to habituation.
- *Pharmacological:* Glutamate antagonists (Caroverine), calcium antagonists (flunarizine, nimodipine), GABA analogues (pregabalin, gabapentin, benzodiazepines, antidepressants, etc.).

"Points to Ponder/Points for Quick revision"

- Meniere's is characterised by an initial loss of low frequency (SN) U/L hearing loss (up sloping audiogram, easy to remember U/L—Up sloping) whereas Presbycusis, Ototoxicity, NIHL are characterised by an initial loss of (SN) B/L high frequency hearing loss (Down sloping audiogram. **Mnemonic:** POND).
- SSCD is characterised by Conductive hearing loss.
- As suggested by their names there is no hearing impairment in BPPV and vestibular neuronitis, they are characterised by vertigo only.
- Meniere's, perilymph fistula and SSCD are all characterised by both deafness and vertigo, but in the later two conditions, vertigo occurs due to external or intra-cranial pressure changes only.
- **Meniere's disease (endolymphatic hydrops):**
  - Dilatation of membranous labyrinth—Idiopathic (MC)/2°/ genetic (Ch 6); U/L, M:F-1:1.
  - Pathogenesis: ↑ endolymph → Scala media dilatation → bulging and rupture of Reissner's membrane → mixing of endo and perilymph → depolarisation block of vestibular and cochlear N.
  - CFs: Triad → 1. Attacks of vertigo (20 min–24 hrs, preceding ear fullness and accompanying vagal symptoms) 2. Fluctuating SNHL (low freq. Bin aural diplacusis) 3. Tinnitus.

- Reverse Meniere's/Lermoyez syndrome: deafness before vertigo—Drop crisis/Tumarkin's crisis—falling while walking; Tullio phenomenon—sound induced vertigo.
- Audiological tests: s/o cochlear pathology—Stapedial reflex threshold and caloric test—↓; ECog—most sensitive–SP/AP > 30%, Glycerol improves ECog—diagnostic.
- T/t: 1st medical—salt, tea/coffee restriction, smoking cessation, diuretics, labyrinthine sedatives, vasodilators (betahistine, etc.). If no response–surgical endolymphatic sac decompression, shunt operation, chemical labyrinthectomy (gentamicin), total labyrinthectomy (once complete SN loss).

- **BPPV:**
  - MC vertigo in clinical practice. Episodic vertigo lasting for seconds, in certain head positions (as per its name).
  - Free floating debris (detached otoconia) from the utricular maculareach the posterior semicircular canal (MC).
  - Diagnosis—'DIX-HALLPIKE test'—a positional test—vertical upbeating geotropical tortional nystagmus.
  - T/t: "Epley's manoeuvre" or canalith repositioning manoeuvre.
- **Vestibular neuronitis:** Viral involvement of the vestibular N.
- **NIHL:** Various sound intensities at 1 metre (*see* Table)—Safe limit of noise–85 dB, 8 hrs, 5 days per week; Auditory fatigue–temporary (< 24 hrs); Acoustic reflex delay–100–200 ms; Initially high frequency hearing loss; Acoustic dip (4000 Hz).
- **Presbycusis:** Age related (>50), slowly progressive, B/L symmetric SNHL—Neural type (MC); Non–curable/preventable.
- **Ototoxicity:** Drugs causing Reversible/irreversible—hearing loss (↑ frequency)/vestibulotoxicity (*see* Table)—Aminoglycosides (most notorious)–cochleotoxic–KAN; vestibulotoxic–NSG-T.
- **SSNHL:** Otological emergency → >30 dB, 3 consecutive frequencies, within 3 days, Rinne's–false –ve, Webers → better ear, Viral aetiology, steroids–mainstay t/t.
- **Tinnitus:** > 5 min, subjective/objective (*see* Table), ↑ glutamate (caroverine), ↑ Ca (flunarizine) ↓ GABA (gabapentin).

PREVIOUSLY ASKED QUESTIONS

1. **Meniere's disease is:** *(Exam 2014)*
   a. Perilymphatic hydrops
   b. Endolymphatic hydrops
   c. Otospongiosis
   d. Coalescent mastoiditis

2. **Endolymphatic Hydrops is seen in:** *(Exam 2013)*
   a. Meniere's disease
   b. Otosclerosis
   c. Acoustic neuroma
   d. Cholesteatoma

3. **Chromosome responsible for hereditary Meniere's disease is:** *(Exam 2012)*
   a. 6
   b. 9
   c. 11
   d. 14

4. **Meniere's disease is characterised by:** *(AI 2004, Exam 2017)*
   a. Vertigo, otalgia and tinnitus
   b. Vertigo, ear discharge and tinnitus
   c. Vertigo, headache and tinnitus
   d. Vertigo, hearing loss and tinnitus

5. **Meniere's disease is manifested by all of the symptoms except:** *(Delhi 96, Exam 2013)*
   a. Tinnitus
   b. Deafness
   c. Vertigo
   d. Otorrhoea

6. **Common presenting manifestations of Meniere's disease are all except:** *(AI 97, Exam 2014)*
   a. Tinnitus
   b. Vertigo
   c. Sensorineural deafness
   d. Loss of consciousness

7. **Meniere's disease is characterised by all except:** *(AIIMS Dec 98, Exam 2015)*
   a. Diplopia
   b. Tinnitus
   c. Vertigo
   d. Fullness of pressure in ear

8. **Which of the following is not a typical feature of Meniere's disease:** *(AIIMS May 2006, Exam 2013)*
   a. Sensorineural deafness
   b. Pulsatile tinnitus
   c. Vertigo
   d. Fluctuating deafness

9. **Fluctuating deafness is seen in:** *(Exam 2013)*
   a. Otosclerosis
   b. Meniere's disease
   c. Acute otitis media
   d. Benign paroxysmal positional vertigo

10. **True about Meniere's disease:** *(PGI June 2003, Exam 2014)*
    a. Tinnitus
    b. Episodic vertigo
    c. Deafness
    d. Diarrhoea
    e. Vomiting

11. **Meniere's disease is characterised by:** *(PGI Dec 2003, Exam 2015)*
    a. Fluctuating hearing loss
    b. Endolymphatic hydrops
    c. Otospongiosis
    d. Coalescent mastoiditis
    e. Paracusis

12. **In a classical case of Meniere's disease which one of the following statements is true:** *(Karnataka 2001, Exam 2017)*
    a. Carhart's notch is a characteristic feature in pure tone audiogram
    b. Schwartze's sign is usually present in the tympanic membrane
    c. Low frequency sensorineural deafness is often seen in pure tone audiogram
    d. Decompression of fallopian canal is the treatment of choice

13. **Recruitment phenomenon is seen in:** *(Exam 2007/Kolkata 2002, Exam 2017)*
    a. Otosclerosis
    b. Meniere's disease
    c. Acoustic nerve schwannoma
    d. Otitis media with effusion

14. **True about Endolymphatic hydrops:** *(PGI June 2006, Exam 2014)*
    a. B/L condition mostly
    b. Females more common
    c. Tullios phenomenon seen
    d. Conductive deafness

15. **Vasodilators in Meniere's disease are useful because they:** *(Kerala 94, Exam 2010)*
    a. Dilate lymphatic vessels
    b. Decrease endolymph secretion
    c. Increase endolymph reabsorption
    d. Are of no use

16. **Vasodilator of internal ear is:** *(AIIMS 2005, Exam 2017)*
    a. Nicotinic acid
    b. Caffeine
    c. Theophylline
    d. Nicotine

17. **Micro Wick and Microcatheter devices are used in:** *(AIIMS 2012)*
    a. Drooling of saliva
    b. Frey's syndrome
    c. Control of epistaxis
    d. Delivering drug to the round membrane

18. **Endolymphatic decompression is done in:** *(Delhi 2006, Exam 2013)*
    a. Tinnitus
    b. Acoustic neuroma
    c. Meniere's disease
    d. Perilymph fistula

Ear

Section I

19. **All are differential diagnosis of Meniere's disease except:** (*UP 2007, Exam 2017*)
    a. Acoustic neuroma   b. CNS disease
    c. Labyrinthitis   d. Suppurative otitis media

20. **Glycerol test is done in:**
    (*AP 95, TN 2000, Exam 2017*)
    a. Otosclerosis
    b. Lateral sinus thrombosis
    c. Meniere's disease
    d. None of the above

21. **Destructive procedures for Meniere's disease are:** (*PGI Nov 2009*)
    a. Fick's procedure
    b. Cody tack procedure
    c. Vestibular neurectomy
    d. Endolymphatic sac decompression
    e. Labyrinthectomy

22. **Third window effect is seen in which of these:** (*AIIMS Nov 2012*)
    a. Perforated tympanum
    b. Dehiscent superior semicircular canal
    c. Round window
    d. Oval window

23. **Features of superior semicircular canal dehiscence are:** (*PGI 2010*)
    a. Positive Romberg's sign
    b. Positive Tullio phenomenon
    c. Positive Hennebert's sign
    d. Oscillopsia
    e. Positive Dix-Hallpike manoeuvre

24. **Positional vertigo is due to stimulation of:** (*UP 2001, Exam 2017*)
    a. Lateral semicircular canal
    b. Superior semicircular canal
    c. Inferior semicircular canal
    d. Posterior semicircular canal

25. **What is the treatment for Benign positional vertigo:** (*APPG 2006, Exam 2017*)
    a. Vestibular exercises
    b. Vestibular sedatives
    c. Antihistamines
    d. Canalith repositioning procedure

26. **Latest treatment in BPPV is:**
    (*Kerala 2003, Exam 2017*)
    a. Intralabyrinthine streptomycin
    b. Intralabyrinthine steroids
    c. Valsalva manoeuvre
    d. Epley's manoeuvre

27. **Epley's manoeuvre:** (*Exam 2013*)
    a. Positional vertigo   b. Otosclerosis
    c. ASOM   d. CSOM

28. **Vertigo, tinnitus and normal hearing is characteristic feature of:** (*Bihar 2004, Exam 2017*)
    a. Acoustic neuroma   b. Meniere's disease
    c. Vestibular neuritis   d. All of the above

29. **All are false regarding vestibular neuronitis except:** (*AI 2006, Exam 2017*)
    a. Caloric test shows diminished response
    b. Neurologic deficit
    c. SN deafness
    d. Conductive deafness

30. **At which level sound is painful:**
    (*Jharkhand 2004, Exam 2017*)
    a. 90–100 dB   b. 120–130 dB
    c. 60–70 dB   d. 20–30 dB

31. **Maximum audible tolerance recommended by WHO is:** (*DPG 2007, Exam 2016*)
    a. 90 dB for 6 hours   b. 85 dB for 8 hours
    c. 85 dB for 6 hours   d. 85 dB for 4 hours

32. **Dip at 4000 Hz is seen in:** (*Exam 2013*)
    a. Otosclerosis   b. Noise trauma
    c. Meniere's   d. Presbycusis

33. **Post-traumatic vertigo is due to:**
    (*PGI 2003/2006/2012*)
    a. Perilymphatic fistula
    b. Vestibular neuronitis
    c. Secondary endolymphatic hydrops
    d. Ossicular discontinuity
    e. Benign paroxysmal positional vertigo

34. **Fluctuating recurring variable sensorineural deafness is seen in:** (*AP 2006, Exam 2017*)
    a. Serous otitis media
    b. Hemotympanum
    c. Perilymphatic fistula
    d. Cholesteatoma

35. **All are ototoxic drugs except:**
    (*RJ 2000, Exam 2017*)
    a. Streptomycin   b. Quinine
    c. Diuretics   d. Propranolol

36. **A patient on ATT develops tinnitus and hearing loss due to:** (*AP 2004, Exam 2017*)
    a. Isoniazid   b. Pyrazinamide
    c. Streptomycin   d. Rifampicin

37. **Ototoxic drugs generally affect the hearing of what frequencies of sound:** (*Exam 2013*)
    a. 250–500 Hz   b. 2000–3000 Hz
    c. 500–1000 Hz   d. 4000–5000 Hz

38. **Ototoxic drugs generally affect the hearing of frequencies more than 4000 Hz. All are ototoxic drugs except:** (*Exam 2012*)
    a. Streptomycin   b. Vancomycin
    c. Furosemide   d. Atropine

39. A case of kidney disease was given repeatedly high doses of frusemide. After 1 week patient started complaining of decreased hearing. Most likely cause of this is damage to: (*AI 2005, Exam 2017*)
    a. Type 1 hair cell
    b. Inner hair cell
    c. Cochlear nerve
    d. Stria vascularis

40. Drugs causing deafness true statements are:
    (*PGI 2006/2013*)
    a. Streptomycin is predominantly vestibulotoxic
    b. Frusemide causes irreversible deafness
    c. Salicylates cause reversible deafness
    d. Kanamycin is mainly vestibulotoxic
    e. Cisplatin causes irreversible deafness

41. A 65-year-old person with B/L SN hearing loss with proportionate speech discrimination is suffering from: (*JIPMER 2005, Exam 2017*)
    a. Noise induced hearing loss
    b. Presbycusis
    c. Ototoxic drug
    d. Acoustic neuroma

42. Virus causing acute onset sensorineural deafness:
    (*PGI Dec 2004/2010*)
    a. Varicella   b. Measles
    c. Mumps   d. Adenovirus
    e. Rota virus

43. Sensorineural deafness is seen in:
    (*PGI June 2002/2011*)
    a. Alport syndrome
    b. Pendred syndrome
    c. Treacher-Collins syndrome
    d. Crouzon disease
    e. Michel aplasia

44. Presbycusis false is: (*Exam 2014*)
    a. Presents as unilateral SNHL mostly
    b. Destruction of small inner hair cells
    c. High frequencies affected first
    d. Corrected well by hearing aid

45. True about Meniere's disease: (*PGI 2014*)
    a. Age of patient 20–40 typically
    b. Presents as hyperacusis, vertigo and tinnitus
    c. Managed with low salt diet and thiazide diuretic
    d. Drop attacks seen
    e. Conductive hearing loss seen

46. Initial mechanism of action of intratympanic Gentamicin micro Wick catheter in treatment of Meniere's disease: (*Exam 2014*)
    a. Direct damage to outer hair cells
    b. Acts on mechanoreceptors of outer hair cells
    c. Bind to Mg channels on stria vascularis
    d. Inactivates Na, K-ATPase channels of type I and type II hair cells

47. Temporary and permanent threshold shift are characteristically seen in: (*Exam 2014*)
    a. Ototoxicity
    b. NIHL
    c. Presbycusis
    d. SSNHL

48. True about Meniere's disease, except: (*Exam 2014*)
    a. Surgery is the mainstay of treatment
    b. Fistula test is negative
    c. Gentamicin can be given in inner ear
    d. Vertigo is the 1st symptom

49. Which is the most common type of presbycusis?
    (*Exam 2013*)
    a. Sensory   b. Neural
    c. Metabolic   d. Mechanical

50. Which one of the following is NOT a feature of Meniere's disease? (*Exam 2016*)
    a. Improvement in hearing with oral glycerol
    b. Fluctuating sensorineural hearing loss
    c. Pulsatile tinnitus
    d. Intolerance to loud sounds due to recruitment phenomenon

51. Ototoxic drugs are all except: (*Exam 2016*)
    a. Kanamycin   b. Gentamicin
    c. Streptomycin   d. Amoxycillin

52. All are treatment of Meniere's disease except:
    (*Exam 2015*)
    a. Surgery is mainstay
    b. Histamine derivative is used
    c. Chemical labyrinthectomy can be done
    d. Prochlorperazine given

53. Selective low frequency sensorineural Hearing loss occurs in: (*Exam 2016*)
    a. Meniere's disease   b. BPPV
    c. Glomus tumour   d. Schwannoma

54. Chemical labyrinthectomy by trans-tympanic route is done in Meniere's disease using which drug:
    (*Exam 2016*)
    a. Amikacin   b. Gentamicin
    c. Amoxicillin   d. Cyclosporine

55. Hearing loss in Meniere's disease is of what type:
    (*Exam 2016*)
    a. Fluctuating SNHL
    b. Progressive retrocochlear
    c. Conductive hearing loss
    d. Mixed Hearing loss

56. A person hearing two different tones in left and right ears when presented with a single tone. This condition is called. (*Exam 2016*)
    a. Diplacusis   b. Paracusis
    c. Presbycusis   d. Hyperacusis

Section I   Ear

57. Hearing loss is not caused by: (*AIIMS 2015*)
    a. Kanamycin b. Vancomycin
    c. Metronidazole d. Quinine

58. A 31-year-old female came to ENT OPD with 6 months H/O ringing in her ear, a feeling of spinning and hearing loss in left ear. Spinning sensation is episodic and lasts for 60 minutes. During these episodes, she has nausea and vomiting. She denies fever, chills, cough, and ear or throat pain. She has H/o hypothyroidism and fibromyalgia and currently on medications—thyroxine and ibuprofen. Her father died of MI at the age of 54. On examination her BP: 128/70; Pulse 60/min; respiration 16/min., left-sided SN hearing loss. Most likely diagnosis is: (*Exam 2015*)
    a. Meniere's disease b. Acoustic neuroma
    c. Migraine d. Multiple sclerosis

IMAGE BASED PRACTICE QUESTIONS BY THE AUTHOR

59. The following audiogram is suggestive of:

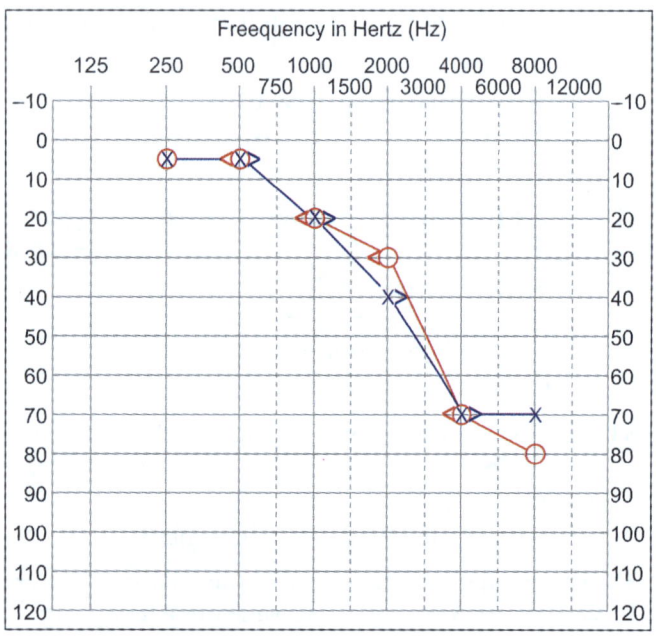

    a. Meniere's b. Otosclerosis
    c. Ototoxicity d. Serous otitis media

60. Which of the following is the most common cause of sensorineural hearing loss in adults? (*Exam 2015*)
    a. Meniere's disease
    b. Presbycusis
    c. Cerebellopontine angle tumour
    d. Trauma

61. True about benign paroxysmal positional vertigo: (*Exam 2013*)
    a. Hearing loss is often present
    b. Hallpike manoeuvre is not helpful in diagnosis
    c. Chemical labyrinthectomy is done for treatment
    d. Disorder of posterior semicircular canal

62. The following audiogram is suggestive of:

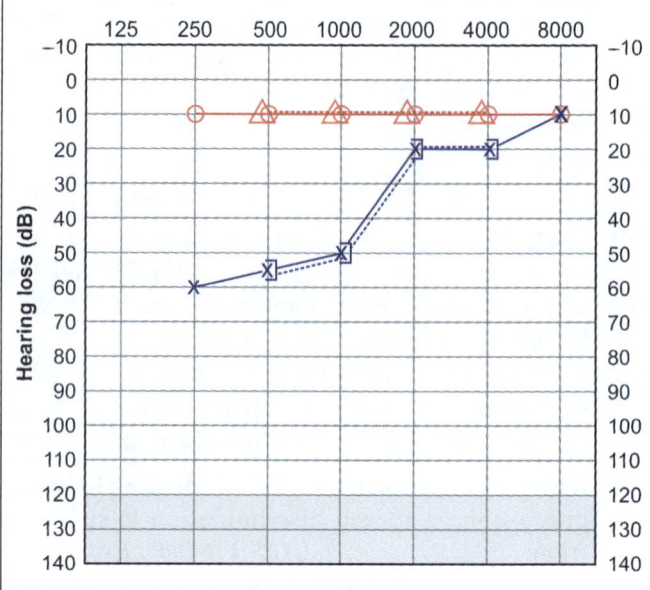

    a. Meniere
    b. Otosclerosis
    c. Ototoxicity
    d. Noise induced hearing loss

63. A 60-year-old male presents with episodes of severe vertigo which lasts for 4 hours, associated with vomiting. O/E he is having right horizontal nystagmus and mild right-sided SN hearing loss during the episode. Diagnosis: (*JIPMER 2015*)
    a. Vertibro-basilar ischemic attacks
    b. Labyrinthitis
    c. Meniere's disease
    d. Benign paroxysmal vertigo

64. The following is the audiogram of a patient presenting with tinnitus. It is suggestive of:

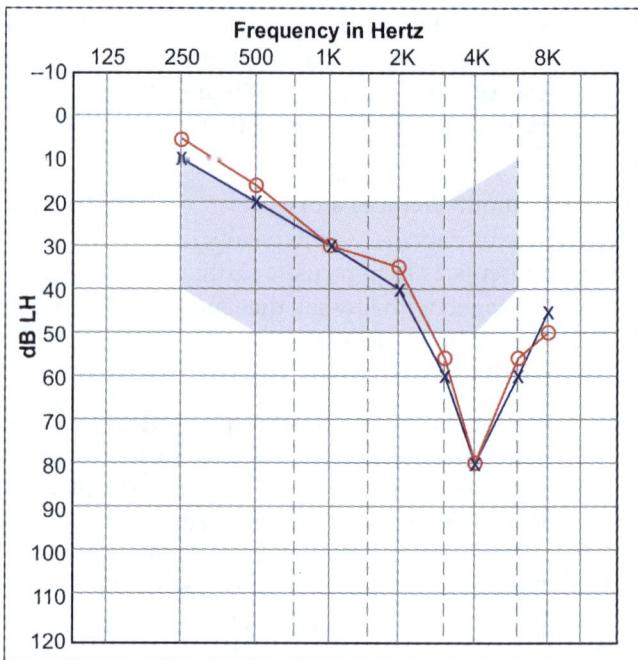

a. Otosclerosis

b. Noise trauma

c. Meniere's disease

d. Presbycusis

65. All the following are features of Meniere's disease except: *(Exam 2016)*

a. No otoscopic abnormality

b. SISI more than 70%

c. Recruitment negative

d. Electrocochleography is diagnostic

66. True about idiopathic sudden sensorineural hearing loss: *(PGI 2009)*

a. Vertigo always present

b. Carbogen (5% carbon dioxide + 95% oxygen) is beneficial

c. Hearing loss occurs within 24 hours

d. Hearing loss occurs within 72 hour

67. MC cause of congenital SNHL: *(Exam 2017)*

a. Parvo virus

b. CMV

c. Rubella

d. Toxoplasmosis

68. For maximum symptomatic relief of intractable vertigo in a patient of Meniere's with complete SN hearing loss, which of the following should be done: *(Exam 2018)*

a. Labyrinthectomy

b. Endolymphatic sac decompression

c. Vestibular neurectomy

d. Sacculotomy

69. A 30-year-male after a fall started experiencing dizziness on loud noise and on blowing the nose. Patient could hear his own footsteps in the ear. Diagnosis: *(Exam 2017)*

a. Superior semi-circular canal dehiscence

b. Meniere's

c. BPPV

d. Vestibular neuronitis

70. All of the following statements about sudden severe sensorineural hearing loss are true except: *(Exam 2018)*

a. Steroids are the mainstay of t/t

b. It is confused with conductive hearing loss

c. It is a medical emergency

d. Rinnes is falsely positive

ANSWERS AND EXPLANATIONS

1. **(b) Endolymphatic hydrops** (*Ref. Cummings, 6th ed., 2331*)
   - Meniere's is also known as endolymphatic hydrops.
   - There is no condition called Perilymphatic hydrops.
   - Otospongiosis also known as otosclerosis is fixation of foot plate of stapes.
   - Coalescent mastoiditis is infection of the mastoid air cells and is a complication following ASOM/ unsafe CSOM.

2. **(a) Meniere's disease** (*Ref. Cummings, 6th ed., 2331*)

3. **(a) 6** (refer to text) (*Ref. Cummings, 6th ed., 2554*)
   - In this regard it is worth mentioning that some authors relate Meniere's disease to the COCH gene ("cochlin" gene) located on chromosome no. 14 q. But studies have proven that the Mutations in the COCH gene are a frequent cause of autosomal dominant progressive cochleovestibular dysfunction, but not of Meniere's disease.

4. **(d) Vertigo, hearing loss and tinnitus** (*Ref. Cummings, 6th ed., 2331*)
   - The presenting triad of Meniere is vertigo followed by deafness (SN) and tinnitus.

5. **(d) Otorrhoea** (*Ref. Scott Brown, 8th ed., Vol 2, 819*)
   - Meniere is manifested as vertigo followed by deafness (SN), tinnitus and a sensation of fullness in the ear but no discharge.

6. **(d) Loss of consciousness** (*Ref. Scott Brown, 8th ed., Vol 2, 819*)
   - The patient is fully conscious and oriented during an attack of Meniere.
   - Meniere being a disturbance of peripheral vestibular system is therefore not characterised by any focal (such as diplopia, dysarthria, paresthesia, etc.) or generalised neurological symptoms like loss of consciousness, seizures, etc.
   - The neurological symptoms accompany a central vestibular disturbance.
   - However, vertigo of Meniere may be associated with vagal symptoms i.e. diaphoresis, pallor, nausea, vomiting, abdominal cramps, diarrhoea and bradycardia.

7. **(a) Diplopia** (*see* the explanation above) (*Ref. Cummings, 6th ed., 2331*)

8. **(b) Pulsatile tinnitus** (*Ref. Cummings, 6th ed., 2331*)
   - The tinnitus in Meniere is subjective (i.e. only the patient can hear).
   - Pulsatile tinnitus is an objective tinnitus (i.e. the examiner also can hear the tinnitus). Pulsatile tinnitus is seen in vascular conditions like Glomus jugulare and aneurysm of internal carotid artery.

9. **(b) Meniere's disease** (*Ref. Cummings, 6th ed., 2331*)
   - In otosclerosis there occurs progressive deafness. AOM shows temporary deafness. There is no deafness in BPPV.

10. **(All)** (*Ref. Cummings, 6th ed., 2556*)
    - Diarrhoea and vomiting along with diaphoresis, pallor, nausea, abdominal cramps, and bradycardia may occur as vagal manifestations associated with vertigo in Meniere.

11. **(a) and (b),** (*Ref. Cummings, 6th ed., 2556*) Refer the text

12. **(c) Low frequency sensorineural deafness is often seen in pure tone audiogram** (*Ref. Cummings, 6th ed., 2331*)
    - Meniere is characterised by endolymphatic hydrops. This dilatation of the membranous labyrinth starts from the apex of membranous cochlea going down, so low frequency sensorineural deafness is seen in pure tone audiogram in the early stages.
    - Carhart's notch, which is a dip at 2000 Hz in BC, is a characteristic feature in pure tone audiogram in otosclerosis.
    - Schwartze's sign or flamingo pink appearance of the tympanic membrane is seen in active otosclerosis.
    - Decompression of fallopian canal is the treatment of choice in facial nerve palsy, *see* chapter on facial nerve palsy. Endolymphatic sac decompression is done in Meniere when the medical management fails.

13. **(b) Meniere's disease** (*Ref. Cummings, 6th ed., 2556*)
    - Recruitment phenomenon, i.e. abnormal growth of loudness on increasing the level of loudness (refer to audiology chapter) is seen in cochlear pathologies like Meniere.
    - Otosclerosis and Otitis media with effusion are middle ear pathologies.
    - Acoustic nerve schwannoma is retro cochlear.

14. **(c) Tullios phenomenon seen** (*Ref. Scott Brown, 8th ed., Vol 2, 819*)

15. **(c) Increase endolymph reabsorption** (*Ref. Cummings, 6th ed., 2558*)

16. **(a) Nicotinic acid** (*Ref. Cummings, 6th ed., 2558*)

17. **(d) Delivering drug to the round membrane** (*Ref. Cummings, 6th ed., 2558*)

18. **(c) Meniere's disease** (*Ref. Cummings, 6th ed., 2559*)
    - Meniere's disease being characterised by endolymphatic hydrops so here endolymphatic sac decompression is done when the medical management fails.
    - Tinnitus is treated as per the underlying cause.
    - Treatment modality of Acoustic neuroma is surgical excision.
    - Perilymph fistula is repaired by grafting the fistula.

19. **(d) Suppurative otitis media** (*Ref. Scott Brown, 8th ed., Vol 2, 833*)
    - The presenting symptom of Meniere is vertigo. So therefore CNS disease, labyrinthitis and Acoustic neuroma are among the differentials.
    - Suppurative otitis media is clearly characterised by ear discharge and perforation of tympanic membrane.

20. **(c) Meniere's disease** (*Ref. Cummings, 6th ed., 2557*)

21. **(c), (e) Vestibular neurectomy, Labyrinthectomy** (*Ref. Cummings, 6th ed., 2559*)

- Fick's procedure and Cody tack procedure were procedures for decreasing the endolymph pressure by doing a sacculotomy (puncturing the saccule through the stapes footplate. They are no longer performed now.
- Endolymphatic sac decompression is not an organ destructive surgery.

22. **(b) Dehiscent superior semicircular canal** (*Ref. Cummings, 6th ed., 2560*)

23. **(b), (c), (d) Positive Tullio phenomenon, Positive Hennebert's sign, Oscillopsia** (*Ref. Scott Brown, 8th ed., Vol 2, 845*)

- Romberg's sign is positive when the patient is able to stand with his feet together while his eyes are open, but sways or falls when they are closed; it is one of the earliest signs of posterior column disease.
- Oscillopsia: patients with nystagmus may notice a constant movement of the objects within the visual field. This subjective manifestation is known as oscillopsia.
- Positive Dix-Hallpike manoeuvre is indicative of BPPV.

24. **(d) Posterior semicircular canal** (*Ref. Scott Brown, 8th ed., Vol 2, 832*)

- Benign paroxysmal positional vertigo (BPPV) is a condition in which there is dislodged otoconia/debris in the posterior semicircular canal. Movement of these particles in certain head positions stimulates the posterior semicircular canal and leads to vertigo.

25. **(d) Canalith repositioning procedure** (*Ref. Scott Brown, 8th ed., Vol 2, 834*)

- Canalith repositioning procedure or the Epley's manoeuvre is the treatment for Benign Paroxysmal Positional Vertigo (BPPV).
- When the vestibular organs are permanently damaged with disease or injury, the brain can no longer rely on them for accurate information about equilibrium and motion. Vestibular exercises promote CNS compensation for these fixed deficits.
- In Benign positional vertigo vestibular exercises are not required, as the cause of BPPV gets treated by Canalith repositioning procedure or the Epley's manoeuvre.
- Vestibular sedatives and antihistamines may be used to control the severe symptoms, though they are not of much benefit and repositioning or Epley's manoeuvre is the treatment of choice in BPPV.

26. **(d) Epley's manoeuvre** (*Ref. Scott Brown, 8th ed., Vol 2, 834*)

27. **(a) Positional vertigo** (*Ref. Scott Brown, 8th ed., Vol 2, 834*)

28. **(c) Vestibular neuritis** (*Ref. Scott Brown, 8th ed., Vol 2, 850*)

- Vestibular neuritis is a viral infection involving the vestibular nerve. The cochlear part is not involved so the hearing remains normal.
- In both Acoustic neuroma and Meniere's disease hearing is affected.

29. **(a) Caloric test shows diminished response** (*Ref. Cummings, 6th ed., 2553*)

30. **(b) 120–130 dB** 1) (*Ref. Dhingra, 6th ed., 19*)

31. **(b) 85 dB for 8 hours** (*Ref. Cummings, 6th ed., 2357*)

32. **(b) Noise trauma** (*Ref. Cummings, 6th ed., 2346*)

- In noise trauma the earliest change seen in a conventional pure tone audiogram is a dip at 4000 Hz in both AC and BC which is known as 'acoustic dip.'
- In otosclerosis the dip is characteristically seen at 2000 Hz in bone conduction and is known as "Carhartz notch".
- In Meniere, the low frequency hearing loss leading to up sloping kind of audiogram is seen in early stages with no particular dip.
- In presbycusis high frequency hearing loss leading to down sloping audiogram is seen with no particular dip.

33. **(a), (c) and (e) All these lead to vertigo and can follow trauma.** (*Ref. Scott Brown, 8th ed., Vol 2 817, 832, 1124*)

- Perilymphatic fistula can follow iatrogenic (stapedectomy) or non iatrogenic trauma (fractures) and can lead to vertigo, SN deafness and tinnitus. Fistula test is positive.
- Secondary endolymphatic hydrops as the name is Meniere's disease secondary to trauma, viral infection, allergy, autoimmune pathology etc. It presents with vertigo, SN deafness, tinnitus and fullness in the ear.
- In Benign paroxysmal positional vertigo (BPPV) history of head trauma may be present which leads to dislodgment of otoconia/debris in the posterior semicircular canal. Movement of these particles in certain head positions stimulates the posterior semicircular canal and leads to vertigo.
- Vestibular neuronitis is characterised by acute onset vertigo with nausea and vomiting but the cause is viral infection.
- Ossicular discontinuity follows trauma but does not lead to vertigo.

34. **(c) Perilymphatic fistula** (*Ref. Scott Brown, 8th ed., Vol 2; 1085*)

- Serous otitis media can lead to Fluctuating conductive deafness.
- In hemotympanum and Cholesteatoma the hearing loss is mainly conductive and not fluctuating.

35. **(d) Propranolol** (*Ref. Cummings, 6th ed., 2378*)

36. **(c) Streptomycin** (*Ref. Cummings, 6th ed., 2371*)

- Streptomycin is predominantly vestibulotoxic. In very high doses they can affect the cochlear system also, leading to hearing loss and tinnitus.

37. **(d) 4000–5000 Hz** (*Ref. Cummings, 6th ed., 2370*)

38. **(d) Atropine** (*Ref. Scott Brown, 8th ed., Vol 2; 722*)

39. **(d) Stria vascularis** (*Ref. Cummings, 6th ed., 2378*)

40. **(a), (c), (e) Streptomycin is predominantly vestibulotoxic, Salicylates cause reversible deafness, Cisplatin causes irreversible deafness** (*Ref. Scott Brown, 8th ed., Vol 2; 723*)

Section I Ear

41. **(b) Presbycusis** (*Ref. Cummings, 6th ed., 2331*)
    - Presbycusis, Noise induced hearing loss and ototoxic drugs all can lead to B/L SN hearing loss (mainly high frequency) with proportionate decrease in speech discrimination as all affect the cochlea. The speech discrimination/word recognition scores are far worse than would be predicted from that ear's pure tone findings in retrocochlear deafness (acoustic neuroma). Moreover acoustic neuroma is U/L.
    - In the above question no history of noise exposure or ototoxic drug intake has been mentioned, ruling out acoustic trauma or ototoxicity. The age here is also suggesting Presbycusis.

42. **(a), (b) and (c) Varicella, Measles and Mumps** (*Ref. Cummings, 6th ed., 2332*)

43. **(a), (b), (d) and (e)** (*Ref. Scott Brown, 8th ed., Vol 2, 84*)
    - Alport syndrome, most commonly an X-linked dominant condition, is the most common hereditary glomerulonephritis. The most common extra-renal manifestation in Alport syndrome is high tone progressive SN hearing loss.
    - Pendred syndrome is autosomal recessive condition characterised by non toxic goitre and SN hearing loss.
    - Treacher–Collins syndrome is autosomal dominant condition characterised by hypoplasia of the first branchial arch which leads to the formation of facial bones. Therefore, this is also known as maxillo-mandibular hypoplasia. In the ear it is associated with malformation of first arch derivatives, i.e. malleus, incus, pinna and meatal atresia. Hence this leads to conductive hearing loss.
    - Crouzon syndrome is autosomal dominant condition characterised by craniofacial dysostosis. It is associated with mixed hearing loss.
    - Michel aplasia is a total non-development of inner ear and therefore is associated with SN hearing loss.

44. **(a) Presents as unilateral SNHL mostly** (*Ref. Scott Brown, 8th ed., Vol 2; 695*)

45. **(a), (c), (d)** (*Ref. Cummings, 6th ed., 2556*)

46. **(d) Inactivates (Na, K-ATPase) channels of type I and type II hair cells** (*Ref. Cummings, 6th ed., 2370*)
    - Gentamicin in the doses given in trans-tympanic injection, affects only the vestibular type I and type II hair cells, sparing the cochlear inner and outer hair cells, it being preferentially a vestibulotoxic drug. The first three choices are about damage to the outer hair cells and stria vascularis in the cochlea so they cannot be the answer.
    - Gentamicin through the transport channels (Na, K-ATPase) on the vestibular hair cells, gets concentrated in these cells leading to their death and ultimately relieving the patient from vertigo, while at the same time preserving hearing as it does not affect the inner and outer hair cells or stria vascularis.
    - In this regard it is also worth mentioning that it is the type 1 hair vestibular hair cells which are more prone to damage by Gentamicin.

47. **(b) NIHL** (*Ref. Cummings, 6th ed., 2346*)

48. **(a) Surgery is the mainstay of treatment** (*Ref. Cummings, 6th ed., 2558*). *See* Chapter 3 for fistula test

49. **(b) Neural** (*Ref. Scott Brown, 8th ed., Vol 2 695*)

50. **(c) Pulsatile tinnitus** (*Ref. Cummings, 6th ed., 2556*)

51. **(d) Amoxycillin** (*Ref. Scott Brown, 8th ed., Vol 2, 722*)

52. **(a) Surgery is mainstay** (*Ref. Cummings, 6th ed., 2395*)

53. **(a) Meniere's disease** (*Ref. Cummings, 6th ed., 2356*)

54. **(b) Gentamicin** (*Ref. Cummings, 6th ed., 2558*)

55. **(a) Fluctuating SNHL** (*Ref. Cummings, 6th ed., 2556*)

56. **(a) Diplacusis** (*Ref. Cummings, 6th ed., 2556*)
    - Paracusis Willisii is paradoxical hearing better in noisy surroundings and is a feature of otosclerosis
    - Presbycusis is age related hearing loss
    - Hyperacusis is normal sounds appearing louder and is a feature of facial nerve palsy

57. **(c) Metronidazole** (*Ref. Cummings, 6th ed., 2379*)

58. **(a) Meniere's disease** (*Ref. Cummings, 6th ed., 2556*) The typical triad of vertigo, deafness and tinnitus in this case is suggestive of Meniere. Acoustic neuroma does not present with vertigo. There is no hearing loss in Migraine. Multiple sclerosis will have other intracranial manifestations also.

59. **(c) Ototoxicity** (*Ref. Scott Brown, 8th ed., Vol 2; 725*)

60. **(b) Presbycusis** (*Ref. Cummings, 6th ed., 2330*)

61. **(d) Disorder of posterior semicircular canal** (*Ref. Scott Brown, 8th ed., Vol 2; 832*)

62. **(a) Meniere** (*Ref. Scott Brown, 8th ed., Vol 2; 819*) The given audiogram shows low frequency sensorineural hearing loss (up sloping audiogram).
    - In otosclerosis there is conductive hearing loss.
    - Ototoxicity and Noise induced hearing loss lead to high frequency hearing loss (downsloping audiogram).

63. **(c) Meniere's disease** (*Ref. Cummings, 6th ed., 2556*)
    - Vertebrobasilar (posterior) circulation constitutes the arterial supply to the brainstem, cerebellum, and occipital cortex.
    - Along with vertigo, nausea and vomiting, the patient presents with loss of vision in one or both eyes, double vision, numbness or tingling in the hands or feet, slurred speech and changes in mental status.
    - In labyrinthitis the vertigo and hearing loss last for a few weeks and not for 4 hours
    - In Benign paroxysmal vertigo there is only vertigo and no hearing loss

64. **(b) Noise trauma** (*Ref. Cummings, 6th ed., 2346*)

65. **(c) Recruitment negative** (*Ref. Cummings, 6th ed., 2556*)

66. **(b), (d), (e)** (*Ref. Scott Brown, 8th ed., Vol 2; 739*)

67. **(b) CMV** (*Ref. Scott Brown, 8th ed., Vol 2; 78*)

68. **(a) Labyrinthectomy** (*Ref. Cummings 6th ed., 2559*)

69. **(a) Superior semi-circular canal dehiscence** (*Ref. Scott Brown, 8th ed., Vol 2; 844*)

70. **(d) Rinnes is falsely positive** (*Ref. Scott Brown, 8th ed., Vol 2; 739*)

Tumours of External and Middle Ear

TUMOURS OF EXTERNAL AUDITORY CANAL

Benign Tumours

1. **Exostosis:** These are the most common benign tumour of the external auditory canal.

   These are B/L, multiple, sessile bony swellings in the deeper (medial) part of bony external auditory canal. They are usually reactive bone formation in response to exposure to cold water. Therefore it is commonly seen in surfer's, hence also known as 'Surfer's ear'.

   Clinical features: If large can cause conductive hearing loss and wax impaction.

   Management: If symptomatic; removal by drill is done.

2. **Osteoma:** This is single, bony pedunculated benign swelling in the lateral part of bony external auditory canal.

   Clinical features and treatment is same as exostosis.

TUMOURS OF MIDDLE EAR

Glomus Tumour

Glomus (tympanicum, read below) is the most common benign tumour of the middle ear. It is **benign but locally invasive tumour**.

Site of Origin

Glomus tumours are slow-growing, encapsulated, highly vascular and locally invasive tumours. These tumours originate from the **paraganglionic cells** or glomus bodies which are cells of neural crest origin. In the temporal bone they are present in relation to the 9th (Jacobson) & 10th (Arnold) nerves. Hence they are **located either at the jugular bulb area (glomus jugulare) or at the tympanic plexus area (glomus tympanicum).**

Other sites where these paraganglionic cells are present and hence where paragangliomas can form are in relation to carotid (carotid body tumours) and adrenal medulla (pheochromocytoma), etc.

10% of these Glomus tympanicum and Glomus Jugulare tumours can be **multicentric,** i.e. they have a tendency towards multiplicity and another Glomus tumour may be present in the patient. The most common combination is a carotid body tumour with an ipsilateral Glomus Tympanicum or Glomus Jugulare tumour.

Though the paraganglionic cells usually contain catecholamines (in the chromaffin cells) and are included in the diffuse neuroendocrine system (DNES), but these tumours are usually non hormone secreting (so these Glomus tympanicum and Glomus Jugulare are **nonchromaffin**, called so as they do not stain positive with chromium salts). But a rare tumour can be chromaffin positive (i.e. secreting hormones like catecholamines, metanephrine, etc.).

Therefore before operating any glomus it is mandatory to get a **urinary VMA** (vanillyl mandelic acid) and serum catecholamine (epinephrine, norepinephrine) done, so that if it is a hormone secreting one, hypertension needs to be managed before and during surgery.

Clinical Features

Glomus jugulare typically occur in **4th or 5th decade**, more commonly in **females**. Since the jugular bulb is related to the floor of the middle ear, this tumour comes into the middle ear from floor leading to **conductive hearing loss** and **pulsatile tinnitus**.

On examination: Since this is a very vascular tumour, this reddish tumourous mass coming from below into the hypotympanum of the middle ear appears like a rising sun through the intact tympanic membrane and is known as **'rising or setting sun appearance'**. This is also known as **'red reflex'**(as the red vascular mass in the middle ear abutting on the tympanic membrane (TM) gives the TM a reddish reflex).

When we introduce a Siegel's speculum in the external auditory canal and increase the pressure of external auditory canal; the tumour blanches and starts pulsating again because of its close proximity to great vessels. This is known as **'pulsation sign'** or **'Brown's sign'**.

Clinical features due to local invasions:

a. This tumour can perforate the TM and come into the external auditory canal presenting like a **bleeding polyp** of external auditory canal.

b. This may go to mastoid. In the middle ear it involves facial nerve (**7th**).

c. Later on the tumour can invade the labyrinth leading to vertigo and SN deafness (**8th**). It may spread infralabyrinthine and involve the **carotid canal**. Patient can also have **multiple cranial nerve palsies (9th, 10th, and 11th)** because of these nerves getting involved in and around the jugular foramen by the enlarging tumour. At the base of the skull, it may involve **12th** cranial nerve also.

d. They may ultimately spread to **middle/posterior cranial fossa leading to focal neurological manifestations**.

A rare chromaffin positive Glomus, i.e. the one secreting hormones may present with symptoms mimicking a pheochromocytoma, e.g. episodic HTN, headache, excessive perspiration, palpitations, pallor and nausea.

Investigation

The best investigation for diagnosis is **CECT**. Normally the jugular fossa is separated from the carotid canal by a crest of bone known as jugular plate. The erosion of the jugular plate occurs upon expansion of this tumour and is seen on CECT and is known as **'Phlep's sign'**.

MRI may be useful to see the intracranial extension of the tumour. MRI shows the characteristic soft tissue mixed intensity with intermixed high intensity signals due to hemorrhage (appearing like salt) and signal voids (appearing like pepper). This is known as salt and pepper appearance. **Magnetic resonance angiography** can be used to evaluate the compression of internal carotid artery. **Magnetic resonance venography** is useful to assess collateral circulation within the dural sinuses of the skull as the tumour blocks the blood flow in the internal jugular vein and in turn leads to blockade of the sigmoid sinus.

Carotid angiography is usually done before surgery to identify and embolise the feeding vessel which is usually the ascending pharyngeal artery.

Management

1. In young patients—**Surgical excision** is done. **Preoperative embolisation** can be done to decrease the vascularity of the tumour. The tumour is supplied by multiple branches of the external carotid, the most common being ascending pharyngeal artery. The surgical approach varies according to the type.

Fisch classified glomus into 4 types:

Type A: Tumour confined to middle ear. These can be approached through external auditory meatus, i.e. transmeatal route.

Type B: Tumour going from middle ear to mastoid also, i.e. tympanomastoid tumours. These tumours can be removed by a combined approach from the external auditory meatus as well from the mastoid (through extended facial recess approach).

Type C: Tumours with labyrinthine and infralabyrinthine spread extending up to petrous apex. These are removed by infratemporal fossa approach.

Type C1: Tumour with limited involvement of the vertical portion of the carotid canal

Type C2: Tumour with significant involvement of the vertical portion of the carotid canal

Type C3: Tumour invasion of the horizontal portion of the carotid canal

(*Mnemonic:* **C** for **C**arotid canal involvement)

Type D: Tumours with intracranial extension. These require a posterior fossa craniotomy.

Type D1: Tumour with an intracranial extension less than 2 cm in diameter

Type D2: Tumour with an intracranial extension greater than 2 cm in diameter.

2. In elderly symptomatic patients—Radiotherapy or stereotactic radio-surgery (in tumours < 3 cm in size), a low morbidity strategy.

3. In elderly infirm patients with minimal symptoms—close follow up, since it is a very slow growing tumour.

 "Points to Ponder/Points for Quick revision"

- Exostosis (Surfer's ear): B/L, multiple, sessile, benign bony growths in the deep EAC in reaction to cold water
- Glomus: MC benign tumour of middle ear (located at jugular bulb–Glomus jugulare, at tympanic plexus–Glomus tympanicum), arises from paraganglionic cells, F (30–40 yrs) MC
  - Encapsulated and slow growing (but locally invasive and highly vascular)
  - 10% multicentric (i.e. additionally carotid body tumours and/or pheochromocytomas)
  - Non-hormone secreting (nonchromaffin)
  - CFs: CHL, pulsatile tinnitus, "rising or setting sun" appearance/red reflex, pulsatile or "Brown's sign"
  - leeding polyp in the EAC, multiple cranial N palsies (7 to 12), focal neurological deficits upon intracranial extension
  - CECT–"Phlep's sign" (erosion of the jugular plate), MRI for intracranial extension–salt and pepper appearance, Carotid angiography–feeding vessel identification
  - Preop embolization and surgical excision (as per Fisch classification). In elderly–radiotherapy or stereotactic surgery (< 3 cm).

PREVIOUSLY ASKED QUESTIONS

1. **Surfers ear is:**   (*AIIMS May 2010*)
   a. Exostosis
   b. Otosclerosis
   c. Otitis externa
   d. Squamous cell carcinoma

2. **Most common benign tumour of middle ear is:**
                                   (*UP 2007, Exam 2017*)
   a. Adeno carcinoma
   b. Squamous cell carcinoma
   c. Glomus tumour
   d. Acoustic neuroma

3. **All are true about Glomus jugulare tumours except:**
                                   (*UP 2003, Exam 2017*)
   a. Common in females
   b. Causes conductive deafness
   c. It is a disease of infancy
   d. It invades labyrinth, petrous pyramid and mastoid

4. **True about Glomus jugulare tumour:**
                            (*PGI June 2004, Exam 2012*)
   a. Most common in male
   b. Arises from non-chromaffin cells
   c. Lymph node metastasis seen
   d. Multicentric
   e. Fluctuating tinnitus and conductive type of hearing loss is seen

5. **Which is the pulsatile tumour found in external auditory meatus which bleeds on touch?**
                                (*AIIMS 95, Exam 2014*)
   a. Squamous cell carcinoma of pinna
   b. Basal cell carcinoma
   c. Adenoma
   d. Glomus tumour

6. **The usual location of Glomus jugulare tumour is:**
                    (*Delhi 2009, UP 2003, Exam 2013*)
   a. Epitympanum
   b. Hypotympanum
   c. Mastoid cell
   d. Promontory

7. **Pulsatile tinnitus in ear is due to:**
                                  (*TN 2001, Exam 2017*)
   a. Malignant otitis media
   b. Osteoma
   c. Mastoid reservoirs
   d. Glomus jugulare tumour

8. **Earliest symptom of Glomus tumour is:**
                                  (*UP 2006, Exam 2017*)
   a. Pulsatile tinnitus   b. SN Deafness
   c. Headache   d. Vertigo

9. **True about Glomus jugulare are all except:**
                                            (*AI 2010*)
   a. Rising sun sign is seen
   b. Involve 9th and 10th cranial nerves
   c. Pulsatile tinnitus is seen
   d. Usually invades epitympanum

10. **Polypoidal mass in ear, on touch bleeding heavily, cause is:**   (*Exam 2001, 2017*)
    a. Glomus jugulare   b. Carcinoma Mastoid
    c. Acoustic neuroma   d. Angiofibroma

11. **Brown sign is seen in:**   (*AI 2007, Exam 2013*)
    a. Glomus tumour   b. Meniere's disease
    c. Acoustic neuroma   d. Otosclerosis

12. **Phlep's sign is seen in:**
                            (*AIIMS May 2002, Exam 2013*)
    a. Glomus jugulare
    b. Vestibular schwannoma
    c. Meniere's disease
    d. Neurofibromatosis

13. **The Glomus jugulare tumour compression of carotid is diagnosed by:**   (*UP 2005, Exam 2017*)
    a. MR angiography   b. CECT
    c. X-ray   d. Jugular venography
    e. MR venography

14. **Fisch classification is used for:**   (*Exam 2014*)
    a. Tonsillar carcinoma
    b. Nasopharyngeal ca
    c. Vestibular schwannoma
    d. Glomus tumour

15. **A patient presents with bleeding from the ear, pain, tinnitus and progressive deafness. On examination there is a red swelling behind the intact tympanic membrane which blanches on pressure with pneumatic speculum. Management includes all except:**   (*AIIMS Nov 2001, Exam 2017*)
    a. Radiotherapy
    b. Surgery
    c. Interferon
    d. Preoperative embolisation

16. **Glomus tumour invading significant vertical part of carotid canal. It is: (Exam 2014)**
    a. Type B   b. Type C1
    c. Type C2   d. Type C3

17. **Which of the following is a cause of pulsatile tinnitus?**   (*Exam 2015*)
    a. Glomus tumour
    b. Cholesterol granuloma
    c. Dehiscent jugular bulb
    d. Carotid artery dissection

18. **A patient presents with pulsatile tinnitus and progressive deafness. Endoscopic picture of his tympanic membrane is given below. The red**

Ear

Section I

swelling blanches on pressure with pneumatic speculum. **All are true about it except:**

(Practice question by Author)

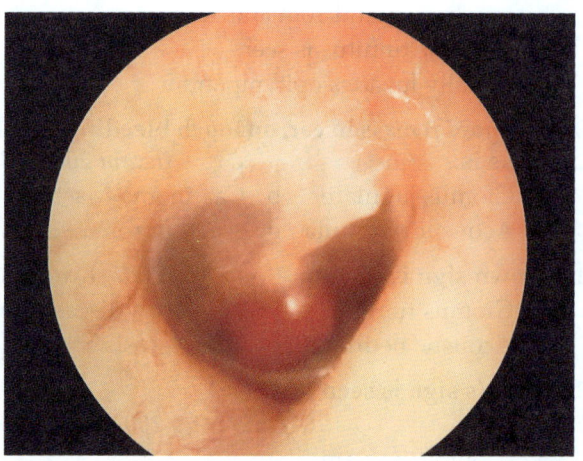

a. Arises from non-chromaffin cells
b. Lymph node metastasis not seen
c. Rising sun sign is seen
d. Fluctuating conductive type of hearing loss is seen

19. **Which of the following is NOT the site of paragangliomas?**   (*MH CET 2015*)
    a. Carotid bifurcation
    b. Geniculate ganglion
    c. Jugular foramen
    d. Promontory of middle ear

20. **Pulsatile tinnitus is a feature of:**   (*Exam 2016*)
    a. Glomus tumour
    b. Acoustic neuroma
    c. Malignant otitis externa
    d. Meniere's disease

ANSWERS AND EXPLANATIONS

1. **(a) Exostosis** (*Ref. Scott Brown, 8th ed., Vol 2 page 964*)
2. **(c) Glomus tumour** (*Ref. Cummings, 6th ed., 2738*)
   - Most common benign tumour of middle ear is glomus tumour.
   - Acoustic neuroma is the most common benign tumour of the CP angle.
   - Squamous cell carcinoma is the most common carcinoma of the middle ear.
   - Adenocarcinoma is an occasional glandular tumour of the middle ear.
3. **(c) It is a disease of infancy** (*Ref. Scott Brown, 8th ed., Vol 2 page 1303*)
   - Glomus is seen most commonly in middle age (40–50 yrs) usually in females. It presents with conductive deafness and pulsatile tinnitus.
   - It is a benign but locally invasive tumour and can invade mastoid, labyrinth, petrous pyramid, jugular foramen, Eustachian tube and middle/posterior cranial fossa.
4. **(b), (d) and (e)** (*Ref. Cummings, 6th ed., 2739*)
   - Since Glomus jugulare is a benign tumour lymph node metastasis is not seen.
5. **(d) Glomus tumour** (*Ref. Cummings, 6th ed., 2739*)
6. **(b) Hypotympanum** (*Ref. Cummings, 6th ed., 2738*)
   - Glomus jugulare arises from the paraganglionic cells in relation to the jugular bulb which is related to the floor of the middle ear. Therefore from the floor it comes into the hypotympanum.
   - Less commonly Glomus may arise from promontory and is called Glomus tympanicum.
     Since it is locally invasive Glomus may later on reach epitympanum, mastoid and other nearby areas.
7. **(d) Glomus jugulare tumour** (*Ref. Scott Brown, 8th ed., Vol 2 page 1283*)
   - For the tinnitus to be pulsatile the cause has to be vascular. Vascular causes to tinnitus are Glomus jugulare and internal carotid aneurysms.
8. **(a) Pulsatile tinnitus** (*Ref. Cummings, 6th ed., 2738*)
   - Earliest presenting symptoms of Glomus tumour are conductive hearing loss and pulsatile tinnitus.

SN deafness and vertigo occur late with labyrinthine spread.

9. **(d) Usually invades epitympanum** (*Ref. Cummings, 6th ed., 2738*)

   From the floor of middle ear glomus jugulare invades into the hypotympanum.
10. **(a) Glomus jugulare** (*Ref. Cummings, 6th ed., 2739*)
11. **(a) Glomus tumour** (*Ref. Scott Brown, 8th ed., Vol 2 page 1215, Dhingra 6th ed., 109*)
12. **(a) Glomus jugulare** (*Ref. Shambaugh, 6th ed., 733*)
13. **(a) MR angiography** (*Ref. Cummings, 6th ed., 2756*)
    - Magnetic resonance angiography is used to evaluate for compression of internal carotid artery.
    - CECT is diagnostic of Glomus jugulare.
    - X-ray has no role in the assessment of Glomus jugulare.
    - MR venography is useful to assess collateral circulation within the dural sinuses of the skull as the tumour blocks the blood flow in the internal jugular vein and in turn leads to blockade of the sigmoid sinus.
    - Jugular venography is no longer used because intravenous tumour extension can be seen with MR venography.
14. **(d) Glomus tumour** (*Ref. Stell and Maran's, 5th ed., 261*)
15. **(c) Interferon** (*Ref. Cummings, 6th ed., 2738*)

    The clinical description suggests Glomus tumour. Please refer the text for its management
16. **(c) Type C2** (*Ref. Current Diagnosis and Treatment Otolaryngology-Lalwani, 3rd ed., 814*)
17. **(a) Glomus tumour** (*Ref. Stell & Maran's, 5th ed., 263*)
18. **(d) Fluctuating conductive type of hearing loss is seen** (*Ref. Stell and Maran's, 5th ed., 263*)
19. **(b) Geniculate ganglion** (*Ref. Cummings, 6th ed., 2738*)
20. **(a) Glomus tumour** (*Ref. Stell & Maran's, 5th ed., 263*)

Acoustic Neuroma/ Vestibular Schwannoma

ACOUSTIC NEUROMA

- Is the most common benign tumour of the cerebello-pontine (CP) angle.
- Is a **benign tumour** but is **locally invasive**.
- Is a well circumscribed but **unencapsulated** tumour.
- Is an extremely slow growing tumour.

Site of Origin

The most common site of origin of acoustic neuroma is from the Schwann cells of the **inferior vestibular nerve** in the zone of transition of central myelin to peripheral myelin. This zone is termed as the Obersteiner-Redlich zone. This zone lies in the **internal acoustic meatus**.

Next most common site of origin of acoustic neuroma is from the Schwann cells of superior vestibular nerve. Rarely, it may originate from the cochlear nerve. Therefore, this tumour is more aptly known as vestibular schwannoma.

Schematic Diagram of IAM

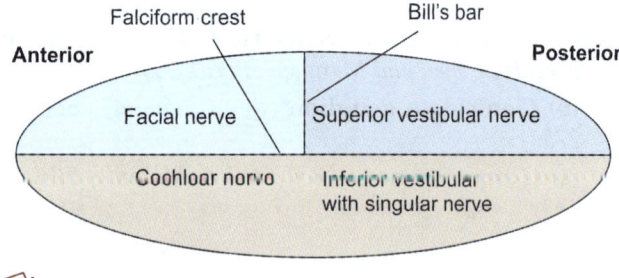

Note:

The most common site of origin of acoustic neuroma is the inferior vestibular nerve in the IAM.

Clinical Features

Acoustic neuroma is usually U/L and occurs in the age group of 40–70 yrs.

If present in young (20–30 yrs), then the patient should be investigated for **neurofibromatosis type 2** where B/L acoustic neuromas are present and neurofibromatosis type 1 where U/L acoustic neuroma may be present (easy to remember type 2 B/L, type 1 U/L).

Since this tumour arises in the internal acoustic meatus, initial symptoms are because of the compression of the adjacent nerves and vessels in the internal acoustic meatus.

Later when the tumour grows into the CP angle, symptoms arise because of compression of structures in the CP angle. Accordingly several stages are described during the progressive growth of tumour.

1. **Otologic stage:** This stage is called so as all the symptoms here are pertaining to the ear. In this stage the symptoms occur because of the compression of the adjacent nerves and vessels in the internal acoustic meatus.

   a. *Cochlear nerve compression symptoms:* The tumour arising in the internal acoustic meatus compresses the cochlear nerve (*see* IAM schematic diagram above) and the **patient presents most commonly with unilateral sensorineural** (retrocochlear) **hearing loss** usually slowly progressive (since the tumour grows very slowly) **and tinnitus.** Hence, it is justifiable to call vestibular schwannoma as acoustic neuroma. Rarely the patient can present with sudden SN hearing loss (if there is sudden increase in size of tumour, due to hemorrhage or cystic enlargement).

   b. *Vestibular nerve compression symptoms:* Compression and destruction of the vestibular nerve usually does not cause severe disturbance of equilibrium and frank vertigo since it is a very slow growing tumour. As the tumour slowly grows and causes involvement of the vestibular function, physiological compensation occurs by the CNS and opposite side vestibular system. Mild disequilibrium however can be present. Like sudden SN deafness, rarely acute vertigo may be there.

   The caloric response is reduced on the side of lesion.

   In this regard it is important to remember that the caloric test is mainly a test for lateral semicircular canal which is innervated by superior vestibular nerve hence small tumours arising from inferior vestibular nerve might not lead to any change in the caloric response. Later on with compression of superior vestibular nerve the caloric response is reduced.,

c. *Facial nerve compression symptoms:* Though facial nerve also lies in the internal acoustic meatus, but it being mainly a motor nerve therefore is resistant to compression and involvement by the tumour. In this regard it is important to remember that the 5th nerve involvement is more common than the 7th, read below. The motor fibres of facial nerve take a very long time to get affected hence facial weakness is seen quiet late in acoustic neuroma.

But sensory fibres of facial may get affected by compression.

This involvement of sensory component of facial (which is known as nervus intermedius or nerve of Wrisberg) leads to anaesthesia over the postero-superior part of external auditory meatus and canal. This is known as **'Hitzelberger's sign'**.

But this 'Hitzelberger's sign' is present only in 25% of patients and it also being subjective, therefore, is clinically less significant than the absent corneal reflex because of involvement of 5th nerve, *see* below.

Less commonly there can also be altered lacrimation or alterations in taste sensation of anterior 2/3rd of tongue due to facial nerve involvement, *see* chapter on facial nerve.

2. **Stage of trigeminal nerve involvement:** From the internal acoustic meatus the tumour grows into the CP angle where it involves the trigeminal nerve, *see* Fig. 14.1.

The 5th (trigeminal) nerve forms the upper boundary of CP angle while traversing the petrous apex to reach the Meckel's cave on the anterior slant of petrous part of temporal bone. It is therefore compressed by the **upper pole of the tumour**.

This involvement of 5th nerve is manifested as a loss of corneal reflex (*see* Chapter on facial nerve for corneal reflex) and this is the **'earliest ocular sign'** of acoustic neuroma. This is also the **'most common sign'** seen in

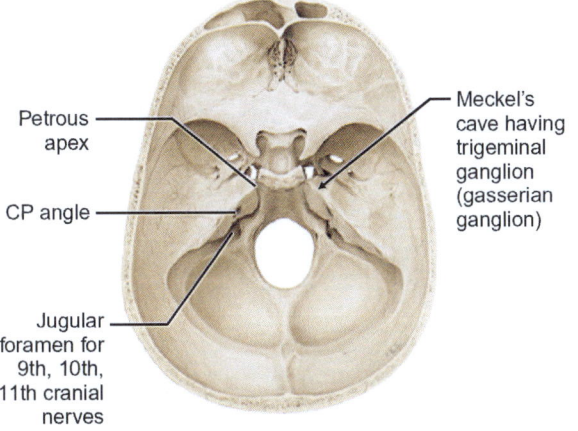

Petrous apex

Meckel's cave having trigeminal ganglion (gasserian ganglion)

CP angle

Jugular foramen for 9th, 10th, 11th cranial nerves

Fig. 14.1: The CP angle and its relations

these patients as Hitselberger sign is seen only in 25% of patients.

If in a patient of acoustic neuroma corneal reflex is absent it means the tumour is at least 2–2.5 cm in size and is outside the internal acoustic meatus, in the CP angle.

With further growth there can be facial numbness.

3. **Stage of Cerebellar compression:** Because of further growth of the tumour in the C P angle there is cerebellar compression leading to ataxia, dysmetria, dyssynergia, dysdiadochokinesia and nystagmus.

There can be multiple cranial nerve palsies. The cranial nerves 9, 10, 11 forming the lower boundary of CP angle are involved by the **lower pole of the tumour** (jugular foramen syndrome).

4. **Stage of increased intracranial pressure and terminal stage:** Hydrocephalus leads to increased intracranial pressure leading to features like headache, nausea, vomiting and papilloedema. Ultimately death can occur due to compression of vital centres in the brain stem.

Investigations (*See* Chapter on Audiology)

The findings are suggestive of a retrocochlear pathology

Rinne +ve

Weber's—Towards normal side

ABC—Shortened

Schwabach—Shortened

PTA shows sensorineural hearing loss

SISI—0–20% (because of negative recruitment)

Tone decay > 30 dB

Acoustic reflex decay—Positive

Speech discrimination score is very poor.

This poor discrimination score becomes poorer when retested at higher speech intensity, i.e. **'Roll over phenomenon'**.

The best audiometric test for acoustic neuroma is **BERA**.

The most diagnostic finding suggestive of acoustic neuroma on BERA is increased interaural latency of wave V of > 0.2 ms. Next important diagnostic finding is increased latency between waves I–V.

Caloric test is reduced on the side of lesion.

VEMP (vestibular evoked myogenic potential) which tests the inferior vestibular nerve is reduced on the side of lesion.

The gold standard investigation for the diagnosis of acoustic neuroma is **gadolinium enhanced MRI**. When the tumour extends from the internal acoustic meatus to CP angle it produces a typical "ice cream cone appearance" (*see* picture of Q 27).

Management

The management of acoustic neuroma is by following modalities:

1. **Surgical excision: Surgical excision is the treatment of choice** for acoustic neuroma. This is done by the

Ear

Section I

following approaches depending upon extent of tumour and residual hearing in the patient:

a. **Translabyrinthine:** This is the **most common approach.** The tumour in the internal acoustic meatus is approached through the labyrinth via the postaural route. Here a mastoidectomy is performed followed by total labyrinthectomy.

b. **Suboccipital/Retrosigmoid:** Here the CP angle is approached through the posterior cranial fossa for tumour resection.

c. **Combined** translabyrinthine and suboccipital approach

d. **Middle cranial fossa approach:**

Here the internal acoustic meatus is approached through the middle cranial fossa by making a craniotomy at the temple without doing labyrinthectomy. So when the hearing of patient is preserved a middle cranial fossa approach is preferred.,

Biopsy: Histologically acoustic neuromas are composed of two patterns; **Antoni A and B.**

Antoni A areas are compact, dense and cellular and contain elongated spindle cells and palisading nuclei aligned in rows (Verocay bodies). Antoni type B are loose, less cellular and cystic. These cystic Antoni B tumours appear hypodense on CT/MRI. Since the cysts can dramatically increase in size they should **not be managed by radiotherapy** and wait and watch policy. They should be excised.

Most acoustic neuromas contain predominantly Antoni type A cells mixed with some areas of type B.

2. **Radiation/Gamma knife:** This is by stereotactic radiotherapy, i.e. by gamma knife. It aims maximum amount of radiation at the tumour site. It retards the growth of tumour but does not destroy it. It is used for small tumours in elderly or medically infirm patients where clinically important tumour growth has been documented (*see* wait and watch policy below).

3. **Observation:** It being a benign and extremely slow growing tumour, if the patient is >65 yrs, and the tumour is very small in size, a wait and watch policy with close observation by yearly MRI should be followed., It can be used for small tumours in elderly or medically infirm patients.

In a patient of neurofibromatosis type 2 operated for B/L acoustic neuromas rehabilitation of hearing is by **auditory brainstem implant (ABI),** which is placed in the lateral recess of 4th ventricle where it directly stimulates the cochlear nuclei.

"Points to Ponder/Points for Quick revision"

- Acoustic neuroma is a benign, uncapsulated, slow growing tumour
- MC site of origin—Schwann cells of the inferior vestibular nerve in the IAM
- CFs (due to growth in the IAM):
  - MC—U/L slowly progressive SNHL and tinnitus
  - Reduced caloric response (with involvement of the superior vestibular N), Hitzelberger's sign (anaesthesia over postero-superior part of EAC)
  - VEMP (tests inferior vestibular N) is reduced on the side of lesion (hence better than caloric test)
- CFs (due to growth in the CP angle):
  - 5th N involvement by the upper pole of the tumour → loss of corneal reflex (earliest and MC sign)
  - Cerebellar involvement
  - 9th, 10th, 11th cranial N involvement by the lower pole of the tumour (jugular foramen syndrome)
- Audiometry: Retro-cochlear pathology, BERA (best test) → increased interaural latency of wave V
- Gold standard investigation: MRI
- Antoni A and B-histological types. A—compact. B—cystic, appear hypodense on MRI
- T/t: Surgical excision (MC—trans-labyrinthine approach). When the hearing is preserved—Middle cranial fossa approach. Radiation/Gamma knife in small sized tumours in elderly.

PREVIOUSLY ASKED QUESTIONS

1. **Most common Cerebellopontine angle tumour is:**
   (Kerala 99, Exam 2014)
   a. Acoustic neuroma   b. Cholesteatoma
   c. Meningioma   d. None of the above

2. **Acoustic schwannoma most common site is:**
   (Exam 2013)
   a. CP angle
   b. Fossa of Rosenmuller
   c. Retropharyngeal space
   d. None

3. **Schwannoma most commonly involves the:**
   (AI 99, 2004, Exam 2017)
   a. Vestibular part of VIII nerve
   b. Cochlear part of VIII nerve
   c. Vagus
   d. Hypoglossal

4. **Acoustic neuroma commonly arise from:**
   (AIIMS Dec 98, AIIMS Nov 2009, J & K 2005 AI 2011)
   a. Superior vestibular nerve
   b. Inferior vestibular nerve
   c. Cochlear nerve
   d. Facial nerve

5. **The earliest symptom of acoustic nerve tumour is:**
   (AI 95/Delhi 2005/Karnataka 2009)
   a. Sensorineural hearing loss
   b. Facial weakness
   c. Vertigo
   d. Otorrhoea

6. **Earliest sign seen in acoustic neuroma is:**
   (UPSC 2005, Exam 2017)
   a. Facial weakness
   b. Unilateral deafness
   c. Reduced corneal reflex
   d. Cerebellar signs

7. **In Acoustic neuroma cranial nerve to be involved earliest is:** *(Exam 2013, AI 2007/UP 2008)*
   a. 5th   b. 6th
   c. 7th   d. 8th

8. **In acoustic neuroma, cranial nerve to be involved earliest is:** *(AI 2007, UP 2008, Exam 2013)*
   a. 5th   b. 7th
   c. 10th   d. 9th

9. **Earliest ocular finding in acoustic neuroma:**
   (PGI 2000, MP 2000, Kerala 2004, Delhi 2006, Exam 2013)
   a. Diplopia
   b. Ptosis
   c. Inability to close eye
   d. Loss of corneal sensation
   e. Papilloedema

10. **True about CP angle tumour:**
    (AIIMS 97, 2002, Exam 2017)
    a. Absent corneal reflex
    b. Superior oblique palsy
    c. Pupillary dilatation
    d. Medial rectus palsy

11. **In acoustic neuroma all are seen except:**
    (MP 2000, Exam 2017)
    a. Loss of corneal reflex
    b. Tinnitus
    c. Facial palsy
    d. Bitemporal hemianopia

12. **Progressive sensorineural loss of hearing, tinnitus and ataxia have been seen in an elderly. This is a case of:** *(SGPGI 2005, Exam 2017)*
    a. Otitis media
    b. Cerebral glioma
    c. Acoustic neuroma
    d. Ependymoma

13. **A 70-year-old male presents with loss of sensation in external auditory meatus (Hitselberger sign positive). The likely diagnosis is:** *(AI 2008)*
    a. Vestibular Schwannoma
    b. Mastoiditis
    c. Bell's palsy
    d. Cholesteatoma

14. **Acoustic neuroma causes:** *(Exam 2011)*
    a. Cochlear deafness
    b. Retrocochlear deafness
    c. Conductive deafness
    d. Any of the above

15. **In a patient with acoustic neuroma all are seen except:** *(SGPGI 2007, Exam 2017)*
    a. Unilateral deafness
    b. Reduced corneal reflex
    c. Cerebellar signs
    d. Acute episode of vertigo

16. **Acoustic neuroma causes the following except:**
    (Exam 2012)
    a. Ptosis   b. Facial numbness
    c. Nystagmus   d. Loss of corneal reflex

17. **Vestibular Schwannoma—not correct:**
    (AP 2005, Exam 2017)
    a. Facial numbness
    b. Sensorineural deafness
    c. Absence of VEMP response
    d. Normal corneal reflex

18. **If in a patient of acoustic neuroma, corneal reflex is absent it implies involvement of cranial nerve:**
    (AIIMS 2006, Exam 2017)
    a. 5th   b. 7th
    c. Both   d. none

Section I   **Ear**

19. **True about acoustic neuroma:** *(Exam 2014)*
    a. Malignant tumour
    b. Arises from vestibular nerve
    c. Upper pole compresses IX,X,XI nerves
    d. Lower pole compresses trigeminal cranial nerve

20. **Acoustic neuroma of 1 cm diameter, the investigation of choice:** *(Kerala 97, AI 2005, Exam 2017)*
    a. CT scan
    b. MRI scan
    c. Plain X-ray skull
    d. Air encephalography

21. **A patient is suspected to have vestibular schwannoma the investigation of choice for its diagnosis is:** *(AIIMS 2004, Exam 2013)*
    a. CECT
    b. Gadolinium enhanced MRI
    c. SPECT
    d. PET Scan

22. **Treatment of choice for acoustic neuroma:** *(Kerala 2008)*
    a. Steroid
    b. Radiotherapy
    c. Anti-neoplastic drugs
    d. Surgical excision

23. **Which of the following would be the most appropriate treatment for rehabilitation of a patient who has bilateral profound deafness following surgery for bilateral acoustic schwannoma:** *(DPG Feb 2009)*
    a. Bilateral powered digital hearing aid
    b. Bilateral cochlear implants
    c. Unilateral cochlear implant
    d. Brain stem implant

24. **Hitzelberger's sign is seen in:** *(Exam 2016)*
    a. Acoustic neuroma
    b. Glomus tumour
    c. Nasal angiofibroma
    d. Acute suppurative otitis media

25. **True about vestibular schwannoma:** *(PGI May 2015)*
    a. U/L hearing loss is commonly present
    b. Mostly malignant
    c. Most common benign tumour of CP angle
    d. Sensorineural deafness
    e. Non-capsulated

26) **BERA is a reliable indicator in the diagnosis of:** *(Kerala PGMEE 2015)*
    a. Otosclerosis
    b. Vestibular neuronitis
    c. Acoustic schwannoma
    d. Vestibular Migraine

27. **A 70-year-old male presents with left sensorineural hearing loss and tinnitus. On examination there is loss of sensation of postero-superior part of external auditory meatus. His MRI is shown below. Most probable diagnosis is:** *(Practice question by Author)*

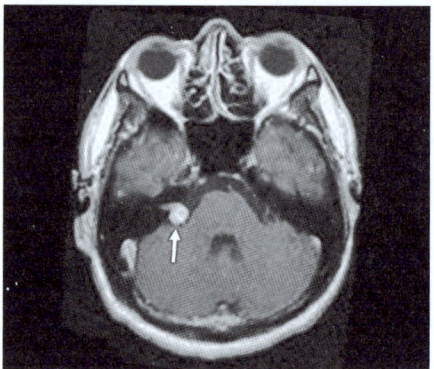

    a. Otitis media with brain abscess
    b. Cerebral glioma
    c. Acoustic neuroma
    d. Ependymoma

28. **The above patient was operated. The biopsy specimen—histopathology will show:** *(Exam 2018)*
    a. Severely increased Mitotic figures
    b. Chromaffin cells
    c. Antoni A or B cells
    d. Reed Sternberg cells

ANSWERS AND EXPLANATIONS

1. **(a) Acoustic neuroma is the most common benign tumour of the CP angle.** (*Ref. Cummings, 6th ed., 2748*)
- The next most common tumour here is meningioma followed by epidermoid, i.e. cholesteatoma.

2. **(a) CP angle** (*Ref. Cummings, 6th ed., 2748*)

3. **(a) Vestibular part of VIII nerve** (*Ref. Shambaugh, 6th ed., 644*)
- Rarely it may originate from the other mentioned options in the question

4. **(b) Inferior vestibular nerve** (*Ref. Shambaugh, 6th ed., 644*)

5. **(a) Sensorineural hearing loss** (*Ref. Scott Brown, 8th ed., Vol 2 page 1371*)
- Mild vertigo and Facial weakness occur late.
- There is no ear discharge in Acoustic neuroma.

6. **(c) Reduced corneal reflex** (*Ref. Scott Brown, 8th ed., Vol 2 page 1371*)
- Facial weakness and cerebellar signs occur late.
- Unilateral deafness is the earliest symptom of Acoustic neuroma.

7. **(d) 8th** (*Ref. Scott Brown, 8th ed., Vol 2 page 1371*)

8. **(a) 5th** (*Ref. Scott Brown, 8th ed., Vol 2 page 1371*)
Of the mentioned choices, 5th cranial nerve is the best answer, please see the text.

9. **(d) Loss of corneal sensation** (*Ref. Scott Brown, 8th ed., Vol 2 page 1371*)
- Involvement of 3rd cranial nerve causing diplopia and ptosis is not described in Acoustic neuroma.
- Motor involvement of facial and thereby inability to close eye occurs uncommonly and that too very late in Acoustic neuroma.
- Papilloedema because of increased intracranial pressure occurs in the terminal stage of Acoustic neuroma.

10. **(a) Absent corneal reflex** (*Ref. Cummings, 6th ed., 2750*)
- Involvement of 3rd and 4th cranial nerve causing pupillary dilatation and medial rectus and superior oblique palsy is not described in Acoustic neuroma.

11. **(d) Bitemporal hemianopia** (*Ref. Cummings, 6th ed., 2750*)
- Bitemporal hemianopia is loss of right and left temporal side of visual fields. It is due to lesions of optic chiasm which is not seen in acoustic neuroma.

12. **(c) Acoustic neuroma** (*Ref. Cummings, 6th ed., 2750*)
- Otitis media presents with ear discharge and conductive hearing loss.
- Glioma is a type of tumour that starts in the brain or spine from glial cells. The three main types of glioma include: ependymoma, astrocytoma and oligodendroglioma The first symptoms of a glioma are likely to be caused by increased intracranial pressure within the skull (headache, nausea, vomiting, seizures, and cranial nerve disorders) in sharp contrast to acoustic neuroma where these usually occur at last. Depending upon the area of brain involved in gliomas, there are focal neurological symptoms, e.g. seizures, hemiparesis, visual field defects, etc.

13. **(a) Vestibular schwannoma** (*Ref. Shambaugh, 6th ed., 647*)
- In vestibular schwannoma the involvement of sensory fibres of facial (i.e. nervus intermedius or nerve of Wrisberg) leads to anaesthesia over the postero-superior part of external auditory meatus and canal. This is known as 'Hitselberger sign'. But this 'Hitselberger sign' is present only in 25% of patients.
- Mastoiditis shows "reservoir sign", *see* Chapter on complications of CSOM.
- Bell's palsy is acute idiopathic lower motor neuron palsy of facial nerve.
- Cholesteatoma is the presence of keratinising stratified squamous epithelium in any part of temporal bone where it is not usually present.

14. **(b) Retrocochlear deafness** (*Ref. Cummings, 6th ed., 2751*)
- Acoustic neuroma arising in the internal acoustic meatus compresses the cochlear nerve and therefore the patient presents most commonly with unilateral retrocochlear hearing loss usually slowly progressive.

15. **(d) Acute episode of vertigo** (*Ref. Cummings, 6th ed., 2750*)
- Though the most common site of origin of acoustic neuroma is from the Schwann cells of the inferior vestibular nerve, compression and destruction of the vestibular nerve usually does not cause severe disturbance of equilibrium and acute episode of vertigo. This is because it is a very slow growing tumour and compensation occurs by the CNS. However mild disequilibrium can be present.
- Acoustic neuroma arising in the internal acoustic meatus compresses the cochlear nerve and therefore the patient presents most commonly with unilateral retrocochlear hearing loss.
- The involvement of 5th nerve is manifested as a loss of corneal reflex and this is the 'earliest ocular sign' of acoustic neuroma. This is also the 'most common sign' seen in these patients.
- Because of the growth of Acoustic neuroma in the CP angle there is cerebellar compression leading to ataxia, dysmetria, dyssynergia, dysdiadochokinesia and nystagmus.

16. **(a) Ptosis** (*Ref. Cummings, 6th ed., 2750*)
- 3rd nerve involvement leading to ptosis does not occur in Acoustic neuroma.
- Facial numbness and loss of corneal reflex is due to the involvement of Vth nerve.
- Nystagmus due to cerebellar involvement occurs late in the course of Acoustic neuroma.

Ear

Section I

17. **(d) Normal corneal reflex** (*Ref. Cummings, 6th ed., 2750*)

- The involvement of 5th nerve is manifested as a loss of corneal reflex and this is the 'earliest ocular sign' of acoustic neuroma. This is also the 'most common sign' seen in these patients.

18. **(a) 5th** (*Ref. Scott Brown, 8th ed., Vol 2 page 1370*)

- In corneal reflex the sensory afferent part of the reflex arc is trigeminal and motor efferent part is facial nerve.
- The involvement of 5th nerve, at the upper pole in CP angle by acoustic neuroma is manifested as a loss of corneal reflex.
- Facial nerve being mainly a motor nerve therefore is resistant to compression. The motor fibres of Facial nerve take a very long time to get affected hence facial weakness is seen quiet late in acoustic neuroma. So loss of corneal reflex in acoustic neuroma, initially and largely, is due to involvement of the sensory efferent element of the reflex arc, i.e. 5th nerve. Technically involvement of motor aspect of facial nerve occurring late in the course of Acoustic neuroma will also contribute to loss of corneal reflex but better signs for looking facial nerve involvement, i.e. the signs eliciting facial muscle movements will now be there.
- Corneal reflex is done primarily to check 5th nerve involvement. This reflex should be elicited carefully avoiding injury to the cornea. *See* Chapter on facial nerve for further details of corneal reflex.

19. **(b) Arises from vestibular nerve** (*Ref. Shambaugh, 6th ed., 645*)

- The most common site of origin of acoustic neuroma is from the Schwann cells of the inferior vestibular nerve followed by superior vestibular nerve.
- Acoustic neuroma is the most common benign tumour of the CP angle.
- When the tumour invades CP angle its upper pole compresses trigeminal nerve which is situated at the upper pole of CP angle.
- 9th, 10th and 11th cranial nerves present at the base of CP angle are compressed by the lower pole of Acoustic neuroma.

20. **(b) MRI scan** (*Ref. Cummings, 6th ed., 2751*)

- The gold standard investigation for the diagnosis of acoustic neuroma is gadolinium enhanced MRI. Even very small asymptomatic lesions can be observed by MRI.

21. **(b) Gadolinium enhanced MRI** (*Ref. Cummings, 6th ed., 2751*)

22. **(d) Surgical excision** (*Ref. Shambaugh, 6th ed., 651*)

23. **(d) Brain stem implant** (*Ref. Shambaugh, 6th ed., 688*)

- Since it is a retrocochlear pathology hearing aid and cochlear implant will not help. Rehabilitation of hearing is by auditory brainstem implant (ABI), which is placed in the lateral recess of 4th ventricle where it directly stimulates the cochlear nuclei.

24. **(a) Acoustic neuroma** (*Ref. Shambaugh, 6th ed., 647*)

25. **(a), (c), (d), (e)** (*Ref. Shambaugh, 6th ed., 644*)

26. **(c) Acoustic schwannoma** (*Ref. Cummings, 6th ed., 2751*)

27. **(c) Acoustic neuroma** (*Ref. Shambaugh, 6th ed., 647*)

28. **(c) Antoni A or B cells** (*Ref. Scott Brown, 8th ed., Vol 2 page 1232*)

Chapter
15

Cochlear Implant, Brainstem Implant and BAHA

Cochlear implant is the first artificial sense organ. It was developed and invented by **Dr. William F House,** who is known as the **father of neuro-otology**.

In most deaf individuals, the main defect lies in the hair cells of the organ of Corti, the auditory nerve being normal.

So the cochlear implant, as the name, bypasses this defect in the hair cells by directly stimulating the auditory nerve fibres.

In other words it **replaces the organ of Corti**. So it will not be useful where the defect is in the auditory nerve (compare from auditory neuropathy, below).

INDICATION OF COCHLEAR IMPLANT

B/L Severe (>70 dB)–profound (>90 dB) SN Hearing Loss

It is important to note that in a patient of significant B/L SN deafness, initially hearing aid is provided. The hearing aid amplifies the sound and send it to the cochlea. So hearing aid requires some functioning of the cochlea. But when the cochlear function is severely compromised, hearing aid of any type will no longer be beneficial. Now the patient is advised for cochlear implant, **provided cochlear nerve is functioning normally**.

The hearing loss can be prelingual or postlingual. Prelingual deafness is deafness before the child has developed speech, i.e. congenitally deaf. Post lingual deafness is either in an adult person or when a child has developed deafness after he has developed speech, e.g. meningitis followed by labyrinthitis and deafness.

In both pre and postlingual deafness the shorter the period of auditory deprivation, the faster and better are the results of implantation.

Note:
- Congenitally absent cochlea is a contraindication to cochlear implant. Please remember that the cochlear implantation is a replacement of the organ of Corti but if there is a complete absence of cochlea, cochlear implantation is not possible.

- Previously the Mondini aplasia (cochlea having only 1 and ½ turns instead of 2 and ½ to 2 and ¾), was a contra-indication. But nowadays with the advancement of cochlear implants, it is no more a contraindication.
- Auditory neuropathy: It is also known as Auditory dyssynchrony. Here there is usually a loss of synchrony of the cochlear inner hair cells or the spiral ganglion nerve synapse leading to a transduction problem, because of which cochlea fails to transmit signals to the auditory nerve. The outer hair cells are normal and the patient presents with mild to severe hearing loss. The speech discrimination score is always out of proportion with the hearing loss, i.e. Patient has great difficulty in understanding speech out of proportion to his pure tone audiometric findings. On examination, the OAE are normal, indicating normal outer hair cells but BERA shows abnormal or absent waves. The patients with severe hearing loss here are also benefited by cochlear implantation.

Prerequisites of Doing Cochlear Implantation

a. Age should be one year and above. The speech centre is maximally active at 3 years. So post implantation the speech development will be easier if implantation has been done early. So implantation should be done as early as possible, the earlier the better. In prelingual deafness the cochlear implant is not much beneficial after 7 years of age as language development will not be possible now. In post-lingual deafness there is no age limit of cochlear implantation.

b. The patients should have an unaided speech discrimination score of 30–50%, indicating severe cochlear pathology, *see* Chapter 2.

c. Minimal or no benefit from hearing aid. Hence, a hearing aid trial of 3–6 months should be given prior to cochlear implant.

d. No evidence of absence of **cochlea, cochlear nerve and central auditory lesions**.

e. The patient should be physically and mentally stable.

PARTS OF COCHLEAR IMPLANT

Cochlear implant has an external component and an internal component.

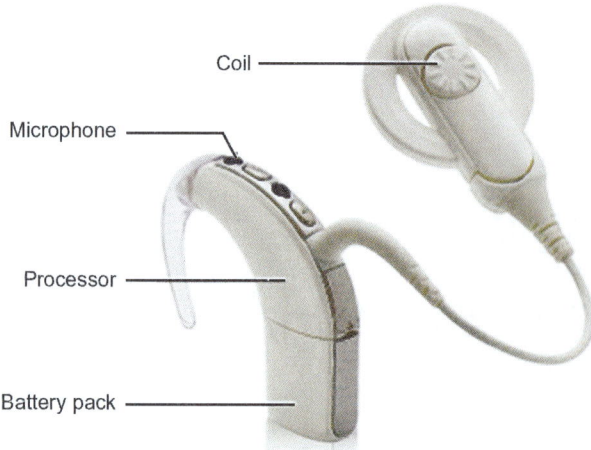

Fig. 15.1

a. **External component:** It comprises a microphone, a speech processor and a transmitter coil which are run by battery.

The microphone and the speech processor (or outer part) looks much like a behind-the-ear hearing aid and is worn on the ear. Attached to the processor is a small transmitter coil that is used to transmit sound from the sound processor to the internal implant. The coil is held in place next to the skin with a small magnet, over the receiver package of internal component, *see* picture on next page.

b. **Internal component:** It consists of a receiver/stimulator package implanted beneath the skin and an electrode array placed in the cochlea.

The internal cochlear implant (or inner part) is placed behind the ear and just under the skin. Attached to the implant is a tiny electrode array, which in the newer devices available comprises 24 electrodes. The surgeon inserts the electrode array into the cochlea in the inner ear, read the procedure below.

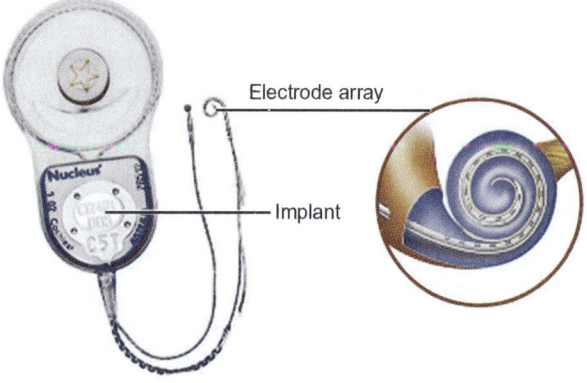

Fig. 15.2

Working of Cochlear Implant

1. The microphone picks up sound from the environment and sends it to the speech processor.
2. The speech processor turns it into a digital signal. The external speech processor then sends this digital signal through the transmitter coil.

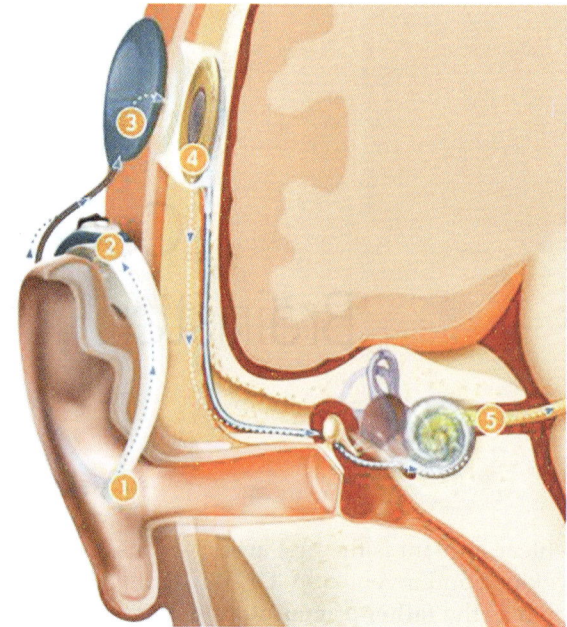

Fig. 15.3

3. The transmitter coil sends this digital signal across the skin (via radio frequency) to the internal cochlear implant system.
4. The internal cochlear implant system changes the digital information into electrical signals and sends them to an electrode array that sits gently inside the inner ear.
5. The electrical signals finally directly stimulate the cochlear nerve. From the cochlear nerve via the auditory pathway, the signal reaches the auditory cortex.

Preoperative Investigations

- **A complete audiological evaluation** is done (PTA, Tympanometry, Speech discrimination tests, OAE, BERA and ASSR, *see* Chapter 2).
- **HRCT and MRI**

These are done to:

a. Study the structure of the cochlea and to find out any cochlear anomalies, or cochlear ossification following meningitis, that may complicate the implantation process. It can also detect the absence of cochlea which is an absolute contraindication to cochlear implantation.

b. Study the cochlear nerve. An absent cochlear nerve is absolute contraindication to cochlear implantation.

c. Find out CNS abnormalities that could adversely affect the outcome of implantation.

PROCEDURE OF IMPLANTATION

Ear selection: B/L cochlear implantation gives better results than U/L implantation as it gives a better sound localisation and better ability to recognise speech. If single ear has to be implanted then the worst ear which benefits least with hearing aid amplification is chosen. This is practised so that if any complication occurs the better ear is still left behind.

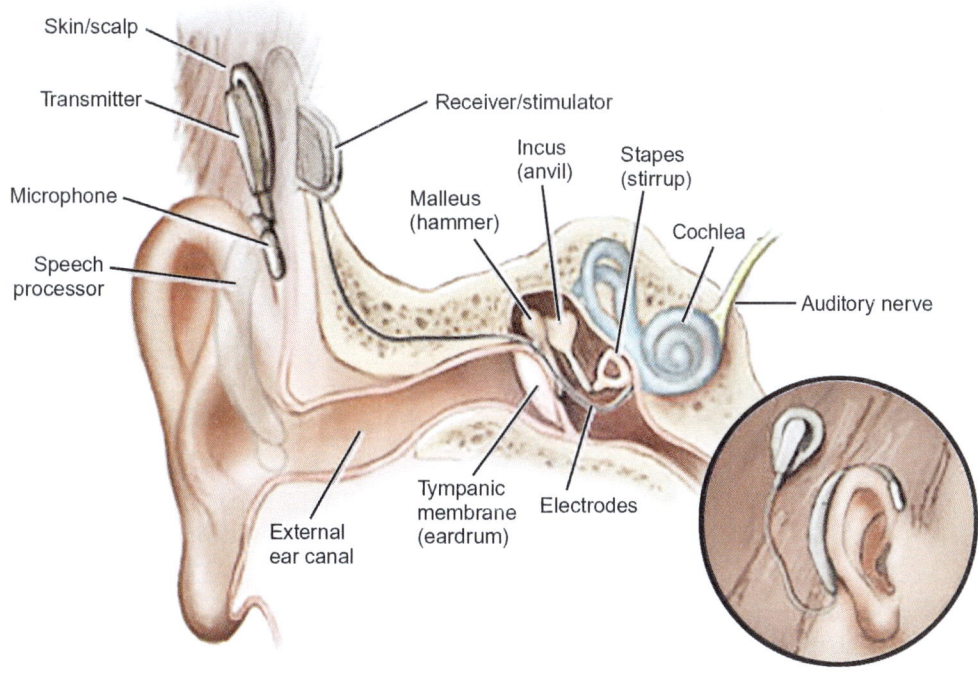

Fig. 15.4

After a postauricular incision, mastoidectomy is done. Posterior to this mastoid cavity a well is drilled where the receiver/stimulator is implanted.,

The electrodes are now passed into the middle ear by making an opening in the **facial recess** area of posterior wall (i.e. **posterior tympanotomy**, *see* Chapter 8).

From the middle ear the electrodes are then introduced into the **scala tympani through the round window**. Insertion of the electrode array can also be done by doing a cochleostomy by widening the anteroinferior lip of round window niche (i.e. opening).

Postoperative Period

Two to four weeks after surgery, when the wound is well healed, the **implant will be activated.**, Activation of the device does not produce "instant" hearing. Initial programming and fine-tuning of the speech processor and auditory training or aural rehabilitation is required.,

Following auditory training, the prelingually deaf children are able to develop good speech and understanding of speech. In patients with cochlear implants in both the ears, localization and discrimination acuity (ability to detect whether sound is arriving from the right or left side) is also improved considerably. Patients of severe to profound hearing loss with tinnitus (which is disturbing perception of noises of different frequencies and intensities in the absence of corresponding sound stimuli) may also have suppression of tinnitus after receiving a cochlear implant. The mechanisms involved in this suppression are not clear.
- Postoperative assessment of the implant is done with an HRCT.
- Postoperative MRI is contraindicated and should, at present, be allowed under restricted conditions only, *see* below.

Some cochlear implants have a removable magnet and specific design characteristics to enable it to withstand MRI of up to 1.5 tesla, but not higher. The magnet must be surgically removed prior to undertaking MRI as tissue damage may occur if the recipient is exposed to MRI with the magnet in place. The patient must take off the sound processor and headset before entering a room where an MRI scanner is located.

Contraindications

As already discussed above Cochlear implantation is contraindicated in the following:
a. Absence of cochlea.
b. Deafness due to an absent cochlear nerve, lesions of the cochlear nerve or central auditory pathway.

AUDITORY BRAIN STEM IMPLANT (ABI)

This implant replaces the auditory nerve and **stimulates the cochlear nucleus directly** so can be used **when both the auditory nerves have been destroyed.**,

It is placed in the lateral recess of 4th ventricle.

It is recommended for rehabilitation of hearing in a patient of B/L acoustic neuromas (as in Neurofibromatosis type 2) whose auditory nerves have been destroyed either by tumour or by surgery. It can also be done in B/L cochlear aplasia or cochlear N aplasia.

Like cochlear implant, ABI also is not recommended in U/L nerve damage as the other ear is functional.

BONE ANCHORED HEARING AID (BAHA)

In patients with conductive or mixed hearing loss with good cochlear function where air conduction hearing aid cannot be used, e.g. atresia of external auditory canal

Section I   Ear

(EAC), microtia, and following MRM with large mastoid cavities, BAHA is a very good option for rehabilitation of hearing.

The BAHA system consists of 3 parts:

1. The **fixture (or implant):** It is a small titanium screw, surgically implanted into the bone behind the ear, with the upper surface exposed outside the skin. As the name, it is fixed into the bone and cannot be removed by the patient. It gets osseo-integrated in the skull bone.

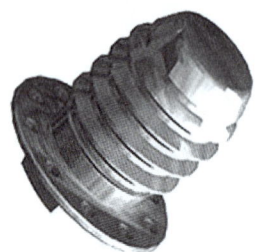

2. The **abutment:** It is a socket attached by screw to the fixture. This socket is shaped to hold the snap-fit coupling of the sound processor, *see* photo below. The abutment can be unscrewed from the fixture for maintenance or replacement.

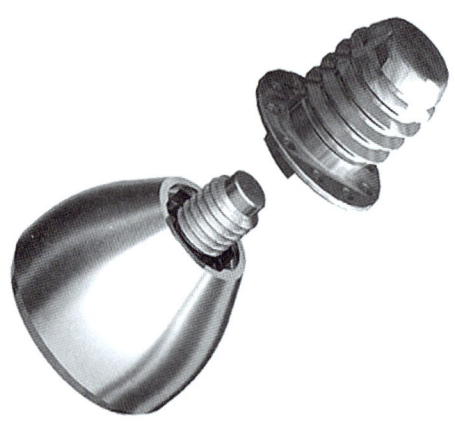

3. The **sound processor:** It is a detachable electronic hearing aid with a snap-fit coupling to the abutment. The user, while washing hair or swimming can remove it.

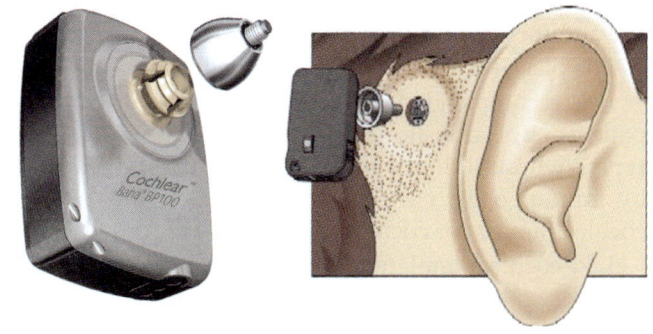

Mechanism of Action

The implant vibrates the skull bone. The bone carries vibrations that bypass the external and middle ear and travel directly to the cochlear nerve.

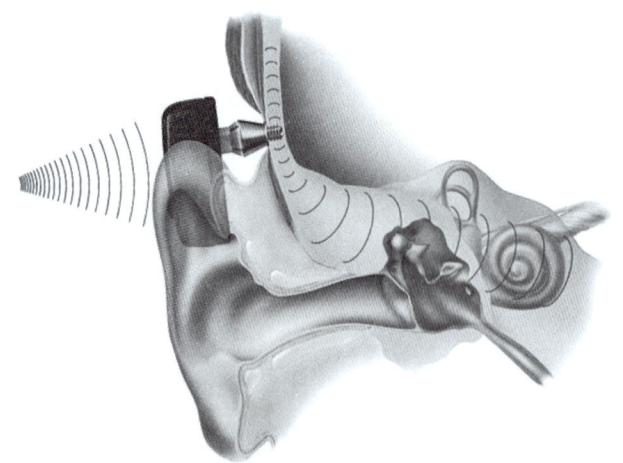

Hence, BAHA bypasses the external auditory canal and middle ear, stimulating the cochlea directly by bone conduction.

Eligibility

BAHA is implanted after 3 years because by this time the skull reaches sufficient thickness to allow osseo-integration. The cochlea and nerve should be functional.

The BC threshold should be better than or equal to 45 dB on PTA.

Indications

1. **Children with atresia of EAC or microtia and anotia:** The reconstructive surgery of pinna (anotia/microtia) is not done before 6 years. This is because the reconstruction is done by autologous costal cartilage, which is sufficiently developed by 6 years for a graft to be taken.

   But these children require hearing augmentation as early as possible for proper speech development. This can be provided by BAHA. In infants with congenital EAC atresias the BAHA can also be fitted to a headband from the age of 3 months till they are old enough for surgery.

2. Patient following MRM with large cavities as a result of which hearing aid is not possible.

3. Patients with chronically discharging ears as a result of which hearing aid is not possible.

4. In **single deaf ear** with no benefit from air conduction hearing aid. As discussed previously cochlear implantation is indicated in B/L severe SN hearing loss not benefited by hearing aids, so in U/L deaf ear cochlear implantation will not be done. When the BAHA is placed on the deaf side, it picks up the sound and transmits it through the bone of the skull (bone conduction) to the inner ear on the hearing side. Hence, it gives better sound localisation of sound coming from the side of deaf ear.

   The utility of BAHA here will be to provide the person an ability to localise the sound coming from the deaf ear's side.

"Points to Ponder/Points for Quick revision"

- Dr William F House—the father of neuro-otology invented cochlear implant
- Cochlear implant—a replacement of the defective organ of Corti (and not complete cochlea)
- Absence of cochlea, defect in cochlear (auditory) nerve or central auditory pathways—contraindications to cochlear implantation
- Indications of cochlear implantation:
  a. B/L severe SNHL (>70 dB) (hearing aid is no longer beneficial and SDS 30–50%)
  b. Mondini aplasia
  c. Auditory neuropathy (this is not cochlear N defect. OAEs are normal. Transduction defect)
- In prelingual (e.g. congenital deafness) cochlear transplantation should be done by 1 year of age so that speech development will be easier
- External components of cochlear implant:
  i. Microphone (picks up sound)
  ii. Speech processor (turns sound into digital signal)
  iii. Transmitter coil (send the digital signal to the receiver/ stimulator part of internal cochlear component)

Internal components:
  iv. Receiver /stimulator package (changes the digital signals into electrical signals) implanted under the skin
  v. Electrode array (24 electrodes) (stimulate the cochlear N with these electrical signals) passed into the middle ear by posterior tympanotomy and then through round window into scala tympani
- Before doing MRI in a person with cochlear implant, the receiver/stimulator package with the magnet has to be removed surgically
- Auditory brain stem implant (ABI): Placed in the lateral recess of 4th ventricle, stimulates cochlear nuclei directly, done in a patient with B/L acoustic neuroma with damage to both the cochlear N, cochlear and cochlear N aplasia.
- Bone anchored hearing aid (BAHA): Bypasses the EAC and middle ear and stimulates the cochlea directly by BC. Used in atresia of EAC, Microtia, Anotia, etc.

Section I Ear

PREVIOUSLY ASKED QUESTIONS

1. Father of Neuro-otology is: *(AIIMS May 2013)*
   a. William F House   b. Julius Lempert
   c. John shea   d. Hayes Martin

2. In a case of bilateral profound hearing loss, what should be done? *(Exam 2013)*
   a. Stapedectomy
   b. Cochlear implant
   c. Hearing aid bone implant
   d. Sodium fluoride

3. Cochlear implant is to be done if the following is intact: *(AIIMS 2007, Exam 2017)*
   a. Outer hair cells   b. Inner hair cells
   c. Auditory nerve   d. All of the above

4. All are true about cochlear implant except: *(AIIMS 2009)*
   a. Minimum age is 1 year
   b. PTA of 70 dB or more
   c. Switch on is done after 3 weeks
   d. MRI has no role in preoperative assessment

5. In cochlear implant electrodes are most commonly introduced through: *(AIIMS 2011)*
   a. Oval window
   b. Round window
   c. Horizontal semi-circular canal
   d. Cochlea

6. In cochlear implantation, which part is placed inside the ear? *(AIIMS Nov 2013)*
   a. Transmitter coil   b. Speech processor
   c. Electrode array   d. Receiver stimulator

7. Cochlear implant electrodes are placed in: *(Bihar 2005, Exam 2017)*
   a. Scala vestibuli   b. Scala tympani
   c. Cochlear duct   d. Endolymphatic duct

8. 3-year-old Rajan is having sensorineural deafness, not benefited by hearing aids. Next best management is: *(AIIMS 2001, Exam 2017)*
   a. Cochlear implant   b. Stapes fixation
   c. Stapedectomy   d. Fenestration

9. Regarding cochlear implant, which of the following is true: *(AIIMS Nov 2010)*
   a. Not contraindicated in cochlear malformation
   b. Contraindicated < 5 years
   c. Indicated in mild to moderate hearing loss
   d. Implanted through oval window

10. All of the following statements about cochlear implants are true, except: *(AI 2012)*
    a. Improved speech and sound perception
    b. Better chance of acquiring normal or near normal verbal skills
    c. Improved sound localization and discrimination is possible
    d. Tinnitus enhancement in patients with tinnitus prior to implantation

11. Which of following would be the most appropriate treatment for rehabilitation of a patient who has bilateral profound deafness following surgery for bilateral acoustic schwannoma: *(AIIMS 2003, Exam 2017)*
    a. Bilateral high powered digital hearing aid
    b. Bilateral cochlear implants
    c. Unilateral cochlear implant
    d. Brain stem implant

12. A 2-year-old child was planned for brain stem implant. All are indications of brain stem implant except: *(AIIMS 2004, Exam 2017)*
    a. B/L neurofibromatosis
    b. Absent auditory nerves
    c. Absent cochlea
    d. Mondini deformity

13. BAHA is used for the conductive hearing loss with the following: *(AIIMS 2013)*
    a. Cochlear malformation
    b. SNHL
    c. B/L acoustic neuroma
    d. Atresia of external ear

14. A newborn presents with bilateral microtia and external auditory canal atresia. Corrective surgery is usually performed at: *(AI 2007, Exam 2017)*
    a. < 1 year of age   b. 5–7 years of age
    c. Puberty   d. Adulthood

15. Internal device of Cochlear implant is: *(AIIMS May 2014)*
    a. Receiver stimulator b. Transmitter Coil
    c. Microphone   d. Speech Processor

16. A cochlear implant is a device designed to create an alternate hearing pathway for people of all ages with bilateral severe profound sensorineural hearing loss. Which of the following normal structures of the ear are directly stimulated by the electrodes: *(Exam 2016)*
    a. Ossicles   b. Oval window
    c. Auditory nerve   d. Intracochlear hair cells

17. Minimum age by which intervention should ideally be in place if a pre-lingually deaf child is to acquire language in a manner as close as possible to normal child in terms of both speed and completeness of development: *(Exam 2016)*
    a. 1 year   b. 4-year
    c. 5-year   d. 6-year

18. Cochlear implants convert which form of energy to which energy: *(Exam 2016)*
    a. Sound energy to mechanical energy to move the hair cells
    b. Electrical energy to mechanical energy to move the hair cells
    c. Sound energy to electrical impulses
    d. Mechanical energy to kinetic energy

19. **Indication of BAHA is:** *(Exam 2016)*
    a. Congenital canal atresia
    b. Bilateral hearing loss
    c. SN hearing loss
    d. All of the above

20. **Electrode of cochlear implant stimulates:** *(UPSC 2015)*
    a. Outer hair cell   b. Inner hair cell
    c. Basilar membrane   d. Auditory nerve

21. **This is showing:** *(Practice question by the Author)*

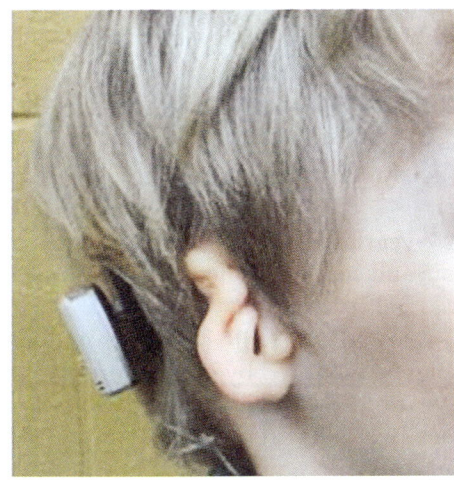

    a. Auditory brain stem implant
    b. Hearing aid
    c. BAHA
    d. Cochlear implant

22. **Modality of rehabilitation for a child with anotia is:** *(Exam 2015)*
    a. In the canal hearing aid
    b. Behind the canal hearing aid
    c. Cochlear implant
    d. BAHA

23. **The below is passed into the inner ear through:** *(Practice question by the Author)*

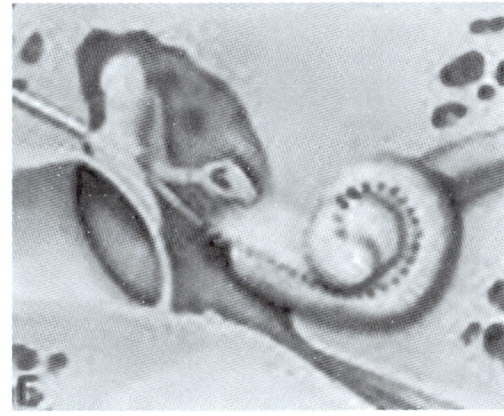

    a. Facial recess   b. Round window
    c. Oval window   d. Bulge of LSC

24. **The below is passed into the middle ear through:** *(Practice question by the Author)*

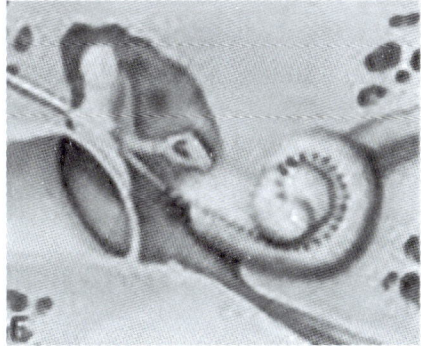

    a. Facial recess   b. Round window
    c. Oval window   d. Aditus

25. **Bone anchored hearing aid (BAHA) can be used for which of the following:** *(Exam 2016)*
    a. A 50-year-old male with bilateral profound hearing loss
    b. A 6-year-old child with bilateral SOM
    c. A 7-year-old child with bilateral microtia, canal atresia and congenital hearing loss
    d. A 25-year-old with bilateral acoustic neuroma planned for surgery

26. **Which device is shown below:** *(Practice question by the Author)*

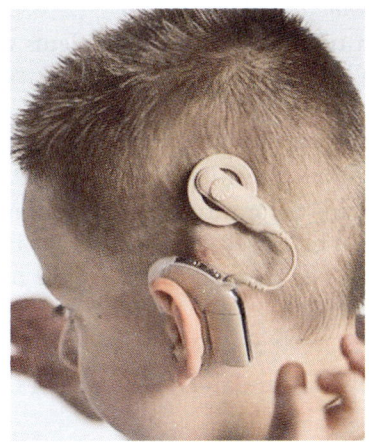

    a. Cochlear implant
    b. Auditory brainstem implant (ABI)
    c. Bone anchored hearing aid (BAHA)
    d. Hearing aid

27. **Total number of electrodes in newer cochlear implants:** *(MAHE 2015)*
    a. 1   b. 10
    c. 24   d. 48

28. **The ABI is placed in which of the following areas?** *(Exam 2015)*
    a. Scala media
    b. CP angle
    c. Lateral recess of 4th ventricle
    d. Pons

29. **Ideal time of treatment of hearing loss for language development is:** *(Exam 2018)*
    a. 6 months   b. 1 year
    c. 2 year   d. 3 year

Ear

Section I

ANSWERS AND EXPLANATIONS

1. **(a) William F House** (*Ref. Scott Brown, 8th ed., Vol 2 page 93*)
2. **(b) Cochlear implant** (*Ref. Cummings, 6th ed., 2432*)
3. **(c) Auditory nerve** (*Ref. Cummings, 6th ed., 2434*)
   - Cochlear implant is done when the defect lies in the Organ of Corti.
4. **(d) MRI has no role in preoperative assessment** (*Ref. Shambaugh, 6th ed., 589; 608*)
   - MRI is contraindicated postoperatively and not pre operatively, please see the text.
5. **(b) Round window** (*Ref. Scott Brown, 8th ed., Vol 2 page 99*)
6. **(c) Electrode array** (*Ref. Scott Brown, 8th ed., Vol 2 page 99*)
7. **(b) Scala tympani** (*Ref. Scott Brown, 8th ed., Vol 2 page 94*)
8. **(a) Cochlear implant** (*Ref. Cummings, 6th ed., 2434*)
   - Stapedectomy is done for otosclerosis.
   - Fenestration operation used to be done previously for otosclerosis, though stapedotomy is done these days.
   - Stapes fixation is no surgery
9. **(a) Not contraindicated in cochlear malformation** (*Ref. Cummings, 6th ed., 2434*)
10. **(d) Tinnitus enhancement in patients with tinnitus prior to implantation.** (*Ref. Scott Brown, 8th ed., Vol 2 page 1158*)
11. **(d) Brain stem implant** (*Ref. Cummings, 6th ed., 2474*)
12. **(d) Mondini deformity** (*Ref. Cummings, 6th ed., 2474*)
    - In Mondini deformity the defect is in the cochlea which can be corrected by a cochlear implant.
13. **(d) Atresia of external ear** (*Ref. Scott Brown, 8th ed., Vol 2 page 1150*)
14. **(b) 5–7 years of age** (*Ref. Cummings, 6th ed., 3000*)
15. **(a) Receiver stimulator** (*Ref. Cummings, 6th ed., 2437*)
16. **(c) Auditory nerve** (*Ref. Scott Brown, 8th ed., Vol 2 page 93*)
17. **(a) 1 year** (*Ref. Cummings, 6th ed., 2434*)
18. **(c) Sound energy to electrical impulses** (*Ref. Cummings, 6th ed., 2429*)
19. **(a) Congenital canal atresia** (*Ref. Cummings, 6th ed., 2425*)
20. **(d) Auditory nerve** (*Ref. Scott Brown, 8th ed., Vol 2 page 93*)
21. **(c) BAHA** (*Ref. Cummings 6th ed., 2423, Scott Brown 8th ed., Vol 2 page 1152*)
22. **(d) BAHA** (*Ref. Scott Brown, 8th ed., Vol 2 page 1150*)
23. **(b) Round window** (*Ref. Scott Brown, 8th ed., Vol 2 page 99*)
24. **(a) Facial recess** (*Ref. Scott Brown, 8th ed., Vol 2 page 1162*)
25. **(c) A 7-year-old child with bilateral microtia, canal atresia and congenital hearing loss** (*Ref. Cummings, 6th ed., 2425*)
    - A 50-year-old male with bilateral profound hearing loss can be managed by cochlear implant
    - A 6-year-old child with bilateral SOM is managed medically and if chronic then by myringotomy and grommet
    - In a 25 year old with bilateral acoustic neuroma planned for surgery rehabilitation of hearing is done with auditory brainstem implant (ABI)
26. **(a) Cochlear implant** (*Ref. Cummings, 6th ed., 2442*)
27. **(c) 24** (*Ref. Scott Brown, 8th ed., Vol 2 page 94*)
28. **(c) Lateral recess of 4th ventricle** (*Ref. Scott Brown, 8th ed., Vol 2 page 1180*)
29. **(a) 6 months** (*Ref. Scott Brown, 8th ed., Vol 2 page 86*)
    - Cochlear implant is done at 1 year but prior to that hearing aid or BAHA soft band is given as early as possible.

Congenital Lesions, Anatomy and Physiology of Nose and Paranasal Sinuses

CHOANAL ATRESIA

During development primitive nasopharynx is separated from the primitive oropharynx by a membrane known as bucconasal membrane which disappears and the nasopharynx starts communicating with the oropharynx.

Persistence of the **bucconasal membrane** leads to the incomplete communication or noncommunication of the nasopharynx with the oropharynx. This condition is known as choanal atresia (choana meaning posterior nares).

There is an increased risk of choanal atresia in children born to hyperthyroid mothers who took **methimazole/ carbimazole** during pregnancy.

Choanal atresia can be unilateral or bilateral with a ratio of 2:1.

It may be mixed, i.e. **bony as well as membranous (70%) or pure bony (30%)**.

U/L choanal atresia is asymptomatic. B/L complete choanal atresia can be life-threatening and the child is born with **respiratory distress.** In such a child, the nasogastric tube does not come into the oropharynx.

Infants are obligatory nasal breathers during the initial 3–5 months. If the nose is obstructed they do not open their mouth and breathe. So the **child is normal while crying** but develops cyanosis and breathlessness when being quiet. Hence for immediate management of this respiratory distress, a wide bore feeding nipple is inserted into the mouth of the infant so that the mouth is actively kept open and the child can respire. This is known as **Mc Govern's technique**.

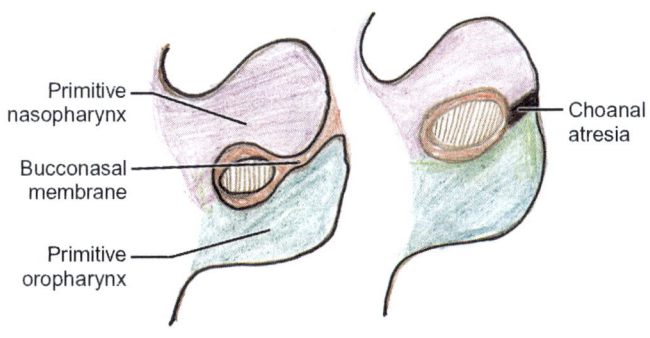

Primitive nasopharynx
Bucconasal membrane
Primitive oropharynx
Choanal atresia

Fig. 16.1: Choanal Atresia

Choanal atresia can be associated with other malformations. The most common of which is "C H A R G E" syndrome which consists of:

C: **C**oloboma of eye (i.e. a hole in iris, choroid or retina) and **C**ranial nerve abnormalities

H: **H**eart abnormalities

A: **A**tresia of nasal choanae

R: **R**etarded growth and development

G: **G**enital (hypogonadism, cryptorchidism) and or urological abnormalities (hypospadias)

E: **E**ar malformations and deafness

Besides the above, other anomalies seen in CHARGE syndrome are facial asymmetry, cleft lip, cleft palate, tracheo-esophageal fistula and impaired cognitive function.

Investigation

As in the majority choanal atresia is bony so CT scan is the best investigation to confirm it.

Management

After initial management with Mc Govern's technique, the child is later taken up for transnasal endoscopic excision or excision by LASER at 1½ years. Post surgery **mitomycin C** can be applied to decrease the chances of re-stenosis.

NASOLABIAL CYST

It is an epithelial inclusion cyst which is extra osseous (i.e. outside the maxillary bone) and located in the region of nasolabial skin fold. It may arise from:

i. Entrapped epithelium at the site of union of medial and lateral nasal process while development of nose and cheek.

ii. Epithelial remnants of nasolacrimal duct.

Since nasolabial cyst is not of odontogenic origin it is also called **non-odontogenic cyst**.

They are present since birth but come into notice once they enlarge or get infected. The **presentation** is usually **late**.

193

They are unilateral and present as swelling in the region of the nasolabial fold raising the upper lip and anterior part of nasal floor (*see* picture below).

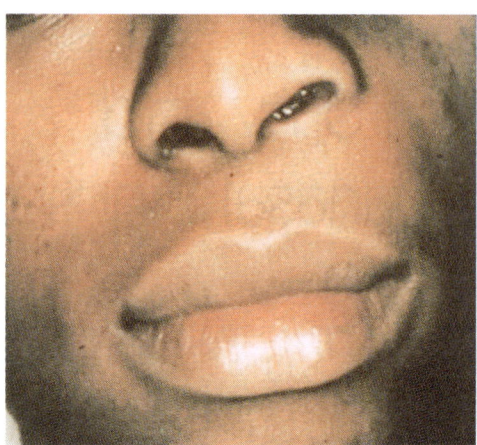

Fig. 16.2

Management is excision by sub-labial approach.

ENCEPHALOCELE

It is a congenital condition where a midline defect in the base of skull leads to herniation of intracranial tissues like meninges (meningocele) alone or along with brain (meningoencephalocele). The **most common location** is occipital followed by frontal. The frontal encephalocele presents at birth as:

i. Subcutaneous **transilluminating, bluish, soft, pulsatile and compressible masses at the root of nose near the glabella** (the glabella is the depressed bone between the eyebrows, above the nasion).

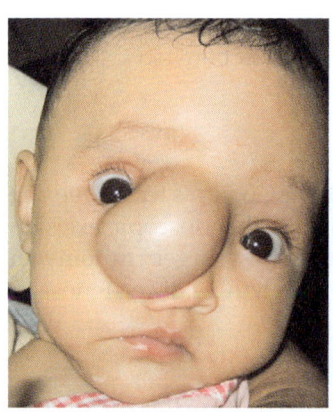 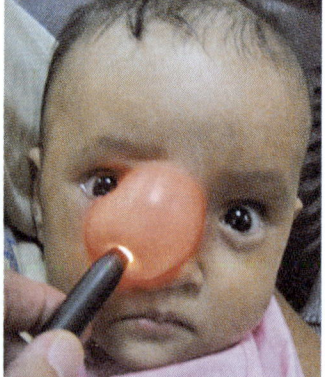

Fig. 16.3

ii. Cystic polypoidal mass inside the nasal cavity leading to nasal obstruction.

iii. CSF rhinorrhoea causing recurrent meningitis.

The mass increases when the child cries or coughs and on bilateral internal jugular venous compression (**positive Furstenberg's test**).

Therefore a small child presenting with nasal polypoid mass should be evaluated by CT and MRI scan for it can be encephalocele. Here CT provides the bony details and soft tissues appear better on MRI. Therefore, both of them

are complimentary to each other and are thus helpful during the reconstruction surgery. Biopsy is contraindicated.

Treatment: It aims at restoring the functional brain tissue in the cranial cavity, performing dural repair and reconstruction of bony defect.

NASAL GLIOMA

It is a misnomer, it is not a tumour. It is similar to encephalocele but with intracranial connection obliterated. It thus presents during infancy as external nasal mass (60%) along the nasal dorsum or intranasal mass (30%) causing intranasal obstruction, or combined (10%).

This mass **is firm, non-compressible, non pulsatile, does not transilluminate and Furstenberg's test** is **negative.** Since their intracranial connection gets obliterated they have low risk for CSF leak and meningitis.

MRI is the best investigation for evaluation and differentiates between glioma and nasal encephalocele. CT scan is also required which provides the bony details
Management is surgical excision.

ANATOMY OF NOSE

The nose is divided into an external nose and an internal nose.

External Nose

The **external nose** is an osteocartilagenous framework of which:

1. The upper 1/3rd is bony.
2. The lower 2/3rd is cartilaginous.

The **bony upper 1/3rd of external nose** is formed by two paired and one unpaired bone. These are:

a. The two **nasal** bones.

b. Lateral to the nasal bones are the two **frontal process of maxilla**.

c. In the centre above nasal bones is the unpaired frontal bone with its two nasal processes on either side of its nasal spine. This intersection of the two nasal bones with the frontal bone above is known as **Nasion**.

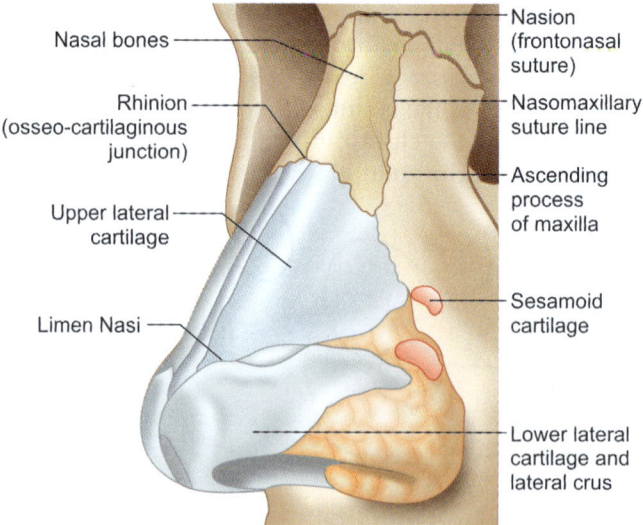

Fig. 16.4: External nose anatomy

The cartilaginous lower 2/3rd of external nose consists of three paired and one unpaired cartilage. These are:
a. Upper lateral cartilage on each side.
b. Lower lateral or alar cartilage on each side.
c. Sesamoid or lesser alar cartilages. The Sesamoid or lesser alar cartilages can also be multiple on each side. They are present just lateral to the lower lateral cartilage or alar cartilage (*see* below).
d. The unpaired cartilage is the antero-superior border of septal cartilage which forms the midline of the lower 2/3rd of the external nose. The complete quadrilateral septal cartilage (*see* below) supports the lower 2/3rd of dorsum of external nose.

Note:

- The two paired cartilages, the upper lateral and lower lateral are called so as they form the lateral part of external nose. The junction of the lower end of the inter nasal suture (i.e. suture in between the two nasal bones) with the lower cartilaginous part of the nose in midline is known as **Rhinion**.
- The two lower lateral cartilages are the lateral crura of the alar crura of both side of which form the columella of the septum.
- The junction of the upper and lower lateral cartilages is known as **limen nasi or limen vestibuli**.
- The limen nasi is the site of intercartilaginous incision in rhinoplasty.
- The limen nasi also forms the lateral boundary of **nasal valve area**. Nasal valve is the **narrowest** part of nasal cavity offering maximum resistance to nasal airflow. The nasal valve is **formed by the limen nasi and anterior end of inferior turbinate laterally and septum medially**.

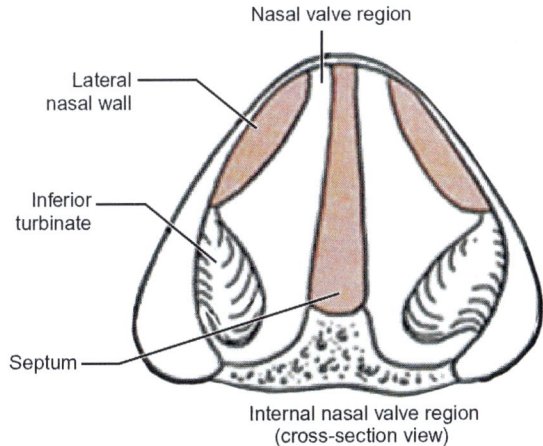

Fig. 16.5

Internal Nose

The internal nose is divided into two nostrils by the septum. Each nostril has a lateral wall, medial wall, a roof and a floor.

Lining membrane of internal nose:
1. **Vestibule:** The antero-inferior part of the nostrils is the continuation of skin and is lined by stratified squamous epithelium with hairs (**vibrissae**), sweat and sebaceous glands and is known as vestibule of nose. A furuncle of the nose arises from the vestibule of nose and hence is known as nasal vestibulitis.

2. **Olfactory epithelium:** This is the lining of the **upper 1/3rd** of the nasal cavity, i.e. the upper 1/3rd of lateral wall, septum and the roof.
3. **Schneiderian membrane:** The main epithelium lining the rest of the nose is **pseudostratified ciliated columnar** containing mucous glands. This is also known as Schneiderian membrane.

Lateral Wall of Nose

In the lateral wall of nose are projections of three bones which are known as **concha** or turbinates. These turbinates increase the surface area of nasal mucosa for better humidification and temperature regulation.

The three turbinates are the **superior, middle and inferior turbinate**. Very rarely above the superior turbinate, there is a **4th turbinate** called **supreme turbinate**.

The largest turbinate is the **inferior turbinate** which occupies **whole of the lateral wall** from anterior to posterior end followed by **middle turbinate** which occupies the **posterior ½** of lateral wall, followed by superior turbinate which occupies only the posterior 1/3rd.

The superior and middle turbinates are parts of ethmoid bone whereas inferior turbinate is an independent separate bone attached to it.

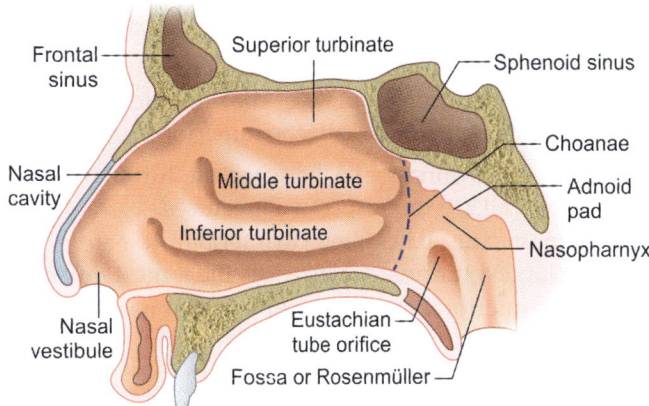

Fig. 16.6: Lateral wall of nose

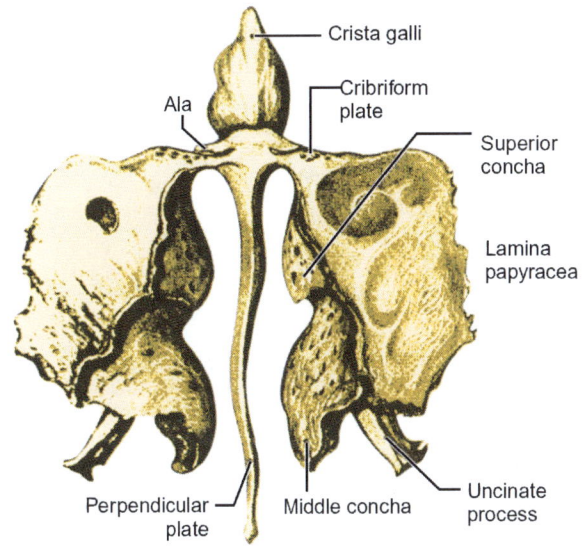

Fig. 16.7

The ethmoid bone is a very important bone of the nose. The various **parts of ethmoid bone** in the nose are:

Laterally

i. Superior and middle turbinate

ii. **Lamina papyracea;** it is a thin papery bone separating nasal cavity from orbit, forming the medial wall of orbit. Hence it is the weakest wall of orbit.

iii. **Uncinate process;** a sickle shaped bone. It forms the lower boundary of hiatus semilunaris (*see* below).

    The lateral wall of the ethmoid bone is pneumatised and contains multiple air cells which constitute **anterior and posterior ethmoid sinuses**.

Medially

iv. **Perpendicular plate of ethmoid;** it forms the bony part of nasal septum (it attaches to quadrilateral septal cartilage on its postero-superior aspect, *see* the septum below).

Superiorly

v. **Cribriform plate:** It is divided into two parts as medial and lateral lamellas. The medial part which forms roof of the nose, separating nasal cavity from anterior cranial fossa is known as medial lamella. The lateral part that forms the roof of ethmoid sinuses is known as lateral lamella. This is the most common site of CSF rhinorrhoea.

vi. The Crista galli is a median ridge of bone that projects from the cribriform plate of the ethmoid bone. It is where the falx cerebri attaches anteriorly to the skull.

Lateral to the turbinates, i.e. between the turbinates and the lateral wall are the respective meatuses.

1. **Inferior meatus:** It lies lateral to inferior turbinate which is the largest turbinate, hence it is the largest meatus.

    In the inferior meatus is the **opening of nasolacrimal duct (NLD)**.

    The nasolacrimal duct begins at the lower end of lacrimal sac and runs **downwards, backwards and laterally** to open just anterior to the highest point (junction of anterior 1/3rd and posterior 2/3rd) of the inferior turbinate. *Mnemonic:* The direction of NLD can be remembered as—we have two, i.e. **DOUBLE** NLDs—**D**ownwards

Backwards, Laterally). This opening of nasolacrimal duct is bounded by a valve known as **valve of Hasner**.

2. **Middle meatus:** It lies lateral to the middle turbinate.

    In the middle meatus is the opening of anterior group of sinuses which are the **maxillary sinus, frontal sinus and the anterior ethmoids** (*see* below). The frontal sinus opens in the antero-superior part of middle meatus via frontonasal duct also called frontal recess. The anterior ethmoids open on the surface of bulla ethmoidalis.

    The **bulla ethmoidalis** is the most prominent anterior ethmoidal sinus cell which appears as a bulge in the middle meatus. Just below the bulla ethmoidalis in the middle meatus is the sickle shaped bone, the **uncinate process** of ethmoid. In between the bulla above and uncinate below there is a semi lunar opening, known as **hiatus semilunaris**.

    Through the hiatus semilunaris we enter into the three dimensional area known as **infundibulum** into which opens the maxillary sinus directly.

    All these structures of the middle meatus together constitute **osteomeatal complex** or **"Picadle's circle"**.

    It is known as a complex as all the three sinuses are opening together into a common area, so any sinusitis of one sinus can lead to the other sinusitis also.

    Also any deformity of the middle turbinate (e.g. concha bullosa, paradoxically curved middle turbinate; *see* below) will predispose to all the three sinusitis.

    The middle turbinate is usually not pneumatised. The pneumatisation of middle turbinate is known as **concha bullosa (bullous turbinate)** (*see* Fig. 16.10).

    This bullous turbinate blocks the drainage of middle meatal area leading to all the three sinusitis. Middle turbinate is usually concave towards middle meatus. A paradoxically curved middle turbinate becomes convex facing the meatus leading to interference with drainage of all the three sinuses.

Agger Nasi: The Agger nasi cell is the anterior most anterior ethmoid sinus cell that is present in almost all individuals just **anterior to the anterior free margin of middle turbinate**.

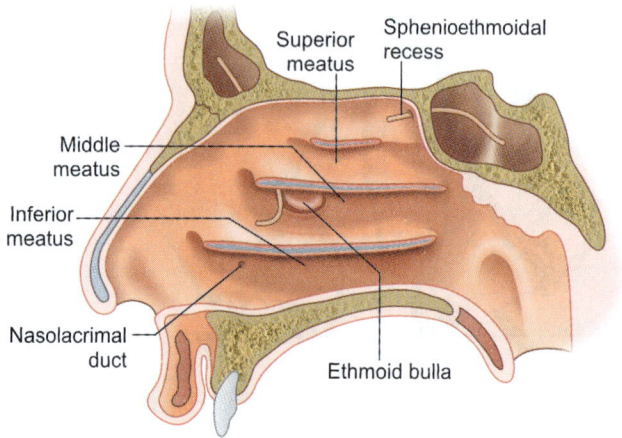

Fig. 16.8: Meatuses in lateral wall of nose

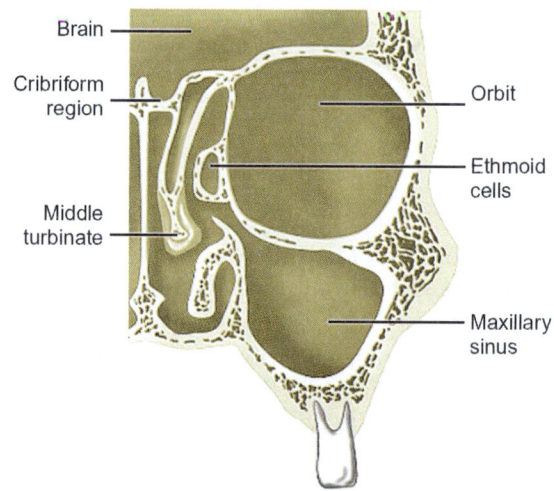

Fig. 16.9: Osteomeatal complex

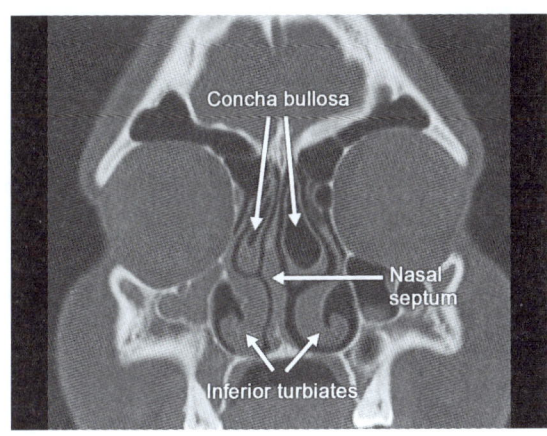

Fig. 16.10: Osteomeatal complex

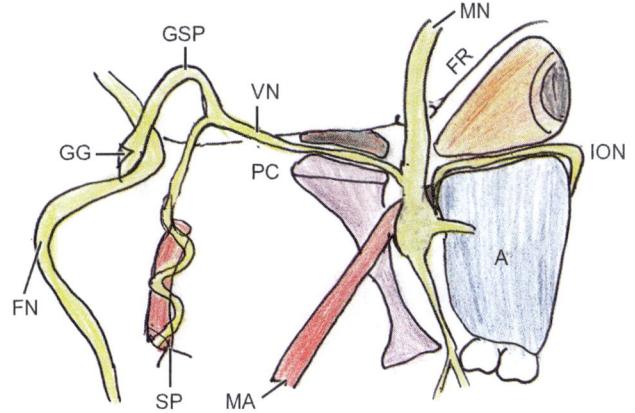

ION: Infraorbital nerve	MN: Maxillary nerve
FR: Foramen rotundum	MA: Maxillary artery
FN: Facial nerve	VN: Vidian nerve
SPG: Sphenopalatine ganglion	PC: Pterygoid canal
GSP: Greater superficial petrosal nerve	A: Antrum of maxilla
SP: Sympathetic plexus around	GG: Geniculate ganglion
internal carotid	DP: Deep petrosal

Fig. 16.11: Sphenopalatine fossa and its contents

Its size may influence patency of frontal recess or fronto-nasal duct and hence drainage of the frontal sinus in the middle meatus.

3. **Superior meatus:** It lies lateral to the superior turbinate. In it opens the **posterior ethmoid sinuses**.

Sphenoethmoidal Recess

This is the area above the superior turbinate. The **sphenoid sinus opens here**. It is known as spheno-ethmoidal recess as it is the recess (deep space) in between the sphenoid superiorly and posterior ethmoids inferiorly.

Important Structures in the Nasopharynx in Relation to the Lateral Wall of Nose

The lateral wall of nose ends at the posterior border of turbinates. **Beyond the turbinates the lateral wall of nose continues as the lateral wall of nasopharynx.**

Eustachian tube: 1.25 cm posterior and just inferior to the posterior end of **inferior turbinate** is the opening of **Eustachian tube (ET)** in the nasopharynx (*Mnemonic:* Behind the Inferior turbinate is ET- sound of vowel **E** = Inferior).

Sphenopalatine foramen: About 1 cm posterior and a little inferior to the posterior end of **middle turbinate** is the opening of the **sphenopalatine foramen** named so as it connects the nasopharynx laterally with sphenopalatine fossa (also known as pterygopalatine fossa).

In the sphenopalatine fossa are present, the **sphenopalatine ganglion** (the largest parasympathetic ganglion), the **maxillary artery** and the **maxillary nerve**.

The sphenopalatine fossa lies just posterior to the maxillary antrum. This fossa can be reached by the **Caldwell Luc** approach (sub labial incision and then drilling the anterior and posterior wall of maxillary antrum).

The boundaries of sphenopalatine fossa are:

1. **Anteriorly:** The posterior wall of the maxillary antrum.
2. **Posteriorly:** The pterygoid plates (part of sphenoid). At the root of pterygoid plate in the base of skull are two foramina:
   i. Foramen rotundum in the base of skull through which the maxillary nerve enters the sphenopalatine fossa
   ii. Foramen leading to pterygoid canal through which the vidian nerve enters the sphenopalatine fossa and relay in the sphenopalatine ganglion, *see* the nerve supply below.
3. **Medially:** The lateral wall of nasopharynx (formed by perpendicular plate of palatine bone on which is the sphenopalatine foramen).
4. **Laterally:** It opens into the infratemporal fossa via the pterygomaxillary fissure.
5. **Floor:** Formed by the palate containing the palatine canal through which the greater palatine artery from the fossa enters the palate.
6. **Roof:** Formed by the floor of orbit containing the inferior orbital fissure

The **sphenopalatine foramen** is important for two reasons:

1. The **main vessel supplying the nose, i.e. sphenopalatine artery** (a branch of maxillary artery present in the sphenopalatine fossa) enters the nose through this foramen. This is known as the artery of epistaxis and can be ligated here. If epistaxis does not get controlled then maxillary artery can be ligated in the sphenopalatine fossa (*see* the section on blood supply of nose below).
2. The sphenopalatine foramen is the **most common site of origin of angiofibroma**.

Medial Wall/Septum

The medial wall of the nose is the septum. It supports the dorsum and divides nose into two nasal cavities.

Septum has Three Parts

a. **Columellar septum:** This is formed by the fusion of the two medial crura of alar cartilages.
b. **Membranous septum:** Just above the columellar cartilage is an area devoid of any cartilage. Only the skin of both sides are meeting here.

Nose

Section II

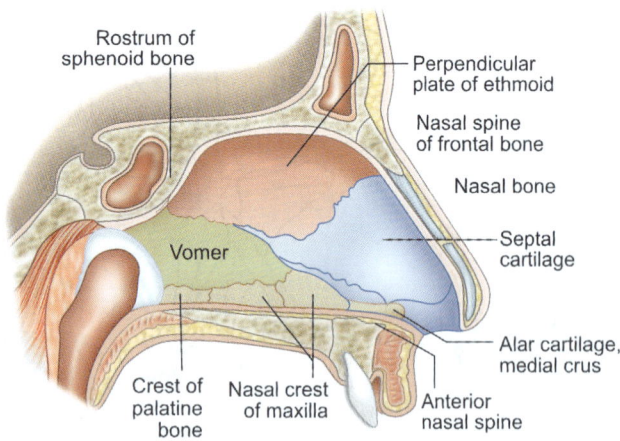

Fig. 16.12: Septum

c. **Septum proper:** Above membranous septum is the septum proper which is an osteocartilagenous framework, i.e. partly bony and partly cartilaginous. It is formed by:
   i. Antero-inferiorly by the **quadrilateral cartilage**, named so because of its quadrilateral shape. **The anterior side of this cartilage forms the lower 2/3rd of the dorsum of external nose**. So one has to be very careful while dealing with this septal cartilage, because if damaged it will lead to the saddling of nose. The **postero-superior, postero-inferior and inferior sides are in contact with the perpendicular plate of ethmoid, vomer and the anterior nasal spine of maxilla** (all bones) respectively.
   ii. Superiorly by the perpendicular plate of **ethmoid bone**.
   iii. Postero-inferiorly by **vomer bone**.

Along with these major components some small bones contribute to the septum e.g. nasal spine of **frontal** bone (anteriorly), rostrum of **sphenoid** (postero-superiorly behind the perpendicular plate of ethmoid), crest of maxilla and crest of **palatine** bones inferiorly.

Roof

The roof of nose is formed mainly by the cribriform plate of the ethmoid. A small sloping part anteriorly is formed by nasal process of frontal bone and posteriorly by body of sphenoid.

Floor

Floor of the nose is the palate formed by the palatine process of maxilla anteriorly (3/4th) and horizontal process of palatine bone posteriorly (1/4th).

BLOOD SUPPLY OF NOSE

Arterial Supply

The nose is supplied by **both external and internal carotid, main arterial supply being the external carotid**. The area below the upper part of middle turbinate of the nose is supplied mainly by external carotid whereas the area above it, is supplied mainly by internal carotid artery.

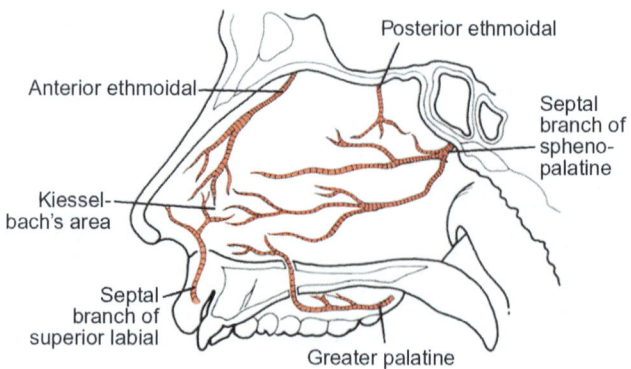

Fig. 16.13: Kiesselbach's plexus

From **external carotid** we have the **maxillary and facial arteries** supplying the nose.

Maxillary artery gives two branches in the sphenopalatine fossa:
   i. **Sphenopalatine**; it enters the nose through the same name foramen, i.e. Sphenopalatine foramen. This is the **main artery** supplying the nose.
   ii. **Greater palatine**; it supplies the palate and then enters the nose to supply it.

From the **Facial**:
• **Septal branch of superior labial** supplies the nose.

From internal carotid we have two branches of ophthalmic:
   i. **Anterior ethmoidal artery**
   ii. **Posterior ethmoidal artery**

The anterior and posterior ethmoidal arteries are given off by the **ophthalmic artery** in the orbital cavity.

Each of these arteries then pierces the medial wall of orbit through the same name foramen to enter the nose.

The anterior ethmoidal foramen lies 24 mm posterior to the lacrimal crest. The posterior ethmoidal foramen lies 12 mm posterior to anterior ethmoidal foramen. The posterior ethmoidal artery acts as a landmark for optic nerve which lies 6 mm posterior to posterior ethmoidal foramen.

All the above arteries **except posterior ethmoidal**, form a plexus on the antero-interior part of nasal septum just above the vestibule in an area known as **"LITTLE'S AREA"**.

This plexus is known as **"KIESSELBACH'S PLEXUS"**.

So the components of Kiesselbach's plexus are:
1. **Sphenopalatine**
2. **Greater palatine**
3. **Superior labial**
4. Septal branches of **anterior ethmoidal**

Little's area is the most common site of epistaxis in young and here epistaxis occurs following trauma due to nose picking. So the epistaxis is usually arterial.

Since **Sphenopalatine** is the main artery supplying the nose, it is also known as the **artery of epistaxis**.

In the posterior part of inferior turbinate is another plexus formed by anastomosis of the posterior nasal branches of sphenopalatine and pharyngeal arterial branches. This is considered as the **most common site of epistaxis in elderly and occurs in hypertension**.

Epistaxis can also be venous from retrocolumellar vein which as per its name, runs behind the columella, crosses the floor of nose and forms a venous plexus on the lateral wall of nose.

VENOUS DRAINAGE

Venous drainage follows the arterial supply:
i. The superior part of nose drains into ophthalmic veins which communicate with cavernous sinus.
ii. Posterior part drains into sphenopalatine veins and then into the pterygoid plexus of veins which also communicate with cavernous sinus and dural venous system.
iii. The **dangerous area of face** and the antero-inferior part of the nose drains into the deep facial vein which communicates with the pterygoid plexus of veins and therefore with cavernous sinus and dural venous system.

So **the venous drainage is a potential vehicle for spread of nasal infections intracranially.**

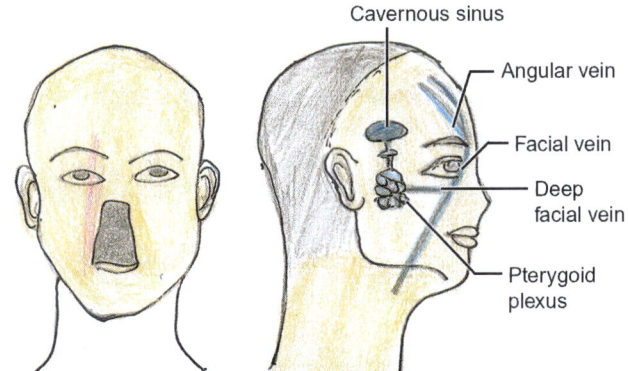

Fig. 16.14: Dangerous area of face

NERVE SUPPLY

The nerve supply of **external nose**:
i. The **Ophthalmic division of trigeminal nerve (V1) supply the root, dorsum and tip of external nose (via nasociliary branch)**.
ii. The side and ala of nose is supplied by **Maxillary division of trigeminal nerve (V2)**. *See* Fig. 20.1a and 20.1b on nerve supply of face in Chapter 20 on Sinusitis.

The nerve supply of **internal nose** is divided into three parts:
i. **Olfactory** nerves; the olfactory epithelium lines the upper 1/3rd and roof of the nasal cavity. From here around 12–20 olfactory nerves pass through the cribriform plate to end in olfactory bulb, read olfaction below.
ii. The rest of the sensory supply of the internal nose is supplied by **ophthalmic V1 (via anterior and posterior ethmoidal nerves) and maxillary V2** division of the trigeminal nerve.

iii. The autonomic supply of the nose is by the **vidian nerve** which is formed by the fusion of **greater superficial petrosal (1st branch of facial nerve, parasympathetic) and deep petrosal (given from the sympathetic plexus around the internal carotid artery)**.

These two fuse in the cranium to form the vidian nerve, which then exits through a foramen in the base of skull at the root of pterygoid plate. This foramen leads to **pterygoid canal (hence vidian nerve is also known as nerve of pterygoid canal)** after passing through which the vidian nerve enters the spheno-palatine fossa. In the sphenopalatine fossa the parasympathetic fibres relay in the sphenopalatine ganglion, which then gives parasympathetic supply to the nasal, nasopharyngeal, palatine mucosal glands and lacrimal gland.

Vidian nerve is sectioned in parasympathetic over activity seen in vasomotor rhinitis, read Chapter 19.

PARA NASAL SINUSES

There are four paired Para nasal sinuses. The horizontal attachment of the middle turbinate to the lateral nasal wall known as ground lamella or basal lamella, divides the paranasal sinuses into anterior and posterior groups.

Anterior group	Maxillary, frontal sinuses and anterior ethmoids
Posterior group	**Sphenoid and posterior ethmoids.**

Since the paranasal sinuses develop as lateral out pouching from the lateral wall of nose, they are also lined by pseudostratified ciliated columnar epithelium. They decrease the weight of the skull and provide resonant chambers for voice.

MAXILLARY SINUS/ANTRUM

(*see* Table 16.1)

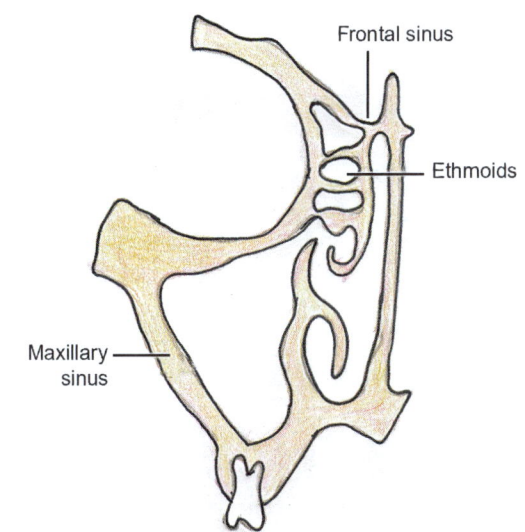

Fig. 16.15: Anterior group of sinuses

It is a pyramidal shaped sinus with its apex lying towards the zygomatic bone. The base (or the medial wall) forms the lateral wall of nose. The roof forms the floor of orbit and is traversed by Infraorbital nerve and vessels.

The floor of the maxillary sinus lies 1 cm below the level of floor of nose and is related to **2nd premolar and 1st molar**. Sometimes it may also be related to 2nd and 3rd molars. Therefore extraction of these teeth can lead to an oro-antral fistula.

The maxillary sinus **opens into the infundibulum of middle meatus**. Since the ostia of middle meatus is much above the floor of the sinus, drainage becomes antigravity leading to collection of secretions and therefore an increased predisposition to sinusitis, making it the **most common sinus to get infected**.

ETHMOID SINUS

The ethmoids are multiple group of air cells present in lateral wall of ethmoid bone and are divided into anterior and posterior groups.

Three cells among anterior ethmoid cells have been named, Bulla ethmoidalis, Agger nasi (*see* above) and Haller cell.

The anterior ethmoidal cells in the **floor of orbit** are known as **"Haller cell" or infra orbital anterior ethmoid cell** (in the CT scan below-the asterisk showing a Haller cell).

The anterior ethmoids open on the surface of bulla ethmoidalis in the middle meatus.

Clinical significance of Haller cell:

i. If infected can cause orbital cellulitis.
ii. While removing disease from Haller cell, there are chances of injury to the orbit during endoscopic surgery.
iii. If large it may narrow the ipsilateral osteomeatal complex (OMC), thereby predisposing to anterior group sinusitis.

The **posterior ethmoids** open into the **superior meatus**.

One posterior ethmoid cell has been named: The posterior most posterior ethmoid cell extending lateral to

the sphenoid sinus is known as **"Onodi cell"**. While removing disease from the Onodi cells there are chances of injury to **optic nerve and internal carotid** artery which lie in the vicinity, read below.

FRONTAL SINUS

This is the superior most placed sinus in the head. The septa that divides the frontal sinuses (of the two sides) is paramedian and obliquely placed so the two frontal sinuses are asymmetrical.

It opens into the **middle meatus** by frontonasal duct or frontal recess (*see* the importance of Agger nasi above).

SPHENOID SINUS

They are situated in the **body of the sphenoid bone**. Like the two frontal sinuses, sphenoid sinuses also do not have symmetrical shape because the dividing bony septum is obliquely placed.

When the sphenoid sinus grows it begins to pneumatise the body of the sphenoid bone. The pattern of pneumatisation of the sphenoid sinus significantly affects the safe access to the pituitary gland in **trans-sphenoidal approach** for pituitary adenomas.

Three types of sphenoid sinus pneumatisation patterns have been found depending upon the position of the sinus in relation to the sella turcica (pituitary fossa) over the body of sphenoid:

a. **Conchal**; no pneumatisation below the sella. Here there is a solid block of bone beneath the sella.
b. **Pre sellar**; pneumatisation does not extend beyond the anterior border of sella turcica.
c. **Sellar/Post sellar**; here pneumatisation is below and posterior to the sella turcica. This is the most common type of sphenoid pneumatisation seen among individuals.

The roof of the sphenoid sinus is related to the pituitary gland and the lateral walls are related to optic nerve, internal carotid artery, cavernous sinus and cranial nerves III, IV, V1, V2 and VI. These can be damaged during surgery on Sphenoid sinus.

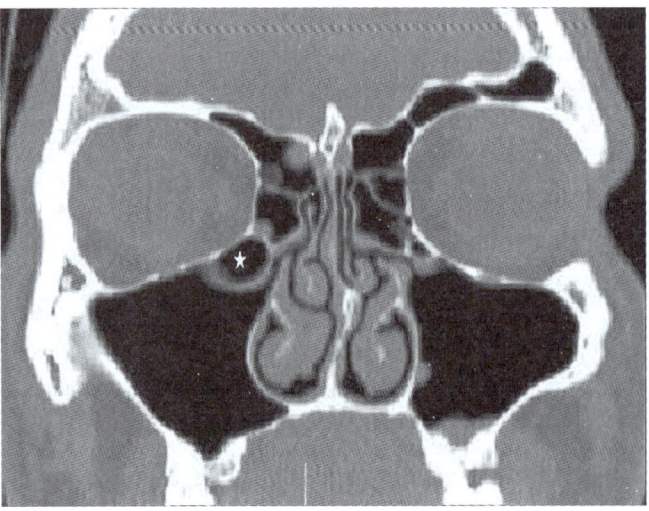

Fig. 16.16

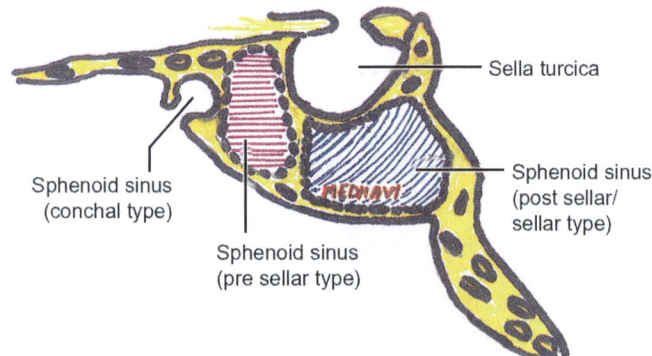

Fig. 16.17: Various pneumatisation patterns of sphenoid sinus in the body of sphenoid bone

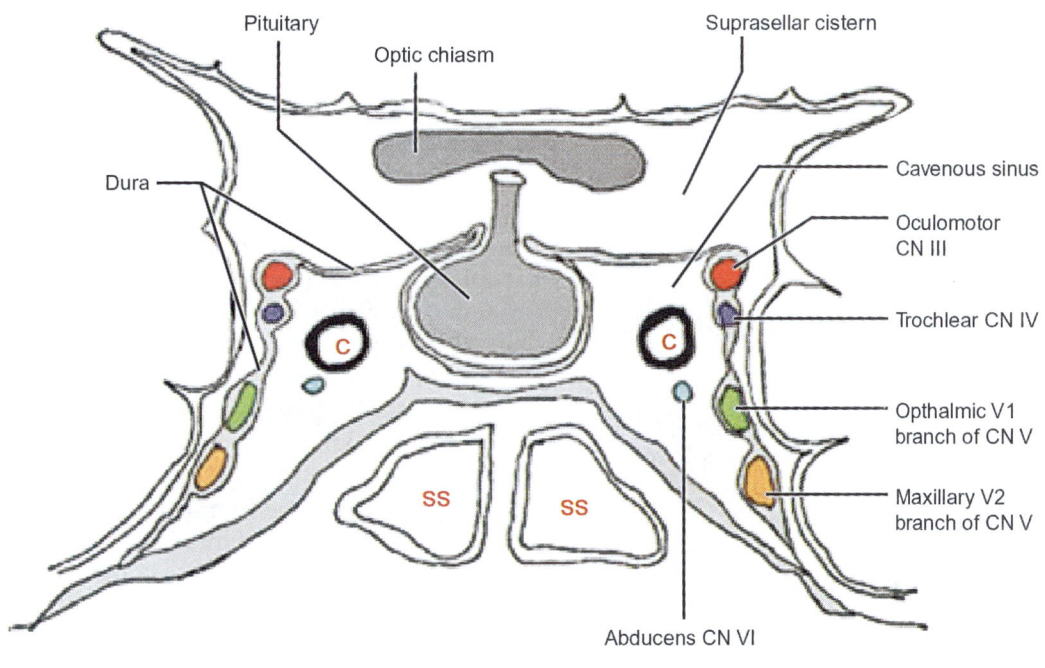

Fig. 16.18: Relations of sphenoid Sinus

Important Features of Para Nasal Sinuses

Table 16.1				
Sinus	*Maxillary*	*Frontal*	*Ethmoids*	*Sphenoid*
Opening	Infundibulum of middle meatus	By Fronto-nasal recess into middle meatus	• Anterior ethmoids—middle meatus • Posterior ethmoids—superior meatus	Spheno-ethmoidal recess above the superior turbinate
At birth	Present Size increases with age becoming almost maximum by the time of completion of secondary dentition (of 2nd premolar and 1st molar), i.e. 12 years, further enlargement coincides with the development of 2nd and 3rd molars till 18 years	**Absent** Attains full size by 19 years	Present Size increases with age reaching a maximum by 15 years	Present (but small) Attains full size by 15 years
X-ray identification at	4–5 months	6 years	1 year	4 years
Capacity	15 ml	7 ml	2–3 ml	0.5–5 ml
Nerve supply	**Maxillary V$_2$ (infra orbital and alveolar nerves)**	Ophthalmic (V$_1$) (supra orbital branch)	Ophthalmic V$_1$ (nasociliary branch) and Maxillary V$_2$ (from sphenopalatine fossa)	**Ophthalmic V$_1$ (nasociliary branch) and Maxillary V$_2$ (from sphenopalatine fossa)**
Remarks	• **Earliest sinus to develop** • **Most common sinusitis in adults** • **Largest paranasal sinus** • Also known as the **antrum of "Highmore"**	**Last sinus to develop**	**Most pneumatised at birth so Most common sinusitis in infants and young children**	**High opening so least commonly infected**

PHYSIOLOGY OF NOSE

Respiration

The main current of airflow passes through the **middle part of the nose** in a parabolic curve **both during inspiration and expiration** (*see* **Fig. 16.9**).

During expiration, the narrowest part of nasal cavity, i.e. the nasal valve area, offers maximum resistance to the nasal airflow leading to the formation of eddy currents which ventilates the sinuses.

So the **ventilation of sinuses occurs during expiration**.

Nasal Cycle

This is a physiological cycle of nasal congestion and decongestion alternating between the two nasal cavities which mean that only one nostril functions at a time. The nasal cycle varies from 2–4 hours.

Humidification

In dry atmospheric conditions the inspired air is humidified to 75% or more in the nose.

Temperature Regulation

However hot or cold the inspired air may be, it is regulated to body temperature in ¼th of a second that the air takes to reach the choana from anterior nares. This is by the radiator mechanism of the **extensive cavernous venous spaces** in the nasal mucosa. Also the turbinates increase the surface area of the nasal mucosa helping in the radiator mechanism.

Therefore, the part of the nose, **maximum affected** by the **hot or cold air is anterior 1/3rd**.

Protection of Lower Airway

Nasal mucosa contains goblet cells responsible for the secretion of mucous. The cilia of nasal mucosa beat 10–20 times per second at room temperature and at a normal nasal pH of 7 making the mucous blanket to move at a speed of **5–10 mm/min**, clearing the complete shed of mucus into the nasopharynx every 10–20 minutes. **The inspired bacteria, viruses and dust particles are entrapped in the mucous blanket.**

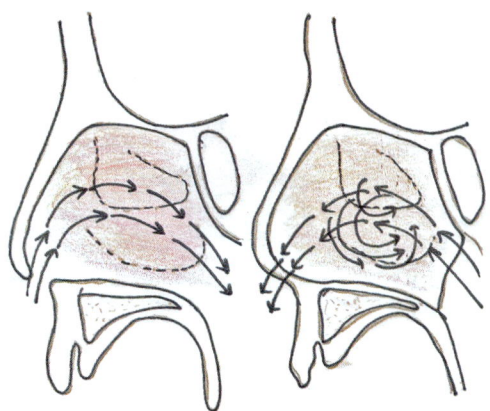

Fig. 16.19

Nasal secretions also contain enzymes, immunoglobulin A, and interferon which provide immunity against upper respiratory infections.

Nasal Resonance

When we speak certain words (nasal consonants m/n/ng), they pass through the nose and acquire a resonance which is known as nasal resonance. When the **nose or nasopharynx is obstructed** these words now cannot pass through the nose and the voice is known as hyponasal, denasal or **rhinolalia clausa**.

When the words which usually do not pass through the nose also starts passing and thus acquiring nasal resonance it is known as **hypernasality** or **rhinolalia aperta**.

The causes of rhinolalia aperta are any condition leading to velopharyngeal insufficiency.

When we eat or when we speak the words, which do not have to pass through the nose, the soft palate moves posteriorly and meets the **passavant's ridge** (*see* the chapter on anatomy of pharynx) to close the nasopharyngeal isthmus. Whenever the palate is not able to move posteriorly a gap is produced through which words and food which usually do not pass through the nose, starts passing through it. This is known as **velopharyngeal** or nasopharyngeal **insufficiency**.

The causes of velopharyngeal insufficiency are: cleft palate, bifid uvula, sub mucus cleft (i.e. cleft palate covered by mucosa so that cleft cannot be seen but palpated) and paralysed palate.

Olfaction

Olfactory epithelium lines the upper 1/3rd and roof of the nasal cavity. During normal respiration, where the main airway passes through the middle part of nose, only around 10% reaches the olfactory epithelium. Hence, whenever we have to smell something properly we sniff to take the air to the olfactory region. Also during swallowing of food there occurs some retro nasal airflow to the upper nasal cavity, further adding flavour to food (i.e. adding smell to taste). In the olfactory epithelium (pseudostratified ciliated columnar) are present the olfactory receptors.

The odorous chemicals after reaching the upper 1/3rd of nasal cavity dissolve in the olfactory mucus and diffuse to olfactory receptors present on the cilia. These olfactory receptors are the dendrites of sensory bipolar cells. These signals are then carried by the axons of these sensory bipolar cells. These axons coalesce to form bundles which are called as olfactory nerves (these are unmyelinated).

There are around 12–20 olfactory nerves which pass through the cribriform plate to end in olfactory bulb. In the olfactory bulb the cell bodies (mitral/tufted cells) of the second order olfactory neurons lie. Axons or Nerve fibres from here now called olfactory tracts project to the primary olfactory cortex (amygdala, piriform and entorhinal cortices) where odour identification occurs.

Note:

Taste related impulses are carried by Facial (anterior 2/3rd of tongue), Glossopharyngeal and Vagus (posterior 1/3rd of tongue) nerves to the olfactory cortex. This further adds flavour to the food.

When the sense of smell is decreased it is known as **hyposmia**. The normal age related decline in the ability to smell is called **presbyosmia**.

Total loss of smell is known as **anosmia**.

Anosmia or hyposmia can be because of:

1. Nasal obstruction leading to impaired transportation to olfactory area (e.g. **DNS, ethmoidal nasal polyps**)
2. Temporary damage to cilia of receptor cells, e.g. rhinitis (**common cold or coryza,** *see* Chapter on rhinitis)
3. Permanent damage to:
   a. Olfactory mucosa, e.g. in **atrophic rhinitis**
   b. Olfactory nerves, e.g. **head trauma** (due to shearing of olfactory nerves as they pass through the cribriform plate, cribriform plate fractures)
   c. Olfactory tract damage owing to tumours involving frontal lobe.

In addition to above, important neurodegenerative diseases are accompanied by olfactory impairment due to central involvements, e.g. Alzheimer's disease, Parkinson's disease and Multiple sclerosis.

Congenital anosmia is seen in "**Kallmann Syndrome**", an X-linked disorder characterised by hypogonadotrophic hypogonadism.

Note:

A patient of anosmia will respond to inhalation of ammonia or alcohol, etc. as these are irritants and the irritation is perceived by trigeminal nerve. Therefore **ammonia** is never used for testing smell sensation, i.e. for testing olfactory nerve.

Parosmia (Cacosmia or Dysosmia)

This is perversion of smell where good smell appears bad to the patient. It occurs due to aberrant regeneration of olfactory nerves following influenza epidemics. It can also follow intracranial tumours.

Phantosmia is perceiving smell in the absence of odourous stimulus. It is seen in temporal lobe seizures, schizophrenia, etc.

Rhinomanometry

It is a diagnostic test to objectively evaluate the respiratory function of the nose. The uses of nasal Rhinomanometry are:

a. It measures nasal airway resistance by measuring pressure and flow during normal inspiration and expiration through the nose. Increased pressure during respiration is a result of increased resistance to airflow through nasal passages, while increased flow is related to better patency. Nasal obstruction leads to increased values of nasal resistance.
b. It can be used to differentiate between anatomical and mucosal abnormalities by performing the tests with a decongestant.
c. It can also be used to check impact of other treatments, like nasal steroid sprays, in conditions causing nasal blockage.

Examination of Nose in the ENT OPD

Anterior Rhinoscopy: Thudichum's speculum (*see* Chapter on instruments at the end) is used to visualise the anterior nasal cavity. This examination is known as anterior rhinoscopy.

Posterior Rhinoscopy: Posterior rhinoscopy is done to examine the post nasal space and nasopharynx. Here the postnasal mirror is warmed and introduced into the oral cavity with the mirror facing upwards to lie behind the uvula while the tongue is depressed with a tongue depressor. Structures visualised on posterior rhinoscopy are:

a. Adenoids in the posterior wall of nasopharynx
b. Eustachian tube openings, torus tubaris and fossa of Rosenmüller in the lateral wall of nasopharynx on both sides (please *see* the chapter on anatomy of pharynx).
c. Choanae with posterior border of nasal septum and posterior ends of inferior and middle turbinates.

Note:

The superior turbinate and the spheno-ethmoidal recess is not visualised on posterior rhinoscopy.

Nasal endoscopy: This is done with the help of 0 degrees or 30 degrees rigid endoscope. It consists of three passes:

i. First pass; here the endoscope is passed along the floor of the nasal cavity between the inferior turbinate and septum. The scope is then advanced into the nasopharynx.
ii. Second pass; here the superior turbinate and its meatus and the spheno-ethmoidal recess is visualised.
iii. Third pass; here the middle meatus is examined.

 "Points to Ponder/Points for Quick revision"

Turbinate/Concha	Meatus	Openings
Inferior (independent bone)	Inferior (largest)	NLD (down, back, lateral)
Middle (part of ethmoid bone)	Middle (posterior half of lateral wall, OMC—MC infected)	Frontal, Ant Ethmoids (Bulla ethmoidalis, Agger Nasi, Haller cell), Maxillary sinus
Superior (part of ethmoid bone)	Superior (smallest)	Posterior ethmoids (Onodi cell)
Above superior	Spheno-ethmoidal recess	Sphenoid sinus (MC—Sellar)

Section II **Nose**

PREVIOUSLY ASKED QUESTIONS

1. **Commonest presentation of an infant with bilateral choanal atresia:** *(AIIMS 96, Exam 2014)*
   a. Difficulty in breathing
   b. Dysphagia
   c. Excessive sneezing
   d. Post-nasal drip (PND)

2. **Choanal atresia is associated with:** *(PGI 93, 2009)*
   a. Colobomatous blindness
   b. Heart disorder
   c. Renal anomaly
   d. Ear disorder
   e. Cranial nerve lesions

3. **A 2-year-old child is brought to the hospital with a compressible swelling at the root of nose, see the clinical picture below, most likely diagnosis is:** *(Practice question by the Author)*

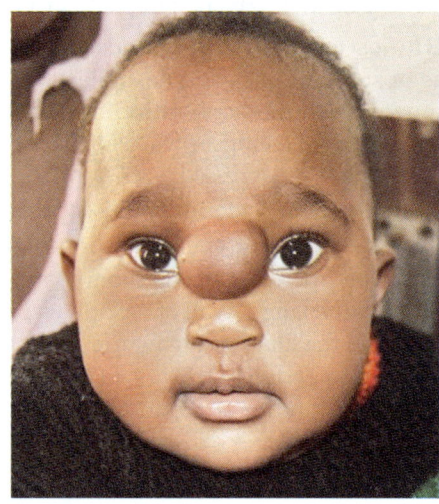

   a. AV malformation
   b. Lacrimal sac cyst
   c. Ethmoid sinus cyst
   d. Meningoencephalocele

4. **True about nasal glioma:** *(PGI June 2009)*
   a. Soft and Compressible
   b. 60% Extranasal
   c. CT provides the bony detail
   d. MRI differentiate between glioma and nasal encephalocele
   e. Present as CSF leak at birth

5. **External nose is formed from:** *(AP 96, 2000, Exam 2017)*
   a. 3 paired + 3 unpaired cartilages
   b. 3 paired + 1 unpaired cartilages
   c. 3 paired + 4 unpaired cartilages
   d. 1 paired + 1 unpaired cartilages

6. **Osseo cartilaginous junction on the dorsum of nose is:** *(Exam 2012)*
   a. Nasion   b. Columella
   c. Rhinion   d. Glabella

7. **Nasal valve is formed by all except:** *(MP 2008, Exam 2017)*
   a. Septum
   b. Middle turbinate
   c. Lower end of upper lateral cartilage
   d. Inferior turbinate

8. **Choana is:** *(TN 2003, Exam 2017)*
   a. Anterior nares   b. Posterior nares
   c. Tonsils   d. Larynx

9. **Ethmoid bone forms all except:** *(Bihar 2005, Exam 2017)*
   a. Superior turbinate   b. Middle turbinate
   c. Inferior turbinate   d. Uncinate process

10. **Inferior turbinate is a:** *(JIPMER 2004, Exam 2017)*
    a. Part of maxilla   b. Part of sphenoid
    c. Separate bone   d. Part of ethmoid

11. **Which of the following is known as 4th turbinate?** *(UP 2001, Exam 2010)*
    a. Superior turbinate   b. Agger nasi
    c. Supreme turbinate   d. Bullous turbinate

12. **Turbinate that articulates with ethmoid is:** *(AP 2002, Exam 2013)*
    a. Superior   b. Middle
    c. Inferior   d. All of the above

13. **All these structures are found in the lateral nasal wall except:** *(MP 2007, Exam 2017)*
    a. Superior turbinate   b. Vomer
    c. Agger nasi   d. Hasner's valve

14. **Nasolacrimal duct opens into:** *(MAHE 2005, Karnataka 2011)*
    a. Superior meatus   b. Middle meatus
    c. Inferior meatus   d. Sphenoethmoidal recess

15. **Direction of nasolacrimal duct is:** *(PGI 98, AI 99, Exam 2013)*
    a. Downwards, backwards and medially
    b. Downwards, backwards and laterally
    c. Downwards, forwards and medially
    d. Downwards, forwards and laterally

16. **Paranasal sinus opening in middle meatus:** *(PGI 2003, 98, 2014)*
    a. Maxillary   b. Anterior ethmoid
    c. Posterior ethmoid   d. Frontal
    e. Sphenoid

17. **All drains into middle meatus except:** *(Exam 2013, 2002)*
    a. Nasolacrimal duct   b. Maxillary sinus
    c. Frontal sinus   d. Ethmoidal sinus

18. **Fronto-nasal duct opens into:** *(Exam 2014)*
    a. Inferior meatus
    b. Middle meatus
    c. Superior meatus
    d. Inferior turbinate

19. **Frontal sinus drain into:** *(Exam 2015)*
    a. Superior meatus   b. Inferior meatus
    c. Middle meatus   d. Ethmoid recess

20. **The maxillary sinus opens into middle meatus at the:** *(Exam 2002, Exam 2017)*
    a. Hiatus semilunaris b. Bulla ethmoidalis
    c. Infundibulum   d. None of the above

21. **Hiatus semilunaris is present in:** *(CUPGEE 2002, Exam 2017)*
    a. Superior meatus   b. Inferior meatus
    c. Middle meatus   d. Spheno-ethmoidal recess

22. **Bulla ethmoidalis is seen in:** *(AIIMS 92, Exam 2013)*
    a. Superior meatus   b. Inferior meatus
    c. Middle meatus   d. Spheno-ethmoidal recess

23. **Osteomeatal complex connects:** *(MH 2002, Exam 2017)*
    a. Nasal cavity with maxillary sinus
    b. Nasal cavity with sphenoid sinus
    c. The two nasal cavities
    d. Nasal cavity with lacrimal sac

24. **Opening of posterior ethmoid sinus is in:** *(Jharkhand 2006, Punjab 2011)*
    a. Middle meatus   b. Inferior meatus
    c. Superior meatus d. None

25. **Sphenoidal sinus opens into:** *(Kerala 98, Exam 2014)*
    a. Superior meatus   b. Inferior meatus
    c. Middle meatus   d. Spheno-ethmoidal recess

26. **Which of the following bones do not contribute to the nasal septum?** *(AI 2003, Exam 2017)*
    a. Sphenoid   b. Lacrimal
    c. Palatine   d. Ethmoid

27. **The shape of the septal cartilage is:** *(Exam 2013)*
    a. Triangular   b. Quadrilateral
    c. Oval   d. Hexagonal

28. **Quadrilateral cartilage is attached to all except:** *(Exam 2001, Exam 2017)*
    a. Ethmoid   b. Vomer
    c. Sphenoid   d. Maxilla

29. **Nasal septum is supplied by:** *(AI 92, Exam 2016)*
    a. Only external carotid artery
    b. Only internal carotid artery
    c. Mainly external carotid artery
    d. Mainly internal carotid artery

30. **Which artery does not contribute to Little's area?** *(Exam 2015, Exam 2018)*
    a. Superior labial branch of facial artery
    b. Anterior ethmoidal artery
    c. Sphenopalatine artery
    d. Posterior ethmoidal artery

31. **Anterior ethmoidal artery arises from:** *(Exam 2013)*
    a. Maxillary artery
    b. Mandibular artery
    c. Superficial temporal artery
    d. Ophthalmic artery

32. **First paranasal sinus to develop at birth is:** *(AIIMS 98, Exam 2013)*
    a. Maxillary   b. Ethmoidal
    c. Frontal   d. Sphenoidal

33. **Sinus not present at birth is:** *(MH 2002, Exam 2017)*
    a. Ethmoid   b. Maxillary
    c. Frontal   d. None

34. **Least common Sinusitis is:** *(UP 2008, Exam 2013)*
    a. Maxillary   b. Ethmoid
    c. Frontal   d. Sphenoid

35. **True about sphenoid sinus:** *(PGI May 2010)*
    a. Lined by stratified Squamous epithelium
    b. Duct open in middle meatus
    c. Open in sphenoethmoidal recess
    d. Present at birth
    e. Present in greater wing of sphenoid

36. **Which sinus is not a part of Para-nasal sinus?** *(MP 2009)*
    a. Frontal   b. Ethmoid
    c. Sphenoid   d. pyriform

37. **Most superior sinus in the face is:** *(Exam 2013)*
    a. Frontal sinus   b. Ethmoid sinus
    c. Maxillary sinus d. Sphenoid sinus

38. **Antral fistula is most common after extraction of:** *(Exam 2000, Exam 2017)*
    a. 2nd incisor   b. 1st premolar
    c. 3rd molar   d. 1st molar

39. **Maxillary sinus achieves maximum size at:** *(Manipal 2006, Exam 2017)*
    a. At birth
    b. At primary dentition
    c. At secondary dentition
    d. At puberty

40. **Onodi cells and Haller cells are seen in relation to:** *(AIIMS Nov 2009)*
    a. Optic nerve and floor of orbit
    b. Optic nerve and frontal sinus
    c. Optic nerve and ethmoid air cells
    d. Optic chiasma and nasolacrimal duct

41. **Pain sensations from the ethmoidal sinus are carried by:** *(AI 2011)*
    a. Supraorbital nerve b. Lacrimal Nerve
    c. Nasociliary Nerve   d. Infraorbital Nerve

42. **Ciliary movement rate of nasal mucosa is:** *(UP 2001, Exam 2017)*
    a. 1–2 mm/min   b. 2–5 mm/min
    c. 5–10 mm/min   d. 10–20 mm/min

Section II   Nose

43. **Function of mucociliary action of upper respiratory tract is:** *(Kerala 94, 2000, Exam 2017)*
    a. Temperature regulation
    b. Increased the velocity of inspired air
    c. Traps the pathogenic organisms in inspired air
    d. Has no physiological role

44. **Movement of mucous in nose is by:** *(Exam 2013)*
    a. Mucociliary action
    b. Inspiration
    c. Expiration
    d. Both Inspiration and expiration

45. **During inspiration the main current of air flow in a normal nasal cavity is through:** *(AI 2007, Exam 2017)*
    a. Middle part of the cavity in a parabolic curve
    b. Lower part of the cavity in a parabolic curve
    c. Superior part of the cavity in a parabolic curve
    d. Through olfactory area

46. **Odour receptors present in:** *(Exam 2013)*
    a. Olfactory epithelium
    b. Olfactory tract
    c. Amygdala
    d. Olfactory bulbs

47. **Anosmia is common in:** *(PGI 2001, 2013)*
    a. Coryza
    b. Atrophic rhinitis
    c. CSF rhinorrhoea
    d. Fracture cribriform plate
    e. Antrochoanal polyp

48. **Parosmia is:** *(MAHE 2001, Exam 2017)*
    a. Perversion of smell sensation
    b. Absolute loss of smell sensation
    c. Decreased smell sensation
    d. Perception of bad smell

49. **Which of the following syndrome is associated with anosmia?** *(Exam 2013)*
    a. Kallmann's syndrome
    b. Turner's syndrome
    c. Bartter syndrome
    d. Klinefelter's syndrome

50. **Nasal cycle is the cyclical alternate nasal blockage occurring:** *(Delhi PG 2009)*
    a. Every 6–12 hours
    b. Every 2 ½ –4 hours
    c. Every 4–8 hours
    d. Every 12–24 hours

51. **All are true about nasolabial cyst except:** *(AIIMS Nov 2008)*
    a. Arises from odontoid epithelium
    b. Presents with a swelling in the anterior nasal floor
    c. unilateral
    d. Usually seen in adults

52. **Thudichum's speculum is used to visualise:** *(AIIMS May 2000, 2014)*
    a. Tonsils
    b. Larynx
    c. Anterior nasal cavity
    d. Posterior nares

53. **Which is not visualised on posterior rhinoscopy?** *(AI 2010, AIIMS May 2008)*
    a. Eustachian tube
    b. Inferior meatus
    c. Middle meatus
    d. Superior concha

54. **Pneumatisation patterns of sphenoid sinus are all except:** *(Exam 2013)*
    a. Pre sellar
    b. Post sellar
    c. Concha bullosa
    d. Conchal

55. **What percentage of total airflow through nose passes through olfactory region?** *(Exam 2014)*
    a. 5–10%
    b. 20–30%
    c. 40–50%
    d. 60–70%

56. **Boundaries of anterior nasal valve are all except:** *(Exam 2014)*
    a. Inferior turbinate
    b. Middle turbinate
    c. Limen nasi
    d. Septum

57. **Lining of maxillary sinus:** *(Exam 2014)*
    a. Stratified squamous keratinised epithelium
    b. Stratified squamous non-keratinised epithelium
    c. Ciliated columnar
    d. Transitional cell epithelium

58. **Sphenopalatine foramen is located at the end of which turbinate:** *(Exam 2014)*
    a. Supreme turbinate
    b. Superior turbinate
    c. Middle turbinate
    d. Inferior turbinate

59. **The narrowest part of the nasal cavity is:** *(Exam 2015)*
    a. Nasal valve
    b. Choanae
    c. Middle turbinate
    d. Vestibule

60. **Ethmoidal bulla is seen in:** *(Exam 2015)*
    a. Middle meatus
    b. Superior meatus
    c. Vestibule
    d. Inferior meatus

61. **Infundibulum lies between:** *(Exam 2015)*
    a. Lateral wall and uncinate process of ethmoid
    b. Middle and inferior turbinate
    c. Hiatus semilunaris and Inferior meatus
    d. Wing of sphenoid and maxillary antrum

62. **The Onodi cell refers to:** *(MH CET 2015)*
    a. Sphenoid sinus
    b. Posterior group of ethmoid cells
    c. Frontal sinus
    d. Anterior group of ethmoid cells

63. **Cause of choanal atresia:** *(Exam 2015)*
    a. Vomero-nasal bone
    b. Bucconasal membrane
    c. Third ethmoidal bone
    d. First branchial arch

Section II Nose

64. Ventilation of Sinuses occurs during: *(Exam 2015)*
    a. Inspiration   b. Expiration
    c. Both   d. None

65. Which turbinate is seen only on nasal endoscopy?
    (Exam 2015)
    a. Superior   b. Middle
    c. Inferior   d. ET

66. Haller cells are present in: *(Exam 2015)*
    a. Roof of maxillary sinus
    b. Floor of maxillary sinus
    c. Lateral wall of Sphenoid
    d. Anterior wall of frontal

67. Lining of maxillary sinus is: *(Exam 2015)*
    a. Stratified squamous keratinized
    b. Stratified squamous non- keratinized
    c. Ciliated columnar
    d. Olfactory epithelium

68. The Onodi cell is in relation to: *(Exam 2016)*
    a. Sphenoid sinus
    b. Anterior group of ethmoid cells
    c. Frontal sinus
    d. Floor of orbit

69. A child is normal while crying but develops cyanosis and breathlessness when being quiet. The most probable diagnosis: *(Exam 2016)*
    a. Laryngomalacia   b. Croup
    c. Choanal atresia   d. Epiglottitis

70. The sphenoethmoidal recess has opening of:
    (Exam 2016)
    a. Maxillary sinus   b. Pituitary
    c. Ethmoid sinus   d. Sphenoid sinus

71. Which sinus is the last sinus to appear radiologically on X-ray?   *(Exam 2008, 2017)*
    a. Maxillary sinus   b. Sphenoid sinus
    c. Frontal sinus   d. Ethmoidal air cells

72. Valve of Hasner is: *(Exam 2016)*
    a. Opening of nasolacrimal duct
    b. Sphenoidal sinus opening
    c. Frontal sinus opening
    d. Ethmoid sinus opening

73. Hiatus semilunaris is present in: *(Exam 2015)*
    a. Superior meatus
    b. Middle meatus
    c. Inferior meatus
    d. Spheno-ethmoidal recess

74. Eustachian tube is located at: *(Exam 2015)*
    a. Posterior to Superior turbinate
    b. Posterior to Middle turbinate
    c. Posterior to Inferior turbinate
    d. At the Spheno-ethmoidal recess

75. All the following are true regarding maxillary sinus except: *(Exam 2015)*
    a. Largest paranasal sinus
    b. Commonest sinus involved in acute bacterial sinusitis
    c. Pain referred to lower premolar and molar teeth via trigeminal nerve
    d. Opens into middle meatus

76. Rhinomanometry is the measurement of:
    (Exam 2015)
    a. Nasal air flow alone
    b. Nasal air flow and nasal airway resistance
    c. Nasal airway resistance alone
    d. Mucociliary blanket

77. Vidian nerve is: *(Exam 2016)*
    a. Auricular branch of Vagus
    b. Nerve of pterygoid canal
    c. Tympanic branch of Glossopharyngeal nerve
    d. Lesser petrosal nerve

78. Roof of nasal cavity is formed by all except:
    (Exam 2015)
    a. Nasal process of Frontal bones
    b. Cribriform plate
    c. Sphenoid bone
    d. Palatine process of maxilla

79. Osteomeatal complex consists of the following except: *(Exam 2015)*
    a. Sphenoidal sinus opening
    b. Frontal sinus opening
    c. Anterior Ethmoidal sinus opening
    d. Maxillary sinus opening

IMAGE BASED PRACTICE QUESTIONS BY THE AUTHOR

80. Where does the given sinus drain into:

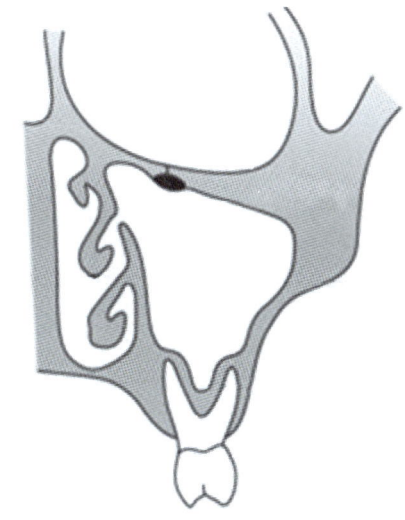

    a. Infundibulum
    b. Sphenoethmoidal recess

Nose

Section II

c. Inferior meatus

d. Superior meatus

81. The shaded area represents:

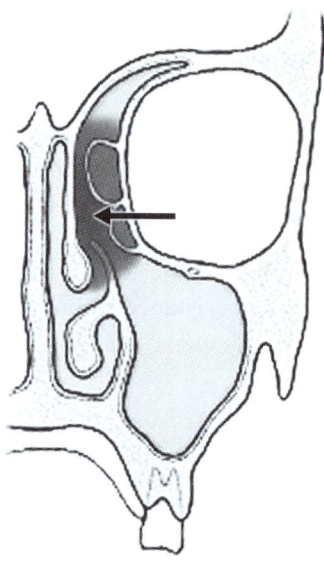

a. Osteomeatal complex

b. Sphenoethmoidal recess

c. Inferior meatus

d. Superior meatus

82. The shaded area (sky blue) is lined by which epithelium:

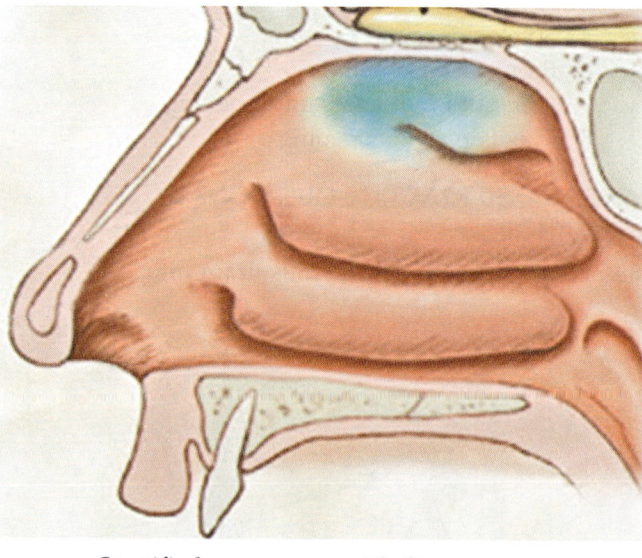

a. Stratified squamous epithelium

b. Ciliated columnar epithelium

c. Olfactory epithelium

d. Simple squamous epithelium

83. The encircled area on the lateral wall of nose in the picture is:

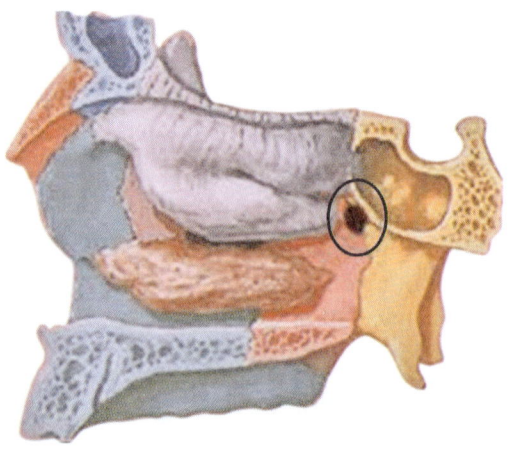

a. Eustachian tube

b. Sphenopalatine foramen

c. Fossa of Rosenmüller

d. Pyriform fossa

84. The marked structure on the X-ray is: *(JIPMER 2018)*

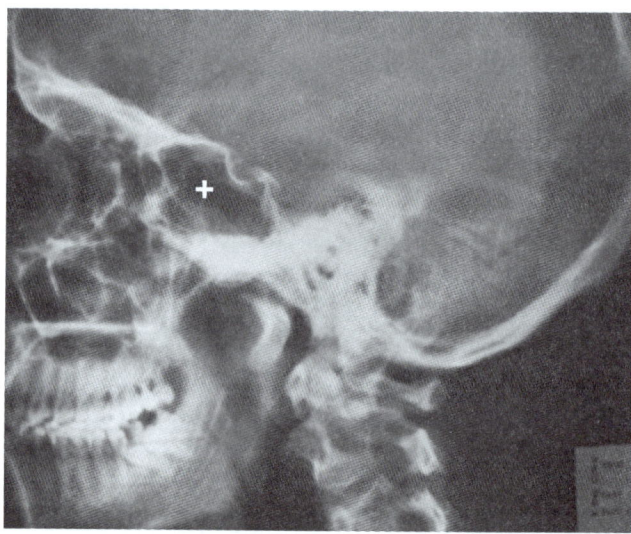

a. Nasopharynx   b. Ethmoidal air cells

c. Sphenoid sinus   d. Pituitary gland

85. Which paranasal sinus is the last to completely develop? *(JIPMER 2018)*

a. Maxillary   b. Sphenoid

c. Frontal   d. Ethmoid

86. Nerve not involved in olfaction while eating is: *(JIPMER 2018)*

a. Facial   b. Glossopharyngeal

c. Vagus   d. Hypoglossal

ANSWERS AND EXPLANATIONS

1. **(a) Difficulty in breathing** (*Ref. Cummings, 6th ed., 2953*)

2. **(a), (b), (d) and (e)** (*Ref. Cummings, 6th ed., 2953*) refer the text. There are urogenital anomalies and not renal.

3. **(d) Meningoencephalocele** (*Ref. Cummings, 6th ed., 2945*)
   - 2 year child with compressible swelling at the root of nose is likely Meningoencephalocele
   - Lacrimal sac cyst occurs as a compressible swelling near the medial canthus.
   - Ethmoid cyst (mucocele) presents as a swelling at the medial quadrant of orbit pushing the orbit forwards and laterally (also see the chapter on sinusitis).
   - AV malformation is a congenital abnormal connection between arteries and veins, bypassing the capillary system. These are largely found in internal organs most commonly brain. It is rare at this site.

4. **(b), (c), and (d) are true** (*Ref. Cummings, 6th ed., 2947*) (refer the text)

5. **(b) 3 paired + 1 unpaired cartilages,** (*Ref. Cummings, 6th ed., 494*) refer the text

6. **(c) Rhinion** (*Ref. Cummings, 6th ed., 493*) refer the text for rhinion, columella nasion and glabella.

7. **(b) Middle turbinate** (*Ref. Cummings, 6th ed., 478; Scott Brown, vol 1; page 1141*)

8. **(b) Posterior nares** (*Ref. Cummings, 6th ed., 659*)
   - The posterior end of each nasal cavity is known as choana.

9. **(c) Inferior turbinate** (*Ref. Cummings, 6th ed., 755*)

10. **(c) Separate bone** (*Ref. Cummings, 6th ed., 755*)

11. **(c) Supreme turbinate** (*Ref. Dhingra, 6th ed., 138*)

12. **(c) Inferior** (*Ref. Cummings, 6th ed., 754*)
    - The superior and middle turbinates are parts of ethmoid bone whereas inferior turbinate is an independent separate bone which articulates with the ethmoid.

13. **(b) Vomer** (*Ref. Cummings, 6th ed., 659*)
    - Vomer is an independent separate bone which forms the postero-inferior part of the septum proper, i.e. the medial wall of nose.
    Rest all are found on the lateral wall, refer the text

14. **(c) Inferior meatus** (*Ref. Cummings, 6th ed., 817*)
    - Nasolacrimal duct opens into Inferior meatus.
    - In the superior meatus open the Posterior ethmoid sinuses.
    - In the middle meatus open the Maxillary sinus, frontal sinus and the anterior ethmoid sinuses.
    - Sphenoid sinus opens in the sphenoethmoidal recess.

15. **(b) Downwards, backwards and laterally** (*Ref. BD Chaurasia, Human Anatomy, 6th ed., Vol 3; 76*)

16. **(a), (b) and (d)** (*Ref. Cummings, 6th ed., 659*)

17. **(a) Nasolacrimal duct** (*Ref. Cummings, 6th ed., 659*)
    - Nasolacrimal duct opens into Inferior meatus.

18. **(b) Middle meatus** (*Ref. Cummings, 6th ed., 757*)

19. **(c) Middle meatus** (*Ref. Cummings, 6th ed., 757*)

20. **(c) Infundibulum** (*Ref. Cummings, 6th ed., 660*) (refer the text)

21. **(c) Middle meatus** (*Ref. Cummings, 6th ed., 753*)

22. **(c) Middle meatus** (*Ref. Cummings, 6th ed., 660*)

23. **(a) Nasal cavity with maxillary sinus** (*Ref. Cummings, 6th ed., 752*)
    - All the structures of the middle meatus together constitutes osteomeatal complex. The osteomeatal complex connects the nasal cavity with maxillary, frontal and anterior ethmoid sinuses.
    - Spheno-ethmoidal recess connects Sphenoid sinus with nasal cavity.
    - Nasolacrimal duct connects nasal cavity with lacrimal sac.
    - The two nasal cavities remain separated by the nasal septum

24. **(c) Superior meatus** (*Ref. Cummings, 6th ed., 659*)

25. **(d) Spheno-ethmoidal recess** (*Ref. Cummings, 6th ed., 659*)
    - The Sphenoid sinus opens into the spheno-ethmoidal recess just above the superior turbinate.

26. **(b) Lacrimal** (*Ref. Cummings, 6th ed., 475*)

27. **(b) Quadrilateral** (*Ref. Scott Brown, 6th ed., 1/5/11*)

28. **(c) Sphenoid** (*Ref. Cummings, 6th ed., 475*) (refer the text)

29. **(c) Mainly external carotid artery** (*Ref. Cummings, 6th ed., 679*)

30. **(d) Posterior ethmoidal artery** (*Ref. Cummings, 6th ed., 679*)

31. **(d) Ophthalmic artery** (*Ref. Cummings, 6th ed., 679*)

32. **(a) Maxillary** (*Ref. Cummings, 6th ed., 2871*)
    - Maxillary sinus is the earliest sinus to develop followed by ethmoid, sphenoid and last to develop is frontal.
    - But the most common sinusitis in infants and young children is ethmoid sinusitis because it is much well pneumatised at birth.

33. **(c) Frontal** (*Ref. Cummings, 6th ed., 2874; Scott Brown, 8th ed., Vol 2, page 262*)
    - This is the last sinus to develop. It is not present at birth.

34. **(d) Sphenoid** (*Ref. Dhingra, 6th ed., 193*)

35. **(c) and (d),** (*Ref. Scott Brown, 6th ed., 1/5/19*) refer the text

36. **(d) Pyriform** (*Ref. Cummings, 6th ed., 659*)
    - Pyriform sinus or pyriform fossa is a part of the hypopharynx.

37. **(a) Frontal sinus** (*Ref. Scott Brown, 6th ed., 4/3/2*)
    - Most superior sinus is the frontal sinus followed by ethmoid, sphenoid and maxillary sinuses.

38. **(d) 1st molar** (*Ref. Scott Brown, 6th ed., 1/5/25*)
    - The floor of the maxillary sinus is related to 2nd premolar and 1st molar. Therefore extraction of these teeth can lead to an oro-antral fistula.

39. **(c) At secondary dentition** (*Ref. Cummings, 6th ed., 2874; Scott Brown, 8th ed., Vol 2; 262*) (refer to text)

40. **(a) Optic nerve and floor of orbit** (*Ref. Cummings 6th ed., 664*) (please refer the text)

41. **(c) Nasociliary Nerve** (*Ref. Cummings, 6th ed., 476*) (refer the table on important features of Para nasal sinuses in the text)
   - Pain sensations from the frontal sinus are carried by supraorbital nerve, a branch of ophthalmic division (V1) of trigeminal.
   - Infra-orbital nerve along with alveolar nerves (branches of the maxillary division of trigeminal) carries pain sensations from the maxillary sinus.
   - Lacrimal nerve (a branch of ophthalmic division of trigeminal) do not supply the paranasal sinuses.

42. **(c) 5–10 mm/min** (*Ref. Dhingra, 6th ed., 141*)

43. **(c) Traps the pathogenic organisms in inspired air** (*Ref. Cummings, 6th ed., 645*)

44. **(a) Mucociliary action** (*Ref. Cummings, 6th ed., 645*)

45. **(a) Middle part of the cavity in a parabolic curve** (*Ref. Cummings, 6th ed., 626*)
   - The main current of airflow passes through the middle part of the nose in a parabolic curve both during inspiration and expiration.

46. **(a) Olfactory epithelium** (*Ref. Cummings, 6th ed., 627*) (refer the text)

47. **(a), (b) and (d)** (*Ref. Cummings, 6th ed., 636*)
   - CSF rhinorrhoea (*see* Chapter on fractures) due to middle cranial fossa fractures will not lead to anosmia.
   - Antrochoanal polyp being unilateral will not lead to anosmia. Here patient can have hyposmia, see chapter on nasal polyposis.

48. **(a) Perversion of smell sensation** (*Ref. Cummings, 6th ed., 639*)
   - Parosmia is perversion of smell sensation. Here good smell appears bad to the patient.
   - Absolute loss of smell sensation is called anosmia, see chapter on nasal polyposis.
   - Decreased smell sensation is called hyposmia. Normal age related decline in smell sensation is presbyosmia.
   - Phantosmia is the perception of a smell in the absence of any physical odours. The odour can range from pleasant to disgusting smells.
   - Cacosmia or an unpleasant phantosmia is the perception of a bad smell without an odorant stimulus.

49. **(a) Kallmann's syndrome** (*Ref. Cummings, 6th ed., 639*)

50. **(b) every 2 1/2–4 hours** (*Ref. Cummings, 6th ed., 647*)

51. **(a) Arises from odontoid epithelium** (*Ref. Scott Brown, 6th ed., 5/23/10*) (refer the text)

52. **(c) Anterior nasal cavity** (*Ref. Scott Brown, 8th ed., Vol 1, 978*)
   - Thudichum's speculum is used to visualise the anterior nasal cavity. This examination is known as anterior rhinoscopy.
   - Tonsils can be visualised by depressing the tongue with a tongue depressor.
   - Larynx can be visualised by indirect laryngoscopic mirror.
   - Posterior nares can be visualised by post nasal mirror on posterior rhinoscopy.

53. **(d) Superior concha** (*Ref. Dhingra, 6th ed., 379*)
   - Superior conchae or turbinates can be visualized only on nasal endoscopy.

54. **(c) Concha bullosa** (*Ref. Scott Brown, 8th ed., Vol 1 963*)
   - Concha bullosa is pneumatised middle turbinate, rest all are the pneumatisation patterns of sphenoid sinus.

55. **(a) 5–10%** (*Ref. Cummings, 6th ed., 626; Scott Brown 8th ed., Vol 1, 1228*)

56. **(b) Middle turbinate** (*Ref. Scott Brown, 8th ed., Vol 1, 963*)

57. **(c) Ciliated columnar** (*Ref. Cummings, 6th ed., 659*)

58. **(c) Middle turbinate** (*Ref. Cummings, 6th ed., 495*)

59. **(a) Nasal valve** (*Ref. Scott Brown, 8th ed., Vol 1, 987*)

60. **(a) Middle meatus** (*Ref. Cummings, 6th ed., 660*)

61. **(a) Lateral wall and uncinate process of ethmoid** (*Ref. Cummings, 6th ed., 753*)

62. **(b) Posterior group of ethmoid cells** (*Ref. Cummings, 6th ed., 756*)

63. **(b) Bucconasal membrane** (*Ref. Cummings, 6th ed., 2953*)

64. **(b) Expiration** (*Ref. Dhingra, 6th ed., 140*)

65. **(a) Superior** (*Ref. Dhingra, 6th ed., 379*)

66. **(a) Roof of maxillary sinus** (*Ref. Cummings, 6th ed., 664*)

67. **(c) Ciliated columnar** (*Ref. Cummings, 6th ed., 659*)

68. **(a) Sphenoid sinus** (*Ref. Cummings, 6th ed., 756*)

69. **(c) Choanal atresia** (*Ref. Scott Brown, 8th ed., Vol 2, 251*)

70. **(d) Sphenoid sinus** (*Ref. Cummings, 6th ed., 659*)

71. **(c) Frontal sinus** (*Ref. Scott Brown, 8th ed., Vol 2, 262*)

72. **(a) Opening of nasolacrimal duct** (*Ref. Cummings, 6th ed., 817*)

73. **(b) Middle meatus** (*Ref. Cummings, 6th ed., 753*)

74. **(c) Posterior to inferior turbinate** (*Ref. Scott Brown, 8th ed., Vol 2; 537*)

75. **(c) Pain referred to lower premolar and molar teeth via trigeminal nerve** (*Ref. Scott Brown, 8th ed., Vol 1; 962, 972*)
   - In maxillary sinusitis pain is referred to upper teeth via trigeminal nerve

76. **(b) Nasal air flow and nasal airway resistance** (*Ref. Cummings, 6th ed., 648*)

77. **(b) Nerve of pterygoid canal** (*Ref. Cummings, 6th ed., 476*)

78. **(d) Palatine process of maxilla** (*Ref. Cummings, 6th ed., 759*)

79. **(a) Sphenoidal sinus opening** (*Ref. Cummings, 6th ed., 659*)

80. **(a) Infundibulum** (*Ref. Cummings, 6th ed., 752*)

81. **(a) Osteomeatal complex** (*Ref. Cummings, 6th ed., 752*)

82. **(c) Olfactory epithelium** (*Ref. Cummings, 6th ed., 627*)

83. **(b) Sphenopalatine foramen** (*Ref. Scott Brown, 6th ed., 1/5/27; 8th ed., Vol 1, 1172*)

84. **(c) Sphenoid sinus** (*Ref. Scott Brown, 6th ed., 4/3/2*)
Shown below are X-ray Waters view (occipito-mental) with open mouth and X-ray Nose & PNS-lateral view. Note the highest sinus in the lateral view is the frontal sinus.

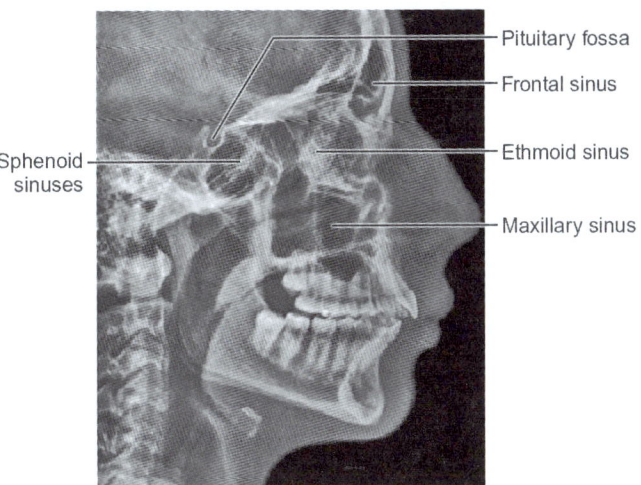

Nose & paranasal sinuses–Lateral view

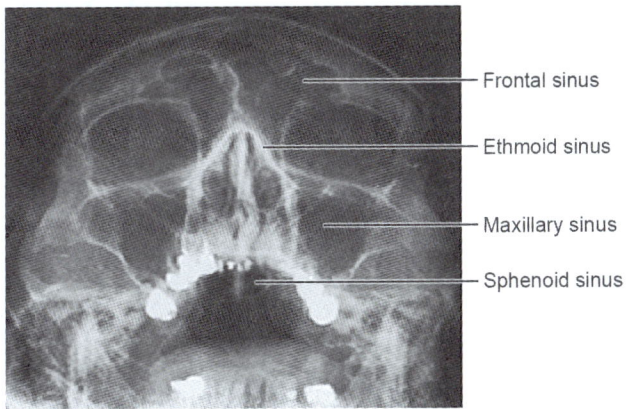

Water's view with open mouth

85. **(c) Frontal** (*Ref. Scott Brown, 8th ed., Vol 2; 262*)
86. **(d) Hypoglossal** (*Ref. Scott Brown, 8th ed., Vol 3; 765*)
   • Hypoglossal is a pure motor nerve.

Section II | Nose

Diseases of External Nose

SADDLE NOSE

This is depressed dorsum.

Conditions causing damage to septal cartilage and thereby loss of support, leading to depressed dorsum:

    i. Iatrogenic/non-iatrogenic trauma,

   ii. Granulomatous conditions,

  iii. Septal hematoma/abscess.

This is managed by **augmentation rhinoplasty** by conchal, tragal, septal or rib cartilage.

HUMP NOSE

Hump over the dorsum of nose. It is managed by **reduction rhinoplasty**.

CROOKED NOSE

The **dorsum is deviated but tip is in midline (C or S shaped)**. It is managed by septo-rhinoplasty.

DEVIATED NOSE

The **dorsum and tip are straight but both deviated to one side**. It is managed by septo-rhinoplasty.

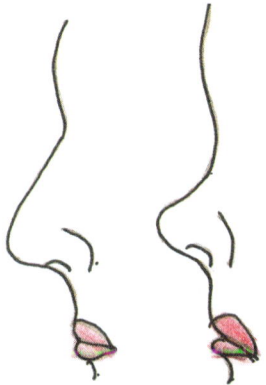

Fig. 17.1: Normal and Saddle nose

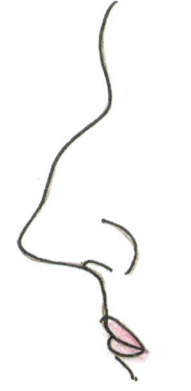

Fig. 17.2: Hump nose

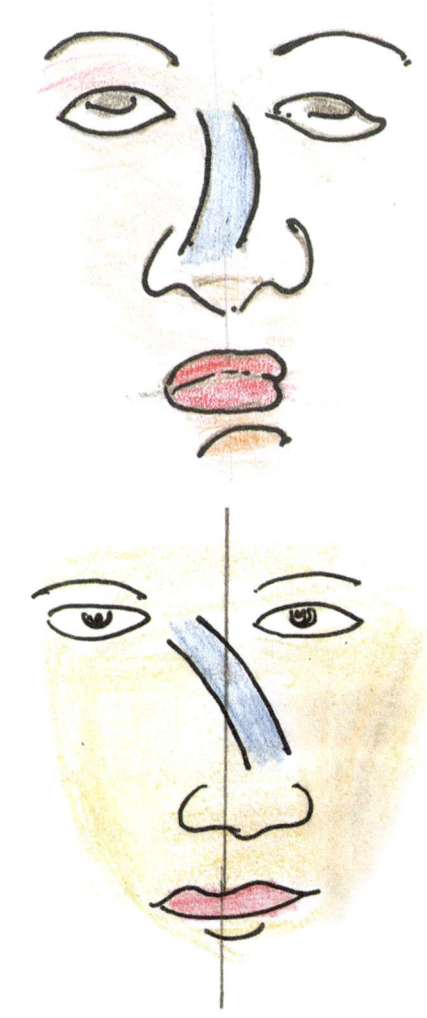

Fig. 17.3: Crooked nose and deviated nose

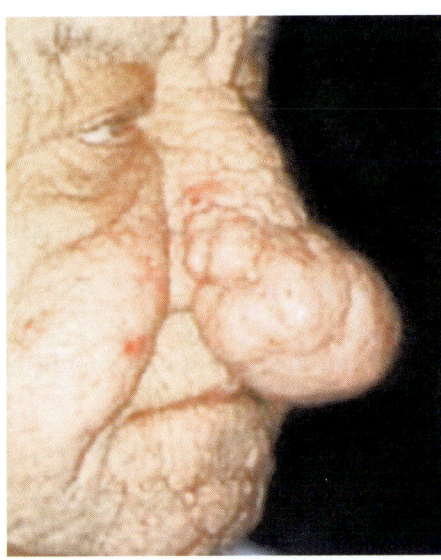

Fig. 17.4: A patient with Rhinophyma

RHINOPHYMA

It is the most common benign tumour of the external nose. It is because of the **hypertrophy of the sebaceous glands of the tip of nose**. It is more commonly seen in **middle aged men** with long standing history of **"acne rosacea"**.

Clinical Features

It causes cosmetic deformity known as **potato nose**. It can lead to difficulty in vision due to the large mass sitting on the tip of nose. If large enough can lead to obstruction of the nostrils.

Management

Excision by CO_2 laser or sharp knife and skin grafting of the raw area.

BASAL CELL CARCINOMA

This is the most common carcinoma of the skin of external nose. It is also known as **"rodent ulcer"**. It can present as pearly nodule or ulcer. Exposure to prolonged sunlight is an important etiological factor.

Management

Excision with a margin of 3–5 mm. Radiotherapy can be used for patients not fit for surgery or postoperatively in patients with aggressive tumour.

"Points to Ponder/Points for Quick revision"

Saddle nose	*Hump nose*
Depressed dorsum (damage to septal cartilage)	Hump over dorsum
Augmentation rhinoplasty	Reduction rhinoplasty

Crooked nose	*Deviated nose*
C shaped–dorsum–deviated, tip-midline	Dorsum and tip-straight line but tip deviation-from midline

- Rhinophyma (potato nose): Hypertrophy of sebaceous (holocrine) glands—Tip; Middle age men; Acne rosacea; Excision and skin grafting.
- Basal cell carcinoma (rodent ulcer): Prolonged sunlight— Wide excision ± radiotherapy.

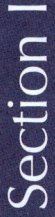

Section II   Nose

PREVIOUSLY ASKED QUESTIONS

1. **Rhinophyma is associated with:**
                                    (*AI 2007, Exam 2015*)
   a. Hypertrophy of the sebaceous glands
   b. Hypertrophy of sweat glands
   c. Hyperplasia of endothelial cells
   d. Hyperplasia of epithelial cells

2. **True about rhinophyma:**   (*AI 2001, Exam 2017*)
   a. Premalignant   b. Common in alcoholics
   c. Acne rosacea   d. Fungal etiology

3. **Depressed bridge of the nose may be due to any of the following except:**   (*AP 2006, Exam 2017*)
   a. Leprosy   b. Syphilis
   c. Septal abscess   d. Acromegaly

4. **True about rhinophyma:**   (*Exam 2013*)
   a. Premalignant
   b. Most commonly due to diabetes mellitus
   c. More common in alcoholics
   d. Hypertrophy of holocrine glands

5. **A crooked nose is due to:**
                                    (*Manipal 2000, Exam 2017*)
   a. Deviated dorsum but tip midline
   b. Depressed dorsum
   c. Humped dorsum
   d. Deviated dorsum and tip

6. **Rodent ulcer is:**   (*RJ 2006, Exam 2017*)
   a. Saddle nose   b. Crooked nose
   c. Rhinophyma   d. Basal cell carcinoma

7. **The following are True regarding the disease shown in the following picture except:**
                                    (*APPG 2016*)

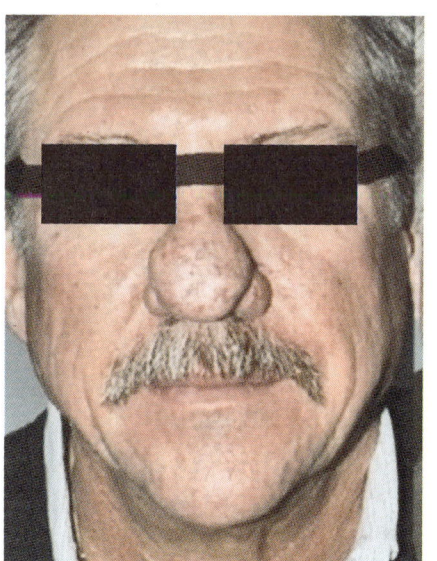

a. It is considered to be the end stage sequel of acne rosacea
b. Also known as potato tumor and rum/whisky nose
c. Hypertrophy of sebaceous glands
d. Treatment is surgical excision of excessive sebaceous tissue and underlying nasal cartilage

IMAGE BASED PRACTICE QUESTION BY THE AUTHOR

8. **The following nose deformity should be treated by:**

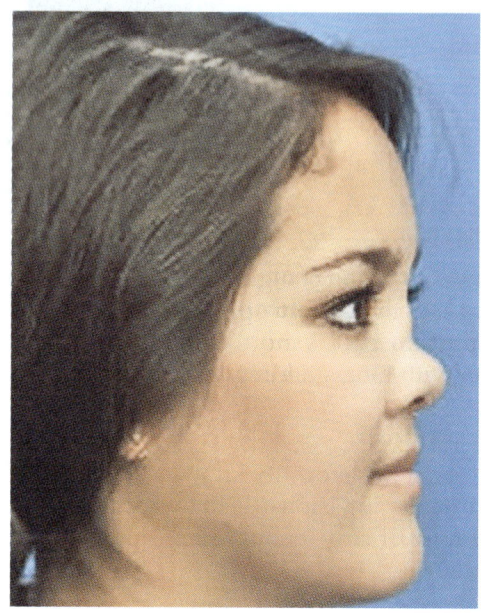

   a. Septoplasty
   b. SMR
   c. Augmentation rhinoplasty
   d. FESS

ANSWERS AND EXPLANATIONS

1. **(a) Hypertrophy of the sebaceous glands** (*Ref. Scott Brown, 6th ed., 4/2/8*)
2. **(c) Acne rosacea** (*Ref. Scott Brown, 6th ed., 4/2/8*)
3. **(d) Acromegaly** (*Ref. Scott Brown, 6th ed., 4/8/29*)
   - Acromegaly occurring due to growth hormone secreting pituitary adenoma is characterised by enlargement of the nose.
4. **(d) Hypertrophy of holocrine glands** (*Ref. Scott Brown, 6th ed., 4/2/8*)
   - Rhinophyma occurs due to hypertrophy of sebaceous glands of tip of nose.
   - Sebaceous glands are holocrine glands (i.e. the entire cell disintegrates while discharging its secretion).
   - Rhinophyma is typically seen in middle aged men with acne rosacea.
5. **(a) Deviated dorsum but tip midline** (easy to remember **C**rooked–**C** shaped) (*Ref. Scott Brown, 6th ed., 4/2/8*)
6. **(d) Basal cell carcinoma** (*Ref. Cummings, 6th ed., 294*)
7. **(d) Treatment is surgical excision of excessive sebaceous tissue and underlying nasal cartilage** (*Ref. Scott Brown, 6th ed., 4/2/8*)
8. **(c) Augmentation Rhinoplasty** (*Ref. Cummings, 6th ed., 506*)
   - Saddle nose deformity is seen in the image. The patient after augmentation rhinoplasty.

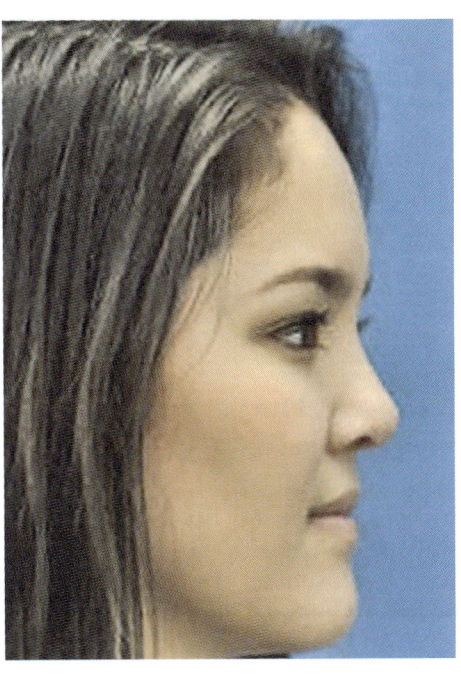

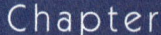

Chapter 18

Diseases of Nasal Septum

DEVIATED NASAL SEPTUM (DNS)

The most common deformity of the nasal septum is deviated nasal septum (DNS).

The most common cause of DNS is **birth trauma** (while passage through the birth canal usually following prolonged labour). Another reason can be differences in rate of growth of base of skull and palate leading to buckling of nasal septum.

About 60% of children are born with some degree of septal deviation. However this is largely asymptomatic and does not require treatment.

Clinical Features

A patient of DNS can present with the following symptoms:

1. **Nasal obstruction:** This is due to septal deviation and later on also due to hypertrophy of turbinate of the opposite side. This hypertrophy on the opposite side occurs to compensate for the increased space here. This hypertrophy is seen most commonly in the **inferior turbinate** (see Fig. 18.1A).

Note:

- Atrophy of turbinate on the side of DNS does not occur as pressure alone does not lead to atrophy.
- The hypertrophy that has occurred on the opposite side does not regress by just correction of the septum. It will have to be dealt separately by partial turbinectomy.

2. **Recurrent sinusitis:** This involves maxillary, ethmoid and frontal sinuses. This is due to interference with drainage of these sinuses leading to Sinusitis, nasal and postnasal discharge.

3. **Acute otitis media:** This may occur due to the infected post-nasal discharge of sinusitis going into middle ear through the Eustachian tube.

4. **Headache:** This is referred pain due to sinusitis or due to pressure of the deviated septum on the lateral wall.

5. **Ethmoidal neuralgia:** This is a rare headache also known as contact point headache, **Sluder's neuralgia** or sphenopalatine ganglion neuralgia. Pressure exerted by the **middle turbinate** (which is a part of ethmoid bone) on adjacent sensory nerves (anterior ethmoidal nerve, see nerve supply in chapter on anatomy of nose) of the deviated septum leads to pain which is known as anterior ethmoidal nerve syndrome or ethmoidal neuralgia.

6. **Epistaxis:** This is due to the deviated part or the septal spur (in DNS, at times there is a sharp deviation at the site of junction of septal cartilage and bone. This sharp deviation is known as septal spur, see Fig 18.1C) getting directly exposed to the drying effect of air and crusting.

7. **Cosmetic problem:** Crooked and Deviated nose.

8. **Hyposmia**

Investigations

A patient coming with the complaint of nasal obstruction should be tested for nasal valve patency.

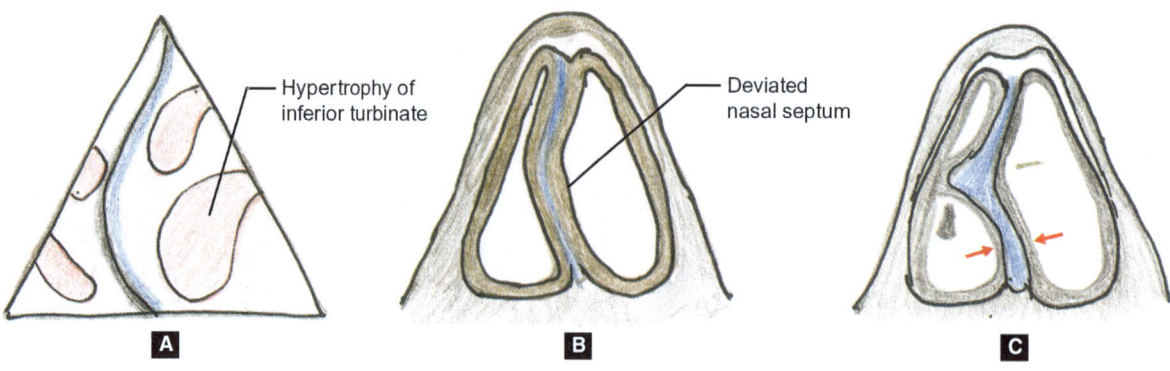

Fig. 18.1A to C

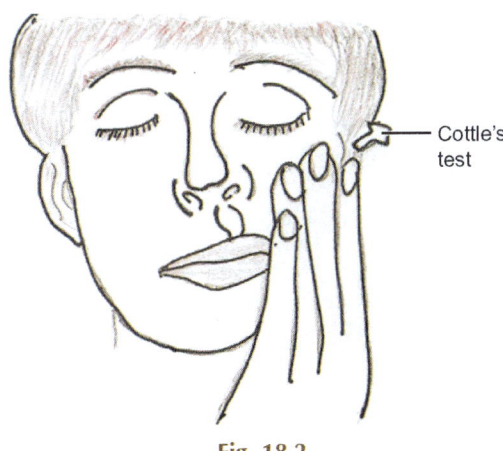

Fig. 18.2

A test for the **patency** of **nasal valve** area is known as "**Cottle's test**". In this test the patient pulls the cheeks upwards and laterally (opening the nasal valve area). If by doing this the nasal obstruction is relieved, an obstruction of nasal valve area by the DNS is confirmed.

This test is done in patients of DNS before doing septoplasty. If the nasal obstruction gets relieved by this test, it is an indication that the correction of septum will relieve the obstruction.

Management

Minor degrees of septal deviation not causing any symptoms do not require any treatment. The patients troubled by the above mentioned symptoms should be operated upon.

If the patient is **more than 17 yrs of age** then the patient is taken up for septal surgery. Any surgery on the septum or on the anterior 1/3rd of nose and adjacent area (e.g. septoplasty, rhinoplasty and Caldwell–Luc) is not done before 17 years of age. This is because in these areas are present the secondary centres of ossification which fuse by 17 years completing the facial development. Their damage will interfere with growth of nasal skeleton.

The two types of surgery on septum are:

a. **Sub-mucous resection of septum (SMR):** It is done under local anaesthesia with 2% xylocaine and adrenaline (cocaine paste alone owing to its anaesthetic and vasoconstricting property is also used in some centres).

Here the incision is given **5 mm above the caudal border of the septal cartilage (Killian's incision)**.

Mucoperichondrial and mucoperiosteal flaps are raised on both sides of the septum, so that the septum is now free on both sides. Leaving a thin (1 cm) dorsal and a caudal strip, the rest of the septum is removed.

Complication: This can lead to loss of support of dorsum and **saddling**. It can also lead to perforation and flapping (free movement) of the septum.

b. **Septoplasty:** It is also done under local anaesthesia. Here the incision is given at the caudal (lower) border of the septal cartilage (**Freer's incision**). **The mucoperichondrial flap is raised only on one side** and **only the deviated part of septum is removed**.

This is more conservative procedure and the **preferred surgery** for DNS.

The incidence of complications of septal perforation, flapping, saddling seen in Septoplasty is much less than SMR.

SEPTAL HEMATOMA

Any **injury** to the nose, iatrogenic or non-iatrogenic can lead to septal hematoma. Here there is collection of blood under the perichondrium on both the sides. Therefore, it leads to **B/L nasal obstruction**.

On examination there is smooth rounded swelling of septum on both its sides.

Management

The blood supply of the septal cartilage is deprived because of its perichondrium being raised on both sides hence a septal hematoma has to be **drained as early as possible** usually within 72 hrs otherwise there will occur necrosis of septal cartilage and loss of support of dorsum leading to saddling of nose. It may get infected and can lead to septal abscess formation.

SEPTAL ABSCESS

Any furuncle of the nose or infection of septal hematoma can lead to septal abscess formation. It leads to B/L nasal obstruction.

A septal abscess has to be drained as early as possible or it will lead to necrosis of septal cartilage and saddling.

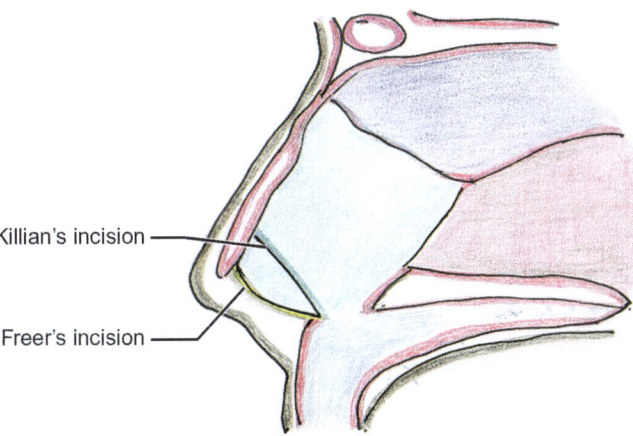

Fig. 18.3: Incision for Septoplasty and SMR

Killian's incision

Freer's incision

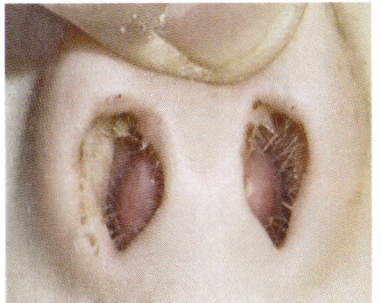 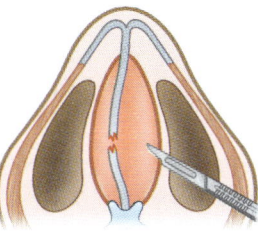

Fig. 18.4: Septal Hematoma

Nose

Section II

Complication: A septal abscess can lead to the following complications:

1. Saddling
2. Perforation
3. Cellulitis of face
4. Meningitis
5. Cavernous sinus thrombosis

A furuncle/septal abscess involves the **dangerous area of face**. This drains into the deep facial vein, which through pterygoid plexus of veins is connected to cavernous sinus and cerebral veins leading to the above complications.

SEPTAL PERFORATION

The causes of septal perforation are as below:

1. **Trauma/Injury (most common):** Iatrogenic (cauterisation of Little's area, septal surgeries, septal piercing for ornaments), non-iatrogenic (habitual nose picking).

2. Septal abscess

3. **Granulomatous conditions** being destructive therefore those involving the nose cause perforation in the cartilaginous part. Some like Syphilis and Wegner's granulomatosis cause additionally bony perforation also.

4. **Nasal myiasis:** Maggots of nose is known as nasal myiasis.

   Any condition leading to foul smelling nasal discharge and putrefied nasal debris (e.g. atrophic rhinitis) attracts flies (commonly chrysomia species) which lay eggs in the nose, its larvae are known as maggots. Management is by killing the maggots with **chloroform water and turpentine oil** and removing them by alkaline nasal douche.

5. **Rhinolith:** Calcium deposition around foreign body of nose is rhinolith which can cause pressure necrosis and perforation of septum. It usually requires removal under general anaesthesia.

6. Cocaine being a vasoconstrictor, in addicts can lead to perforation.

7. **Tumours**

Clinical features: Small perforations cause whistling sound during respiration and large perforation causes excessive crusting and nasal obstruction.

Management: Perforations can be closed by flap. In case of larger perforations where surgery is not possible, silastic button can be worn.

SMR	Septoplasty
Killian's incision	Freer's incision
Flaps raised on both sides	On one side only
Almost all of the cartilaginous septum is removed	Only the deviated part of the cartilaginous septum is removed
Therefore extensive procedure and hence more complications	Conservative procedure, less complications
Less preferred	More preferred

 "Points to Ponder/Points for Quick revision"

DNS:

- Birth trauma (60%)
- CFs: U/L or B/L Nasal obstruction (deviation + opposite side hypertrophied turbinates (MC–inferior)—interference with sinus drainage (except sphenoid) → sinusitis → ± AOM.
- Headache (Sluder's neuralgia; middle turbinate → ant. Ethmoidal N)—septal spur crust → epistaxis; Hyposmia.
- Cottle's test-nasal valve patency.
- Management: If CFs +, Cottle's test + ve and age > 17 → surgical correction (*see* table SMR *vs* Septoplasty) ↓ LA (2% xylocaine + adrenaline or cocaine paste).

Septal hematoma:

- Blood collection on both sides of septum ↓ the perichondrium → B/L nasal obstruction. O/E–B/L rounded swelling; Complications–saddle nose, septal abscess; Drainage (<72 hrs).

Septal abscess:

- Dangerous area → meningitis, cavernous sinus thrombosis— Saddle nose, septal perforation; I & D (asap).

Septal perforation:

- Trauma (MC), septal abscess, granulomatous conditions (syphilis and WG → bony septum perf.), nasal myiasis, rhinolith, cocaine abuse.
- Excessive crusting → nasal obstruction—closure by flap/ silastic button.

PREVIOUSLY ASKED QUESTIONS

1. **Percentage of newborns with deviation of nasal septum:** *(Karnataka 2000, Exam 2017)*
   a. 2%
   b. 10%
   c. 30%
   d. 60%

2. **Features associated with DNS include all of the following except:** *(AI 2005, Exam 2017)*
   a. Epistaxis
   b. Atrophy of turbinate
   c. Hypertrophy of turbinate
   d. Recurrent sinusitis

3. **DNS may be associated with all the following except:** *(AI 2002, Exam 2017)*
   a. Recurrent sphenoiditis
   b. Acute otitis media
   c. Hypertrophy of the inferior turbinate
   d. Recurrent maxillary sinusitis

4. **The aetiology of anterior ethmoidal neuralgia is:** *(AIIMS 2003, Exam 2017)*
   a. Inferior turbinate pressing on the nasal septum
   b. Middle turbinate pressing on the nasal septum
   c. Superior turbinate pressing on the nasal septum
   d. Causing obstruction of sphenoid opening

5. **For DNS, surgery is required for:** *(PGI 2001, 2014)*
   a. Septal spur with epistaxis
   b. Septal deviation
   c. Nasal obstruction
   d. Recurrent sinusitis
   e. Prolonged DNS

6. **Cottle's test is for the patency of the nares in:** *(JIPMER 2000, Exam 2017)*
   a. Atrophic rhinitis
   b. Rhinosporidiosis
   c. Deviated nasal septum
   d. Hypertrophied inferior turbinate

7. **Improvement in nasal patency by retracting the lateral part of the cheek and thus testing the valvular component of the nose is:** *(MH 2008, Exam 2016)*
   a. Epley's manoeuvre
   b. Cottle's test
   c. Schwartz manoeuvre
   d. Heimlich manoeuvre

8. **All of the following are true of septoplasty operation for DNS except:** *(UPSC, Exam 2017)*
   a. Indicated in septal deviation
   b. Mucoperichondrium removed
   c. Preferably done after 17 years of age
   d. Done in cases of epistaxis

9. **Which of the following surgery is not contraindicated below 12 years of age?** *(MH 2003, Exam 2017)*
   a. Rhinoplasty
   b. SMR
   c. Septoplasty
   d. FESS

10. **Alternative for SMR:** *(Exam 2001, Exam 2017)*
    a. Tympanoplasty
    b. Septoplasty
    c. Caldwell-Luc operation
    d. Turboplasty

11. **Common indication of septoplasty:** *(PGI June 2004, Exam 2014)*
    a. DNS with symptoms
    b. Anosmia
    c. Sluder's neuralgia
    d. Septal spur

12. **Killian's incision is used for:** *(TN 2004, Exam 2017)*
    a. SMR operation
    b. Intranasal antrostomy
    c. Caldwell-Luc operation
    d. Myringoplasty

13. **Local anaesthetic used for nasal surgery:** *(Exam 2013)*
    a. Cocaine paste
    b. Xylocaine
    c. Both
    d. None of the above

14. **True about septal hematoma:** *(PGI 2002, 2015)*
    a. Occurs due to trauma
    b. Can lead to saddle nose deformity
    c. Conservative treatment
    d. May lead to abscess formation
    e. Surgical drainage has to be done immediately

15. **After laparoscopic appendicectomy, patient had fall from bed on her nose after which she had swelling in nose and difficulty in breathing. Next step in management:** *(AIIMS May 2013, 2007)*
    a. I/V antibiotics for 7–10 days
    b. Observation in hospital
    c. Surgical drainage
    d. Discharge after 2 days and follow-up of the patient after 8 weeks

16. **Most common cause of perforation of cartilaginous part of nasal septum:** *(Kolkata 2006, Exam 2017)*
    a. Syphilis
    b. Tuberculosis
    c. Trauma
    d. Septal abscess

17. **Bony septal perforation occurs in:** *(Karnataka 95, Exam 2016)*
    a. TB
    b. Syphilis
    c. Leprosy
    d. Sarcoidosis

Nose

Section II

18. **Nasal septum perforation occurs in all the following except:** *(UP 2004, Exam 2017)*
    a. Tuberculosis
    b. Nasal surgery
    c. Syphilis
    d. Allergic rhinitis

19. **Septal perforation is not seen in:**
    (Exam 2002, Exam 2017)
    a. Septal abscess
    b. Leprosy
    c. Rhinophyma
    d. Trauma

20. **Bony Nasal septal perforation is characteristically seen in:** *(TN 2004, Exam 2017)*
    a. Wegener's granulomatosis
    b. Leprosy
    c. Sarcoidosis
    d. Tuberculosis

21. **Maggots in nasal cavity are most commonly treated by:** *(AI 98, Exam 2015)*
    a. Chloroform diluted with water
    b. Liquid paraffin
    c. Systemic antibiotics
    d. Lignocaine spray

IMAGE BASED PRACTICE QUESTION BY THE AUTHOR

22. **A patient presents with nasal obstruction after being hit on face from front. On examination, a boggy swelling of the septum is seen on either sides (*see* picture below), which is fluctuant on palpation with a swab or blunt probe. He should be managed by:**

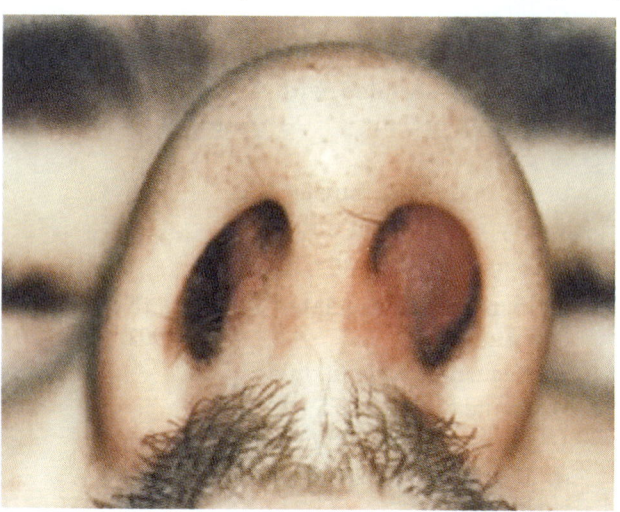

    a. Incision and drainage
    b. Nasal packing
    c. Antibiotics
    d. Nasal decongestants

ANSWERS AND EXPLANATIONS

1. **(d) 60%** (*Ref. Scott Brown, 6th ed., Paediatric, 6/15/5; Cummings, 6th ed., 2879*)

2. **(b) Atrophy of turbinate** (*Ref. Cummings, 6th ed., 474*)
   There is no pressure atrophy of the turbinates on the side of deviation of septum. In DNS there occurs hypertrophy of turbinate of opposite site.

3. **(a) Recurrent sphenoiditis** (*Ref. Cummings, 6th ed., 474*)
   - The sphenoid sinus opens in the spheno-ethmoid recess near the roof of the nasal cavity and this opening is not affected by DNS.
   - DNS predisposes to all the other sinusitis, i.e. maxillary, frontal and ethmoid, by interfering with their drainages.
   - The post nasal discharge of sinusitis, through the Eustachian tube, leads to acute Otitis media.

4. **(b) Middle turbinate pressing on the nasal septum** (*Ref. Scott Brown, 6th ed., Paediatric, 4/11/5*) (refer the text)

5. **(a), (c) and (d)** (*Ref. Scott Brown, 8th ed., Vol 1; 1140*)
   - Minor degrees of septal deviation not causing any symptoms do not require any treatment. The cases producing symptoms, e.g. epistaxis, nasal obstruction, recurrent sinusitis should be operated upon.

6. **(c) Deviated nasal septum** (*Ref. Cummings, 6th ed., 477*)

7. **(b) Cottle's test** (*Ref. Cummings, 6th ed., 477; Scott Brown, 8th ed., Vol 1; 987*)
   - Epley's manoeuvre is the repositioning manoeuvre done for the management of BPPV (benign paroxysmal positional vertigo).
   - Heimlich manoeuvre is the initial immediate management of accidental inhalation of foreign body. In Heimlich manoeuvre multiple thrusts are given with the wrist in the upper epigastrium while standing behind the patient.
   - There is no Schwartz manoeuvre

8. **(b) Mucoperichondrium removed** (*Ref. Cummings, 6th ed., 2880*)
   - Mucoperichondrium is neither removed in septoplasty nor in SMR.

9. **(d) FESS** (*Ref. Cummings, 6th ed., 2879*)
   - Rest of the surgeries mentioned above are done after complete facial development, i.e. 17 years of age
   - Rhinoplasty is a cosmetic surgery aimed at correcting the external deformity of the nose.

10. **(b) Septoplasty** (*Ref. Cummings, 6th ed., 481*)
    - Septoplasty is more conservative procedure than SMR and is the preferred surgery for DNS.

11. **(a), (c) and (d)** (*Ref. Scott Brown, 6th ed., Paediatric, 4/11/6*) (refer the text)

12. **(a) SMR operation** (*Ref. Cummings, 6th ed., 482; Scott Brown, 8th ed., Vol 1; 1137*)

13. **(c) Both** (*Ref. Cummings, 6th ed., 482*)
    - Most common local anaesthetic used for nasal surgery (septoplasty) is 2% xylocaine (along with adrenaline) for local infiltration and 4% xylocaine for nasal packing (for doing nasal endoscopy).
    - Cocaine is one of the most potent anesthetic agent and vasoconstrictor. These two characteristics make it an ideal medication for use during nasal surgery (here there is no need to give adrenaline) to decrease bleeding and pain. However because of its toxicity Cocaine paste use in nasal surgeries has decreased.

14. **(a), (b), (d) and (e)** (*Ref. Cummings, 6th ed., 2964*) (refer to text)

15. **(c) Surgical drainage** (*Ref. Scott Brown, 6th ed., Paediatric, 4/11/1*)
    - She has possibly developed septal hematoma which has to be drained as early as possible.

16. **(c) Trauma** (*Ref. Scott Brown, 8th ed., Vol 1; 1149*)

17. **(b) Syphilis** (*Ref. Scott Brown, 6th ed., Paediatric, 4/11/19*)
    - Syphilis leads to perforation of the bony part of nasal septum. Another important cause of bony septal perforation is Wegener's granulomatosis.
    - Rest options may lead to perforation of the cartilaginous part of the septum.

18. **(d) Allergic rhinitis** (*Ref. Scott Brown, 8th ed., Vol 1; 1150*)
    - Rhinosporidiosis is a Protistan Protozoa infection and does not lead to septal perforation.

19. **(c) Rhinophyma** (*Ref. Scott Brown, 8th ed., Vol 1; 1150*)
    - Also known as potato nose Rhinophyma is due to hypertrophy of the sebaceous glands of the tip of nose. It does not involve the septum.

20. **(a) Wegener's granulomatosis** (*Ref. Scott Brown, 6th ed., Paediatric, 4/11/19*)

21. **(a) Chloroform diluted with water** (*Ref. Scott Brown, 6th ed., Paediatric, 4/8/45*)

22. **(a) Incision and drainage** (*Ref. Cummings, 6th ed., 2964*)
    - The history is suggestive of septal hematoma. Image shows the bulging of the septum on the sides.

Acute and Chronic Rhinitis

ACUTE RHINITIS

The most common acute infection of the nose is viral rhinitis also called coryza or common cold.

Common cold is the most common illness in humans. Rhinovirus (most commonly), Influenza, parainfluenza, Coronavirus, respiratory syncitial virus, etc. all lead to common cold.

CHRONIC SIMPLE RHINITIS

If any patient is chronically exposed to infection from adjacent areas (e.g. sinusitis, adenoiditis), he develops chronic simple rhinitis.

Clinical Features

Patient presents with nasal obstruction, nasal discharge and postnasal discharge.

On examination, the nasal mucosa appears congested and swollen which pits on pressure and decongests by decongestants.

Management

Treatment of the underlying cause and nasal decongestants to relieve nasal obstruction. Nasal decongestants should not be given continuously **for more than 7 days** because they can lead to rhinitis medica mentosa.

RHINITIS MEDICA MENTOSA

The prolonged use of nasal decongestants, e.g. oxy and xylometazoline (alpha 1 agonists) lead to a condition called Rhinitis medicamentosa. It is characterised by a progressive increase in dose and frequency of nasal decongestants and despite using higher doses there occurs progressively severe nasal obstruction, once the effect of the decongestant dissipates. This is due to rebound congestion.

Proposed Mechanisms of Rhinitis Medicamentosa

1. Down regulation of alpha 1 receptors leading to requirement of higher doses.

2. Higher dosage leads to severe vasoconstriction leading to local hypoxia and release of ischemic toxic metabolites which in turn leads to rebound congestion. This can also result in atrophic changes (loss of cilia and squamous metaplasia).

Rhinitis medicamentosa is managed by withdrawal of the drug and a short course of preferably local steroids and if required systemic steroids. Steroids by modulating the gene transcription restore the alpha 1 receptors.

HYPERTROPHIC RHINITIS

If a patient of chronic simple rhinitis is not treated he will go into the sequelae, i.e. hypertrophic rhinitis. As the name, because of repeated infection submucosal fibrosis occurs leading to hypertrophy of turbinates.

The turbinate to get hypertrophied most commonly is the **inferior turbinate**. This gives **mulberry appearance** to the inferior turbinate.

The main complaint here is nasal obstruction.

Management

Here since the nasal obstruction is because of fibrosis, the turbinate will neither pit on pressure nor will it decongest with decongestants. So to relieve the nasal obstruction, the size of hypertrophic turbinates will have to be reduced, by doing **turbinectomy** either partial or total.

Turbinectomy is done by laser, cryosurgery, diathermy, radiofrequency ablation or surgically by submucous resection of turbinate.

ATROPHIC RHINITIS

It is a form of chronic rhinitis associated with atrophy of nasal mucosa, mucous glands, nerves and vessels.

It can be primary or secondary.

Primary atrophic rhinitis is idiopathic, however many theories have been postulated for its causation, *see* below

Secondary atrophic rhinitis is secondary to some of the destructive granulomatous conditions of the nose, e.g. leprosy, rhinoscleroma, syphilis, SLE or secondary to excessive tissue destruction following surgery or trauma.

Primary atrophic rhinitis postulated causes:

a. Hereditary

b. Endocrinal—**oestrogen deficiency**. It is typically seen at puberty in those females who are oestrogen deficient.

c. Racial—white and yellow races more prone

d. Nutritional deficiency—vitamin A, D and iron

e. Autoimmune

f. Infective—infection with *Klebsiella ozanae*, *Cocobacillus Ozanae* and Diphtheroids are associated with atrophic rhinitis, because of which atrophic rhinitis is also known as **Ozanae**.

Pathology

Everything in the nose atrophies. The normal pseudostratified ciliated columnar epithelium undergoes metaplasia to stratified squamous epithelium. The mucous glands atrophy. Arteries undergo obliterative endarteritis and atrophy. Nerves undergo atrophy. The turbinates undergo atrophy.

When everything in the nose becomes atrophic, both the nasal cavities become **roomy**. Because of the cavities becoming roomy and also due to mucus gland destruction they get exposed to the drying effects of air and crusting.

In spite of roomy cavities the patient has nasal obstruction. This is because of:

a. Excessive crusting

b. Loss of sensory nerves: The sensory nerves sense the flow of air mainly through the nasal valve area. These nerve endings are destroyed in patients with atrophic rhinitis. In the absence of these sensations the nose feels blocked.

Because the defence mechanisms of cilia and mucous glands is no more there, nose becomes more prone to get severely secondarily infected leading to tissue destruction and anaerobic infection resulting in a **very foul smelling discharge from the nose**.

The patient is brought by his family or friends, with the complaint of very foul smelling discharge from the nose of the patient which the patient himself is unaware of. This is because the patient has anosmia because of atrophy of nerves and whatever mucosa and nerves is left is covered by crust preventing air contact. This is known as **merciful or blissful anosmia**.

On removal of crusts there is bleeding. The nasal mucosa appears pale due to obliterative endarteritis.

A patient of atrophic rhinitis can have atrophic pharyngitis and atrophic laryngitis (laryngitis sicca) also.

Management

The **principle of medical management** of atrophic rhinitis is removal of crusts, treatment of the infection and prevention of further formation of crusts thereby relieving nasal obstruction. For the above we use:

1. **Alkaline nasal douche:** This is sodium chloride, sodium bicarbonate and sodium biborate in 280 ml of distilled water in the ratio of 2 : 1 : 1. This is for removal of crusts.

2. **25% glucose in glycerine spray:** Glucose on fermentation produces lactic acid and an acidic pH that inhibits proteolytic bacteria. Glycerine helps as a lubricant and hygroscopic agent (adsorbs water from the atmosphere and moistens mucosa, and hence impedes crust formation).

3. **Kemicetine solution:** This contains chloramphenicol (C), oestradiol (O), propylene glycol (P), and vitamin D2 (D) (*Mnemonic:* COPD).

4. **Submucosal placental extract and oestradiol spray** have shown to increase the blood supply of nasal mucosa.

5. **Potassium iodide:** It increases the nasal secretions.

The **surgical options** aim to reduce the size of the roomy cavities to prevent the exposure to drying effects of air and crusts formation and thus help regeneration of nasal mucosa.

Young's Operation

In this surgery a mucosal flap is raised from the lateral wall and another flap is raised from the medial wall, i.e. the septum and they are sutured in the midline so as to close the nostril completely. When the nostril is opened after 6 months to 1 year, the nasal mucosa has got regenerated.

This procedure was not tolerated by some as it led to mouth breathing and a de-nasal voice. So a modification of the above procedure is to leave a 3 mm opening in the centre of the two flaps. This is known as **modified Young's operation**.

Lautenslager's Operation

This surgery also aims at narrowing the nasal cavities to decrease the drying effects and crusting. This can be done by displacing the lateral wall of nose medially by insertion of Teflon or cartilage.

RHINITIS SICCA

It is a condition seen in people exposed to hot dry climate like bakers, iron smiths.

The anterior rhinoscopic appearance resembles atrophic rhinitis with the only difference that it affects **only the anterior 1/3 of the nose**, the posterior part of nasal cavities appearing normal. This is because, as discussed in chapter 16, one of the function of the nose is temperature regulation and however hot or cold the air may be, the temperature gets regulated to body temperature in ¼th of a second that the air takes to reach the choana. So the ill effects of the hot air is maximum in the anterior 1/3rd.

Management is removal of crusts and application of lubricants and antibiotic ointments.

RHINITIS CASEOSA (NASAL CHOLESTEATOMA)

Collection of cheesy material in the nose following chronic sinusitis or any obstruction is known as rhinitis caseosa. It has been named cholesteatoma just because of its appearance like cholesteatoma of the ear. It is a unilateral condition seen more commonly in males. Management is by scooping the discharge and treating the associated cause.

Nose

Section II

ALLERGIC RHINITIS

Allergic rhinitis is an IgE mediated **Type 1 hypersensitivity** reaction to one or more allergens. It can be seasonal where the most common cause of allergy is pollens, or perennial, where it is caused by house dust, animal dander or mould spores.

Clinical Features

Patients present with rhinorrhoea, postnasal drip, paroxysmal episodes of sneezing, nasal obstruction, lacrimation, itching of eyes and nose. There is usually dark discolouration and puffiness below lower eyelids (allergic shiners); creases in the lower eyelid skin (Dennie Morgan lines). These are due to venous stasis due to chronic nasal obstruction.

Also because of repeated pushing upwards of the nasal tip with hands there appears a crease. This skin crease is known as allergic salute.

Diagnosis

A family history of allergy is generally present.

On examination, anterior rhinoscopy shows pale boggy (swollen) sometimes bluish mucosa.

Investigations

All the tests of allergy are positive, e.g. skin prick tests, intradermal testing, peripheral eosinophilia, absolute eosinophil count (AEC), RAST (Radio Allergosorbent test) which tests the IgE in the serum.

Management

1. Avoidance of allergens
2. Antihistaminics (Fexofenadine, Cetirizine, Loratadine, etc.) and decongestants (Pseudoephedrine, Phenylephrine)
3. Intranasal steroids which are used in the form of nasal spray or systemic steroids in severe cases
4. Mast cell stabilizers
5. Leukotriene antagonists (Montelukast)
6. Immunotherapy may be considered. It may increase the threshold of appearance of symptoms.

VASOMOTOR RHINITIS/NON-ALLERGIC RHINITIS/INTRINSIC RHINITIS

Non Allergic Rhinitis is the name given to a group of rhinitis where the symptoms resemble allergic rhinitis but the tests of allergy, as mentioned above, are negative. It can be hormone related, medications, irritants or chemical induced.

When no clear aetiology of non-allergic rhinitis is found it is called idiopathic orintrinsic or vasomotor rhinitis. It is the most common form of non-allergic rhinitis.

Vasomotor rhinitis is thought to be due to **parasympathetic over-activity**. The parasympathetic supply of the nose is by vidian nerve (*see* the Chapter on anatomy). Its over activity leads to vasodilatation and congestion.

Here the patient presents exactly like allergic rhinitis, i.e. paroxysmal sneezing, rhinorrhoea, postnasal drip, nasal obstruction but there is no history of allergy and the symptoms persist throughout the year.

On examination, anterior rhinoscopy shows congested (due to vasodilatation) nasal mucosa and hypertrophic turbinate.

Management

The medical management consists of oral (e.g. phenylephrine) and local nasal decongestants (e.g. xylometazoline) and steroids in the form of nasal spray.

If the patient does not benefit by medical management, **vidian neurectomy** (section of parasympathetic fibres can be done).

The nasal obstruction due to hypertrophic turbinate (inferior turbinate) can be managed by partial or total turbinectomy by laser, cryosurgery and cautery or submucosal resection.

 Note:

A type of non-allergic rhinitis where as usual the blood and skin tests of allergy are negative but the cytological examination of nasal secretions shows marked eosinophilia is known as non allergic rhinitis with eosinophilia (NARES).

 "Points to Ponder/Points for Quick revision"

Acute rhinitis: Common cold/coryza–viral–Rhinovirus (MC).

Rhinitis medicamentosa: Prolonged nasal decongestants oxy and xylometazoline $\rightarrow$ $\downarrow$ $\alpha1$ rec $\rightarrow$ $\uparrow$ dose requirement $\rightarrow$ ischemic damage; t/t—local steroids (modify gene transcription $\rightarrow$ restoration of $\alpha1$ rec.

Chronic simple rhinitis: If untreated $\rightarrow$ Hypertrophic rhinitis (MC-inferior turbinate fibrosis); Mulberry appearance; t/t—turbinectomy.

Atrophic rhinitis (ozanae): B/L, young females (*mnemonic*: Young's operation in the t/t)

- 1°–hereditary, pubertal oestrogen deficiency, Klebsiella ozanae; 2°–Granulomatous diseases, trauma.
- CFs: Nasal obstruction (despite B/L roomy nasal cavities) due to $\uparrow$ crusting; 2° infections $\rightarrow$ very foul nasal discharge; Merciful anosmia; Atrophic pharyngitis/laryngitis.
- T/t: Medical–Alkaline douche (Na Cl/HCO$_3$/biborate), 25% glucose-glycerine, Kemicetine (COPD), KI, oestrogen spray
- Young's operation/modified Young's operation (preferred-with 3 mm opening left).

Rhinitis sicca: Resembles atrophic rhinitis (but involves only anterior 1/3 of nose), bakers, iron smiths.

Allergic rhinitis: IgE Type 1 hypersensitivity; Seasonal (pollens–MC), Perennial-dust mites, animal dander, etc.

- CFs: Rhinorrhoea, paroxysmal sneezing, lacrimation, itching, "allergic shiners", "Dennie Morgan lines", "allergic salute"; Pale and swollen mucosa.
- T/t: Avoidance of allergens, Antihistaminics, Mast cell stabilisers, Leukotriene antagonists, Intra-nasal steroids, Immunotherapy.

Vasomotor rhinitis: Parasympathetic overactivity; CFs like allergic rhinitis but congested nasal mucosa; Inferior turbinate hypertrophy; T/t–decongestants and steroids, if no relief $\rightarrow$ Vidian neurectomy.

PREVIOUSLY ASKED QUESTIONS

1. **Common cold is caused primarily by:**
   (Karnataka 2002, Exam 2017)
   a. Viruses
   b. Bacteria
   c. Fungi
   d. Allergy

2. **Prolonged and repeated use of nasal decongestants leads to:** *(CUPGEE 95, 2015)*
   a. Rhinitis medicamentosa
   b. Bronchitis
   c. Both
   d. None

3. **Rhinitis medica mentosa is due to:**
   (Exam 2013, 2016, 2018)
   a. Nasal decongestants
   b. Steroids
   c. Antihistamines
   d. Surgery

4. **A man using xylometazoline nasal drops continuously for long period of time. What can be the possible adverse effect?** *(Exam 2013)*
   a. Mulberry turbinate
   b. Allergic rhinitis
   c. Vasomotor rhinitis
   d. Rhinitis medicamentosa

5. **All of the following surgical procedures are used for hypertrophic rhinitis except:**
   (AIIMS 2004, Exam 2017)
   a. Radiofrequency ablation of the inferior turbinate
   b. Laser ablation of the inferior turbinate
   c. Sub-mucosal placement of silastic in inferior turbinate
   d. Inferior turbinectomy

6. **Mulberry appearance of nasal turbinate is seen in:** *(MP 2006, Exam 2017)*
   a. Coryza
   b. Atrophic rhinitis
   c. Maxillary sinusitis
   d. Hypertrophic rhinitis

7. **Which of the following organism is known to cause atrophic rhinitis?** *(MP 2007, Exam 2017)*
   a. *Klebsiella pneumoniae*
   b. *Klebsiella ozanae*
   c. *Streptococcus pneumoniae*
   d. *Streptococcus foetidis*

8. **Ozaena is also known as:** *(Exam 2013)*
   a. Hypertrophic rhinitis
   b. Vasomotor rhinitis
   c. Allergic rhinitis
   d. Atrophic rhinitis

9. **All are implicated in aetiology of atrophic rhinitis except:** *(Exam 2002, Exam 2017)*
   a. Surgical excessive tissue destruction
   b. Granulomatous conditions
   c. DNS
   d. Strong hereditary factors

10. **Regarding atrophic rhinitis which is incorrect?**
    (AP 98, Exam 2011)
    a. Common in females
    b. Seen at 50–60 years of life
    c. Can occur secondary to syphilis
    d. Anosmia

11. **All are true about ozanae except:**
    (UP 2003, Exam 2017)
    a. Common in female
    b. It is usually unilateral
    c. Nasal cavity is filled with crusts
    d. Atrophic pharyngitis

12. **All are true regarding atrophic rhinitis except:**
    (AP 2004, Exam 2017)
    a. More common in males
    b. Crusts are seen
    c. Anosmia is noticed
    d. Young's operation is useful

13. **Most common cause of obstruction in atrophic rhinitis is:** *(PGI 97, 2000, 2014)*
    a. Excessive formation of crust
    b. Polyp
    c. Synechiae
    d. Hypertrophy of turbinate

14. **Alkaline douche solution of nose does not contain:** *(MH 2006, Exam 2017)*
    a. NaCl
    b. Na biborate
    c. $NaHCO_3$
    d. Glucose

15. **Young's operation is done for:**
    (JIPMER 2002, MP 2003, Jharkhand 2006, MH CET 2015)
    a. Allergic rhinitis
    b. Atrophic rhinitis
    c. Vasomotor rhinitis
    d. Viral rhinitis

16. **In allergic rhinitis nasal mucosa is:**
    (MP 2003, Exam 2017)
    a. Pale and swollen
    b. Congested and swollen
    c. Pale and atrophied
    d. Any of the above

17. **Allergic rhinitis treatment include all except:**
    (Exam 2013)
    a. Mast cell stabilisers
    b. Avoiding allergen
    c. Corticosteroids
    d. Surgery

18. **Vidian neurectomy is done for:**
    (CUPGEE 97, Exam 2015)
    a. Vasomotor rhinitis
    b. Rhinitis sicca
    c. Allergic rhinitis
    d. Atrophic rhinitis

Section II Nose

19. **What is the treatment of rhinitis medicamentosa?**
                                         (*Exam 2016*)
   a. Withdrawal of nasal drops with short course of steroids
   b. Antibiotics
   c. Polypectomy
   d. Increasing the dose of the nasal drops

20. **Which of the following drugs is linked with rhinitis medicamentosa?**   (*MH CET 2015*)
   a. Intranasal steroid spray
   b. Ipratropium bromide
   c. Xylometazoline
   d. Cocaine

21. **Feature of atrophic rhinitis includes:**
                                  (*Kerala PGMEE 2015*)
   a. Watery nose
   b. Anosmia
   c. Swelling of turbinates
   d. Swelling over dorsum of nose

22. **True about vasomotor rhinitis:**   (*PGI May 2015*)
   a. It is a type of allergic reaction
   b. Clinically simulate nasal allergy
   c. Nasal mucosa generally congested and hypertrophic
   d. Hypertrophy of inferior turbinate is commonly present
   e. Oral nasal decongestant are used in treatment

23. **Management of rhinitis medicamentosa is:**
                                         (*UPSC 2015*)
   a. Local steroids   b. Systemic steroids
   c. Xylometazoline   d. FESS

RECENT EXAM PATTERN IMAGE BASED PRACTICE QUESTION BY THE AUTHOR

24. **A patient presents with nasal obstruction and anosmia. His nasal endoscopy picture is given below. All the following constitute the treatment except:**

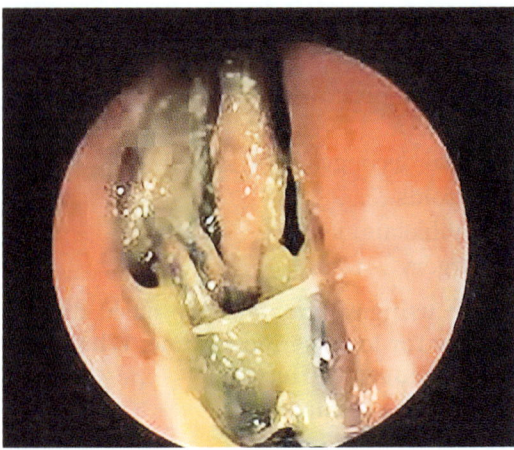

   a. Nasal douching
   b. Inferior turbinectomy
   c. Young's operation
   d. Glucose in glycerine solution

ANSWERS AND EXPLANATIONS

1. **(a) viruses** (*Ref. Cummings, 6th ed., 725*)
2. **(a) Rhinitis medicamentosa** (*Ref. Cummings, 6th ed., 695*)
3. **(a) Nasal decongestants** (*Ref. Scott Brown, 8th ed., Vol 1; 1006*)
4. **(d) Rhinitis medicamentosa** (*Ref. Cummings, 6th ed., 695; Scott Brown, 8th ed., Vol 1; 1006*)
5. **(c) Submucosal placement of silastic in inferior turbinate** (*Ref. Cummings, 6th ed., 700; Scott Brown, 8th ed., Vol 1; 1146*)
   - Submucosal placement of silastic will aggravate the condition, refer the text.
6. **(d) Hypertrophic rhinitis** (*Ref. Cummings, 6th ed., 491*) (refer the text)
7. **(b) *Klebsiella ozanae*** (*Ref. Cummings, 6th ed., 695*)
8. **(d) Atrophic rhinitis** (*Ref. Cummings, 6th ed., 695*)
9. **(c) DNS** (*Ref. Cummings, 6th ed., 695*)
   - In DNS there occurs physiologic hypertrophy of the nasal turbinates on the opposite side of deviation.
10. **(b) Seen at 50–60 years of life** (*Ref. Cummings, 6th ed., 695*)
    - Though estrogen deficiency has been implicated in the causation of atrophic rhinitis, but it is not seen at menopause. It is seen in females with low estrogen at puberty.
11. **(b) It is usually unilateral** (*Ref. Scott Brown, 6th ed., 4/8/27*)
    - Here both the nasal cavities are filled with crusts.
12. **(a) More common in males** (*Ref. Scott Brown, 6th ed., 4/8/27*)
13. **(a) Excessive formation of crust** (*Ref. Cummings, 6th ed., 695*)
    - The excessive crusting leads to nasal obstruction in spite of roomy cavities.

- On removal of crusts there is bleeding. But there is no synechiae formation. There is no polypoidal change [for the mucosa is not oedematous (*see* chapter on nasal polyps), it is atrophied].
14. **(d) Glucose** (*Ref. Scott Brown, 6th ed., 4/8/27*) (refer to text)
15. **(b) Atrophic rhinitis** (*Ref. Scott Brown, 6th ed., 4/8/27*)
    - Allergic rhinitis is managed by antihistaminics, decongestants and steroid nasal spray.
    - Vasomotor rhinitis is managed by local and systemic decongestants and if required vidian neurectomy.
    - In viral rhinitis only symptomatic treatment is given.
16. **(a) Pale and swollen** (*Ref. Cummings, 6th ed., 618; Scott Brown, 8th ed., Vol 1; 1001*)
    - In allergic rhinitis nasal mucosa on anterior rhinoscopy appears pale, boggy (swollen) and sometimes bluish.
    - Congested and swollen appearance is seen in infective rhinitis, vasomotor rhinitis and sinusitis.
    - Pale and atrophied mucosa is seen in Atrophic rhinitis.
17. **(d) Surgery** (*Ref. Cummings, 6th ed., 619*)
18. **(a) Vasomotor rhinitis** (*Ref. Cummings, 6th ed., 700*)
19. **(a) Withdrawal of nasal drops with short course of steroids** (*Ref. Cummings, 6th ed., 621*)
20. **(c) Xylometazoline** (*Ref. Cummings, 6th ed., 695*)
21. **(b) Anosmia** (*Ref. Cummings, 6th ed., 695*)
22. **(b), (c), (d), (e)** (*Ref. Cummings, 6th ed., 694*)
23. **(a) Local steroids** (*Ref. Cummings, 6th ed., 621*)
24. **(b) Inferior turbinectomy** (*Ref. Scott Brown, 6th ed., 4/8/27*)
    - The history is suggestive of atrophic rhinitis. Nasal endoscopy showing nasal cavity filled with infected crusts.

Section II Nose

Sinusitis

Sinusitis is an acute or chronic inflammation of the paranasal sinuses (PNS).

Since the nose and PNS are in continuity, they get involved together hence sinusitis is nowadays termed as rhinosinusitis.

Rhinosinusitis can be acute or chronic (if lasting > 12 weeks).

Pathophysiology of acute rhinosinusitis: Secondary to allergy or acute viral infection there occurs inflammatory oedema leading to obstruction of the sinus ostium. This results in impairment of the sinus ventilation and drainage and negative pressure resulting in transudation of fluid into the sinuses. Subsequently there may occur secondary bacterial infection in this retained fluid.

Pathophysiology of chronic rhinosinusitis: Chronic rhinosinusitis results from ongoing microbial colonisation and chronicity due to:

i. High virulence of the organisms
ii. Low host immunity and high allergic tendency in the host
iii. Due to microbial biofilm formation (due to wrong selection or under treatment with antibiotics) or
iv. Due to persistence of infected secretions due to unfavourable ostial anatomy, DNS, mucociliary dysfunction, ostial obstruction due to infective or allergic oedema, etc.

Chronic rhinosinusitis is often associated with polyps (*see* Chapter 21).

Rhinosinusitis can be viral (most common), bacterial or fungal. The same viruses which cause acute rhinitis (*see* Chapter 19) cause acute sinusitis.

The bacteria causing acute sinusitis:

1. *Streptococcus pneumoniae* (**most common**)
2. *H. influenzae*
3. *Moraxella catarrhalis*
4. *Streptococcus pyogenes*
5. *Staph. aureus.*

- In chronic bacterial sinusitis there is a mixed aerobic (MC being *Staph. aureus* here) and anaerobic infection.

Symptoms in acute or chronic sinusitis:

i. Nasal obstruction
ii. Nasal discharge
iii. Postnasal discharge
iv. Headache (referred pain to the respective division of trigeminal as per the nerve supply of the respective sinus)
v. Facial pain and congestion
vi. Hyposmia and anosmia
vii. Fever (usually in case of acute rhinosinusitis).

MAXILLARY SINUSITIS

This is the **most common sinusitis in adults** (because its floor is much lower than its ostia in middle meatus, *see* chapter on anatomy)

The patient complains of pain over upper jaw (in the territory of Infraorbital nerve, (maxillary V2, *see* Fig. 20.1a and 20.1b) which increases with jaw movement and

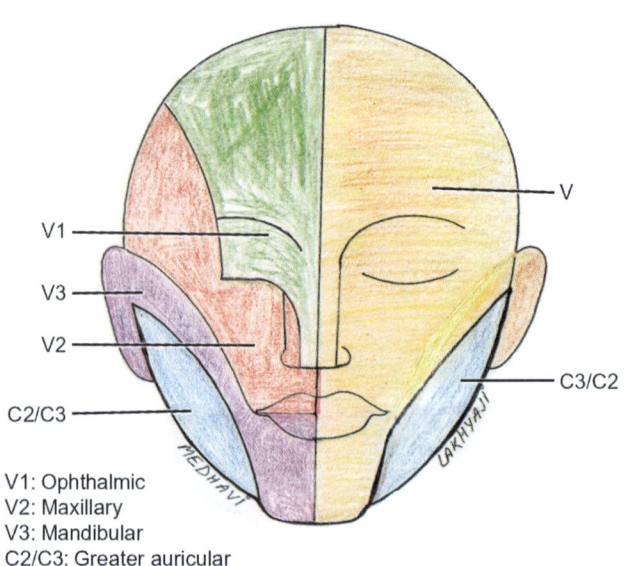

V1: Ophthalmic
V2: Maxillary
V3: Mandibular
C2/C3: Greater auricular
     at angle of mandible

Fig. 20.1a: Anterior view of face showing segmental innervation

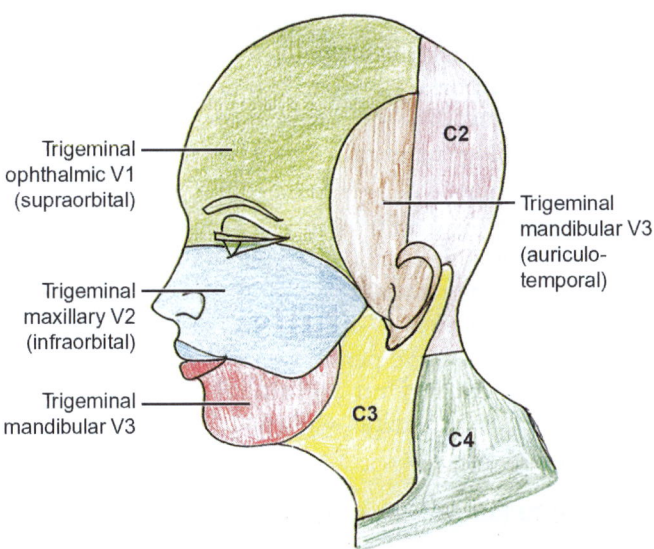

Trigeminal
ophthalmic V1
(supraorbital)

Trigeminal
maxillary V2
(infraorbital)

Trigeminal
mandibular V3

C2

Trigeminal
mandibular V3
(auriculo-
temporal)

C3

C4

Fig. 20.1b: Lateral view: Segmental innervation of face and head

stooping. There is tenderness over the anterior wall of maxillary sinus or antrum.

ETHMOID SINUSITIS

Since this is the most well pneumatised sinus at birth, this is the **most commonly infected sinus in infants and children**.

The patient complains of pain and tenderness over the root of nose and medial and deep to eye (involvement of nasociliary branch of ophthalmic division of trigeminal, *see* Chapter on Anatomy) which is aggravated by movements of eyeball.

FRONTAL SINUSITIS

The patient complains of headache which is maximum in the morning and subsides by evening. It is known as **periodic headache**, **office headache** or **early morning headache**. This may be due to the sinus secretions getting drained out gradually as the day progresses with gravity assistance as the person gets up. The headache here is frontal (in the territory of the supraorbital branch of ophthalmic division of trigeminal nerve) with the tenderness on the floor of frontal sinus just above the medial canthus.

SPHENOID SINUSITIS

This is the **least common sinusitis** as the sphenoid sinus opens high up in the spheno-ethmoidal recess which is not affected by most of the conditions of the nose. The headache here is occipital or at the vertex (referred pain) (Table 20.1).

FUNGAL SINUSITIS

Most common cause is **Aspergillus fumigatus**.

Fungal sinusitis can be non-invasive or invasive. Whereas anti-fungals are usually required in the invasive fungal sinusitis, surgical management is done for both the varieties, read below (Table 20.2).

1. Non-invasive Fungal Sinusitis

This is seen in immunocompetent individuals.
  i. **Fungal ball:** It is the collection of fungal hyphae to form a mass. The most common site of fungal ball formation is in the maxillary sinus. The patient may

Table 20.1

Sinusitis	Pain territory	Additional features
Maxillary (most common sinusitis in adults)	Cheek and upper jaw	Pain aggravated by stooping and jaw movements
Ethmoid (most common sinusitis in children)	Root of nose and medial and deep to eye	Pain aggravated by eye movements
Frontal	Frontal headache	Periodic, maximum in the morning (office headache)
Sphenoid (least common sinusitis)	Occipital or vertex	—

Table 20.2

Non-invasive fungal sinusitis	Invasive fungal sinusitis
Occur in immunocompetent Caused by *Aspergillus* and Dermataceous species	Invasion occur in **immunocompromised patients** Caused by: i. *Aspergillus fumigatus* ii. Rhizopus, mucor
Presents as: i. Fungal ball and ii. Allergic fungal rhinosinusitis	Presents acutely as: i. Invasive aspergillosis, and ii. Mucormycosis Presents chronically as: Chronic invasive sinusitis
Antifungals usually not required in the management	Antifungals are required

Nose

Section II

be asymptomatic or may present with features of chronic rhinosinusitis.

Management is removal of the fungal mass by FESS.

ii. **Allergic fungal rhinosinusitis (AFRS):** This occurs in individuals genetically predisposed to **fungal allergy (atopy).** During respiration the fungal spores get entrapped in the sinuses (most commonly **ethmoid**) because of disruption of mucociliary transport or large inoculum or dryness leading to inspissation of the fungal elements.

This leads to type I hypersensitivity reaction leading to formation of allergic mucin characterised by presence of eosinophils, Charcot laden crystals (a by-product of eosinophilic degranulation), necrotic inflammatory cells and hyphal elements.

The fungus continues to grow in the allergic mucin eliciting more hypersensitivity reaction and more production of allergic mucin.

The sticky allergic mucin does not get cleared leading to obstruction of the osteomeatal complex and nasal polyp formation. There can be expansion of sinus walls but no invasion of sinus mucosa.

Since the fungus can randomly get lodged in only one of the nostrils, AFRS is usually U/L leading to U/L multiple polyps. It is caused by Dermataceous fungal species or by *Aspergillus*.

NCCT here shows the characteristic diffuse opacification of the sinuses along with **heterogeneous opacities,** known as **double density sign.** These heterogenous opacities are due to the accumulation of iron, calcium and manganese within the mucin.

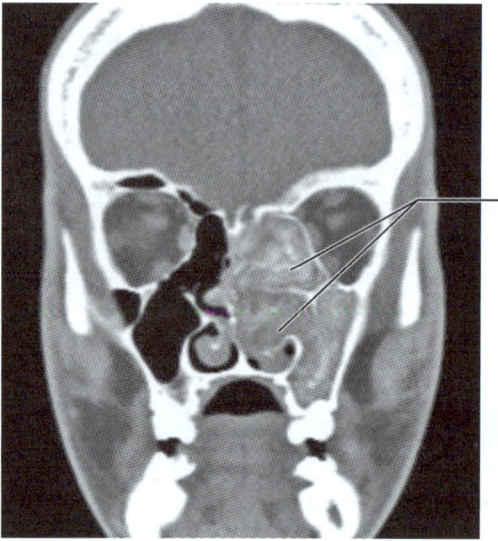

NCCT Nose and PNS showing double density sign (heterogeneous opacities) in a patient of allergic fungal sinusitis

Bent and Kuhn Diagnostic Criteria of Allergic Fungal Rhinosinusitis

i. Type I hypersensitivity (raised IgE levels)
ii. Nasal polyps,
iii. Positive fungal stain

iv. Biopsy showing fungal elements, and eosinophilic mucin or allergic mucin which is Hallmark of ARFS having a peanut butter/axle grease appearance without invading sinus mucosa and

v. CT showing hazy sinuses with heterogeneous opacities.

Treatment is primarily surgical by FESS. All the antigenic fungal elements, nasal polyps and inspissated allergic mucin is removed and drainage of the affected sinus is re-established.

In the postoperative period oral or local (nasal spray) steroids are given. Oral antifungal (Itraconazole) is restricted only to patients with poor response to oral/topical steroids.

2. Invasive Fungal Sinusitis

It can be acute/rapidly invasive or chronic (indolent) invasive.

Acute invasive is usually seen in diabetics or other immunocompromised individuals where the fungus invades the mucosa and even bone leading to bone erosion. It follows a rapidly fatal course.

It can be due to:

a. Invasive aspergillosis

or

b. Mucormycosis.

Invasive Aspergillosis

It is caused by Aspergillus fumigatus and less commonly by Aspergillus flavus and niger.

It invades cheek and orbit and leads to local destruction and proptosis.

It is managed by **FESS and oral/IV antifungal drugs (voriconazole).**

Mucormycosis/Rhinocerebral Phacomycosis

- It is caused by Rhizopus and Mucor.
- There occurs anaesthesia of nasal mucosa and cheeks.
- This fungus invades the endothelium of blood vessels (**angio-invasive**) and spreads through blood very rapidly from the nose and sinuses to the orbit and intracranially.
- On examination **black necrotic turbinates** and debris is seen which is due to arterial and venous thrombosis (leading to ischemia and necrosis) due to direct fungal infection. Black necrotic eschar can also be seen in other involved areas.
- CT shows sinus opacification with bony erosion and tissue infiltration.
- It is a **life-threatening condition** and has to be managed aggressively with:
  i. Amphotericin B
  ii. Surgical debridement of all the involved tissues. If orbit is involved, orbital exenteration should be done.
  iii. Reversal of underlying cause of immunosuppression.

Chronic invasive: It is rare. It is seen in patients without or with limited immunosuppression. It is caused by Aspergillus fumigatus and flavus. Patients usually present with painless proptosis or with cranial neuropathies. It is slowly progressive. It is managed by exenteration by FESS and antifungal therapy with voriconazole or itraconazole.

Investigations in a Patient with

1. **Chronic sinusitis:** The Ist evaluation to be done in chronic sinusitis is **nasal endoscopy** to visualise the various sinus meatuses, mucopus or any other pathology. If mucopus is seen in the meatus, it is confirmatory of sinusitis.

   If any pathology is found the **best investigation** is **NCCT nose and PNS**. CT shows air-fluid levels and mucosal thickening. CT also provides excellent detail of sinus and osteomeatal complex anatomy as good anatomic definition is desirable before surgical intervention.

   These days NCCT has largely replaced X-ray paranasal sinuses for evaluating various sinus pathologies.

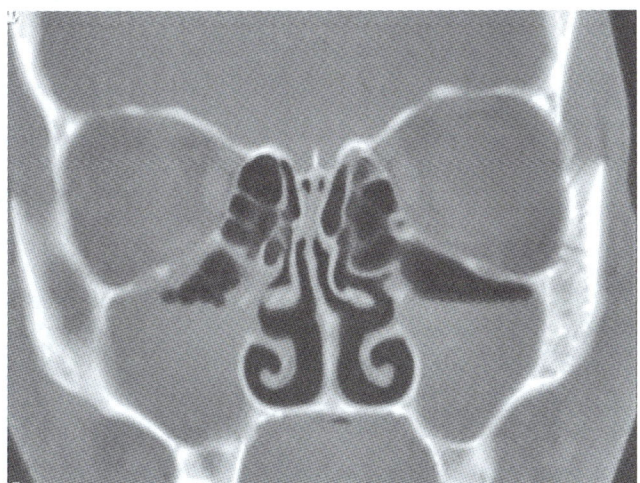

Fig. 20.2: NCCT of the nose and PNS (coronal view) showing hazy maxillary sinuses suggestive of B/L maxillary sinusitis

2. **Acute sinusitis:** It is a clinical diagnosis based on history and anterior rhinoscopic examination with Thudiculum speculum.

   In a patient of acute sinusitis if any complication is suspected then CT scan is done after an initial endoscopic assessment. In this regard X-ray of the sinuses was formerly the standard method but now, since a computed tomography (CT) scan shows a much clearer picture of the sinuses and other structures and thus is of great utility in assessing the complications of sinusitis, the use of standard X-rays has declined.

   Two important X-ray PNS:
   a. **Waters' view:** This is an Occipitomental view X-ray in which maxillary, frontal and ethmoid sinuses are seen. In water's view with open mouth, additionally sphenoid can also be seen, *see* the practice question in the end of this Chapter.

   b. **Caldwell's view:** This is occipitofrontal view for the better visualisation of frontal sinuses.

Management

The medical management of acute bacterial sinusitis includes:
   i. Antibiotics
   ii. Decongestants and
   iii. Saline irrigation.

Note:

- In patients of chronic rhino-sinusitis in addition to the above, topical nasal steroids are also given: Since all the forms of chronic rhino-sinusitis are characterised by persistent mucosal inflammation, topical steroids which have broad anti-inflammatory effects are used here.
- In patients of chronic sinusitis not responding to medical management the treatment of choice is FESS (functional endoscopic sinus surgery).

COMPLICATIONS OF SINUSITIS

The complications of sinusitis arise when the infection goes out of the sinuses through bony dehiscences, osteitic bony erosions or hematogenously through valveless ophthalmic or facial veins. The complications of sinusitis can be acute or chronic.

1. **Acute**
   i. *Orbital complications:* This is overall the **most common complication** of sinusitis. Orbital complications occur most commonly following **ethmoid sinusitis** as the ethmoid sinus is separated from the orbit by a thin papery bone known as lamina papyracea. Also the venous supply of orbit and ethmoid sinuses is same and additionally these veins are valveless (superior and inferior ophthalmic veins).

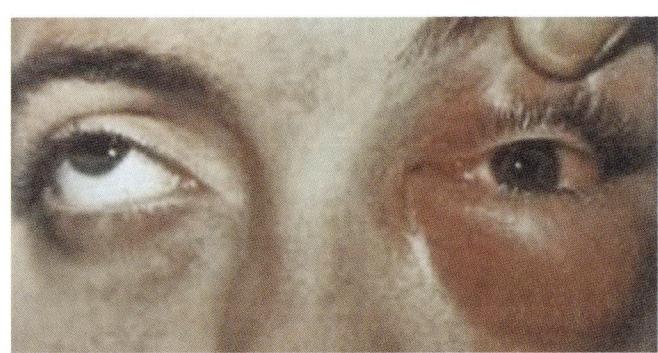

Orbital cellulitis: Periorbital edema, chemosis, restriction of ocular movement

The orbital complications are the following:
   a. **Periorbital oedema:** It involves only the pre-septal space. There is edema and erythema of eyelid. The ocular movements and vision are normal.

b. **Orbital cellulitis:** It gradually progresses from lid oedema to conjunctival chemosis, proptosis, restricted ocular movements, ophthalmoplegia and partial or total loss of vision. The cranial nerves 3rd, 4th, and 6th are involved concurrently. It is potentially dangerous and has to be managed by i/v antibiotics. Orbital cellulitis should be differentiated from cavernous sinus thrombosis.

Orbital cellulitis	Cavernous sinus thrombosis
Slow onset	Abrupt onset
Unilateral involvement	Bilateral
Concurrent involvement of the 3rd, 4th and 6th nerves	Sequential involvement of 6th, 3rd and 4th nerves (*see* below)
No stimulation of sympathetic plexus	Stimulation of sympathetic plexus.

c. **Subperiosteal abscess**
d. **Orbital abscess**
e. **Cavernous sinus thrombosis**
   - *Superior orbital fissure syndrome*: This is a rare complication and usually follows sphenoid sinusitis. There is progressive paralysis of structures passing through the superior orbital fissure, i.e. the 6th, 3rd, 4th and the ophthalmic branch of 5th cranial nerve.
   - *Orbital apex syndrome*: Here there is involvement of the optic nerve and the maxillary branch of 5th cranial nerve along with the involvement of the structures passing through the superior orbital fissure.

ii. *Osteomyelitis:* This involves either maxillary or frontal sinuses.

Osteomyelitis of maxillary sinus affects only the children since there is no marrow in the adult maxilla.

Osteomyelitis following frontal sinusitis affects only the anterior table of frontal bone since presence of marrow is limited to the anterior table. It is seen mainly in adults as frontal sinus is not developed in children.

The subperiosteal abscess following osteomyelitis of frontal bone presents externally as a soft doughy swelling known as **Pott's puffy tumour**.

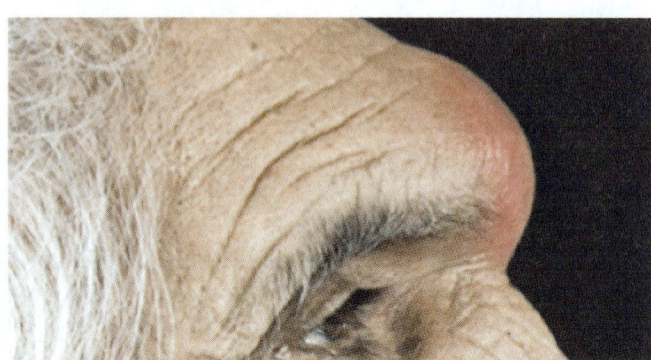

Pott's puffy tumour

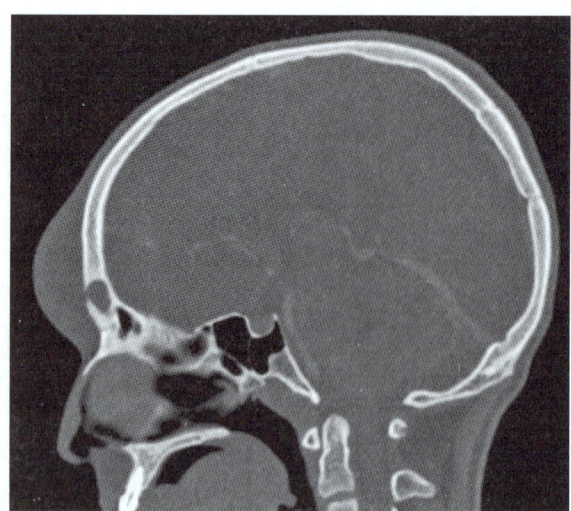

CT showing pott's puffy tumour (osteomyelitis of frontal sinus leading to subperiosteal abscess)

iii. *Intracranial complication:* These can be the following:
   a. Subdural empyema (most common)
   b. Brain abscess (2nd most common complication. MC site of brain abscess is frontal lobe and it usually follows frontal sinusitis)
   c. Meningitis
   d. Extradural abscess
   e. Cavernous sinus thrombosis

Cavernous sinus thrombosis can follow:

a. Any infection of the dangerous area of face. This area drains into the deep facial vein which is a deep connection of facial vein (facial vein is a continuation of angular vein from the medial angle of the eye). The deep facial vein communicates with the pterygoid plexus of veins which in turn communicate with cavernous sinus.

b. Ethmoid Sinusitis or orbital complications of sinusitis (via superior and inferior ophthalmic veins and central vein of retina which drain into cavernous sinus).

Clinical presentation of cavernous sinus thrombosis: The patient presents **abruptly** with fever with associated chills and rigor. Eye swelling begins as a unilateral process and spreads to the other eye within 24–48 hours via the intercavernous connection. This presentation is suggestive of Cavernous sinus thrombosis.

In the eye periorbital edema may be the earliest physical finding. Conjunctival chemosis occurs and results from occlusion of the ophthalmic veins.

Lateral gaze palsy (due to isolated cranial nerve VI palsy involving the lateral rectus muscle) is usually **seen first** since CN VI lies freely within the cavernous sinus in contrast to CN III and IV, which lie within the lateral walls of the cavernous sinus, *see* Fig. 16.18 in Chapter 16.

Ptosis, and mydriasis (dilatation of pupil), results from cranial nerve III dysfunction. With the involvement of IVth CN there occurs complete ophthalmoplegia.

The retrobulbar pressure increases (following cavernous sinus thrombosis) leading to exophthalmos.

Because of stimulation of sympathetic plexus around the internal carotid artery which passes through the cavernous sinus, the pupils are further dilated and fixed.

iv. *Descending infections:* The infected secretions of sinusitis going as postnasal drip can lead to the following:
   a. Otitis media
   b. Pharyngitis and tonsillitis
   c. Laryngitis

2. **Chronic complications of sinusitis**
   i. *Mucocele:* This occurs because of chronic obstruction of the ostia of sinuses or cystic dilatation of the mucous glands of sinuses.

The most common site of mucocele formation is frontal followed by ethmoid, maxillary and sphenoid.

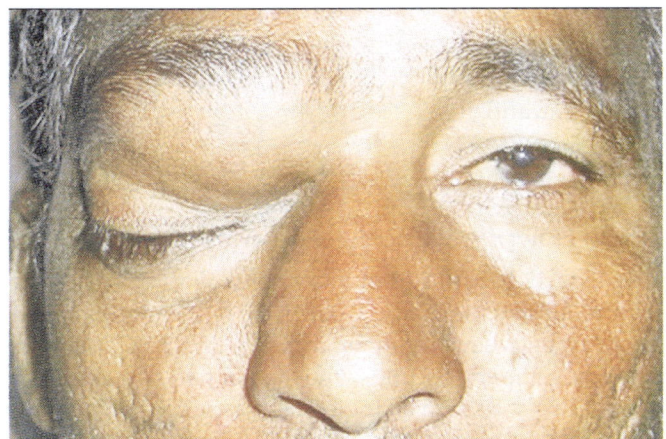

Fig. 20.3: Right-sided frontal mucocele

The mucocele of the frontal sinuses presents as a firm non tender swelling in the superomedial quadrant of the orbit pushing the orbit downwards, forwards and laterally whereas ethmoidal mucocele pushes the orbit forwards and laterally. So with the displacement of the orbit the site of origin of mucocele can be found.

   ii. *Pyocele:* It is infection of the mucocele leading to pus formation.

Another condition which should be considered here is pneumocele, though it may not be a direct complication of sinusitis.

Pneumocele (also called pneumatocele, hyperpneumatisation, sinus ectasia, and ***aerocele***):

It is the abnormal enlargement of the paranasal sinuses due to further air entrapment causing increased sinus pressure leading to focal or generalized thinning of their bony walls.

Again **frontal sinus is the most commonly affected sinus**. Like mucocele it presents as a firm non tender swelling.

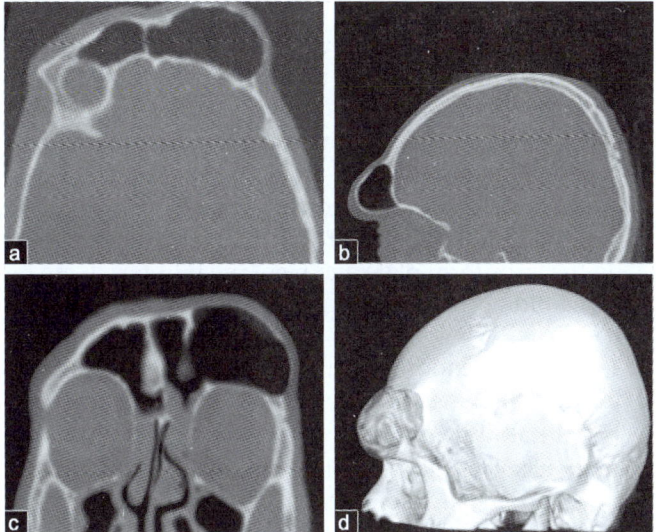

Fig. 20.4a to d: CT scan showing left pneumocele

Underlying causes of pneumocele:
   i. Infection by a gas-forming organism
   ii. Trauma
   iii. Spontaneous drainage of a mucocele
   iv. Increased sinus pressure caused by a one-way-valve obstruction of the nasofrontal duct which allows air to enter into the sinus but prevents its return.

FESS (FUNCTIONAL ENDOSCOPIC SINUS SURGERY)

It is an endoscope guided surgery and is called functional as we try to restore the normal function of the sinuses. Here we preserve everything healthy and remove only the unhealthy tissue and re-establish physiologic ventilation and drainage of the sinuses.

Indications of FESS and Endoscopic Nasal Surgeries

Among the below, only the surgeries on sinuses which are done to reverse the pathology and restore the normal function are considered as functional. The rest are the conditions which are approached endoscopically through the nose.

1. **In conditions of nose**, e.g.
   a. Chronic sinusitis (bacterial or fungal)
   b. Sinonasal polyposis
   c. Fronto-ethmoidal mucocele
   d. Endoscopic septoplasty and Turbinate reduction surgery/cauterisation
   e. Endoscopic sphenopalatine arterial ligation in epistaxis
   f. Endoscopic repair of choanal atresia
   g. Excision of sino-nasal tumours.

While approaching the middle meatus in FESS, the first step is to remove the uncinate process **(uncinectomy)**. By doing this the space available for surgery and the ease to approach the sinuses increases. Since this uncinectomy opens the infundibulum it is also known as infundibulotomy (*refer* to chapter on anatomy).

Nose

Section II

This is followed by middle meatal antrostomy (widening of maxillary sinus ostium), anterior ethmoidectomy (opening up of anterior ethmoid cells), clearing frontal recess, and if required posterior ethmoidectomy and sphenoidotomy (widening of sphenoid ostium).

The nose is separated from the orbit by a thin papery bone (lamina papyracea), from the anterior cranial fossa by the cribriform plate and from the pituitary fossa by sphenoid so these can also be approached from the nasal cavity.

Therefore, endoscopic nasal surgery can also be used for the following:

2. **In orbital indications:**
   a. In nasolacrimal duct obstruction, the lacrimal sac is approached and opened directly into the nose endoscopically by a procedure which is known as endoscopic dacryocystorhinostomy (DCR).
   b. Endoscopic orbital decompression and optic nerve decompression
   c. Drainage of orbital abscess
3. **Repair of CSF leaks**
4. In pituitary surgeries through sphenoid, e.g. endoscopic **Trans-sphenoidal hypophysectomy.**

Complications of FESS

Since nose is related to important structures superiorly (cranium) and laterally (orbit), these can be injured during FESS. So the complications of FESS can be:

1. Orbital injuries
2. Injury to nasolacrimal duct.
3. CSF leak, meningitis, injury to brain parenchyma.
4. Injury to optic nerve and internal carotid (**most dreaded complication of FESS**) and cranial nerves III, IV, V and VI (while surgery to sphenoid sinus and "Onodi cell", see chapter on anatomy).
5. Hemorrhage (**MC complication**) from sphenopalatine and ethmoidal arteries: Injury to the ethmoidal artery carries potential risk of intra-orbital bleed also and hematoma formation, as it enters the nose from the orbit. Immediate orbital decompression has to be done here.
6. Synechiae formation in between the middle turbinate and lateral wall of nose, or in between the middle turbinate and septum. If synechiae forms then they have to be excised. **To reduce the synechiae formation** here **mitomycin-C** is used. Mitomycin-C is an antineoplastic agent having anti-fibroblastic activity.

OTHER SURGICAL PROCEDURES TO APPROACH SINUSES

Caldwell–Luc Operation

It is a procedure of opening the **maxillary antrum** by making an opening on its anterior wall by giving a sub-labial

incision. Following the procedure a naso-antral window/opening is made in the inferior meatus for drainage or packing of maxillary antrum.

Caldwell-Luc operation was used to be done in the past for chronic maxillary sinusitis and excision of recurrent antrochoanal polyp (*see* Chapter on nasal polyposis).

With the advent of FESS it is no longer done for chronic maxillary sinusitis and antrochoanal polyp. Its present **indications** are:

   a. Reduction of maxillary fracture
   b. Elevation of fracture of floor of orbit in blow out fracture of orbit.
   c. Opening of posterior wall of maxillary sinus for approaching sphenopalatine fossa to ligate maxillary artery or to do vidian neurectomy.
   d. Taking a biopsy in suspected malignancy of maxilla.

Complications

   a. Facial swelling (most common)
   b. Anaesthesia or paresthesia of the cheek, teeth and gingiva because of stretch injury of infraorbital nerve (2nd most common)
   c. Trauma to tooth
   d. Oro-antral fistula
   e. Haemorrhage
   f. Injury to orbit

Lynch Howarth Procedure

It is external fronto-ethmoidectomy. To approach the frontal sinus externally a curvilinear incision starting midway between the inner canthus and nasal dorsum extending superiorly under the medial part of eyebrow is given. This is known as Lynch Howarth approach.

Indications

   a. Drainage of frontoethmoidal mucocele/pyocele which cannot be approached endoscopically.
   b. Excision of frontal osteoma (MC benign sino nasal tumour)
   c. Approach to anterior ethmoidal artery for ligation in epistaxis.

Antral Puncture

Antral puncture is also known as proof puncture as it was used to confirm maxillary sinusitis by collecting material for diagnosis.

Antral puncture or proof puncture is a procedure of puncturing the medial wall of maxillary sinus with Lichtwitz trocar and cannula in the region of inferior meatus to irrigate the sinus. Once the antrum is opened, irrigation with normal saline is done with the cannula. Insufflation of air into the antrum during lavage can lead to air embolism and death.

With the advent of FESS antral puncture is no more done now.

"Points to Ponder/Points for Quick revision"

- Sinusitis—inflammation of PNS
- Often seen as—rhinosinusitis
- Acute or chronic (>12 weeks)
- Central pathogenetic mechanism—sinus ostium obstruction
- Acute rhino-sinusitis—viral (MC), *Strept. pneumoniae* (MC among bacteria)
- Chronic—mixed aerobic and anaerobic bacteria
- Imp CFs: Nasal obstruction, PND and headache
- MC sinusitis in adults—maxillary
- MC sinusitis in children—ethmoid
- Least common sinusitis—sphenoid (occipital headache)
- Periodicity (office headache)—frontal
- Fungal sinusitis—aspergillus fumigatus (MC)
  1. Non-invasive—immunocompetent
     a. Fungus ball: Maxillary (MC)—T/t (FESS)
     b. AFRS: Ethmoid (MC)—Type 1 hypersensitivity, multiple polyps, Bent and Kuhn diagnostic criteria, T/t-FESS, steroids in postoperative
  2. Invasive (usually acute-immunocompromised, rapidly fatal)
     a. Invasive Aspergillosis: Cheek invasion, proptosis, T/t-FESS, Voriconazole

  b. Mucormycosis: Angio-invasive, black necrotic eschar, T/t-debridement, AmB.
- Nasal endoscopy—muco-pus → Confirmatory of sinusitis.
- NCCT Nose and PNS—Best investigation in providing the detailed anatomy before surgical intervention.
- Acute sinusitis—clinical diagnosis, if complications-CT.
- Acute sinusitis—T/t-antibiotics, decongestants, saline sprays.
- Chronic sinusitis—T/t-additionally topically steroids. If no response → FESS.
- MC acute complication of sinusitis—orbital (MC-Ethmoid).
- Orbital cellulitis *vs* Cavernous Sinus thrombosis—*see* table in the text.
- Pott's puffy tumour—osteomyelitis of the frontal sinus → Subperiosteal abscess.
- MC intracranial complication—subdural empyema.
- Frontal lobe brain abscess—2nd MC intracranial complication.
- MC chronic complication—mucocele (MC frontal sinusitis).
- FESS: 1st step—uncinectomy; MC complication—haemorrhage (like any other surgical procedure); Most dreaded complication-injury to internal carotid artery.

Section II Nose

PREVIOUSLY ASKED QUESTIONS

1. **In sinusitis the sinus most often involved in children is:** *(UPSC 2007, 2014)*
   a. Maxillary
   b. Sphenoid
   c. Ethmoid
   d. Frontal

2. **Most common organism causing acute sinusitis:** *(AI 2001, Exam 2017)*
   a. Pseudomonas
   b. *Moraxella catarrhalis*
   c. *Streptococcus pneumoniae*
   d. *Staph. epidermidis*

3. **Common organisms causing acute sinusitis:** *(PGI 2001, 2012)*
   a. Pseudomonas
   b. *Moraxella catarrhalis*
   c. *Streptococcus pneumonia*
   d. *Staph. epidermidis*
   e. *H. influenzae*

4. **Symptoms of sinusitis are all except:** *(MP 2000, Exam 2017)*
   a. Rhinorrhoea
   b. Headache
   c. Nasal blockade
   d. Diplopia

5. **Periodicity is a characteristic feature in which sinus infection:** *(COMED 2006, Exam 2017)*
   a. Maxillary sinus infection
   b. Frontal sinus infection
   c. Sphenoid sinus infection
   d. Ethmoid sinus infection

6. **Sphenoid sinusitis pain is referred most commonly to:** *(AP 2005, Exam 2017)*
   a. Occiput
   b. Root of nose
   c. Frontal
   d. Temporal region

7. **Pathognomonic feature of chronic maxillary sinusitis is:** *(UP 2007, Exam 2016)*
   a. Muco-pus in the middle meatus
   b. Inferior turbinate hypertrophy
   c. History of early morning headache
   d. Atrophic sinusitis

8. **All sinuses are seen in which view?** *(Exam 2013)*
   a. Caldwell's view
   b. Luc's view
   c. Water's view
   d. None of these

9. **Caldwell view is done for:** *(AIIMS 2011)*
   a. Sphenoid sinus
   b. Maxillary sinus
   c. Ethmoid sinus
   d. Frontal sinus

10. **Best view for evaluating frontal sinus is:** *(Exam 2003, Exam 2017)*
    a. Water's with open mouth
    b. Schuller's view
    c. Towne's view
    d. Caldwell view

11. **Most definitive diagnostic of sinusitis is:** *(Exam 2015)*
    a. X-ray PNS
    b. Proof puncture
    c. Nasal endoscopy
    d. Transillumination test

12. **A 35-year-old male presented with h/o nasal discharge, facial pain and fever which did not subside with few course of antibiotics and antihistaminics for 3 months. His symptoms have aggravated again. On endoscopy mucopurulent discharge from middle meatus and inflamed sinus openings, investigation of choice:** *(AIIMS Nov 2007, Exam 2016)*
    a. X-ray PNS
    b. NCCT PNS
    c. MRI of the face
    d. Inferior meatal puncture

13. **Which of the following is the most common etiological agent in paranasal sinus mycosis?** *(AIIMS May 2006, Exam 2016)*
    a. *Aspergillus* species
    b. Histoplasma
    c. *Conidiobolus coronatus*
    d. *Candida albicans*

14. **All of the following are diagnostic criteria of allergic fungal sinusitis except:** *(AI 2008, Exam 2017)*
    a. Heterogeneous opacities on CT scan
    b. Orbital invasion
    c. Allergic eosinophillic mucin
    d. Type 1 hypersensitivity

15. **Which among the following is true regarding fungal sinusitis?** *(PGI 2001, 2015)*
    a. Surgery is required for treatment
    b. Most common organism is *Aspergillus niger*
    c. Amphotericin B is used for invasive fungal sinusitis
    d. Hazy appearance on NCCT with heterogeneous radio-opaque densities
    e. Seen only in immunodeficient conditions

16. **Allergic fungal sinusitis:** *(Exam 2013)*
    a. Immunocompetent patient
    b. Immunocompromised patient
    c. Diabetic patient
    d. None

17. **Type 1 diabetes mellitus patient presents with nasal septal and palatal perforation with brownish black nasal discharge probable diagnosis is:** *(Rajasthan 2006, Exam 2017)*
    a. Rhinosporidiosis
    b. Aspergillus
    c. Leprosy
    d. Mucormycosis

18. **68-year-old Chandu is a diabetic and presented with black, foul smelling discharge from the nose.**

Examination revealed blackish discoloration of the inferior turbinates. The diagnosis is:
(AIIMS 99, 2012)
a. Mucormycosis
b. Aspergillosis
c. Infarct of inferior turbinate
d. Foreign body

19. The best surgical treatment for chronic maxillary sinusitis is: *(MP 2002, Exam 2017)*
a. Repeated antral washout
b. Functional endoscopic sinus surgery
c. Caldwell-Luc operation
d. Horgan's operation

20. FESS means: *(Exam 2014)*
a. Factual endoscopic sinus surgery
b. Functional endonasal sinus surgery
c. Factual endonasal sinus surgery
d. Functional endoscopic sinus surgery

21. Sinusitis—most common complication:
(Exam 2013)
a. Orbital cellulitis   b. Meningitis
c. Brain abscess   d. Septicemia

22. Orbital cellulitis most commonly occurs after which sinus infection? *(Exam 2013)*
a. Maxillary   b. Frontal
c. Ethmoidal   d. Sphenoidal

23. Complication of sinus disease includes:
(AIIMS 93, Exam 2012)
a. Orbital cellulitis
b. Cavernous sinus thrombosis
c. Superior orbital fissure syndrome
d. All of the above

24. Complications of acute sinusitis: *(PGI 2003, 2014)*
a. Orbital cellulitis
b. Pott's Puffy tumour
c. Conjunctival chemosis
d. Subdural abscess
e. All of the above

25. A patient with sinus infection develops acute onset bilateral conjunctival chemosis, bilateral proptosis and fever, the diagnosis goes in favour of:
(Exam 2011)
a. Lateral sinus thrombosis
b. Frontal lobe abscess
c. Cavernous sinus thrombosis
d. Meningitis

26. Infection within the right cavernous sinus results in the following signs except: *(AIIMS 2003, 2012)*
a. Constricted pupils in response to light
b. Engorgement of retinal veins
c. Ptosis of right eyelid
d. Right ophthalmoplegia

27. A young female with a long history of sinusitis presents with frequent episodes of fever, headache of recent onset along with personality changes. Fundus examination revealed papilloedema. Most likely diagnosis is: *(AIIMS 2004, 2013)*
a. Frontal lobe abscess
b. Meningitis
c. Orbital cellulitis
d. Encephalitis

28. Unilateral proptosis and bilateral 6th nerve palsy is seen in: *(Exam 2013)*
a. Cavernous sinus thrombosis
b. Meningitis
c. Hydrocephalus
d. None

29. Angular vein infection may cause thrombosis of:
(DPG 2008, Exam 2017)
a. Cavernous sinus
b. Sphenoidal sinus
c. Petrosal sinus
d. Sigmoid sinus

30. A 2-year-old child with a long history of purulent nasal discharge now presents with fever and right-sided conjunctival congestion and edema for the past 3 days, *see* picture below. His fever is 103°F and WBC count is 12000/µL. The culture of eye discharge was negative. X-ray shows opacification of ethmoid sinus. Which of the following should be the next step in evaluating this patient?
(Exam 2007, MH 2011)

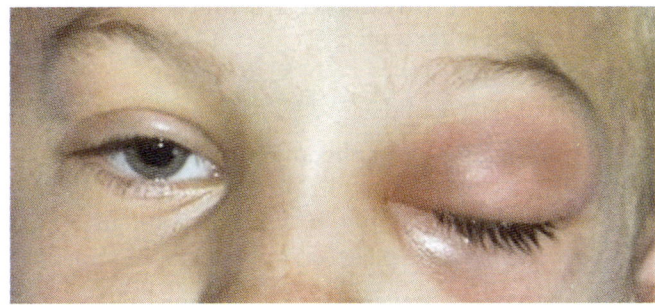

a. CT Scan
b. FESS
c. Blood culture
d. Repeat culture of eye discharge

31. Mucocele is commonly seen in which sinus?
(Exam 2007, 2012)
a. Frontal   b. Maxillary
c. Ethmoid   d. Sphenoid

32. Pneumatocele/Aerocele is seen most commonly in:
(ASSAM 95, Exam 2013)
a. Maxillary sinus
b. Frontal sinus
c. Ethmoid sinus
d. Sphenoid sinus

Nose

Section II

33. **Which of the following is the very first step in functional endoscopic sinus surgery?** (*MH 2010*)
    a. Opening of bulla ethmoidalis
    b. Uncinectomy
    c. Middle meatal antrostomy
    d. Middle turbinectomy

34. **Infundibulotomy is done for:** (*Exam 2013*)
    a. Approaching middle meatus
    b. Approaching nasolacrimal duct
    c. Rhinoplasty
    d. Choanal atresia repair

35. **Indications of FESS:** (*PGI Nov 2010*)
    a. Inverted papilloma
    b. Nasal allergic polyposis
    c. Mucocele
    d. Carcinoma maxilla
    e. Chronic maxillary sinusitis

36. **Endoscopic surgery is used for the following:** (*PGI 2014*)
    a. Inverted papilloma
    b. Orbital abscess
    c. Nasal polyposis
    d. Optic nerve decompression
    e. CSF rhinorrhoea repair

37. **Endoscopic nasal surgery is indicated in:** (*MP 2003, Exam 2017*)
    a. Chronic sinusitis   b. Epistaxis
    c. Both   d. None

38. **Endoscopic intranasal approach is used for accessing all except:** (*AIIMS Nov 2010*)
    a. Lacrimal sac   b. Cerebellum
    c. Pituitary gland   d. Optic nerve

39. **Complications of sphenoid sinus surgery are all except:** (*Kerala 2010*)
    a. CSF leak   b. Optic nerve injury
    c. Lateral rectus palsy d. Orbital emphysema

40. **Endoscopic nasal surgery is not done in:** (*MH 2001, Exam 2017*)
    a. Optic nerve compression
    b. CSF rhinorrhoea
    c. Dacryocystic carcinoma
    d. Ethmoidal polyps

41. **To reduce synechiae formation after nasal surgery which one of the following packing is most useful:** (*AIIMS Nov 2004, May 2013*)
    a. Mitomycin C   b. Ribbon gauze
    c. Liquid paraffin   d. Steroids

42. **In Caldwell-Luc operation the nasoantral window is made through:** (*TN 2004, Exam 2017*)
    a. Superior meatus   b. Inferior meatus
    c. Middle meatus   d. None of the above

43. **Caldwell-Luc approach opens:** (*Exam 2013*)
    a. Maxillary sinus   b. Frontal sinus
    c. Sphenoid sinus   d. Ethmoid sinus

44. **Commonest complication of Caldwell-Luc operation is:** (*AP 2000, Exam 2017*)
    a. Oroantral fistula
    b. Infra-orbital nerve injury
    c. Haemorrhage
    d. Orbital cellulitis

45. **Lynch Howarth surgery is for:** (*Exam 2013*)
    a. Nasal septal perforation
    b. Sinonasal tumours
    c. Acoustic neuroma
    d. Otosclerosis

46. **Antral puncture is done through:** (*RJ 2006, Exam 2017*)
    a. Superior meatus
    b. Inferior meatus
    c. Middle meatus
    d. All

47. **Proof puncture is done for:** (*Exam 2013*)
    a. Ethmoid sinus   b. Sphenoid sinus
    c. Maxillary sinus   d. None

48. **During maxillary wash sudden death is due to:** (*Exam 2013*)
    a. Air embolism
    b. Maxillary artery thrombus
    c. Meningitis
    d. Bleeding

49. **A 49-year-old diabetic patient presents with black necrotic mass filling the nasal cavity and diplopia of the affected side, management should be:** (*AIIMS 2013*)
    a. Endoscopic DCR
    b. Steroids
    c. I/V Amphotericin B with orbital exenteration
    d. Antibiotics

50. **Which one of the following is FALSE regarding Chronic maxillary sinusitis?** (*APPG 2015*)
    a. Normal X-ray effectively excludes hypertrophic mucosa
    b. FESS is indicated for failure of medical treatment or presence of sino-nasal polyp
    c. Patient complains of postnasal discharge
    d. Headache is absent except during exacerbation of acute sinusitis

51. **Most feared complication of FESS is:** (*Exam 2015*)
    a. Retroorbital hematoma
    b. CSF rhinorrhoea
    c. Internal carotid injury
    d. NLD injury

52. **FESS is not done for:** *(Exam 2015)*
    a. Chronic maxillary sinusitis
    b. Blow out fracture
    c. Ethmoidal polyp
    d. Allergic fungal sinusitis

53. **Nerve supplying the angle of mandible:** *(Exam 2015)*
    a. Auriculotemporal
    b. Lingual
    c. Facial
    d. Greater auricular

54. **True about allergic fungal sinusitis are all except:** *(Exam 2016)*
    a. Fungal hyphae are present in allergic mucin which is the pathologic hallmark
    b. Invasion of the sinus mucosa with fungus
    c. Allergic reaction to fungus
    d. Surgical clearance is the mainstay of treatment

55. **In Caldwell-Luc operation, the approach is through:** *(Exam 2015)*
    a. Opening of maxillary antrum through inferior orbital rim
    b. Opening of maxillary antrum through the sphenopalatine recess
    c. Opening of maxillary antrum through gingivolabial sulcus by sublabial approach
    d. Opening of maxillary antrum through superior meatus

56. **Which agent is used to prevent synechiae after nasal surgery?** *(Exam 2015)*
    a. Mitomycin
    b. Tacrolimus
    c. Cyclosporine
    d. Doxycycline

57. **What is Pott's puffy tumour:** *(Exam 2015)*
    a. Osteosarcoma of the frontal bone
    b. Adamantimoma of the mandible
    c. Osteomyelitis of frontal bone causing subperiosteal abscess
    d. Proliferative aspergillosis of maxillary sinus

58. **Treatment of choice for nasal synechiae:** *(Exam 2015)*
    a. Surgical removal of adhesions
    b. Topical mitomycin
    c. Nasal stent
    d. None of the above

59. **Most common cause of fungal sinusitis:** *(Exam 2016)*
    a. *A. fumigatus*
    b. *A. niger*
    c. *A. fiavus*
    d. Candida

60. **A 45-year-old male with history of nasal blockade for 6 months. On examination, the patient had a nasal mass with mucin discharge. What is the probable diagnosis based on the CT scan:** *(AIIMS May 2016)*

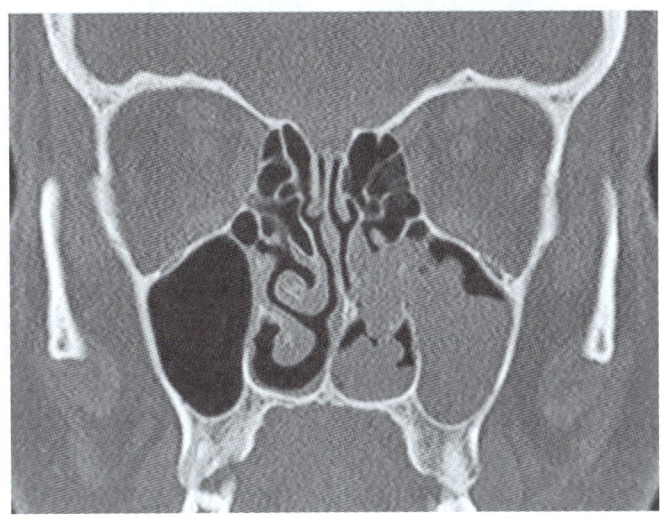

    a. Antrochoanal polyp
    b. Ethmoidal polyp
    c. Maxillary carcinoma
    d. Allergic fungal sinusitis

IMAGE BASED PRACTICE QUESTIONS BY THE AUTHOR

61. **A 35-year-old male presented with nasal discharge, facial pain and fever which persisted with several courses of antibiotics and antihistaminics over a period of 3 months. On nasal endoscopy mucopurulent discharge from middle meatus and inflamed sinus openings seen. His NCCT nose and PNS is given below. He should be best managed by:**

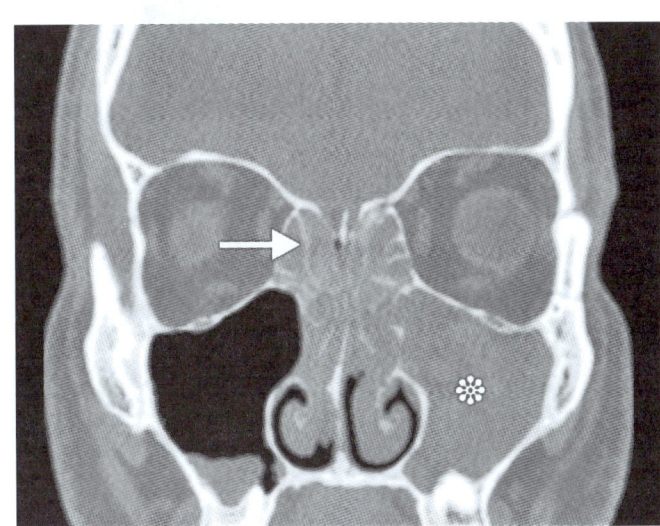

    a. Repeated antral washout
    b. Functional endoscopic sinus surgery
    c. Caldwell-Luc operation
    d. Lynch Howarth operation

62. Which view of X-ray is shown below:

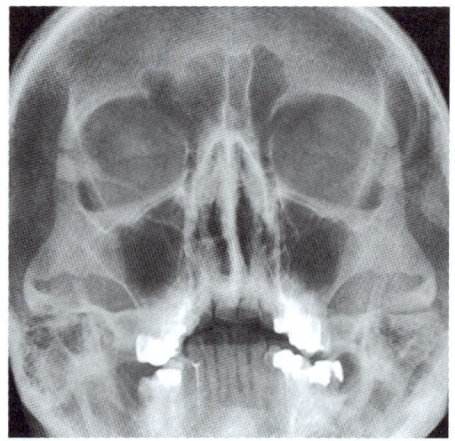

    a. Water's view   b. Schuller's view
    c. Towne's view   d. Caldwell view

63. A Type-I diabetic presents with fever, left-sided facial oedema, periorbital oedema, diplopia and acidotic breath. On examination there were necrotic areas on the upper lip and black necrotic mass in the nasal cavity, see the patient below. Random blood sugar 450 mg/dl. Ketones were detected on urine examination. She should be managed by:

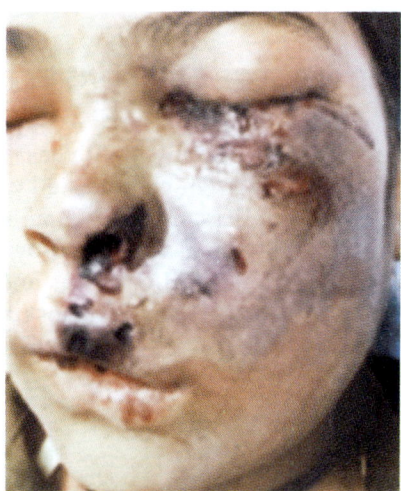

    a. FESS
    b. Local debridement and I/V amphotericin B
    c. Cisplatin
    d. Steroids

64. Which surgery is shown below?

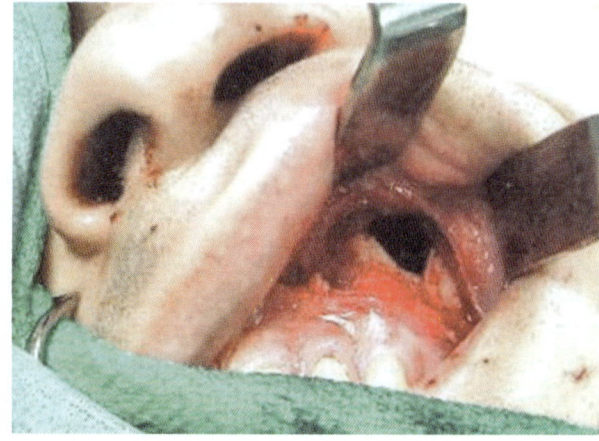

    a. Antral washout
    b. Functional endoscopic sinus surgery
    c. Caldwell-Luc operation
    d. Lynch Howarth operation

65. A 35-year-old male presents with nasal polyp and mucinous nasal discharge. His CT scan is given here. This radiological sign is: (*Exam 2019*)

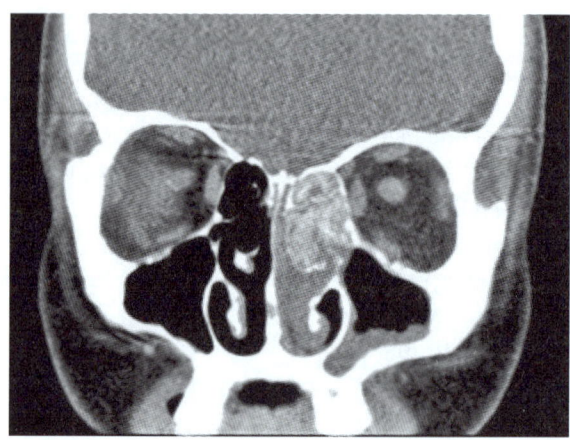

    a. Honey comb   b. Ground glass
    c. Double density   d. Onion peel

66. Pott's puffy tumour is: (*Exam 2019*)
    a. Subperiosteal abscess of frontal sinus
    b. Subperiosteal abscess of ethmoid sinus
    c. Mucocele of frontal sinus
    d. Mucocele of ethmoid sinus

Section II   Nose

ANSWERS AND EXPLANATIONS

1. **(c) Ethmoid** (*Ref. Cummings, 6th ed., 2871*)
   - The maxillary sinus develops earlier to the ethmoid though both are present at birth.
   - But since ethmoid is the more well pneumatised sinus at birth; this is the most commonly infected sinus in infants and young children.
   - Maxillary is the most common sinusitis in adults.
   - Sphenoid sinusitis is the least common sinusitis.

2. **(c) *Streptococcus pneumoniae*** (*Ref. Cummings, 6th ed., 665, 725*)

3. **(b), (c) and (e)** (*Ref. Cummings, 6th ed., 665, 725*)

4. **(d) Diplopia** (*Ref. Cummings, 6th ed., 725*)
   - Diplopia can occur in orbital complications following sinusitis.

5. **(b) Frontal sinus infection** (*Ref. Scott Brown, 6th ed., 4/8/19*)

6. **(a) Occiput** (*Ref. Scott Brown, 6th ed., 4/8/19*)

7. **(a) Muco-pus in the middle meatus** (*Ref. Cummings, 6th ed., 697*)

8. **(c) Water's view** (*refer* to text) (*Ref. Scott Brown, 6th ed., 4/3/2*)
   There is no view named Luc's view.
   - These days NCCT has largely replaced X-ray paranasal sinuses for evaluating various sinus pathologies.

9. **(d) Frontal sinus** (*Ref. Scott Brown, 6th ed., 4/3/2*)

10. **(d) Caldwell view** (*Ref. Scott Brown, 6th ed., 4/3/2*)
    - Caldwell view is the occipitofrontal view. The frontal sinuses are seen very clearly here
    - Water's with open mouth is the occipitomental view. All the four sinuses the maxillary, frontal, ethmoid and sphenoid sinuses are clearly visible.
    - Schuller's view is lateral oblique view of mastoid.
    - Towne's view is the antero-posterior view to *see* both the petrous pyramids and posterior cranial fossa.

11. **(c) Nasal endoscopy** (*Ref. Cummings, 6th ed., 726*)

12. **(b) NCCT PNS** (*Ref. Cummings, 6th ed., 760*)

13. **(a) *Aspergillus* species** (*Ref. Cummings, 6th ed., 732*)
    - The most common etiological agent in paranasal sinus mycosis is *Aspergillus fumigatus*.

14. **(b) Orbital invasion** (*Ref. Cummings, 6th ed., 736*)
    - Orbital invasion leading to proptosis is a feature of invasive aspergillosis
    - Refer to the text for the diagnostic criteria of allergic fungal sinusitis

15. **(a), (c) and (d)** (*Ref. Cummings, 6th ed., 735*)
    - The most common organism causing fungal sinusitis is *Aspergillus fumigatus*.
    - Hazy appearance on NCCT with heterogeneous radio-opaque densities is characteristic of allergic fungal sinusitis.

- Fungal ball and allergic fungal sinusitis are the non-invasive fungal sinusitis conditions which can be seen even in immunocompetent individuals.
- Invasive fungal sinusitis is seen in immunodeficient conditions.
- Surgical management by FESS is treatment of choice for all types of fungal sinusitis.

16. **(a) Immunocompetent patient** (*Ref. Scott Brown, 8th ed., Vol 1; 1048*)
    - Invasive fungal sinusitis is seen in immunodeficient conditions (most common of them being diabetes mellitus).

17. **(d) Mucormycosis** (*Ref. Cummings, 6th ed., 733*)
    - Diabetic patient (immunocompromised), with local tissue destruction with brownish black nasal discharge is suggestive of mucormycosis. The black discharge is due to the angioinvasive nature of mucormycosis (leading to vascular thrombosis and gangrene formation).
    - Invasive aspergillosis and leprosy also present with nasal septal and palatal perforation but black discharge does not occur.
    - Rhinosporidiosis presents with blood tinged nasal discharge from red polypoid mass of sporangia (mulberry or strawberry appearance) and there is no local destruction.

18. **(a) Mucormycosis** (*Ref. Cummings, 6th ed., 732*)
    - Diabetic patient (immunocompromised) with foul smelling black nasal discharge and black necrotic turbinates on examination is suggestive of mucormycosis. This is due to arterial and venous thrombosis due to direct fungal invasion causing local vascular insufficiency leading to gangrene.
    - Invasive aspergillosis lead to local destruction but black discharge does not occur.
    - Foreign body nose presents with foul smelling U/L nasal discharge.
    - Infarct of inferior turbinate is no condition.

19. **(b) Functional endoscopic sinus surgery** (*Ref. Cummings, 6th ed., 760*)
    - In patients of chronic sinusitis not responding to medical management the treatment of choice is FESS (functional endoscopic sinus surgery).
    - Caldwell-Luc operation and antral wash are no longer done for the treatment of chronic maxillary sinusitis.
    - Horgan's operation which is a combination of Caldwell-Luc and external ethmoidectomy has become obsolete.

20. **(d) Functional endoscopic sinus surgery** (*Ref. Cummings, 6th ed., 760*)

21. **(a) Orbital cellulitis** (*Ref. Cummings, 6th ed., 728; Scott Brown, Vol 1; 1114*)

22. **(c) Ethmoidal** (*Ref. Cummings, 6th ed., 728*)

23. **(d) All of the above** (*Ref. Cummings, 6th ed., 728*)
    (Please refer to the text for complications of sinusitis)

Nose

Section II

24. **(e) All of the above** (*Ref. Cummings, 6th ed., 729*) (Please refer to the text for complications of sinusitis)

25. **(c) Cavernous sinus thrombosis** (*Ref. Cummings, 6th ed., 728*)
    - Fever along with acute onset bilateral ocular manifestations point towards cavernous sinus thrombosis.
    - Lateral sinus thrombosis presents with fever, jugular vein tenderness and oedema of the mastoid in a patient of unsafe CSOM.
    - Frontal lobe abscess presents with:
        i. Headache, nausea and vomiting, papilloedema, drowsiness and confusion (due to raised ICT)
        ii. Fever
        iii. Focal neurological deficit (contralateral hemiparesis, personality changes)
    - Meningismus (neck rigidity) is generally not present in brain abscess unless the abscess has ruptured into the ventricle or the infection has spread to the subarachnoid space.
    - Meningitis presents with fever, headache and neck rigidity

26. **(a) Constricted pupils in response to light** (*Ref. Cummings, 6th ed., 174*)
    - In cavernous sinus thrombosis pupils are dilated and fixed due to the involvement of 3rd nerve and stimulation of sympathetic plexus.

27. **(a) Frontal lobe abscess** (*Ref. Cummings, 6th ed., 729*)
    - Long history of sinusitis and personality changes, fundus showing papilloedema favours the diagnosis of frontal lobe abscess.
    - Viral encephalitis which is usually meningoencephalitis is characterised by fever, headache, neck rigidity and altered sensorium. Please see the above explanation also.

28. **(a) Cavernous sinus thrombosis** (*Ref. Cummings, 6th ed., 729*)
    - In this patient the cavernous sinus of the other side has started getting involved leading to the 6th nerve palsy. Bilateral proptosis will soon follow.
    - Meningitis and hydrocephalus do not lead to proptosis though both of them can involve B/L 6th nerve involvement (this being the most common nerve involved in CNS pathologies)

29. **(a) Cavernous sinus** (*Ref. Scott Brown, 8th ed., Vol 1; 965*)
    - Angular vein (from the medial angle of the eye) continues as the facial vein which through the deep facial vein communicates with the cavernous sinus through the pterygoid plexus of veins.

30. **(a) CT Scan** (*Ref. Cummings, 6th ed., 729*)
    The child has probably developed orbital cellulitis or orbital abscess following ethmoid sinusitis for which a CT scan should be done. CT scan will differentiate orbital cellulitis from orbital abscess and also helps to see the extent of involvement of sinuses. In case of orbital cellulitis, after initial stabilisation

with antibiotics, FESS should be performed later on for chronic sinusitis. If orbital abscess is there it will require antibiotics along with orbital decompression and FESS.

31. **(a) Frontal** (*Ref. Cummings, 6th ed., 761*)

32. **(b) Frontal sinus** (*Ref. Cummings, 6th ed., 799*) (please *refer* to text)

33. **(b) Uncinectomy** (*Ref. Cummings, 6th ed., 766*)

34. **(a) Approaching middle meatus** (*Ref. Cummings, 6th ed., 766*)

35. **(b), (c), and (e) Nasal Allergic polyposis, Mucocele, and Chronic maxillary sinusitis** (*Ref. Cummings, 6th ed., 760*)

    Inverted papilloma is benign but locally invasive tumour hence here a wide excision is done by a lateral rhinotomy approach. Maxillectomy in carcinoma maxilla is done by an open (Weber Fergussen incision) approach (*see* Chapter on tumours of nose and PNS).

36. **All** (*Ref. Cummings, 6th ed., 760*)

37. **(c) Both** (*Ref. Cummings, 6th ed., 760*)

38. **(b) Cerebellum** (*Ref. Cummings, 6th ed., 760*)

39. **(d) Orbital emphysema** (*Ref. Cummings, 6th ed., 778*)
    Orbital complications will follow maxillary, ethmoid and frontal sinus surgeries due to close proximity.

40. **(c) Dacryocystic carcinoma** (*Ref. Cummings, 6th ed., 760*)

    Endoscopic dacryocystorhinostomy can be done by Endoscopic nasal surgery but dacryocystic carcinoma has to be excised by an external approach.

41. **(a) Mitomycin C** (*Ref. Scott Brown, 8th ed., Vol 2; 253*)
    - Mitomycin C is an antineoplastic agent with antifibroblastic activity. It is used to decrease the chances of adhesions and fibrosis following surgery.
    - In ENT it is used in functional endoscopic sinus surgery (FESS) (as any adhesion between the middle meatus and lateral wall of nose will again block the drainage of sinuses), after correction of choanal atresia and laryngotracheal stenosis (as any fibrosis or adhesion of this area will lead to re stenosis leading to stridor).

42. **(b) Inferior meatus** (*Ref. Cummings, 6th ed., 775*)

43. **(a) Maxillary sinus** (*Ref. Cummings, 6th ed., 780*)

44. **(b) Infra-orbital nerve injury** (*Ref. Cummings, 6th ed., 781*)

45. **(b) Sinonasal tumours** (*Ref. Cummings, 6th ed., 800*)
    Frontal osteomas can be excised by Lynch Howarth surgery.

46. **(b) Inferior meatus** (*Ref. Scott Brown, 6th ed., 4/12/18*)

47. **(c) Maxillary sinus** (*Ref. Scott Brown, 6th ed., 4/12/7*)

48. **(a) Air embolism** (*Ref. Scott Brown, 6th ed., 4/12/9*)

49. **(c) I/V Amphotericin B with orbital exenteration** (*Ref. Scott Brown, 8th ed., Vol 1; 1055*)
    This is a case of mucormycosis

50. **(d) Headache is present in both acute and chronic sinusitis** (*Ref. Scott Brown, 8th ed., Vol 1; 1025*)
51. **(c) Internal carotid injury** (*Ref. Cummings, 6th ed., 778*)
52. **(b) Blow out fracture** (*Ref. Cummings, 6th ed., 760*)
53. **(d) Greater auricular** (*see* Fig. 20.1a) (*Ref. Scott Brown, 8th ed., Vol 3; 559*)
54. **(b) Invasion of the sinus mucosa with fungus** (*Ref. Cummings, 6th ed., 736*)
55. **(c) Opening of maxillary antrum through gingivolabial sulcus by sublabial approach** (*Ref. Cummings, 6th ed., 780*)
56. **(a) Mitomycin** (*Ref. Scott Brown, 8th ed., Vol 2; 253; Cummings, 6th ed. 2954*)
57. **(c) Osteomyelitis of frontal bone causing subperiosteal abscess** (*Ref. Cummings, 6th ed., 799*)
58. **(a) Surgical removal of adhesions** (*Ref. Scott Brown, 8th ed., Vol 2; 253*)
59. **(a) *A. fumigatus*** (*Ref. Cummings, 6th ed., 732*)
60. **(d) Allergic fungal sinusitis** (*Ref. Cummings, 6th ed., 736*)
    - The NCCT shows haziness of the left maxillary sinus and mass in the left nasal cavity without any bony erosion.

- Fungal sinusitis presents as U/L nasal mass (ployp) with mucinous discharge in adults. Antrochoanal polyp is seen in young as U/L nasal mass, patient presents here mainly with nasal obstruction, discharge if at all present is purulent and not mucinous. Ethmoidal polyps are B/L. Maxillary carcinoma is U/L nasal mass, presenting with blood tinged nasal discharge, CT here shows bony erosion.

61. **(b) Functional endoscopic sinus surgery** (*Ref. Scott Brown, 8th ed., Vol 1; 1072*)
    NCCT shows left maxillary sinus (asterisk) haziness s/o sinusitis.
62. **(a) Water's view** (*Ref. Scott Brown, 6th ed., 4/3/2*)
63. **(b) Local debridement and I/V amphotericin B** (*Ref. Scott Brown, 8th ed., Vol 1; 1055*)
    A case of Mucormycosis is being shown
64. **(c) Caldwell-Luc operation** (*Ref. Cummings, 6th ed., 780*)
65. **(c) Double density** (*Ref. Scott Brown, 8th ed., Vol 1; 1050*)
66. **(a) Subperiosteal abscess of frontal sinus** (*Ref. Scott Brown, 8th ed., Vol 1; 1088*)

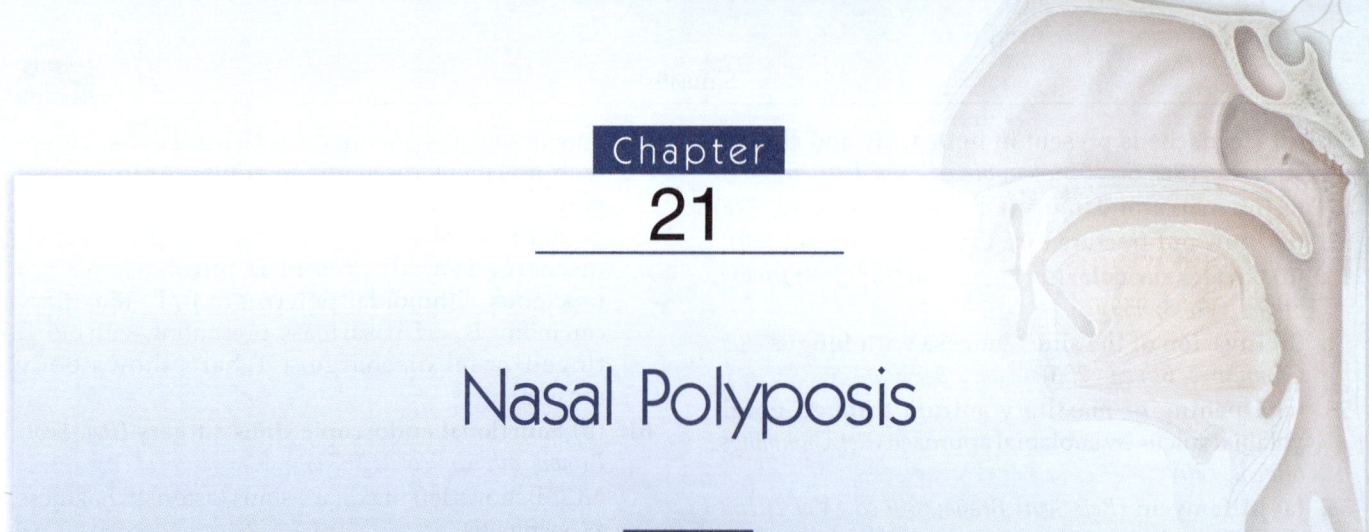

Chapter

21

Nasal Polyposis

Nasal polyposis is not a disease in itself. It is the end stage local manifestation of certain chronic inflammatory diseases of the nose and paranasal sinuses.

Nasal polyps are the polypoidal nasal masses arising from the oedematous nasal mucosa and can follow the following:

1. **Infection:** If localised only to maxillary sinus; leads to **antrochoanal** polyp, *see* below. If generalised in the nose (due to conditions like cystic fibrosis, primary ciliary dysfunction, read below); leads to ethmoidal polyps.
2. **Allergy:** Allergic rhinitis; leads to **ethmoidal** polyps, *see* below. Many patients with allergic rhinitis also have asthma (as one airway one disease). If nasal polyposis and asthma is associated with aspirin hypersensitivity it is termed as **"Samter's triad"**.
3. **Mucoviscidosis/Cystic fibrosis:** By causing chronic bacterial rhinosinusitis presents with **nasal polyposis in the first decade** of life.
4. **Ciliary dysfunction: Kartagener's syndrome** (recurrent sinusitis, bronchiectasis and situs inversus) and **Young's syndrome** (recurrent sinusitis, bronchiectasis and infertility due to azoospermia). There can be associated polyps.
5. **Bernoulli's phenomenon:** It states that when air passes through a constriction it attains high velocity leading to the development of an area of negative pressure in its vicinity. Here in the nose when the inhaled air crosses the narrowest part (nasal valve area), it attains high velocity. This air then passes in a parabolic curve through the middle meatus area (*see* chapter on anatomy) which is already edematous (because of infection and allergy). Hence the velocity of air passing through this constricted area remains high and creates a negative pressure. This sucks the mucosa of the sinuses into the nasal cavity leading to polyp formation.

Whatever the cause may be, it ultimately leads to oedema of the mucosa and polypoidal change. These polyps to begin with are sessile and become pedunculated due to gravity and excessive sneezing (in allergy).

NASAL POLYPS ARE OF TWO TYPES

1. Ethmoidal

Ethmoidal polyps are mainly **allergic** in aetiology. They are **multiple** and **bilateral** (multiple because they arise from multiple ethmoid air cells and bilateral since the aetiology is allergic). They are seen at **middle age**.

If **B/L ethmoidal polyps** are seen in young **(5–20 years)**, the patient should be investigated for **cystic fibrosis** which is a generalised dysfunction of the exocrine glands. Here there is a genetic defect in the chloride ion transport leading to thick and inspissated secretions causing mucous stasis predisposing to infection which in turn leads to inflammation and oedema (and subsequently polypoidal change).

Cystic fibrosis is associated with recurrent pulmonary airways infections, bronchiectasis, intestinal obstruction, pancreatic insufficiency and malabsorption.

A **raised sweat chloride is diagnostic (>70 mEq/L)**. Further confirmatory tests are raised nasal transepithelial electric potential difference and DNA analysis.

Another systemic condition associated with B/L multiple polyps is Churg Strauss Syndrome (Eosinophilic granulomatosis with polyangiitis) which is an ANCA mediated small vessel vasculitis additionally characterised by bronchial asthma, eosinophilia and rapidly progressive Glomerulonephritis (RPGN).

Investigation

The ethmoidal polyps can be seen on anterior rhinoscopy. Endoscopy gives better visualisation. *See* below the nasal endoscopic picture of middle meatus showing nasal polyps.

The best investigation in ethmoidal polyps is **NCCT of the nose and paranasal sinuses**, to know the complete extent of disease.

Management

Since the ethmoidal polyps are allergic in origin they are **highly recurrent**. Medical management with steroids and antihistaminics is done in the preoperative period to decrease their size and in the postoperative period to

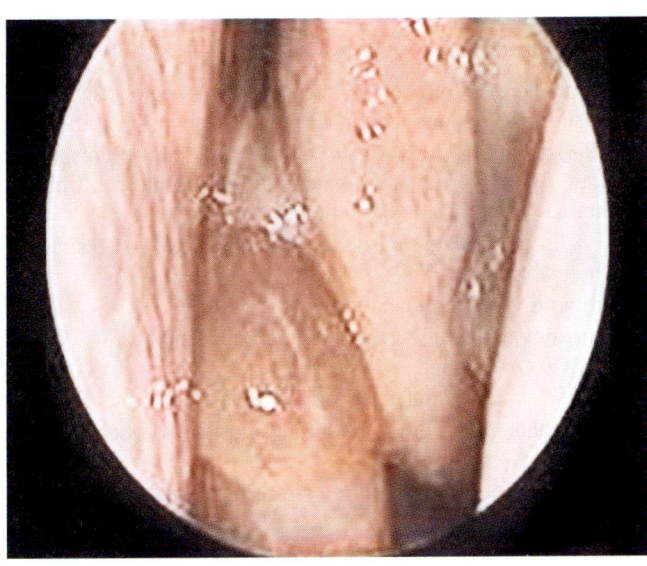

Fig. 21.1

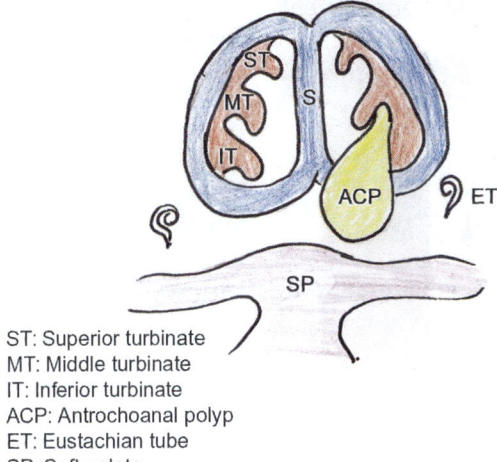

ST: Superior turbinate
MT: Middle turbinate
IT: Inferior turbinate
ACP: Antrochoanal polyp
ET: Eustachian tube
SP: Soft palate

Fig. 21.2: Antrochoanal Polyp hanging into the Choana

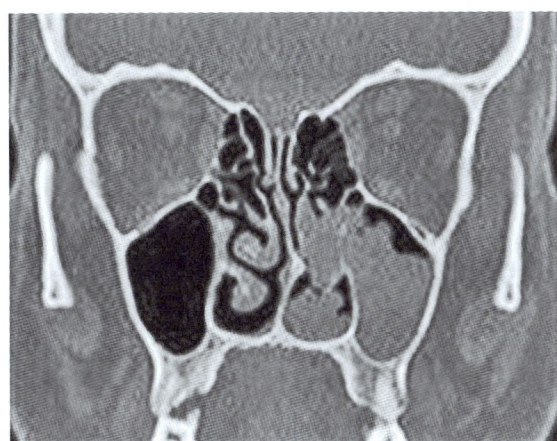

Fig. 21.3

decrease their chances of recurrence. If they do not regress by medical management then surgical management is carried out.

The surgical management is by functional endoscopic sinus surgery (**FESS)** where all the polyps and unhealthy mucosa are removed.

Recurrent cases are also managed by FESS.

2. Antrochoanal Polyp/Killian's Polyp

Localised U/L nasal polyposis can occur following obstruction to the osteo-meatal complex due to anatomical variation (e.g. Haller cell, Concha bullosa, DNS, etc.). Though uncommon, when it involves only the maxillary sinus leading to the formation of **single, U/L** polyp, it is known as antrochoanal polyp. It is seen in young.

The main aetiology of antrochoanal polyp is infection.

Antrochoanal polyp arises from the **maxillary antrum** and as the name antro (antrum) choanal (posterior nares) it grows through the nasal cavity posteriorly into the choana and nasopharynx. Hence it is large and in spite of this it might not be visible on anterior rhinoscopy. It can be seen on **posterior rhinoscopy**. It can even hang down behind soft palate into oropharynx.

Though it is unilateral but once the polyp grows into the nasopharynx it can cause bilateral **nasal obstruction.**

Differential Diagnosis

a. Polypoidal mass in the nostril of an infant should be investigated for **encephalocele or meningo-encephalocele** as nasal polyps do not occur at this age. These appear as soft compressible masses that transilluminate. They demonstrate a positive **Furstenberg test,** i.e. they expand when the child cries or on bilateral internal jugular venous compression.

b. Nasal polyp can be confused with **concha bullosa** (pneumatised middle turbinate). Probe test can be used to differentiate the two. **A polyp neither bleeds nor does it pain** on probing because of its poor vascular as

well as nerve supply (it being oedematous polypoidal nasal mucosa). A probe can be passed all around a polyp but not a turbinate.

c. U/L polypoidal mass in a young boy with recurrent epistaxis should be investigated for angiofibroma.

d. U/L polypoidal mass in an elderly should be investigated for malignancy.

Investigation

The best investigation here is **NCCT** nose and paranasal sinuses. Figure 21.3 shows the NCCT nose and PNS coronal view showing a mass filling the left maxillary antrum and extending into the nasal cavity s/o antrochoanal polyp.

CT/X-ray lateral view of the nose and nasopharynx will show a column/crescent of air between the mass, i.e. the antrochoanal polyp and the pharyngeal wall (known as **crescent or Dodd sign,** *see* the practice question in the end) which will be absent in any mass arising from the pharyngeal wall itself, e.g. angiofibroma (which also occurs in young).

Management

Previously antrochoanal polyp used to be removed by avulsion and nasal snare. Now it is also best managed by **FESS**.

Nose

Section II

Previously for recurrent cases Caldwell-Luc used to be done. But now recurrent cases are also managed by FESS.

Ethmoidal	Antrochoanal
Mainly allergic etiology	**Infective**
Common	**Uncommon**
Middle age	Young
Multiple	**Single**
Bilateral	Unilateral
Seen on anterior rhinoscopy	**Posterior rhinoscopy**
Steroids and antihistaminics are used in t/t	No role
Highly recurrent	**Recurrence is uncommon**

Note:

U/L multiple polyps with allergic mucin should be investigated for allergic fungal sinusitis (*see* Chapter 20).

FOREIGN BODY NOSE

This is mainly seen in **children**. Inanimate foreign body is more common than animate.

Foreign body of nose in a child presents with:

  i. **Unilateral fetid (foul smelling) nasal discharge**
 ii. Epistaxis (mild)
iii. Unilateral nasal obstruction.

Button batteries as foreign bodies in the nasal cavities are dangerous because if they leak, they can cause liquefaction necrosis with severe local tissue destruction leading to septal perforations or nasal meatus stenosis. Hence batteries found in the nasal cavities should be removed immediately.

Removal of foreign body is done using a foreign body hook without any anaesthesia. Impacted foreign body may require removal under general anaesthesia.

"Points to Ponder/Points for Quick revision"

- Nasal Allergy or Infection → Mucosal oedema → Polyp (initially sessile later pedunculated)—Bernoulli's phenomenon.
- Allergic rhinitis (MC), Cystic fibrosis (infection predisposition), Ciliary dysfunction (infection predisposition) & Churg Strauss (vasculitis) → B/L ethmoidal polyps.
- Localised maxillary sinusitis (bacterialinfection) → U/L antrochoanal polyp.
- Ethmoid *vs* antrochoanal polyp—*see* Table.
- One airway one disease—allergic rhinitis and asthma being often seen together.
- Samter's triad—Nasal polyposis + asthma + Aspirin sensitivity.
- Kartagener's syndrome—recurrent sinusitis + bronchiectasis + situs inversus.
- Young's syndrome—recurrent sinusitis + bronchiectasis + infertility (azoospermia).
- Cystic fibrosis: Ethmoidal polyps in young age, recurrent bronchitis → bronchiectasis and intestinal obstruction—Pancreatic insufficiency–malabsorption; ↑ sweat chloride (>70 mEq/L), ↑ transepithelial potential difference.
- Churg Strauss syndrome—classical triad → RPGN + asthma + eosinophilia.
- Nasal polyps—endoscopy gives better visualisation than rhinoscopy; NCCT (Nose & PNS) shows complete extent–important to know before FESS.
- D/D:
   i. Polypoidal mass in an infant—encephalocele/meningoencephalocele (Furstenberg test +).
  ii. Polypoidal mass in an elderly—malignancy (crescent or Dodd sign absent on NCCT).
 iii. Concha bullosa—bleeding and pain upon Prob test, also probing cannot be done all around.
  iv. U/L polypoidal mass with profuse and recurrent epistaxis in a young boy—angiofibroma.
- T/t of nasal polyps—FESS (also for recurrent cases).
- FB nose: U/L foul discharge/obstruction/mild epistaxis—removal by FB hook without anaesthesia (urgent in case of button batteries).

PREVIOUSLY ASKED QUESTIONS

1. **Which of the following statements is not correct for ethmoidal polyp?** *(AIIMS 2002, Exam 2016)*
   a. Allergy is an etiological factor
   b. Occur in the first decade of life
   c. Are bilateral
   d. Are often associated with bronchial asthma

2. **Most common nasal mass:** *(Exam 2013)*
   a. Polyp
   b. Papilloma
   c. Angiofibroma
   d. None

3. **Regarding ethmoidal polyp, which one of the following is true:** *(Kolkata 2005, Exam 2016)*
   a. Epistaxis
   b. Unilateral
   c. Less than 10 years
   d. Associated with bronchial asthma

4. **Ethmoidal polyp, true is:** *(Exam 2013)*
   a. Children   b. Solitary
   c. Unilateral   d. Adults

5. **Recurrent polypi are seen in:** *(UP 2007, Exam 2016)*
   a. Antrochoanal polyp
   b. Ethmoidal polyp
   c. Concha bullosa
   d. Hypertrophic turbinate

6. **Which of the following best differentiates antrochoanal polyp from ethmoidal polyp?** *(MH 2008, Exam 2016)*
   a. They are multiple
   b. Best seen on posterior rhinoscopy
   c. Recurrence on polypectomy
   d. They are bilateral

7. **In a patient with multiple bilateral nasal polyps with X-ray showing opacity in the para-nasal sinuses. The treatment consists of all of the following except:** *(AIIMS 2002, Exam 2016)*
   a. FESS   b. Corticosteroids
   c. Amphotericin B   d. Antihistaminics

8. **Patient with ethmoidal polyp undergoes polypectomy, presents 6 months later with ethmoid polyp, correct treatment:** *(AIIMS 95, Exam 2011)*
   a. FESS
   b. External ethmoidectomy
   c. Caldwell-Luc procedure
   d. Intranasal polypectomy

9. **Samter's triad includes:** *(PGI May 2010, 2013)*
   a. Bronchiectasis   b. Asthma
   c. Aspirin sensitivity   d. Nasal polyposis
   e. Tinnitus

10. **Samter's triad is related to:** *(Exam 2013)*
    a. Ethmoid polyp   b. Nasopharyngeal
    c. Angiofibroma   d. Nasal glioma

11. **Young's syndrome is:** *(Exam 2013)*
    a. Neutrophilia with red papular rash
    b. Mitral stenosis with atrial septal defect
    c. Infertility with bronchiectasis
    d. Multiple enchondromas with phleboliths

12. **All are seen in Kartagener's syndrome except:** *(DPG 2007, Exam 2016)*
    a. Ciliary dysfunction
    b. Azoospermia
    c. Aspirin sensitivity
    d. Situs inversus

13. **"Bernoulli's theorem" explains:** *(UP 2007, Exam 2016)*
    a. Nasal polyp
    b. Thyroglossal cyst
    c. Zenker's diverticulum
    d. Laryngomalacia

14. **Killian term is used for which of the following polyp:** *(UP 2005, Exam 2016)*
    a. Ethmoidal
    b. Antrochoanal polyp
    c. Tonsillar cyst
    d. Tonsillolith

15. **All of the following are true of antrochoanal polyp except:** *(AI 94, Exam 2016)*
    a. Common in young
    b. Single and unilateral
    c. Bleeds on touch
    d. Treatment involves FESS

16. **Regarding antrochoanal polyp which one is true:** *(Kolkata 2005, Exam 2016)*
    a. Origin from maxillary sinus and goes to nasopharynx
    b. Present with severe bleeding
    c. Bilateral
    d. Seen in elderly person

17. **Antrochoanal polyp:** *(Exam 2013)*
    a. Single and grows posteriorly
    b. Multiple
    c. Bleeding
    d. None

18. **Recurrent epistaxis is not a common feature of:** *(AI 96, Exam 2014)*
    a. DNS
    b. Rhinosporidiosis
    c. Nasal polypi
    d. Maxillary carcinoma

19. Antrochoanal polyp is characterised by:
                              (*PGI Dec 2003, 2014*)
    a. Usually bilateral
    b. It is of allergic in origin
    c. It arises from maxillary antrum
    d. Caldwell-Luc operation is the treatment of choice in recurrent cases
    e. Recurrence is common

20. All of the following are true about antrochoanal polyp except: (*TN 2007, Exam 2016*)
    a. Single
    b. Unilateral
    c. Premalignant
    d. Arises from maxillary antrum

21. Treatment for recurrent antrochoanal polyp:
                              (*MP 2007, Exam 2016*)
    a. Caldwell-Luc operation
    b. FESS
    c. Simple polypectomy
    d. Both A and B

22. The current treatment of choice for a large antro-choanal polyp in a 10-year-old is:
                      (*AIIMS Nov 2005, 2002, May 2014*)
    a. Intranasal polypectomy
    b. Caldwell-Luc operation
    c. FESS
    d. Lateral rhinotomy and excision

23. A 2-year-old child presents with B/L polypoidal nasal masses. Most important investigation prior to undertaking surgery is: (*AI 97, Exam 2015*)
    a. Ultrasound   b. FNAC
    c. Biopsy   d. CECT

24. About foreign body nose in a child true is:
                              (*PGI June 2003, 2011*)
    a. Unilateral fetid discharge
    b. Presents with unilateral nasal obstruction
    c. Has torrential epistaxis
    d. Inanimate is more common than animate
    e. Always removed under GA

25. The commonest cause of U/L mucopurulent rhinorrhoea in a child: (*Kolkata 2001, Exam 2016*)
    a. Antrochoanal polyp
    b. Foreign body
    c. Angiofibroma
    d. Rhinosporidiosis

26. A child presented with history of unilateral purulent nasal discharge with occasional bloody discharge from the same side, the diagnosis is:
                              (*SGPGI 2005, Exam 2016*)
    a. Antrochoanal polyp
    b. Foreign body
    c. Angiofibroma
    d. Rhinosporidiosis

27. Topical steroid has no role after sinus surgery in:
                              (*AIIMS Nov 2013, Exam 2014*)
    a. Ethmoidal polyp
    b. Antrochoanal polyp
    c. Allergic fungal sinusitis
    d. None of the above

28. Child with battery as foreign body in nose. Which of the following is an important concern?
                              (*AIIMS Nov 2014*)
    a. Refer to specialist and plan for elective removal
    b. Local release of chemical from battery and destruction of tissue
    c. Rhinolith formation
    d. Septal abscess formation

29. All of the following are features of ethmoidal polyp except: (*Exam 2016*)
    a. Common in adults
    b. Commonly singular
    c. Commonly bilateral
    d. Is usually allergic

30. Which of the following is true about Killian's polyp?   (*Exam 2016*)
    a. Common in adults
    b. Singular
    c. Commonly bilateral
    d. Is usually allergic

31. True about antrochoanal polyp: (*PGI 2011*)
    a. Starts as edema of maxillary sinus mucosa
    b. Steroid drops beneficial
    c. Grows towards posterior nares
    d. More common in adults
    e. Excised by FESS

32. Treatment of choice in bilateral ethmoidal polyp is: (*Exam 2016*)
    a. Maxillectomy   b. FESS
    c. Caldwell Luc   d. Chemotherapy

33. The combination of nasal polyps, bronchial asthma and aspirin sensitivity is referred to as:
                              (*APPG 2016*)
    a. Virchow's triad   b. Trotter's triad
    c. Samter's triad   d. Saint's triad

34. Postoperative steroids are not used for: (*Exam 2015*)
    a. Post antrochoanal surgery
    b. Allergic rhinosinusitis
    c. Post fungal sinusitis surgery
    d. Multiple ethmoidal polyps

35. All are true about antro-choanal polyp except:
                              (*Exam 2015*)
    a. Bleeds on touch
    b. Insensitive to pain
    c. Probing can be done all around
    d. Pale in appearance

Nose

Section II

36. **A 12-year-old child presents with bilateral nasal polyps. He should be investigated for:** (*Exam 2016*)
    a. Rhinosporidiosis   b. Mucoviscidosis
    c. Angiofibroma   d. Antrochoanal polyp

IMAGE BASED PRACTICE QUESTIONS BY THE AUTHOR

37. **A 35-year-old male presented with nasal obstruction. His nasal endoscopy finding of one nostril is given. Which one is true regarding this condition?**

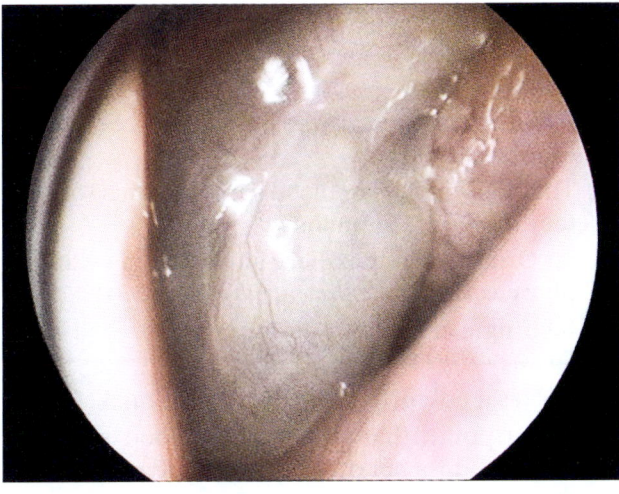

    a. Best managed by intranasal polypectomy with snare
    b. It bleeds on probing

    c. Caldwell-Luc operation is the treatment of choice in recurrent cases
    d. It originates from maxillary sinus and goes to nasopharynx

38. **A 20-year-old male presents with nasal obstruction and nasal discharge. Nasal endoscopy shows a large polyp in the right nostril extending into the nasopharynx. His NCCT nose and PNS axial view is given. He should be managed by:**

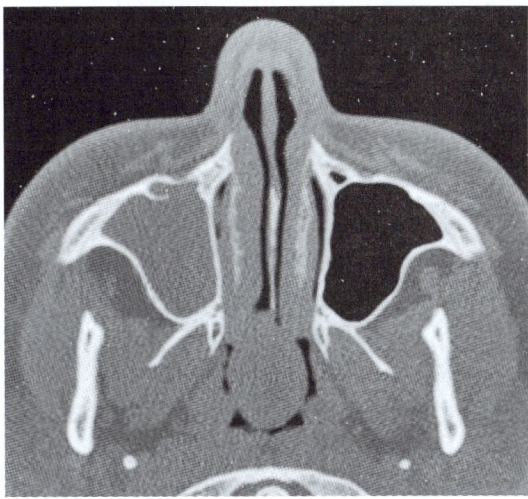

    a. Intranasal polypectomy
    b. Steroids
    c. FESS
    d. Caldwell Luc

Section II   Nose

ANSWERS AND EXPLANATIONS

1. **(b) Occur in the first decade of life** (*Ref. Scott Brown, 6th ed., 4/10/5*)
   - Ethmoidal polyps are usually seen at middle age. If they occur early in life, the patient should be investigated for cystic fibrosis.

2. **(a) Polyp** (*Ref. Scott Brown, 6th ed., 4/10/5*)

3. **(d) Associated with bronchial asthma** (*Ref. Scott Brown, 6th ed., 4/10/3*) (refer the text)
   - Polyps (being oedematous change in nasal mucosa) does not present with epistaxis because of their poor vascular supply. They present with nasal obstruction.

4. **(d) Adults** (*Ref. Scott Brown, 6th ed., 4/10/5*)

5. **(b) Ethmoidal polyp** (*Ref. Scott Brown, 6th ed., 4/10/13*)
   - As the ethmoidal polyps are allergic in etiology they are highly recurrent.
   - Antrochoanal polyp can also recur though their recurrence is uncommon.
   - Concha bullosa is pneumatised middle turbinate. It does not recur after surgical correction.
   - Hypertrophic turbinate also does not recur after turbinectomy.

6. **(b) Best seen on posterior rhinoscopy** (please refer the table in the text) (*Ref. Scott Brown, 6th ed., 4/10/14*)

7. **(c) Amphotericin B** (*Ref. Scott Brown, 8th ed., Vol 1; 1043*)
   - The clinical description is suggestive of ethmoidal polyps. Here there is no role of anti-fungal agent Amphotericin B.

8. **(a) FESS** (*Ref. Scott Brown, 6th ed., 4/10/11; Cummings, 6th ed., 760*)
   - The surgical management of recurrent ethmoidal polyps is excision by FESS.
   - External ethmoidectomy used to be done for recurrent ethmoidal polyps before the advent of FESS.
   - Caldwell-Luc procedure which is a sub labial approach for the maxillary sinus used to be done for recurrent antrochoanal polyps previously. Nowadays FESS is done for the same.
   - Intranasal polypectomy which is avulsion of polyp using a nasal snare is no more done.

9. **(b), (c), and (d)** (*Ref. Scott Brown, 8th ed., Vol 1; 1039*)

10. **(a) Ethmoid polyp** (*Ref. Scott Brown, 8th ed., Vol 1; 1039*)
    - Allergic nasal polyposis (ethmoidal polyp) and asthma with aspirin hypersensitivity is termed as Samter's triad.

11. **(c) Infertility with bronchiectasis** (*Ref. Scott Brown, 8th ed., Vol 1; 1040*)

12. **(b) Azoospermia** (refer the text) (*Ref. Scott Brown, 8th ed., Vol 2; 273*)

13. **(a) Nasal polyp** (please *see* the text) (*Ref. Scott Brown, 6th ed., 4/10/2*)
    - Thyroglossal cyst and laryngomalacia are the congenital malformations (see chapters on anatomy of oral cavity and pharynx and congenital lesions of larynx).
    - Zenker's diverticulum occurs due to neuromuscular incoordination (*see* Chapter on pharyngeal pouch).

14. **(b) Antrochoanal polyp** (*Ref. Scott Brown, 6th ed., 4/10/14*)
    - Killian polyp is another name for antrochoanal polyp.

15. **(c) Bleeds on touch** (refer the text) (*Ref. Scott Brown, 6th ed., 4/10/14*)
    - They have very poor blood supply because of which they do not bleed on touch.

16. **(a) Origin from maxillary sinus and goes to nasopharynx** (*Ref. Scott Brown, 6th ed., 4/10/14*)

17. **(a) Single and grows posteriorly** (*Ref. Scott Brown, 6th ed., 4/10/14*)

18. **(c) Nasal polypi** (*Ref. Scott Brown, 8th ed., Vol 1; 1038*)
    - Nasal polypi have very poor blood supply so epistaxis does not occur in nasal polyposis.

19. **(c) It arises from maxillary antrum** (please refer the text) (*Ref. Scott Brown, 6th ed., 4/10/14*)

20. **(c) Premalignant** (*Ref. Scott Brown, 6th ed., 4/10/14*)
    - Nasal polyps arise due to edema of the nasal mucosa. They are not premalignant.

21. **(b) FESS** (*Ref. Cummings, 6th ed., 760*)

22. **(c) FESS** (*Ref. Cummings, 6th ed., 760*)
    - Antrochoanal polyp arise from the maxillary antrum and grow into the nasopharynx, hence they are always large at presentation and management is excision by FESS.

23. **(d) CECT** (*Ref. Scott Brown, 8th ed., Vol 2; 255*)
    - In such a small child nasal polyps are not there, so we have to rule out a meningocele or a meningomyelocele and have to go for a CECT before proceeding further.

24. **(a), (b), and (d)** (*Ref. Scott Brown, 6th ed., 6/14/4*)

25. **(b) Foreign body** (*Ref. Scott Brown, 8th ed., Vol 2; 386*)
    - Antrochoanal polyp usually presents with unilateral nasal obstruction. Nasal discharge if occurs is mucoid.
    - Angiofibroma presents with repeated torrential or profuse epistaxis in pubertal males.
    - Rhinosporidiosis presents with epistaxis and a mulberry nasal mass.

26. **(b) Foreign body** (*Ref. Scott Brown, 8th ed., Vol 2; 243*)
    Please *see* the above explanations.

27. **(b) Antrochoanal polyp** (*Ref. Cummings, 6th ed., 760*)

28. **(b) Local release of chemical from battery and destruction of tissue** (*Ref. Scott Brown, 8th ed., Vol 2; 386*)

29. **(b) Commonly singular** (*Ref. Scott Brown, 6th ed., 4/10/1*)

30. **(b) Singular** (*Ref. Scott Brown, 6th ed., 4/10/14*)

31. **(a), (c), (e)** (*Ref. Scott Brown, 6th ed., 4/10/14*)

32. **(b) FESS** (*Ref. Cummings, 6th ed., 760*)

33. **(c) Samter's triad** (*Ref. Scott Brown, 8th ed., Vol 1; 1039*)

34. **(a) Post antrochoanal surgery** (*Ref. Scott Brown, 6th ed., 4/10/14*)

35. **(a) Bleeds on touch** (*Ref. Scott Brown, 6th ed., 4/10/14*)

36. **(b) Mucoviscidosis** (*Ref. Scott Brown, 8th ed., Vol 2; 272*)

37. **(d) It Originates from maxillary sinus and goes to nasopharynx** (*Ref. Scott Brown, 8th ed., Vol 1; 1029*)

38. **(c) FESS** (*Ref. Cummings, 6th ed., 760*)
   - The NCCT nose and PNS axial view shows the right maxillary sinus filled with mass, going to the nasal cavity and extending into the nasopharynx, suggestive of antrochoanal polyp. Also notice the crescent of air in the nasopharynx, between the mass and the posterior pharyngeal wall known as Dodd/crescent sign.

Granulomatous Conditions of the Nose

The granulomatous conditions of the nose are:
a. Bacterial
b. Fungal
c. Protozoal
d. Systemic diseases.

They are destructive conditions and may progress to cause atrophic rhinitis.

BACTERIAL

Rhinoscleroma

It is caused by *Klebsiella rhinoscleromatis*, a gram-negative bacteria also known as **Frisch bacillus** (named after Von Frisch who discovered it). It is seen more commonly in northern parts of India.

Clinical Features

There are three stages in the course of the Rhinoscleroma:
  i. **Atrophic stage:** Due to tissue destruction here the patient has lots of crusting and foul smelling nasal discharge.
 ii. **Granulomatous stage:** Here extensive granuloma formation occurs leading to a very **hard nose** also described as **woody nose or Hebra nose,** shown below.
iii. **Cicatricial stage:** In this stage extensive fibrosis leads to deformity or stenosis of the nose. This deformed

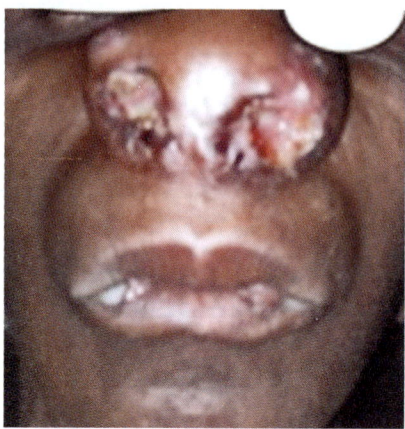

Fig. 22.1

nose is known as tapir nose (Tapir is a mammal with a big snout).

Along with the nose, rhinoscleroma involves the nasopharynx, oropharynx and larynx also.

Diagnosis

Biopsy is diagnostic. It shows granulomas with plasma cells and macrophages. The large macrophages containing the phagocytosed bacteria are known as Mikulicz cells. The eosinophilic inclusion bodies present in the plasma cells are known as Russell bodies.

The **Mikulicz cells and Russell bodies** are diagnostic of rhinoscleroma.

A positive culture is diagnostic, but cultures come positive only in 50–60% of cases.

Management

1. **Streptomycin, tetracycline, rifampicin and ciprofloxacin:** These antibiotics form the different treatment regimes which are given for at least 6 weeks till cultures become negative. They constitute the mainstay of management (easy to remember, most of them we use in TB—the commonest granulomatous condition in day to day clinical practice).
2. **Steroids:** These are given to reduce the fibrosis.
3. **Surgery:** Surgery is done only in cases where nasal deformity needs to be corrected or to maintain airway. Granulations are removed with cautery or LASER. In case of cicatrisation, the airway is dilated and polythene spacers are placed for 6 weeks. Plastic reconstruction is considered at a later stage with complete control of infection.

SYPHILIS

Both congenital and acquired syphilis can be seen in the nose.

Congenital syphilis either presents early (3 weeks to 3 months) after birth as **snuffles** (catarrhal rhinitis) or late as **gummas** (solitary lesions showing granulomatous inflammation).

Acquired Syphilis

a. Primary; it presents as chancre (painless, non-tender, indurated ulcer) of nasal vestibule.

b. Secondary; it presents as mucous patches and snail track ulcers.

c. Tertiary; **the most common** syphilis seen in the nose is **tertiary syphilis**. Here gummas are seen on the nasal septum. Later on **perforations** occur in both **bony** and cartilaginous part of septum and hard palate. Saddling of nose may result.

Management

Injection benzathine penicillin 2.4 MU I/M is given every week for 3 weeks or cap Doxycycline 100 mg twice daily for 4 weeks.

TUBERCULOSIS

TB of the nose is usually secondary to pulmonary TB. It involves the anterior part of the nasal septum and anterior end of inferior turbinate. Hence, it causes **perforation** in the anterior **cartilaginous part of septum**.

Diagnosis: Biopsy and AFB stain

Management: ATT

LUPUS VULGARIS

It is a low grade tuberculous infection of the skin in the nose, i.e. the nasal vestibule. Brownish nodules not blanching on pressure described as **Apple jelly nodules** are seen in the nasal vestibule.

Diagnosis: Biopsy

Treatment: ATT

LEPROSY

Like tuberculosis, it also involves anterior part of nasal septum and anterior end of inferior turbinate causing perforation in the cartilaginous part. It can progress to cause atrophic rhinitis, depression of nasal bridge and retrusion of collumella.

Diagnosis: Biopsy

Treatment: Rifampicin, dapsone and others.

ASPERGILLOSIS AND MUCORMYCOSIS

The fungal infections of the nose (*Aspergillus fumigates, Aspergillus flavus, Aspergillus niger*, Mucor & Rhizopus) can lead to granuloma formation (refer to chapter on sinusitis for the various other clinical presentation of fungal infections).

RHINOSPORIDIOSIS

It is a **granuloma** caused by *Rhinosporidium seeberi*. This organism was previously considered to be a fungus. It is now identified to be an **aquatic protistan protozoa** (unicellular) parasite belonging to the class Mesomycetzoea.

It is seen more commonly in the **southern parts** of India especially towards the costal belt of Kerala and Tamil Nadu.

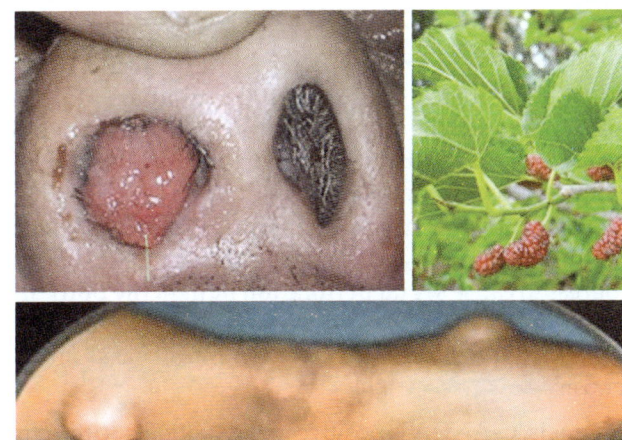

Fig. 22.2

Clinical Features

The patient of Rhinosporidiosis is **immunocompetent**. There is a history of taking **bath in ponds frequented by animals** as these sporangia (A **sporangium** or spore case is an enclosure in which spores of the infecting organisms are formed) are present in the cattle dung. It affects the previously traumatized mucous membrane of nose, nasopharynx, oropharynx, conjunctiva, rectum, external genitalia and skin. **Cutaneous/subcutaneous nodular lesions** can also develop due to contact by contaminated finger nails (e.g. following nose picking).

The patient presents with blood tinged nasal discharge, epistaxis and nasal obstruction. Anterior rhinoscopy shows a **red polypoidal mass** appearing like a **mulberry or strawberry with white dots** (sporangia) studded on the surface. Figure 22.2 shows the mulberry mass (resembling the ripe mulberry) with white dots and subcutaneous nodules on the legs of the patient.

Diagnosis: Nasal smear or biopsy shows sporangia.

Treatment: Wide excision and cauterisation of base. **Recurrence** may occur if sporangium is left behind.

Dapsone is given in the postoperative period to decrease the chances of recurrence.

Rhinoscleroma	Rhinosporidiosis
Caused by gram-negative bacteria *Klebsiella rhinoscleromatis*	Caused by aquatic protistan protozoa *Rhinosporidium seeberi*
Endemic in north India	Endemic in south India
Woody/Hebra and Tapir nose	Polypoid mulberry or strawberry nasal mass with white dots
Additionally involves naso and oropharynx and larynx	Additionally involves naso and oropharynx, larynx, skin, eyes, external genitalia and rectum
Biopsy—Mikulicz cells and Russell bodies are diagnostic	Biopsy showing sporangia is diagnostic
Primary management is medical (Streptomycin, tetracycline, rifampicin and ciprofloxacin along with steroids)	Primary management is surgical (wide excision and cauterisation of base)

Section II **Nose**

GRANULOMATOSIS WIH POLYANGIITIS/WEGNER'S GRANULOMATOSIS

It is the necrotising granulomatous vasculitis affecting most commonly the **upper and lower respiratory tract** (multiple B/L cavitary lesions in the lungs) **and the kidneys** (glomerulonephritis).

Nasal involvement causes rhinitis, sinusitis, anosmia, crusting, blood tinged nasal discharge which might progress to cause septal **perforation both in the bony and cartilaginous part** (like syphilis) ultimately leading to whole septal destruction, saddle nose or nasal airway stenosis.

Diagnosis: C-ANCA is positive in 85% patients with active systemic disease. C-ANCA being negative in 15% of patients with Wegner's, therefore, the diagnosis is made on lung biopsy which shows necrotising granulomatous vasculitis.

Treatment: Steroids and cyclophosphamide.

SARCOIDOSIS

It is a chronic granulomatous disease which may involve any organ, though lung involvement is most common. The sino-nasal symptoms are nonspecific like nasal obstruction, crusting, friable mucosa, diffuse thickening and violaceous affection of skin of the tip of nose known as **lupus pernio**. Examination shows red nodules within the nasal mucosa appearing like **strawberry**.

Septal perforation in the cartilaginous part may be present and saddle deformity may result.

Diagnosis: Made on biopsy (characterised by non-caseating granulomas). For patients with negative pathology, an important supportive test for the diagnosis of sarcoidosis is serum ACE levels which are found to be elevated here.

Treatment: Steroids

MIDLINE MALIGNANT RETICULOSIS/MIDLINE LETHAL GRANULOMA/ T-CELL LYMPHOMA/ NATURAL KILLER (NK) LYMPHOMA

It is also called Stewart's granuloma. This extra nodal natural killer (NK)/T-cell lymphoma (nasal type) is an aggressive lymphoma characterised by extensive necrosis and angioinvasion. It most often presents in extra nodal sites, in particular the nasal or paranasal sinus region.

The tumour cells usually show the presence of **Epstein-Barr virus.**

Patient presents with nasal obstruction and epistaxis. Later on ulceration, perforation and necrosis of septum and palate occurs. It is highly invasive locally and invades paranasal sinus, orbit and skin leading to the destruction of nose and **mid-facial structures**.

A biopsy is necessary for a definitive diagnosis. The lymphoma cells **express T-cell antigens (CD 56 expression)**.

Management is by a combination of chemotherapy and radiotherapy. Surgical management is limited to reconstruction of bony and soft tissue defects after treatment. Prognosis is very poor.

 "Points to Ponder/Points for Quick revision"

- **Rhinoscleroma:**
- *Klebsiella rhinoscleromatis* (gram-ve Frisch bacillus)—North India.
- CFs: Excessive crusts → nasal obstruction, foul discharge. Hard/woody/Hebra nose. Fibrosis → Tapir nose.
- Biopsy—diagnostic → granulomas with plasma cells (with eosinophilic inclusion bodies—Russell bodies), macrophages with phagocytosed bacteria–Mikulicz cells.
- T/t—antibiotics till 6 weeks (Strepto, tetra, R cin & Cipro) and steroids.

Syphilis:
- Congenital: 3 weeks–3 months after birth–snuffles.
- Acquired: 1°—chancre (painless, non-tender, indurated ulcer), 2°—snail track ulcer, 3°—(MC)—Gummas, bony septal perforation also.
- T/t: Inj Benzathine penicillin or Cap doxycycline.

Tuberculosis:
- 2° to pulmonary—anterior nose–perforation of cartilaginous septum; nasal vestibule; lupus vulgaris (apple jelly nodules).

Leprosy:
- Like TB, anterior nose—perforation of cartilaginous septum.

Rhinosporidiosis:
- Granuloma—*Rhinosporidium seeberi* (protozoa); South India; Immunocompetent; Bathing in ponds frequented by cattle.
- CFs: Bloody nasal discharge, obstruction, red polypoidal mass (mulberry or strawberry with white dots)—Cutaneous nodules.
- Biopsy—diagnostic shows sporangia.
- T/t—wide excision and cauterisation of base, dapsone–postoperatively.

Granulomatosis with polyangiitis (WG):
- CFs: ENT (nasal crusts, sinusitis, bony and cartilaginous septal perforation + Lungs (B/L cavitary lesions) + Kidney (RPGN).
- Diagnosis: C—ANCA (+ 85%), Hallmark; Lung Biopsy–necrotising granulomatous vasculitis.
- T/t: Steroids + cyclophosphamide.
- **Sarcoidosis:** Non caseating granulomas, multisystem (MC-Lungs)—skin of nose tip; Lupus pernio, cartilaginous septal perforation.
- **Midline lethal/T cell/NK cell Lymphoma (Stewart's granuloma):** Aggressive, Angio-invasive, extensively destructive—EBV; CD 56; Chemo + radiotherapy; Poor prognosis.

PREVIOUSLY ASKED QUESTIONS

1. **Rhinoscleroma is caused by:** *(PGI 99, Exam 2013)*
   a. Klebsiella
   b. Autoimmune
   c. Spirochetes
   d. Rhinosporidium

2. **Mikulicz cell and Russell bodies are characteristic of:** *(JIPMER 2002,Bihar 2006, Exam 2013)*
   a. Rhinoscleroma
   b. Rhinosporidiosis
   c. Lupus vulgaris
   d. Lethal midline granuloma

3. **Atrophic dry nasal mucosa, extensive crustations with woody hard external nose is suggestive of:** *(MH 2005, Exam 2017)*
   a. Rhinosporidiosis
   b. Rhinoscleroma
   c. Atrophic rhinitis
   d. Carcinoma nose

4. **All the following are true about rhinoscleroma except:** *(PGI June 2009, 2015)*
   a. Biopsy is diagnostic
   b. Causative organism can be cultured
   c. Occur in endemic areas
   d. Medical management is done
   e. Surgical intervention is treatment of choice

5. **About nasal syphilis true:** *(PGI 2002, 2014)*
   a. Perforation occurs in septum
   b. Saddle nose deformity may occur
   c. In newborn, it presents as snuffles
   d. Atrophic rhinitis is a complication
   e. Secondary syphilis is the commonest association

6. **Apple jelly nodules on the nasal vestibule are found in cases of:** *(MP 2005, Exam 2017)*
   a. Rhinosporidiosis
   b. Syphilis
   c. Lupus vulgaris
   d. Rhinoscleroma

7. **Rhinosporidiosis is caused by:** *(Exam 2013)*
   a. HPV
   b. *Klebsiella rhinoscleromatis*
   c. *R. seeberi*
   d. EBV

8. **Rhinosporidiosis is caused by:** *(PGI 99, UP 2000, Exam 2013)*
   a. Fungus
   b. Virus
   c. Bacteria
   d. Protozoa

9. **True statement about Rhinosporidiosis is:** *(AI 99, Exam 2011)*
   a. Most common organism is *Klebsiella rhinoscleromatis*
   b. Seen in immunocompromised patients
   c. Presents as a nasal polyp
   d. Can be diagnosed by identification on biopsy

10. **Which of the following is not a feature of rhinosporidiosis?** *(JIPMER 2000, Exam 2016)*
    a. Bleeding polypoid mass
    b. Russell bodies are seen
    c. Oral dapsone is useful in treatment
    d. Excision with the knife is the treatment

11. **Bleeding nasal polypoidal mass with subcutaneous nodules on skin are seen in:** *(MP 2001, Exam 2017)*
    a. Zygomycosis
    b. Rhinosporidiosis
    c. Sporotrichosis
    d. Aspergillosis

12. **Ideal treatment of rhinosporidiosis is:** *(AIIMS 97, Exam 2015)*
    a. Rifampicin
    b. Excision with cautery at base
    c. Tetracycline
    d. Laser

13. **In rhinosporidiosis the following is true:** *(PGI 99, Exam 2016)*
    a. Fungal granuloma
    b. Greyish mass
    c. Surgery is the treatment
    d. Radiotherapy is treatment

14. **Strawberry appearance of nasal mucosa is seen in:** *(AI 2002, Exam 2016)*
    a. Wegener's granulomatosis
    b. Sarcoidosis
    c. Kawasaki disease
    d. Rhinosporidiosis

15. **True about nasal T-cell lymphoma:** *(PGI June 2009)*
    a. Presents with nasal obstruction and epistaxis
    b. Association with EBV
    c. Cell express T-cell marker
    d. Wide local excision is treatment of choice
    e. Locally invasive

16. **All of the following are causes of perforation of only cartilaginous part of nasal septum except:** *(Exam 2015)*
    a. Tuberculosis
    b. Leprosy
    c. Lupus
    d. Syphilis

17. **Frisch bacillus is the causative agent of:** *(Exam 2016)*
    a. Rhinoscleroma
    b. Rhinosporidiosis
    c. Rhinophyma
    d. Atrophic rhinitis

18. **Features of Granulomatosis with Polyangitis:** *(PGI May 2015)*
    a. Nasal polyp
    b. Perforated nasal septum
    c. Persistent sinusitis
    d. Crusting of nasal mucosa
    e. Collapse of nasal bridge

Section II **Nose**

19. Which of the following statements are true regarding the disease depicted here?

   i. The histopathology shows foamy macrophges with intracytomplasmic bacilli and plasma cells with Russel bodies

   ii. It is case of granulomatosis with polyangitis

   iii. It is caused by a gram-positive bacillus

   iv. Nasal obstruction is a common complaint

   v. Streptomycin and tetracycline for 4–6 weeks are used in treatment   (*APPG 2016*)

a. i, iv, v

b. i, ii, iii

c. i, iii, v

d. iii, iv, v

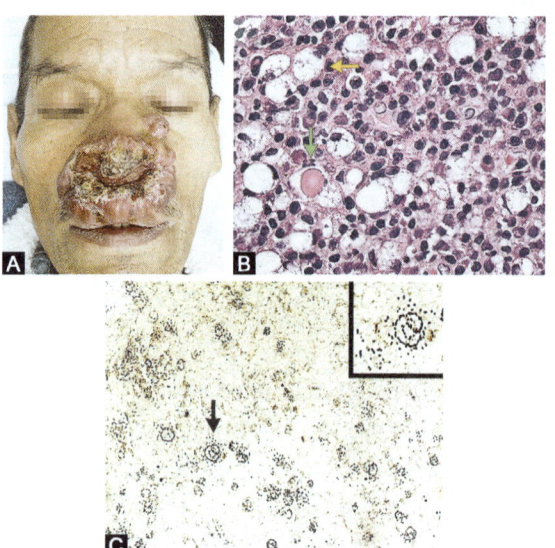

20. A 30-year-old male presents with right-sided nasal obstruction and recurrent epistaxis. On examination, a mulberry mass with white dots seen in the right nostril. Following is true about the disease: (Image-based practice question by the author)

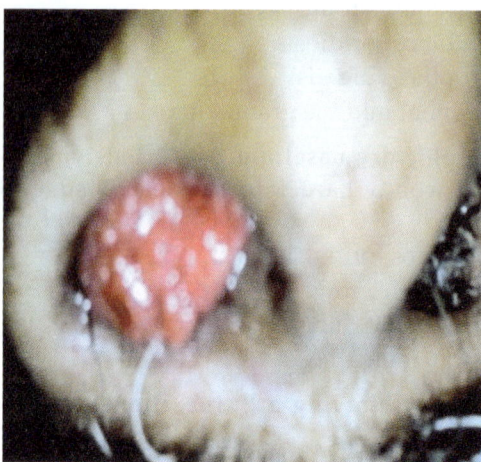

a. Should be managed by excision with cautery at base

b. Caused by fungus Rhinosporidium

c. Biopsy shows Miculicz cells

d. Rifampicin is given here

ANSWERS AND EXPLANATIONS

1. **(a) Klebsiella** (*Ref. Scott Brown, 8th ed., Vol 1; 1212*)
- Rhinoscleroma is a bacterial granuloma caused by *Klebsiella rhinoscleromatis* also known as Frisch bacillus.
- *Rhinosporidium seeberi*, an aquatic protistan protozoa (unicellular) parasite, causes a granulomatous condition called rhinosporidiosis.
- Spirochete (syphilis) and autoimmune conditions (e.g. Wegener's granulomatosis) are the other nasal granulomatous conditions.

2. **(a) Rhinoscleroma** (*Ref. Scott Brown, 6th ed., 4/8/34*)
- Definitive diagnostic test of rhinoscleroma is biopsy
- Biopsy in rhinoscleroma shows granulomas with plasma cells containing Russell bodies and large macrophages containing the phagocytosed bacteria are known as Mikulicz cells.

3. **(b) Rhinoscleroma** (*Ref. Scott Brown, 6th ed., 4/8/34*)
Woody hard nose is diagnostic of Rhinoscleroma.

4. **(e) Surgical intervention is treatment of choice.** Rest are true. Refer to text (*Ref. Scott Brown, 6th ed., 4/8/34*)

5. **(a), (b), (c) and (d)** (*Ref. Scott Brown, 6th ed., 4/8/29*)
Syphilis and some other granulomatous conditions can lead to secondary atrophic rhinitis; refer to Chapter 19 on acute and chronic rhinitis. The most common syphilis seen in the nose is tertiary syphilis.

6. **(c) Lupus vulgaris** (please refer the text) (*Ref. Scott Brown, 6th ed., 4/8/31*)

7. **(c) R. seeberi** (*Ref. Scott Brown, 8th ed., Vol 1; 208*)

8. **(d) Protozoa** (*Ref. Scott Brown, 8th ed., Vol 1; 208*)
- Rhinosporidiosis is a granuloma caused by *Rhinosporidium seeberi*. This organism was previously considered to be a fungus. It is now considered to be an aquatic protistan protozoa (unicellular) parasite.

9. **(d) Can be diagnosed by identification on biopsy** (*Ref. Scott Brown, 8th ed., Vol 1; 208*)
- Rhinosporidiosis is caused by an aquatic protozoa parasite *Rhinosporidium seeberi*. *Klebsiella rhinoscleromatis* is a bacteria leading to rhinoscleroma.
- The patient of rhinosporidiosis is immunocompetent. There is a history of taking bath in ponds frequented by animals.
- There is a red polypoid (polyp like but not true polyp. A true polyp arises because of nasal mucosal edema) mass on anterior rhinoscopy appearing like a mulberry or strawberry with white dots (sporangia). Nasal smear or biopsy shows sporangia which is diagnostic.

10. **(b) Russell bodies are seen** (*Ref. Scott Brown, 6th ed., 4/8/40*)

- Russell bodies which are the eosinophilic inclusion bodies present in the plasma cells are seen in Rhinoscleroma. Rest all are features of rhinosporidiosis (refer the text)

11. **(b) Rhinosporidiosis** (*Ref. Scott Brown, 6th ed., 4/8/40*)
- Anterior rhinoscopy in a patient of rhinosporidiosis shows a red polypoidal mass.
- Subcutaneous lesions in rhinosporidiosis can occur due to contact by contaminated finger nails.
- Zygomycosis group contain the fungus Mucor and Rhizopus which lead to mucormycosis (*see* Chapter on sinusitis). Skin lesions are not seen here.
- Sporotrichosis (also known as rose thorn or "Rose gardener's disease) is a disease caused by the infection of the **fungus *Sporothrix schenckii***. This fungal disease affects the **skin**. It does not affect the nose.
- In aspergillosis nasal polyps can occur but skin lesions are not seen (*see* Chapter on sinusitis).

12. **(b) Excision with cautery at base** (*Ref. Scott Brown, 6th ed., 4/8/40*)
- Rhinosporidiosis is managed by wide excision and cauterisation of base. Recurrence may occur if sporangium is left behind. Dapsone is given in the postoperative period to decrease the chances of recurrence.

13. **(c) Surgery is the treatment** (*Ref. Scott Brown, 6th ed., 4/8/40*)
Please refer to above explanations.

14. **(b) Sarcoidosis** (*Ref. Scott Brown, 8th ed., Vol 1; 1213*)
- Strawberry appearance of nasal mucosa is seen in sarcoidosis whereas strawberry mass is seen in the nasal cavity in rhinosporidiosis.

15. **(a), (b), (c) and (e)** (*Ref. Scott Brown, 8th ed., Vol 1; 1222*)
- Management is by a combination of chemotherapy and radiotherapy.

16. **(d) Syphilis** (*Ref. Scott Brown, 6th ed., 4/8/29*)

17. **(a) Rhinoscleroma** (*Ref. Scott Brown, 6th ed., 4/8/34*)

18. **(b), (c), (d), (e)** (*Ref. Scott Brown, 8th ed., Vol 1; 1215*)

19. **(a)** (*Ref. Scott Brown, 6th ed., 4/8/34*)
- This is a patient of Rhinoscleroma caused by *Klebsiella rhinoscleromatis* which is a gram-negative bacteria.
- Granulomatosis with polyangitis is Wegner's granulomatosis.

20. **(a) Should be managed by excision with cautery at base** (*Ref. Scott Brown, 6th ed., 4/8/39*)
- The description and picture is suggestive of rhinosporidiosis.

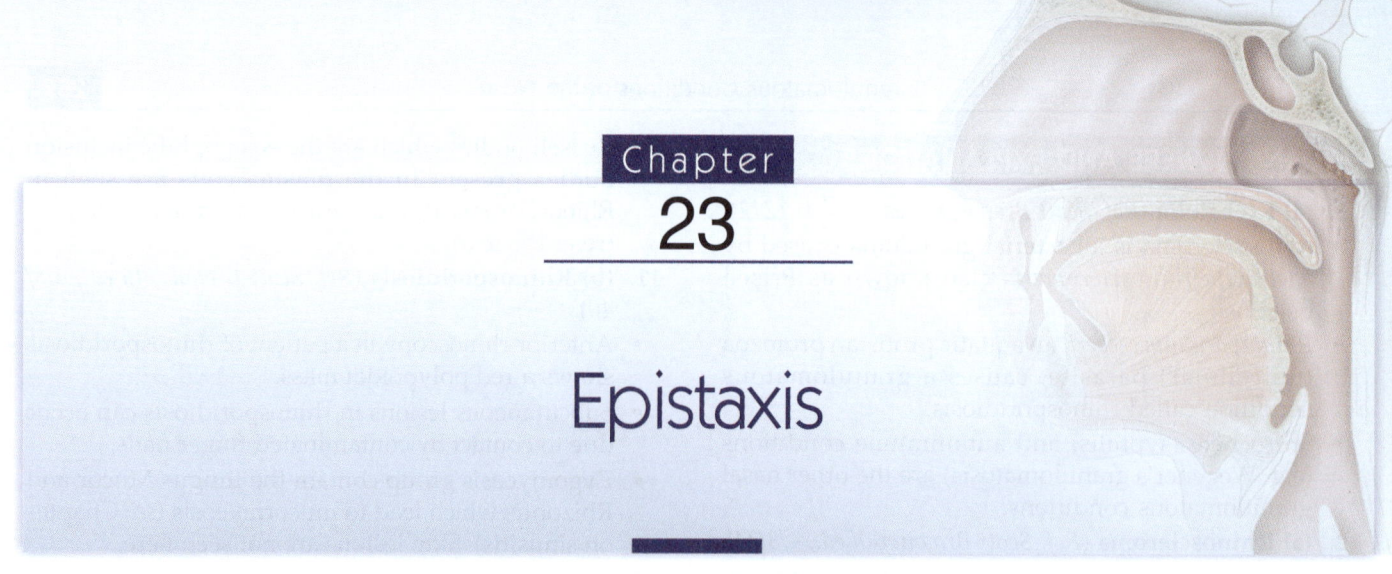

Epistaxis

Epistaxis means bleeding from inside of nose.

IMPORTANT CAUSES OF EPISTAXIS

1. The overall MC cause of epistaxis is idiopathic. In children the MC cause is traumatic after **nose picking**. Upper respiratory tract infections (coryza, sinusitis) lead to dryness, crusting and irritation which on removal by nose picking lead to epistaxis.
2. In any child with **unilateral epistaxis, foreign body** should be ruled out.
3. Any young adolescent male with profuse and recurrent epistaxis should be investigated for **angiofibroma**.
4. The most common cause of epistaxis in an elderly person is hypertension.
5. Other causes of epistaxis are:
   - Blunt trauma
   - Anatomical deformities, e.g. DNS with septal spur predisposing the deviated part to drying effects of air and crusting
   - Antiplatelet and anticoagulant drugs
   - Topical nasal drugs such as antihistamines and corticosteroids may cause mucosal dryness and irritation leading to epistaxis
   - Granulomatous diseases such as sarcoidosis, Wegener granulomatosis, tuberculosis, syphilis, and rhinoscleroma often lead to crusting and friable mucosa and may be a cause of recurrent epistaxis.
   - Intranasal tumours
   - Bleeding disorders: Thrombocytopenia, haemophilia, von Willebrand disease, liver diseases.
   - Hereditary hemorrhagic telangectasia or Osler-Rendu-Weber syndrome. This is an autosomal dominant condition characterised by telangiectasia (small vessel malformations) of the skin and mucosal lining. The most common complaint here is recurrent epistaxis.

SITES OF EPISTAXIS

Epistaxis can be either anterior or posterior. Bleeding from a source anterior to the plane of pyriform aperture (the bony anterior limit of nasal skeleton in the skull)/maxillary sinus ostium is known as anterior epistaxis and bleeding posterior to it is called posterior epistaxis.

1. Overall **90%** of epistaxis occurs from **Little's area**, *see* below.

   The MC site in children and young is the Little's area (Kiesselbach's plexus) present in the anteroinferior septum just above the vestibule.

   Four arteries contribute to Kiesselbach's plexus:
   i. Septal branch of Sphenopalatine; this is the main artery of Kiesselbach's plexus hence also known as "**artery of epistaxis**". Sphenopalatine is a branch from the maxillary artery which in turn is a branch of external carotid.
   ii. Septal branch of greater palatine; greater palatine is also a branch of maxillary artery.
   iii. Septal branch of superior labial (superior labial is a branch of facial artery which is a branch of external carotid)
   iv. Anterior ethmoidal artery (it is a branch of ophthalmic artery which is a branch of internal carotid).

   So most commonly epistaxis is arterial.
2. Anterior Epistaxis can sometimes be venous from the retrocolumellar vein which runs behind collumella of septum.
3. The majority of **posterior epistaxis** occur from septal branch of **sphenopalatine artery**. In **elderly** epistaxis is usually posterior. It occurs in response to **hypertension**.
4. Posterior epistaxis can also occur from **Woodruff's plexus**. The site of this plexus is on the lateral wall of nose inferior to posterior end of inferior turbinate. It was thought to be arterial however micro dissection has now shown it to be a **venous plexus**.

MANAGEMENT OF EPISTAXIS

The first step of management of epistaxis is to pinch the nose tightly for 10–15 minutes and sit bending forwards to prevent the blood from dripping post-nasally and getting swallowed. This is known as **Trotter's method/**

Hippocratic technique. Phenylephrine has a significant decongestant effect and is used here. If not controlled and if bleeding site can be recognised, it can be cauterised by chemical (silver nitrate) or bipolar-cautery.

If bleeding continues anterior nasal packing is done. If bleeding still not controlled then posterior nasal packing is done. Anterior nasal packing is done in both the nostrils for better pressure on the nasal septum, where the Little's area is present. Anterior nasal packing can be done by 1 meter long roller gauze soaked in antibiotic cream or by gelatin sponge, merocel or balloon tamponade.

Posterior nasal packing is done by putting a large gauze pack into the choanae and nasopharynx from behind the soft palate or by inserting a Foley's catheter and inflating its bulb in the nasopharynx or by pneumatic nasal tamponade which is by a balloon inflated in the postnasal space (all these putting pressure on the lateral wall of nasopharynx).

Figure 23.1 shows anterior nasal pack with gauze and posterior nasal pack with Foley's catheter.

Figure 23.2 is the picture of a nasal pack which contains a balloon covered by biocompatible self lubricating fabric. The first picture is the deflated state in which it is inserted into the nose. The second picture shows the inflated (with air using syringe) state which is done once it is fully inserted in the nose.

If epistaxis is not getting controlled by the above, arterial ligation has to be done. Preferred technique is **TESPAL** (transnasal endoscopic sphenopalatine artery ligation). This is done where sphenopalatine artery enters the nasal cavity from the sphenopalatine foramen, i.e. 1 cm behind the posterior end of middle turbinate.

TESPAL has now largely replaced maxillary and external carotid ligation. If required the maxillary artery can be ligated in the sphenopalatine/pterygopalatine fossa which lies just behind the posterior wall of maxillary antrum (via Caldwell-Luc operation) and the external carotid can be ligated in the neck above the superior thyroid artery.

If in a patient epistaxis is from the internal carotid branch supplying the Little's area, i.e. **anterior ethmoidal artery**, it can be ligated in the medial wall of orbit 24 mm posterior to the lacrimal crest by a medial canthal incision.

**Note:**

Hierarchy of ligation: Sphenopalatine → Maxillary → External carotid → Anterior ethmoidal artery.

In an elderly patient epistaxis is managed by controlling the hypertension first.

The underlying cause of epistaxis should be found and managed accordingly.

Patients of **Hereditary hemorrhagic telangiectasia,** besides the usual management of epistaxis as discussed above, can be treated by LASER (Argon, KTP, Nd: YAG). Some cases require septodermoplasty where septal mucosa from the Little's area is excised and replaced by a split skin graft.

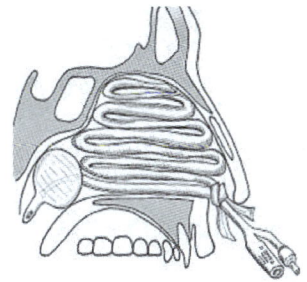

Fig. 23.1: Anterior and posterior nasal pack

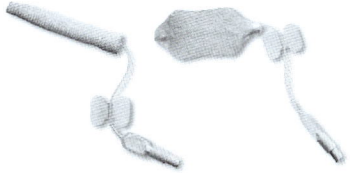

Fig. 23.2

 "Points to Ponder/Points for Quick revision"

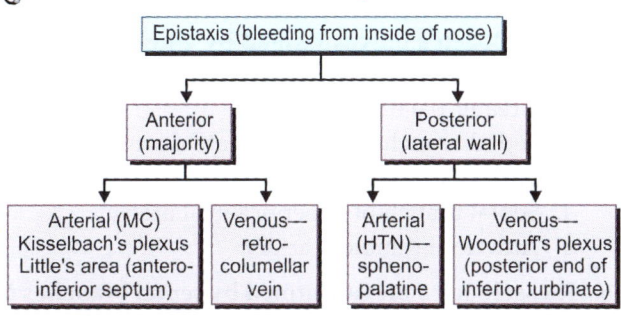

- **4 Arteries to Little's area:** Septal branches of sphenopalatine, greater palatine and superior labial (external carotid) and anterior ethmoidal artery (internal carotid).
- **Artery of Epistaxis:** Sphenopalatine (main artery at Little's area as well in HTN bleed).
- **Causes:** Nose picking (MC), HTN, Foreign body (U/L), Angiofibroma (profuse and recurrent), trauma, DNS with septal spur, drugs (antiplatelet, anticoagulants, topical antihistamines and corticosteroids), granulomatous diseases, tumours, bleeding disorders, hereditary hemorrhagic telangectasia or Osler-Rendu-Weber syndrome.
- **Management:**

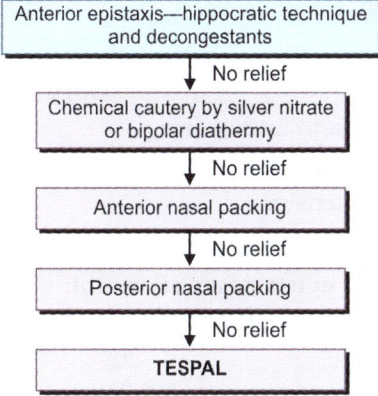

- Posterior epistaxis—HTN—antihypertensives.
- Hereditary hemorrhagic telangectasia (Osler-Rendu-Weber syndrome): LASER, septodermoplasty.

PREVIOUSLY ASKED QUESTIONS

1. **Commonest site of epistaxis in young is:**
   (Exam 2014)
   a. Bony septum   b. Little's area
   c. Superior turbinate   d. Lateral wall of nose

2. **Little's area is situated in nasal cavity in:**
   (Delhi PG 2009, Exam 2016)
   a. Antero-inferior septum
   b. Antero-superior septum
   c. Postero-inferior septum
   d. Postero-superior septum

3. **Main vascular supply of Little's area is all, except:**
   (PGI Dec 2008, 2015)
   a. Septal branch of superior labial artery
   b. Septal branch of sphenopalatine artery
   c. Anterior ethmoidal artery
   d. Palatal branch of sphenopalatine
   e. Greater palatine

4. **Kiesselbach's plexus formed by all except:**
   (Manipal 2008, Exam 2016)
   a. Greater palatine artery
   b. Septal branch of sphenopalatine artery
   c. Posterior ethmoidal artery
   d. Septal branch of superior labial artery
   e. Anterior ethmoidal artery

5. **Kiesselbach's plexus formed by septal branches of all except:**
   (PGI 2008, 2012)
   a. Posterior ethmoidal artery
   b. Anterior ethmoidal artery
   c. Sphenopalatine artery
   d. Greater palatine artery
   e. Facial

6. **Which artery does not contribute to Little's area?**
   (PGI 98, Exam 2013)
   a. Anterior ethmoidal artery
   b. Septal branch of facial artery
   c. Sphenopalatine artery
   d. Posterior ethmoidal artery

7. **Most common cause of nose bleeding is:**
   (AIIMS 95, Exam 2015)
   a. Trauma to Little's area
   b. AV aneurysm
   c. Hypertension
   d. Angiofibroma

8. **Causes of epistaxis are all except:**   *(Exam 2014)*
   a. Allergic rhinitis   b. Foreign body
   c. Tumour   d. Hypertension

9. **Commonest cause of epistaxis in children is:**
   (UP 2007, Exam 2013)
   a. Trauma   b. Foreign body
   c. Nasal diphtheria   d. Enlarged adenoids

10. **Most common cause of bleeding in children:**
    (Exam 2013)
    a. Nose picking   b. Hypertension
    c. Tumour   d. None

11. **MC cause of epistaxis in 3 years old child:**
    (Exam 2013)
    a. Nasal polyp
    b. Foreign body
    c. Upper respiratory catarrh
    d. Atrophic rhinitis

12. **In a 5-year-old child, cause of unilateral epistaxis is:**   *(Exam 2015)*
    a. Foreign body   b. Polyp
    c. Atrophic rhinitis   d. Maggot's

13. **Recurrent epistaxis in a 15-year-old female the probable cause is:**   *(JIPMER 90, Exam 2013)*
    a. Juvenile nasopharyngeal fibroma
    b. Rhinosporidiosis
    c. Foreign body
    d. Haematological disorder

14. **Epistaxis in elderly person is most commonly due to:**   *(Exam 2015)*
    a. Foreign body
    b. Bleeding disorder
    c. Hypertension
    d. Nasopharyngeal carcinoma

15. **A 70-year-old patient with epistaxis, on examination BP 200/100 mm Hg, no active nasal bleeding noted. Next step of management is:** *(DPG 2006, Exam 2016)*
    a. Observation with BP management
    b. Internal maxillary artery ligation
    c. Anterior and posterior nasal pack
    d. Anterior nasal pack

16. **Common sites of bleeding:**   *(PGI 2008, 2016)*
    a. Woodruff plexus
    b. Olfactory area
    c. Little's area
    d. Vestibular area
    e. Superior meatus

17. **Woodruff plexus is seen at:**
    (AP 95, TN 99, Exam 2013)
    a. Antero-inferior part of superior turbinate
    b. Middle turbinate
    c. Posterior part of inferior turbinate
    d. Anterior part of inferior turbinate

18. **Source of epistaxis after ligation of external carotid artery is:**   *(AIIMS 93, Exam 2013)*
    a. Maxillary artery
    b. Greater palatine artery
    c. Superior labial artery
    d. Ethmoidal artery

19. **If posterior epistaxis cannot be controlled which artery is ligated:** *(Kolkata 2000, Exam 2016)*
    a. Posterior ethmoidal artery
    b. Maxillary artery
    c. Sphenopalatine artery
    d. External carotid artery

20. **In case of uncontrolled epistaxis ligation of internal maxillary artery is to be done in the:** *(Kolkata 2001, Exam 2016)*
    a. Maxillary antrum
    b. Pterygopalatine fossa
    c. In the neck
    d. Medial wall of orbit

21. **Treatment of choice in recurrent epistaxis in a patient with hereditary hemorrhagic telangiectasis:** *(Kolkata 2005, Exam 2016)*
    a. Rhinoplasty
    b. Posterior ethmoidal artery ligation
    c. Septal dermoplasty
    d. Internal carotid artery ligation

22. **Posterior epistaxis true is:** *(PGI 2014)*
    a. Controlled by posterior nasal packing
    b. Is managed by ligation of anterior ethmoidal artery
    c. Is less dangerous than anterior bleeds
    d. Seen in hypertensives
    e. Seen in syphilitic perforation of palate

23. **Location of Woodruff's plexus is:** *(Exam 2014)*
    a. Posterior end of middle turbinate
    b. Posterior end of inferior turbinate
    c. Posterior end of superior turbinate
    d. Anterior end of septum

24. **The artery which leads to bleeding in posterior epistaxis is:** *(Exam 2016)*
    a. Anterior ethmoidal artery
    b. Sphenopalatine artery
    c. Greater palatine artery
    d. Superior labial artery

25. **Kiesselbach's plexus is situated in:** *(Exam 2016)*
    a. Anteroinferior part of nasal septum
    b. Woodruff's area
    c. On the lateral wall
    d. Posterior nasal cavity

26. **Woodruff's area is situated in:** *(Exam 2016)*
    a. Posterior end of inferior turbinate
    b. Anterior end of middle turbinate
    c. Near hiatus semilunaris
    d. Below superior turbinate

27. **All of the following are true about nasal myiasis except:** *(Exam 2016)*
    a. Common in vasomotor rhinitis
    b. Intense nasal irritation present
    c. Caused by maggots
    d. Chloroform water is one of the modes of treatment

28. **A 7-year-old child presents with unilateral nasal obstruction with foul smelling nasal discharge. The diagnosis is:** *(Exam 2016)*
    a. Foreign body
    b. Rhinophyma
    c. Rhinosporidiosis
    d. Angiofibroma

29. **All of the following are features of a nasal foreign body except:** *(Exam 2016)*
    a. Foul smelling discharge
    b. Epistaxis
    c. Nasal obstruction
    d. Saddling of nose

30. **Endoscopic sphenopalatine artery ligation is done in:** *(Exam 2016)*
    a. Severe epistaxis
    b. Rhinophyma
    c. CA Maxillary sinus
    d. Multiple antrochoanal polyps

31. **Which of the following is TRUE regarding anterior epistaxis?** *(APPG 2015)*
    a. Patient is kept in sitting and slight leaning forward position while compressing the nares
    b. Topical phenylephrine is contraindicated as it increases blood pressure
    c. Commonly from Kiesselbach venous plexus in the anterior septum
    d. Foley's nasal tamponade is a treatment option

32. **The artery of epistaxis is:** *(Kerala PGMEE 2015)*
    a. Anterior ethmoidal artery
    b. Posterior ethmoidal artery
    c. Sphenopalatine artery
    d. Greater palatine artery

IMAGE BASED PRACTICE QUESTIONS BY THE AUTHOR

33. **The following device is used for the management of:**

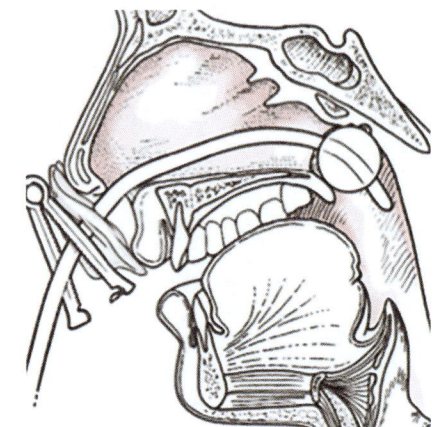

    a. CSF rhinorrhoea
    b. Velopharyngeal insufficiency
    c. Posterior epistaxis
    d. Adenoid hypertrophy

34. The given picture shows:

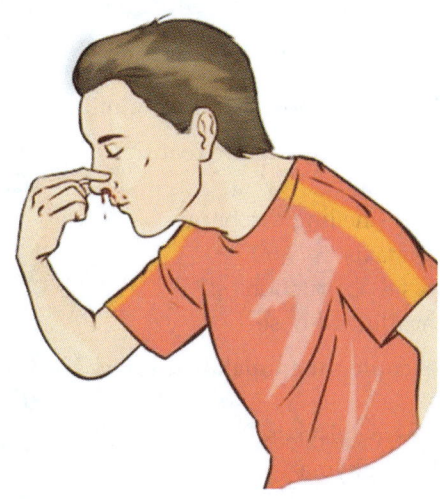

a. McGovern's technique
b. Hippocratic technique
c. Epley's manoeuvre
d. Reservoir sign

35. The vessel marked with arrow in the given picture is:

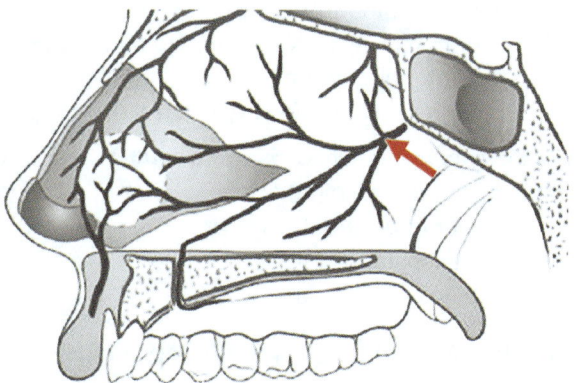

a. Anterior ethmoidal artery
b. Septal branch of facial artery
c. Sphenopalatine artery
d. Posterior ethmoidal artery

36. The circle area in blue in the given picture is:

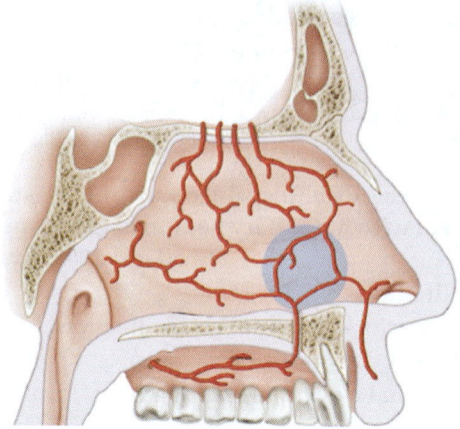

a. Woodruff's plexus
b. Retrocolumellar anastomosis
c. Kiesselbach plexus
d. Sphenopalatine ganglion

37. Injury to which artery leads to orbital hematoma:
(Exam 2017)

a. Sphenopalatine
b. Anterior ethmoidal
c. Maxillary
d. Facial

38. Which of the following artery is never ligated to control epistaxis? *(Exam 2017)*

a. Maxillary
b. External carotid
c. Internal carotid
d. Anterior ethmoidal

ANSWERS AND EXPLANATIONS

1. **(b) Little's area** (*Ref. Cummings, 6th ed., 678*)
2. **(a) Antero-inferior septum** (*Ref. Cummings, 6th ed., 678*)
3. **(d) Palatal branch of sphenopalatine** (*Ref. Cummings, 6th ed., 679*)
4. **(c) Posterior ethmoidal artery** (*Ref. Cummings, 6th ed., 678*)
5. **(a) Posterior ethmoidal artery** (*Ref. Cummings, 6th ed., 679*)
6. **(d) Posterior ethmoidal artery** (*Ref. Cummings, 6th ed., 679*)
7. **(a) Trauma to Little's area** (*Ref. Cummings, 6th ed., 680*)
8. **(a) Allergic rhinitis** (*Ref. Cummings, 6th ed., 680*)
   - Allergic rhinitis presents with paroxysmal episodes of sneezing, itching, rhinorrhoea, post nasal drip and not with epistaxis.
9. **(a) Trauma** (*Ref. Cummings, 6th ed., 680*)
   - The MC cause of epistaxis in children and young is trauma by nose picking.
   - Foreign body is the most common cause of unilateral foul smelling nasal discharge in children.
   - Nasal diphtheria presents with fever, generalised toxaemia and rhinitis. On nasal examination, membrane is seen which bleeds on removal.
   - Adenoid hypertrophy presents with nasal obstruction, recurrent sinusitis, sleep apnoea and serous otitis media.
10. **(a) Nose picking** (*Ref. Scott Brown, 8th ed., Vol 1; 242*)
11. **(c) Upper respiratory catarrh** (*Ref. Scott Brown, 8th ed., Vol 1; 242*)
    - Upper respiratory catarrh leads to dryness, crusting and irritation which on removal by nose picking lead to epistaxis.
12. **(a) Foreign body** (*Ref. Scott Brown, 8th ed., Vol 1; 243*)
    - Trauma to Little's area is the most common cause of epistaxis in children.
    - In this age group foreign body can be a cause of unilateral epistaxis, though foreign body usually presents with unilateral foetid (foul smelling) discharge.
    - Polyps and atrophic rhinitis do not show epistaxis moreover both of them do not occur in this age group.
    - Maggots present with blood stained nasal discharge which is bilateral.
13. **(d) Haematological disorder** (*Ref. Cummings, 6th ed., 680*)
    - Juvenile nasopharyngeal fibroma is seen typically in adolescent males.
    - In Rhinosporidiosis there is nasal obstruction along with epistaxis and a history of taking bath in ponds frequented by animals is present (see chapter on granulomatous conditions of nose).
    - Foreign body is not seen at this age.

- So the probable cause here is haematological disorder. In this regard the patient should be asked regarding bleeding from any other site also.
- Characteristically haematological disorders present with bleeding from multiple sites.

14. **(c) Hypertension** (*Ref. Cummings, 6th ed. 680*)
    - The most common cause of epistaxis in an elderly person is hypertension.
    - Foreign body is not seen at this age.
    - Bleeding disorder will present with bleeding from multiple sites.
    - Nasopharyngeal carcinoma presents with upper deep cervical lymph node. Nasal obstruction and blood tinged nasal discharge can occur later on.
15. **(a) Observation with BP management** (*Ref. Cummings, 6th ed., 682*)
    - Since no active bleed at present so here the main management should aim at lowering of BP.
16. **(a) and (c)** (*Ref. Scott Brown, 8th ed., Vol 1; 1170*)
    - Vestibular area is not the site of bleeding. Little's area, Woodruff's plexus and retrocolumellar venous plexus all lie above the vestibule beneath the mucosa, refer the text.
17. **(c) Posterior part of inferior turbinate** (*Ref. Scott Brown, 8th ed., Vol 1; 1170*)
18. **(d) Ethmoidal artery** (*Ref. Cummings, 6th ed., 679*)
19. **(c) Sphenopalatine artery** (*Ref. Cummings, 6th ed., 685*)
    - The main artery of anterior as well as posterior epistaxis is sphenopalatine, please see text. So if epistaxis is not getting controlled sphenopalatine arterial ligation has to be done.
20. **(b) Pterygopalatine fossa** (*Ref. Scott Brown, 8th ed., Vol 1; 1178*)
    - The maxillary artery which is also called internal maxillary artery along with sphenopalatine and greater palatine artery lies in the sphenopalatine/pterygopalatine fossa just behind the posterior wall of maxillary antrum.
    - In uncontrolled epistaxis ligation of internal maxillary artery is to be done in the sphenopalatine fossa via Caldwell-Luc operation.
21. **(c) Septal dermoplasty** (*Ref. Scott Brown, 8th ed., Vol 1; 1178*)
22. **(a) and (d)** (*Ref. Scott Brown, 8th ed., Vol 1; 1177*)
23. **(b) Posterior end of inferior turbinate** (*Ref. Scott Brown, 8th ed., Vol 1; 1170*)
24. **(b) Sphenopalatine artery** (*Ref. Scott Brown, 8th ed., Vol 1; 1177*)
25. **(a) Anteroinferior part of nasal septum** (*Ref. Cummings, 6th ed., 678*)
26. **(a) Posterior end of inferior turbinate** (*Ref. Scott Brown, 8th ed., Vol 1; 1170*)
27. **(a) Common in vasomotor rhinitis, refer to Chapter 18** (*Ref. Scott Brown, 6th ed., 4/8/45*)
28. **(a) Foreign body, refer to Chapter 21** (*Ref. Scott Brown, 8th ed., Vol 2; 243*)

Section II **Nose**

29. **(d) Saddling of nose, refer to Chapter 21** (*Ref. Scott Brown, 8th ed., Vol 2; 243*)

30. **(a) Severe epistaxis** (*Ref. Scott Brown, 8th ed., Vol 1; 1172*)

31. **(a)** (*Ref. Cummings, 6th ed., 684*)
   - Phenylephrine being a decongestant is used to prepare the nose before cauterization.
   - Foley's nasal tamponade is done in posterior nasal space in posterior epistaxis.

32. **(c) Sphenopalatine artery** (*Ref. Scott Brown, 8th ed., Vol 1; 1170*)

33. **(c) Posterior epistaxis** (*Ref. Scott Brown, 8th ed., Vol 1; 1177*)

The picture shows posterior nasal pack with balloon tamponade.

34. **(b) Hippocratic technique** (*Ref. Scott Brown, 8th ed., Vol 1; 1175*)

Trotter's method is the first step for the management of epistaxis

35. **(c) Sphenopalatine artery** (*Ref. Cummings, 6th ed., 684; Scott Brown, 8th ed., Vol 1; 1170*)

36. **(c) Kiesselbach plexus** (*Ref. Cummings, 6th ed., 682*)

37. **(b) Anterior ethmoidal** (*Ref. Scott Brown, 8th ed., Vol 1; 1171, 1179*)

38. **(c) Internal carotid** (*Ref. Scott Brown, 8th ed., Vol 1; 1177*)

Section II **Nose**

Fractures of Face and CSF Rhinorrhoea

In any patient of craniofacial trauma it is critically important to follow **the ABC of trauma**, i.e.

A → Airway management

B → Breathing

C → Circulation

NASAL FRACTURES

The MC fracture of the face is the fracture involving the nose as it is the most prominent part of the face. It is best diagnosed on clinical examination. X-ray may not show the fracture.

While evaluating nose injuries, 3 things are evaluated:

a. Nasal bones deformity

b. Septal deviation

c. Septal hematoma, which if present needs immediate drainage (*see* Chapter on DNS).

Fractures of Nose are of 3 Types

Class 1

It is the simplest of nasal fractures. It involves the nasal bones with the fracture line running parallel to the dorsum of nose. There may be a vertical fracture involving the septum but there is no septal deviation. So there is minimal deformity here.

This injury occurs by a blow from below. This is known as **Chevallet fracture**.

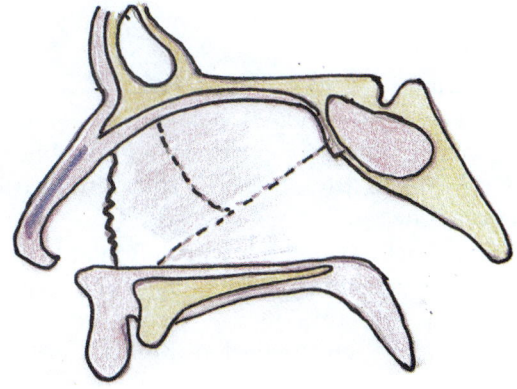

Fig. 24.1: Chevallet fracture

Class 2

It results from a blow from front. The nasal bone is fractured with gross deviation.

Here the septal fracture is horizontal or C-shaped leading to septal deviation. This fracture causes significant cosmetic deformity. It is known as **Jarjavay fracture**.

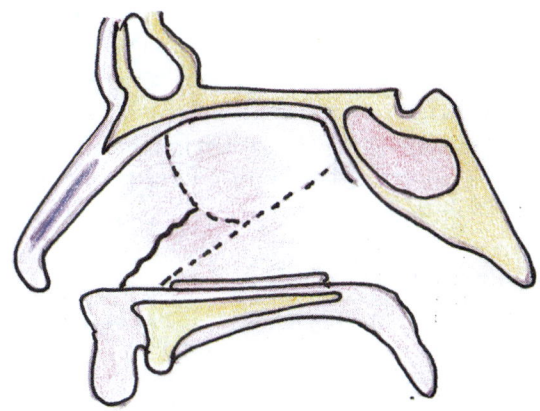

Fig. 24.2: Jarjavay fracture

Class 3

It is the most severe nasal injury and occurs due to high velocity trauma, e.g. in road traffic accidents (RTA). It is also known as **naso-orbito-ethmoid fracture**.

The perpendicular plate of ethmoid is crushed leading to depression of upper part of nasal dorsum and pulling of the tip of nose upwards because of which the nostrils start facing anteriorly. This appearance is known as pig nose. Because of the involvement of other parts of ethmoid bone (*see* chapter on anatomy), i.e. the cribriform plate and lamina papyracea. This type of fracture is associated with CSF rhinorrhoea and orbital involvement.

Treatment

The management of **class 1 and 2** fractures is closed reduction after the oedema subsides (usually after 5–7 days). It is important for the oedema to subside in a nasal fracture as reduction of fracture is required only if deformity is there and how much is the deformity can be found out

Table 24.1: Management of Class 1 and 2 fractures	
Presentation	*Management*
Patient presents initially	Closed reduction after 5–7 days
Patient presenting late (> 3 weeks)	Rhinoplasty/septorhinoplasty (after the attainment of 17 years of age)

only when the oedema has gone so as to prevent over-reduction or under reduction.

In closed reduction two types of forceps are used. To reduce the bone we use **Walsham** forceps and for the reduction of septum we use **Asche's** forceps (please *see* Chapter 41 on Important instruments in ENT). The fracture segments are disimpacted and re-aligned.

If the septal deformity does not get corrected by closed reduction then open reduction of septal deformity, i.e. septoplasty can be done in the same sitting if the patient is more than 17 years of age (*see* chapter on DNS for details of septoplasty).

If the patient of nose injury presents late, i.e. anytime **after 3 weeks** of injury, closed reduction will not be possible because in 3 weeks callus formation starts and fibrous and bony reunion occurs. If the patient is above 17 years of age he is now taken up for open reduction, i.e. rhinoplasty or septo-rhinoplasty (correction of external deformity of nose is called rhinoplasty whereas correction of septal deformity is known as septoplasty).

Class 3 fractures should be treated immediately by open surgery exposing all the fractured bones and internal fixation **(Table 24.1)**.

FRACTURE OF ZYGOMATIC BONE

This is the second most common fracture of the face.

The zygomatic bone is a pyramidal bone articulating with three bones:

1. Frontal (superiorly at zygomatico-frontal suture)
2. Temporal (posteriorly at zygomatico-temporal suture)
3. Maxilla (anteriorly at zygomatico-maxillary suture in the infraorbital region).

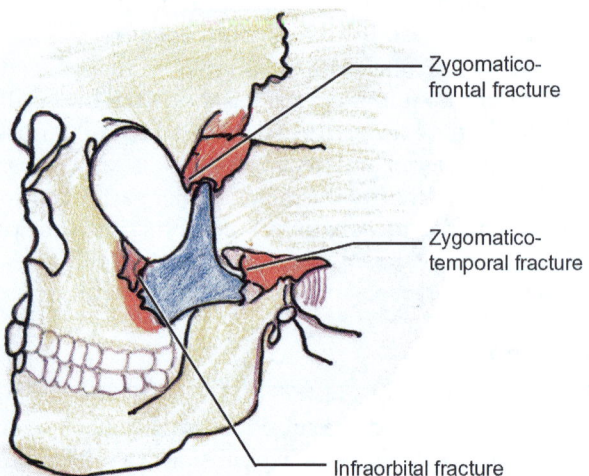

Fig. 24.3: Tripod fracture

Fracture at all the above three sutures is known as **tripod fracture**. The features of tripod fractures are as follows:

Cheek Findings

1. **Flattening of malar eminence**.
2. **Trismus** due to the zygoma impinging on the coronoid process of mandible behind.
3. Anaesthesia in the territory of **infraorbital nerve** (the maxillary nerve exits the orbit through the infraorbital foramen below the infraorbital margin, ending as Infraorbital nerve. It is prone to injury here in fractures involving infraorbital region, also *see* blow out fractures of orbit and Le Fort II fractures below). *See* the diagram in sinusitis chapter showing the sensory nerve supply of face.

Orbital findings:

1. Periorbital emphysema
2. Step deformity of Infraorbital margin (zygomatico-maxillary suture) and lateral orbital margin (zygomatico-frontal suture).
3. Restricted ocular movements due to entrapment of inferior rectus or inferior oblique leading to **diplopia**.
4. **Enophthalmos**

Management: If undisplaced nothing has to be done. If displaced these fractures have to be reduced by open reduction and internal wire fixation.

BLOW OUT FRACTURE

Any severe blow from front on the **orbit** with blunt object leads to an increase in the intraorbital pressure leading to giving way of the inferior wall or floor of orbit and herniation of orbital contents into the maxillary antrum. This appears like a tear drop on X-ray or CT (**tear drop sign, please** *see* **Fig. 24.4**). This is known as blow out fracture. The medial wall of orbit is also usually involved here. In spite of the medial wall of orbit being the thinnest wall (lamina papyracea), the blow out fracture most commonly involves the orbital floor. This is because in the medial wall there are multiple ethmoidal air cells which distribute the increase in pressure evenly because of which the medial wall is able to withstand the force better than the floor.

Clinical Features

1. Orbital ecchymosis
2. Step deformity of infraorbital margin (zygomatico-maxillary suture)
3. Enophthalmos
4. Diplopia due to restricted ocular movements due to entrapment of inferior rectus and inferior oblique
5. Anaesthesia of the cheek in the distribution of infraorbital nerve

The other fractures involving infra-orbital margin are the zygomatic (*see* above) and Le Fort II fractures (*see* below).

If enophthalmos and persistent diplopia are present these fractures have to be reduced usually by a transantral route.

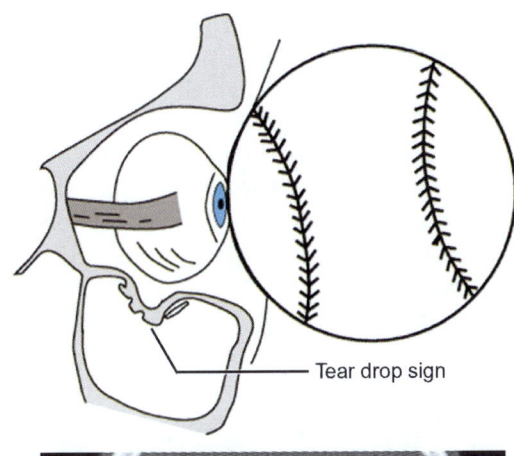

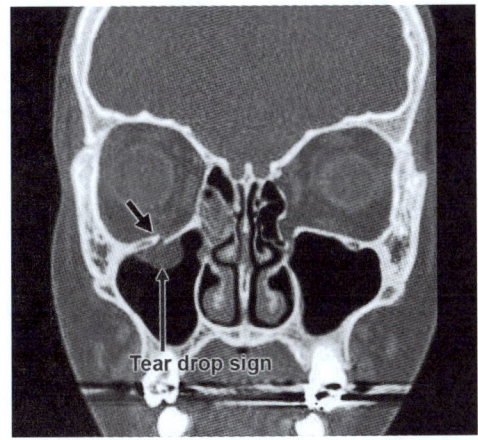

Fig. 24.4: CT of blow out fracture

MAXILLARY FRACTURES

These are known as **Le Fort fractures**. These are caused due to high velocity injury (RTA).

They are of 3 types:

1. **Le Fort I:** This fracture runs parallel to the palate. The fracture line passes from the lower part of maxillary antrum and floor of nose anteriorly to pterygoid plates posteriorly.

    This separates palate from the rest of the face above appearing on X-ray or CT as floating palate or floating teeth.

2. **Le Fort II:** This is a pyramidal fracture. Fracture line runs on both sides from floor of maxillary sinus going superiorly to infraorbital margin (zygoma), lacrimal bone, nasal bone and nasion meeting the fracture line of the other side. This on CT or X-ray appears like hanging maxilla. This is associated with CSF rhinorrhoea.

3. **Le Fort III:** This leads to **cranio-facial dysjunction** passing anteriorly through the superior orbital fissure going posteriorly disconnecting the cranial base from the facial skeleton. This is also associated with CSF rhinorrhoea.

FRACTURES OF MANDIBLE

Two important fractures involving mandible are:
1. Sub-condylar fracture
2. Guardsman fracture

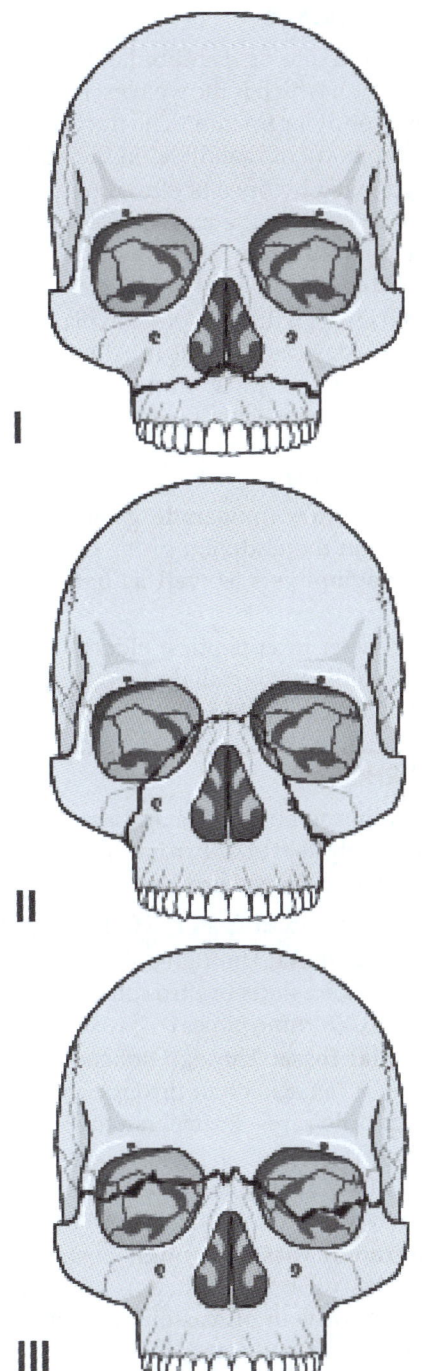

Fig. 24.5: Le Fort fractures

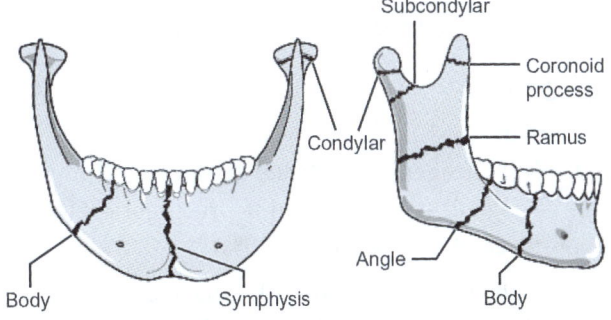

Fig. 24.6: Various sites of mandibular fractures

Section II   Nose

Sub-condylar Fracture

The **most common** site of mandibular fracture is at its neck (sub-condyle), which is the weakest site of mandible and called sub-condylar fracture. The fracture occurs due to trauma to the body of mandible on the opposite side.

It can be managed by open or closed reduction. When closed reduction is done the mandible should never be immobilised for more than 3 weeks as it can lead to Temporomandibular (TM) joint ankylosis.

Open rigid fixation with compression plates (titanium) is preferred these days as it allows functional mastication immediately after surgery preventing prolonged immobilisation and hence iatrogenic TM joint fixation.

Guardsman Fracture

A **guardsman fracture** (or **parade ground fracture**) is caused by a fall on the midpoint of the chin resulting in fracture of the **symphysis as well as both condyles** of mandible.

It is usually seen in epileptics, elderly patients and occasionally in soldiers who fall down during parade (so it is called Guardsman fracture).

CSF RHINORRHOEA

Any disruption in the bone, dura and arachnoid of base of skull leading to the exit of CSF from subarachnoid space to the nose is called CSF rhinorrhoea.

CSF rhinorrhoea can occur from the following sites:

1. **Anterior cranial fossa:** Through cribriform plate (most common), ethmoid sinus or through posterior wall of frontal sinus (CSF rhinorrhoea).
2. **Middle cranial fossa:** Through sphenoid sinus (CSF rhinorrhoea). It can also occur through roof of mastoid air cells → middle ear → Eustachian tube → nose (CSF otorhinorrhoea)
   Or directly from roof of middle ear (tegmen tympani) → Eustachian tube → nose (CSF Otorhinorrhoea)
3. **Posterior cranial fossa:** Through posterior wall of sphenoid sinus (CSF rhinorrhoea). It can also occur through posterior wall of mastoid air cells → middle ear → Eustachian tube → nose (CSF Oto-rhinorrhoea)
   In short there are 3 routes for CSF rhinorrhoea:
   i. Via damaged cribriform plate (most common).
   ii. Via the upper three sinuses (ethmoid, frontal, sphenoid).
   iii. From middle ear via Eustachian tube.

ETIOLOGY

1. Traumatic (95%);
   i. **Non-iatrogenic/accidental (80%)**
   ii. Iatrogenic (e.g. nasal and neurosurgeries) (15%)
2. Non-traumatic/spontaneous (5%)

1. **Traumatic CSF rhinorrhoea:** The most common site of traumatic CSF rhinorrhoea is fracture of the part (lateral lamella) of the cribriform plate that forms the medial part of roof of ethmoid sinus. The roof of ethmoid sinus is formed medially by lateral part of cribriform plate (known as lateral lamella), which is a very thin bone and laterally by frontal bone (known as fovea ethmoidalis), which in contrast is a thicker bone.

Traumatic CSF otorhinorrhoea can also occur following transverse fracture of temporal bone.

The facial fractures causing CSF rhinorrhoea are class 3 nasal fractures and Le Fort II and III maxillary fractures, *see* above.

Traumatic CSF rhinorrhoea can also be classified as:
1. Immediate
2. Delayed

Immediate occurs immediately after injury.

Delayed CSF rhinorrhoea occurs usually within 3 months of injury although it has been known to occur even after 20 years after trauma.

Delayed CSF rhinorrhoea occurs because of:
   i. Resolution of oedema or lysis of clots in and around the injury site which were temporarily obstructing the CSF flow.
   ii. Loss of vascularity due to injury with resultant necrosis of soft tissue and bone.

2. **Non-traumatic/spontaneous CSF rhinorrhoea** can be:
1. High pressure leak
2. Normal pressure leak

High pressure leak

This can occur following any condition leading to prolonged increase in intracranial pressure leading to continued erosion and weakening of bone the most common site (again) being the cribriform plate. For example:
   i. Any intracranial tumour, e.g. pituitary neoplasms, posterior fossa tumours.
   ii. Pseudo tumour cerebri (also known as idiopathic intracranial hypertension); Here there are features of increased intracranial pressure without any intracranial tumour, hence the name.

Normal pressure CSF leak; can occur from:
   i. Congenital/potential pathways (90%); i.e. prolongation of the subarachnoid space along the olfactory nerves and stalk of hypophysis.
   ii. Congenital defects in the skull base leading to meningo-encephalocele.
   iii. Empty sella syndrome: Ischemic necrosis can lead to atrophy of pituitary. The empty space becomes a pouch filled with CSF. The normal pulse pressure causes this pouch to exert a focal erosive effect leading to formation of excavations, thinning and ultimately CSF fistula.
   iv. Direct erosion by tumour from below, e.g. nasopharyngeal carcinoma, angiofibroma.
   v. Direct erosion by infection, e.g. osteomyelitis occurring as a complication of sinusitis.

Complication

Any patient of repeated attacks of meningitis should be investigated for dural defect with CSF leakage leading to ascending infection.

Diagnosis

History: CSF rhinorrhoea should be suspected if there is U/L watery rhinorrhoea increasing on leaning forward. History of head trauma or surgeries involved in skull base should be taken.

Diagnosis of CSF rhinorrhoea is a two-step process. First we need to confirm that the fluid is CSF. Second the site of leak has to be determined.

To distinguish CSF rhinorrhoea from simple rhinorrhoea of rhinitis the following tests can be done in the OPD:

1. **Sniff test:** Patient is not able to sniff CSF back.
2. **Handkerchief test:** Mucus stiffens the handkerchief but CSF does not.
3. **Halo sign/Target sign/Double ring sign:** This test is useful when CSF rhinorrhoea is associated with epistaxis (in the immediate period after trauma). A drop is put on Whatman's filter paper. The blood in the drop produces a central circle and if CSF is present in the drop it produces a halo around the blood circle.
4. **Reservoir sign:** The patient after being made to lie supine for some time is brought to upright position with neck flexed. If this leads to a sudden gush of clear fluid from the nose it is indicative of CSF.
5. Valsalva or compression of both jugular veins increases CSF leak.

Biochemical Tests

Glucose estimation: CSF glucose concentration is 45–85 mg/dl (approximately 60% of blood glucose). In nasal mucous secretions glucose is <10 mg/dl. This is not a very useful test as there is decrease in CSF glucose in meningitis which can lead to false negative result. Also contamination with blood makes the test invalid.

β_2 **transferrin:** β_2 transferrin on electrophoresis is pathognomonic of CSF as this protein is present only in CSF. Presence of β trace protein that is synthesized primarily in the arachnoid cells and choroid plexus is also being commonly used to diagnose CSF rhinorrhoea.

HRCT: This is done once the fluid has been confirmed to be CSF through β_2 transferrin. This is the imaging modality of choice for identifying skull base defect associated with CSF rhinorrhoea. HRCT will show the fracture or underlying pathology of CSF rhinorrhoea.

If the HRCT shows fracture, the patient is first advised conservative management. If in spite of conservative management CSF rhinorrhoea persists then surgical repair has to be done for which the exact site of leak should be localised.

The localising tests are as follows:

Localising tests

1. **Intrathecal dye administration:** 1 ml of 5% Fluorescein is injected intrathecally by lumbar puncture. This stains the CSF bright yellow green colour. This is followed by nasal endoscopy to see the site of leakage.
2. **CT Cisternography:** Here HRCT using contrast media is done after putting a dye in the CSF by lumbar puncture, to delineate the site of leakage. This is the best investigation to localise active CSF rhinorrhoea. Patients with intermittent CSF rhinorrhoea may have false negative CT cisternograms. Radionucleotide cisternography, which is performed by administering Indium 111 DTPA in the lumbar subarachnoid space, following which images are taken at 2, 6, 12, 24, 48 and 72 hours is useful in the detection of intermittent leaks.

MRI: MRI is the investigation of choice for visualizing potential brain anomalies such as encephaloceles.

Management: For traumatic causes conservative management has to be followed initially for 10–14 days.

It includes:

a. Bedrest in propped up position
b. Diuretics
c. Avoidance of straining (coughing, sneezing, nose blowing)
d. Prophylactic antibiotics
e. Stool softeners

If the patient does not benefit by medical management, surgical repair either endoscopic (preferred) or external is done. Non traumatic CSF rhinorrhoea is managed by direct operative repair with treatment of the cause.

"Points to Ponder/Points for Quick revision"

- **ABC of trauma**

Fracture #	Mechanism	Findings	Management
Nasal (MC # of face) 1. Chevallet	Blow from below or lateral blow	• Vertical septal # • No deformity	• Closed reduction after 1 week. • If no relief/> 3 weeks & age > 17 years–septoplasty/septo-rhinoplasty
2. Jarjaway	Blow from front	• Horizontal or C-shaped septal # • with deformity	As above • To reduce bone—Walsham. To reduce cartilage—Asche's forceps
3. Naso-orbito-ethmoid	↑velocity RTA	• CSF rhinorrhoea • Deformity • Orbital complications	• ORIF
Zygomatic bone (Tripod) #	Direct blow	• Flattened malar eminence • Trismus • Infra orbital N injury • Diplopia • Enophthalmos	• ORIF (in displaced/diplopia)
Blow out #	Blow on the orbit from front	• Tear drop sign • Infra orbital N injury • Diplopia • Enophthalmos	• ORIF (in displaced/diplopia)
Maxillary # 1. Le fort I	↑velocity RTA	• Floating palate	• ORIF
2. Le fort II	As above	• Hanging maxilla • Pyramidal # • CSF rhinorrhoea	• ORIF
3. Le fort III	As above	• Cranio-facial dysjunction • CSF rhinorrhoea	• ORIF
Mandibula # • Sub Condylar (MC)	Trauma to the mandibular body from opposite side	• # mandibular neck	Open rigid fixation
• Guardsman #	Fall on the mid-point of the chin	• Symphysis as well as both the condyles #	Open rigid fixation

- CSF Rhinorrhoea: Traumatic (MC)/Spontaneous.
- MC Site of traumatic CSF rhinorrhoea: Cribriform plate (Lateral lamella).
- Facial # → CSF rhinorrhoea: Class 3 nasal fractures, Le Fort II & III maxillary fractures.
- CSF rhinorrhoea *vs* Rhinitis rhinorrhoea: Sniff test, Reservoir sign, Valsalva & Jugular vein compression tests.
- Traumatic CSF rhinorrhoea Vs epistaxis: Halo sign/Target sign.
- Biochemical tests for CSF rhinorrhoea: β_2 transferrin (diagnostic).
- HRCT—IOC–Site of Skull base # → CSF rhinorrhoea.
- Localisation for active leak: CT Cisternography, intrathecal dye.
- T/t—Traumatic CSF Rhinorrhoea: Initially conservative (bed rest-propped up for 2 weeks). If no benefit-endoscopic repair.

PREVIOUSLY ASKED QUESTIONS

1. **Most important primary care in Faciomaxillary trauma is to:** *(MP 2002, Exam 2017)*
   a. Asses the level of consciousness
   b. Ensure adequate airway
   c. Look for CNS injury
   d. Immediate fracture reduction

2. **Most common fractured bone in the face is:** *(Exam 2013)*
   a. Nasal
   b. Maxillary
   c. Zygomatic
   d. Temporal

3. **Ideal time for correction of fracture of nasal bone is:** *(Kolkata 2000, Exam 2017)*
   a. Immediately
   b. After 1 week
   c. After 3 weeks
   d. After 6 weeks

4. **Vertical and horizontal fractures of nasal septum are called:** *(Exam 2010)*
   a. Chevallet and Jarjavay fracture
   b. Arnold fracture
   c. Citelli fracture
   d. Thudicum fracture

5. **In Jarjavay fracture of nasal septum the fracture line is:** *(MH 2007, Exam 2013)*
   a. Comminuted
   b. Vertical
   c. Horizontal
   d. None of the above

6. **In Chevallet fracture of nasal septum the mechanism of trauma is:** *(MH 2008, AI 2013)*
   a. Blow from above
   b. Blow from below
   c. Blow directly from front
   d. Any of the above

7. **While playing football an 18-year-old boy was hit on the nose and developed deviation of nose. O/E the septum was not deviated. The following about the patient is true:** *(JIPMER 2007, Exam 2014)*
   a. He should be taken up for open reduction one week later
   b. He should be taken for closed reduction as soon as overlying edema subsides
   c. Septoplasty should be done in the same sitting
   d. He is having Jarjavay fracture

8. **Nasal bone fracture is corrected by:** *(MH 2007, Exam 2017)*
   a. Citelli's forceps
   b. Luc's forceps
   c. Tilly's forceps
   d. Walsham's forceps

9. **Tripod fracture is seen in:** *(MP 2008, Exam 2013)*
   a. Mandible
   b. Maxilla
   c. Nasal bone
   d. Zygoma

10. **Fracture zygoma shows all the features except:** *(AI 2007, Exam 2017)*
    a. Diplopia
    b. CSF rhinorrhoea
    c. Enophthalmos
    d. Trismus

11. **Fracture zygoma shows all the features except:** *(PGI June 2009)*
    a. Cheek swelling
    b. Trismus
    c. Nose bleeding
    d. Infraorbital anaesthesia
    e. Diplopia

12. **A patient presents with enophthalmos after a trauma to face by blunt object. Diagnosis is:** *(Exam 2013)*
    a. Fracture maxilla
    b. Fracture zygoma
    c. Fracture nasal bone
    d. Fracture ethmoid

13. **Tear drop sign is seen in:** *(SGPGI 2005, Exam 2017)*
    a. Fracture of floor of orbit
    b. Fracture of lateral wall of nose
    c. Fracture of roof of nose
    d. Le Fort's fracture

14. **Blow out fracture refers to:** *(Exam 2013)*
    a. Fracture of orbit
    b. Fracture of nasal septum
    c. Fracture base of skull
    d. Fracture of mandible

15. **Nerve damage in zygomatic fracture:** *(AIIMS 2006, Exam 2017)*
    a. Supraorbital nerve
    b. Infraorbital nerve
    c. Facial nerve
    d. Lingual nerve

16. **Le Fort classification is for fractures involving which bone:** *(Exam 2013)*
    a. Maxilla
    b. Mandible
    c. Zygomatic arch
    d. Nasal bone

17. **Le Fort's fracture does not involve:** *(AI 2006, Exam 2017)*
    a. Zygoma
    b. Maxilla
    c. Nasal bone
    d. Mandible

18. **Craniofacial dissociation is seen in:** *(SGPGI 2005, TN 2006, Exam 2017)*
    a. Le Fort I fracture
    b. Le Fort II fracture
    c. Le Fort III fracture
    d. Tripod fracture

19. **Most common site of fracture of mandible is:** *(AI 2004, Exam 2017)*
    a. Sub-condylar
    b. Angle
    c. Body
    d. Symphysis

20. **Guardsman fracture involves:** *(Manipal 2013)*
    a. Symphysis with condyles
    b. Angle and body
    c. Ramus and body
    d. None of the above

21. **CSF rhinorrhoea occurs most commonly due to fracture of:** *(AI 2007, Exam 2017)*
    a. Tegmen tympani
    b. Cribriform plate
    c. Frontal sinus
    d. Sphenoid sinus

Nose

Section II

22. **The most common site of leak in CSF rhinorrhoea is:** *(AI 2005, Exam 2013)*
    a. Ethmoid
    b. Frontal
    c. Petrous part of temporal bone
    d. Sphenoid

23. **Most common cause of traumatic CSF rhinorrhoea:** *(AI 2011)*
    a. Injury to ethmoidal sinus
    b. Injury to maxillary sinus
    c. Injury to frontal bone
    d. None

24. **CSF rhinorrhoea is seen in:** *(Exam 2011)*
    a. Le Fort's fracture type I
    b. Blow out fracture
    c. Naso-orbito-ethmoid fracture
    d. Frontozygomatic fracture

25. **Spontaneous CSF rhinorrhoea is associated with all except:** *(AIIMS 2008, Exam 2017)*
    a. Transverse fracture temporal bone
    b. Partial or complete empty sella syndrome
    c. Pseudo tumour cerebri
    d. Encephalocele

26. **CSF rhinorrhoea is diagnosed by:** *(AI 2007, Exam 2017)*
    a. β_2 microglobulin   b. β_2 transferrin
    c. Thyroglobulin   d. Transthyretin

27. **True about CSF rhinorrhoea:** *(PGI 2002, 2011)*
    a. Seen in fracture of cribriform plate
    b. Contains glucose
    c. Contains β_2 transferrin proteins
    d. Requires immediate surgery
    e. Halo sign is absent

28. **All of the following statements about CSF leak are true, except:** *(AI 2012)*
    a. Commonest site of CSF leak is lateral lamella of Cribriform plate
    b. β_2 transferrin estimation is highly specific for diagnosis
    c. Fluorescein Dye can be used intrathecally for diagnosis of site of leak
    d. MRI (Gadolinium chanced) T1 images are best for diagnosis of site of active leak

29. **A young male is brought to the hospital after RTA. Patient is stable but has clear water-like fluid coming from nose, management of choice is:** *(Exam 2014)*
    a. Conservative   b. MRI
    c. Immediate repair   d. Nasal packing

30. **Halo sign and handkerchief test are positive in:** *(Exam 2016)*
    a. CSF Rhinorrhoea   b. Deviated nasal septum
    c. Nasal Myiasis   d. Choanal atresia

31. **Intrathecal Fluorescein with endoscopic visualization is useful in diagnosis of:** *(Exam 2014)*
    a. Deviated nasal septum
    b. Multiple ethmoidal polyps
    c. Rhinitis medicamentosa
    d. CSF rhinorrhoea

32. **The pathognomonic test for CSF in suspected CSF rhinorrhoea is:** *(MH CET 2016)*
    a. Glucose concentration
    b. Handkerchief test
    c. Halo sign
    d. β_2 transferrin

33. **Infraorbital nerve is injured commonly in:** *(APPG 2015)*
    a. Mandibular fracture b. Blow out fracture of orbit
    c. Le Fort III fracture   d. Le Fort I fracture

34. **Head injury, patient conscious, CT is showing fracture, CSF leakage through right nostril-management:** *(Exam 2015)*
    a. Head low position
    b. Wait for two weeks for spontaneous stoppage of leakage
    c. Immediate Cisternography and transcranial operation to close the defect
    d. Endoscopically stop leakage

35. **In CSF rhinorrhoea CSF from middle cranial fossa reaches the nose via:** *(Exam 2014)*
    a. Sphenoid sinus   b. Frontal sinus
    c. Cribriform plate   d. Fovea ethmoidalis

IMAGE BASED PRACTICE QUESTIONS BY THE AUTHOR

36. **A 25-year-old player got hit on the nose and developed deviation of nose. He should be managed by:**

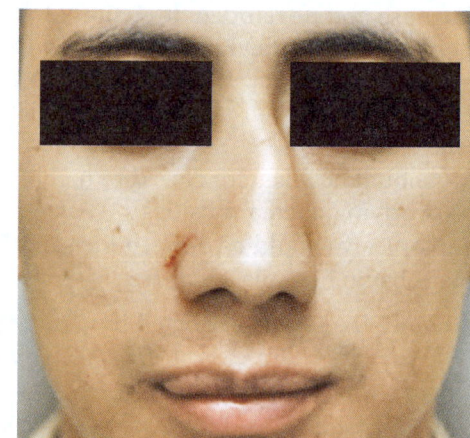

    a. He should be taken up for open reduction one week later
    b. He should be taken for closed reduction as soon as overlying edema subsides
    c. Septoplasty should be done in the same sitting if septum deviated
    d. He should be taken up for rhinoplasty one week later

37. **The following instruments are used in which surgery:**

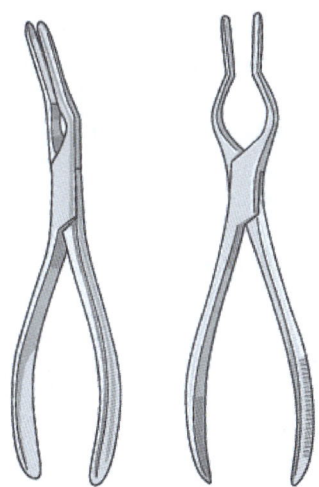

   a. Closed reduction of nasal bone fracture
   b. FESS
   c. Nasal packing for epistaxis
   d. Intranasal polypectomy

38. **The following test is done for:**

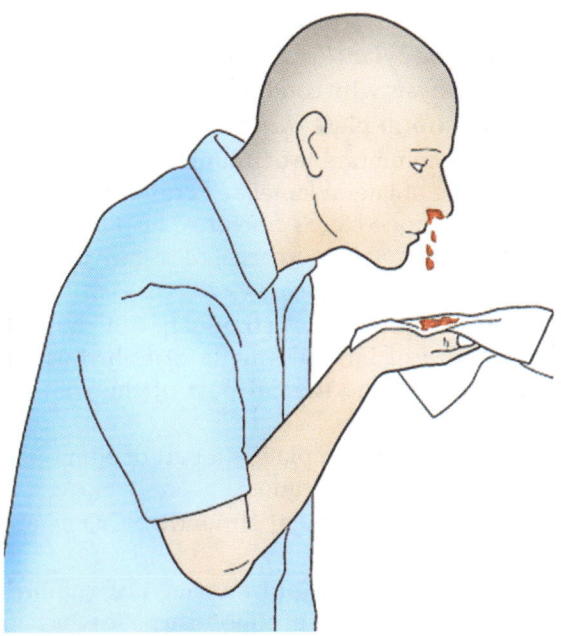

   a. Allergic rhinitis
   b. CSF rhinorrhoea
   c. Epistaxis
   d. Anosmia

39. **The given picture shows:**

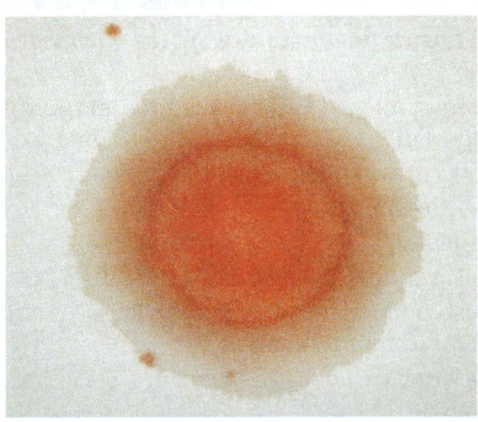

   a. Tear drop sign   b. Halo sign
   c. Crescent sign   d. Antral sign

40. **Target sign is most likely suggestive of:** (*Exam 2018*)
   a. Traumatic CSF rhinorrhoea
   b. Spontaneous CSF rhinorrhoea
   c. Angiofibroma
   d. Glomus tympanicum

41. **Blow out fracture most commonly involves:**
   (*Exam 2018*)
   a. Floor of orbit
   b. Lateral wall of orbit
   c. Superior wall of orbit
   d. Medial wall of orbit

42. **A patient presents to the casualty following injury on the face. His CT is given below. Most probable diagnosis is:** (*Exam 2019*)

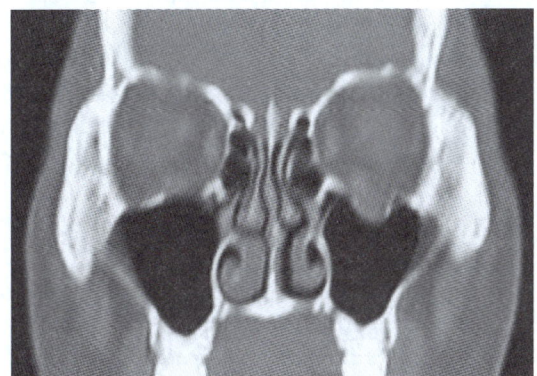

   a. Le Fort fracture I fracture
   b. Blow out fracture
   c. Tripod fracture
   d. Chevallet fracture

Nose

Section II

ANSWERS AND EXPLANATIONS

1. **(b) Ensure adequate airway** (*Ref. Cummings, 6th ed., 498*)

   In any patient of craniofacial trauma it is critically important to follow the ABC of trauma, i.e.

   A → Airway management
   B → Breathing
   C → Circulation

2. **(a) Nasal** (*Ref. Cummings, 6th ed., 693*)
   - Most common fractured bone in the face is nasal bone followed by zygomatic bone.

3. **(b) After 1 week** (*Ref. Cummings, 6th ed., 501*) (refer to text)

4. **(a) Chevallet and Jarjavay fracture** (*Ref. Scott Brown, 6th ed., 4/16/6*)
   - The other given fractures do not involve the human body.

5. **(c) Horizontal** (*Ref. Scott Brown, 6th ed., 4/16/7*)
   - Vertical fracture line in nasal septum is seen in Chevallet fracture.
   - Comminuted fracture of nasal septum is seen in class 3 fractures of nose.

6. **(b) Blow from below** (*Ref. Scott Brown, 8th ed., Vol 3; 1127*) (refer to text)
   - Blow directly from front will cause Jarjavay fracture.
   - Blow from side may depress only one nasal bone. Side force can cause severe septal displacement, which can twist or buckle the nose.

7. **(b) He should be taken up for closed reduction as soon as overlying edema subsides** (*Ref. Cummings 6th ed., 501; Scott Brown, 6th ed., 4/16/9*)
   - Since the septum is not deviated he is most likely having class 1 Chevallet fracture. Hence, he should be managed by closed reduction as soon as overlying edema subsides which generally takes around 5–7 days.
   - Since the septum is not deviated so septoplasty will not be required.
   - If the patient presents after 3 weeks then the management is open reduction.

8. **(d) Walsham's forceps** (*Ref. Scott Brown, 8th ed., Vol 1; 1187*)
   - Luc's forceps is used in septoplasty and Caldwell-Luc operation
   - Citelli's forceps is used for punching out holes in bones or other tissues
   - Tilly's forceps is used for dressing in EAC and doing anterior nasal packing in epistaxis

9. **(d) Zygoma** (*Ref. Scott Brown, 8th ed., Vol 1; 1196*)

10. **(b) CSF rhinorrhoea** (*Ref. Scott Brown, 8th ed., Vol 1; 1196*)
    - Fracture of zygoma presents with orbital and cheek findings (refer to text above). CSF rhinorrhoea does not occur here.

- In facial fractures, CSF rhinorrhoea is seen in class 3 nasal fracture and Le Fort II and III fractures.

11. **(a), (c)** (*Ref. Scott Brown, 8th ed., Vol 1; 1196*)
    Flattening of malar eminence is seen in zygomatic fracture. Also epistaxis is not seen (please refer text).

12. **(b) Fracture zygoma** (*Ref. Scott Brown, 8th ed., Vol 1; 1196*)
    - Enophthalmos can be present in fracture zygoma or blow out fracture of orbit.
    - Fracture maxilla, i.e. Le Fort fracture are caused by high velocity injuries.
    - Fracture nasal bone class 3, i.e. including ethmoid are also caused by high velocity injuries and will cause predominantly nasal manifestations which are not mentioned.

13. **(a) Fracture of floor of orbit** (*Ref. Dhingra, 6th ed., 184*)

14. **(a) Fracture of orbit** (*Ref. Cummings, 6th ed., 329*)

15. **(b) Infraorbital nerve** (*Ref. Cummings, 6th ed., 328*) (please see the text)

16. **(a) Maxilla** (*Ref. Cummings, 6th ed., 334*)

17. **(d) Mandible** (*Ref. Cummings, 6th ed., 334*)
    Le Forte fractures do not involve the mandible.

18. **(c) Le Fort III fracture** (*Ref. Cummings, 6th ed., 334*)

19. **(a) Sub-condylar** (*Ref. Cummings, 6th ed., 330*)

20. **(a) Symphysis with condyles** (*Ref. https://maxfacts.uk*)

21. **(b) Cribriform plate** (*Ref. Cummings, 6th ed., 805*)
    - The most common site of traumatic CSF rhinorrhoea is fracture of lateral lamella of cribriform plate. The other mentioned site's fractures can also cause CSF rhinorrhoea/otorhinorrhoea, please *see* the text.

22. **(a) Ethmoid** (*Ref. Cummings, 6th ed., 805*)
    - The most common site of traumatic CSF rhinorrhoea is fracture of lateral lamella of cribriform plate which forms the medial part of the roof of the ethmoid.
    - Since the cribriform plate is a part of ethmoid bone the answer here is ethmoid.

23. **(a) Injury to ethmoidal sinus** (*Ref. Cummings, 6th ed., 805*)
    - Most common cause of traumatic CSF rhinorrhoea is fracture of that part of cribriform plate which forms the roof of the ethmoid sinus.

24. **(c) Naso-orbito-ethmoid fracture** (*Ref. Cummings, 6th ed., 804*)
    - Naso-orbito-ethmoid fracture, i.e. Class III nasal fracture, Le Fort II and Le Fort III are associated with CSF rhinorrhoea among facial fractures.

25. **(a) Transverse fracture temporal bone is the traumatic cause** (*Ref. Cummings, 6th ed., 805*)
    Rest are causes of Non-traumatic/spontaneous CSF rhinorrhoea, please *see* the text.

26. **(b) β_2 transferrin** (*Ref. Cummings, 6th ed., 807*)
    - β_2 transferrin on electrophoresis is pathognomonic of CSF as this protein is present only in CSF.

27. **(a), (b) and (c)** (*Ref. Cummings, 6th ed., 807*)

28. **(d) MRI (Gadolinium enhanced) T1 images are best for diagnosis of site of leak** (*Ref. Cummings, 6th ed., 809*)
    - HRCT Cisternography is the best for diagnosis of site of active CSF leak (please see the text)

29. **(a) Conservative** (*Ref. Cummings, 6th ed., 811*)

30. **(a) CSF rhinorrhoea** (*Ref. Cummings, 6th ed., 807*)

31. **(d) CSF rhinorrhoea** (*Ref. Cummings, 6th ed., 809*)

32. **(d) β$_2$ transferrin** (*Ref. Cummings, 6th ed., 809*)

33. **(b) Blow out fracture of orbit** (*Ref. Cummings, 6th ed., 328*)

34. **(b) Wait for two weeks for spontaneous stoppage of leakage** (*Ref. Cummings, 6th ed., 811*)

35. **(a) Sphenoid sinus** (*Ref. Cummings, 6th ed., 805*)

36. **(b) He should be taken for closed reduction as soon as overlying edema subsides (after 5 to 7 days)** (*Ref. Cummings, 6th ed., 500*)

37. **(a) Closed reduction of nasal bone fracture** (*Ref. Scott Brown, 8th ed., Vol 1; 1187*)

    Asch forceps (Left) and Walsham forceps (right), *see* Chapter on ENT instruments in the end.

38. **(b) CSF rhinorrhoea** (*Ref. Cummings, 6th ed., 807*)

    The picture shows handkerchief test for CSF rhinorrhoea

39. **(b) Halo sign** (*Ref. Cummings, 6th ed., 807*)
    - Halo sign is seen in CSF rhinorrhoea (refer to text)
    - Tear drop sign is seen in blow out fracture of orbit
    - Crescent sign is seen in antrochoanal polyp
    - Antral sign is seen in angiofibroma

40. **(a) Traumatic CSF rhinorrhoea** (*Ref. Cummings, 6th ed., 807*)

41. **(a) Floor of orbit** (*Ref. Cummings, 6th ed. 329*)

42. **(b) Blow out fracture** (*Ref. Cummings, 6th ed. 329*)

Section II

Nose

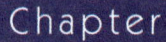

Tumours of Nose and PNS

BENIGN SINO-NASAL TUMOURS

Inverted Papilloma/Schneiderian Papilloma/ Transitional Cell Papilloma/Ringertz Tumour

This is the **MC benign tumour of the nasal cavity**. It is a benign but locally invasive tumour.

Clinical Features

- It is seen more commonly in **men**.
- It is seen mostly in the age group of **40–70 years**.
- Association with HPV (human papillomavirus) has been found.
- It arises from the **lateral wall of nose** and is usually unilateral. The patient presents with unilateral nasal obstruction and unilateral epistaxis. On examination, it appears like a pale polypoidal lesion with papillary appearance that protrudes from the middle meatal area.
- On histopathologic examination there is proliferation of epithelium with finger-like inversions into the underlying stroma because of which it is known as inverted papilloma.
- It is **premalignant** with 5–15% risk of developing squamous cell carcinoma.

Treatment

Treatment consists of **wide excision** of the tumour by lateral rhinotomy (by giving incision in the naso-facial crease) or midfacial degloving approach (by giving sub-labial incision from one molar to the other and raising the skin flap over the cheek and nose).

Chances of its **recurrence** are **very high**.

Osteomas

The **MC benign tumour of the paranasal sinuses** is osteoma. Osteomas are osteogenic tumours composed of mature bone.

PNS osteomas are seen **most commonly** in the **frontal sinus** followed by ethmoid, maxillary and sphenoid.

They can lead to obstruction of ostia (i.e. sinus opening) leading to chronic sinusitis and mucocele formation. They can also lead to mass effect causing headache, diplopia and facial deformity.

The most common histological pattern recognised is:
Ivory osteoma: It is composed of dense bone lacking Haversian canal system.

They can be present in association with other osteomas, soft tissue tumours and intestinal polyposis when it constitutes Gardner's syndrome.

The radiographic appearance is that of a dense well circumscribed mass.

Removal of frontal and ethmoidal osteoma is by external fronto-ethmoidectomy. This is known as **Lynch Howarth approach** (please *see* Chapter on sinusitis).

Fibrous Dysplasia

This is an idiopathic benign condition where medullary bone is replaced by poorly organised fibro-osseous tissue. Most common site of involvement is **maxilla**. It presents with painless asymmetrical enlargement of one sided maxilla. The fibrous tissue expands to fill the maxillary sinus also. It is more commonly seen in young age.

CT is the best investigation and characteristically shows a **ground glass appearance**.

Management is correcting the deformity by surgical re-sculpting of the maxilla.

MALIGNANT TUMOURS OF NOSE

Basal Cell Carcinoma

The most common malignancy of skin of external nose is Basal cell carcinoma. It arises from keratinocytes of epidermis and adnexal structures.

Prolonged exposure to sunlight (UV radiation) is important etiological factor.

It is seen more commonly in males, 40–80 years of age.

Besides nose the basal cell carcinoma also involves the other areas of face, site of predilection being a line joining the angle of mouth to ear lobule. It is a locally invasive tumour causing local erosion (burrowing) because of which it is also known as **Rodent ulcer**.

Dangerous anatomic sites are embryonal fusion planes such as naso-facial sulcus, medial canthus and postauricular areas. Here the neoplasm can proliferate deeply before becoming clinically apparent.

Metastasis is very rare.

Treatment

It is managed by wide excision.

Moh's micrographic surgery (a technique in which precise surgical margins are obtained by using frozen section during the surgery) is ideal for recurrent cases, poorly defined or in high risk areas.

Squamous Cell Carcinoma

MC carcinoma of the nasal cavity is squamous cell carcinoma, most commonly arising from the lateral wall. It can also arise from the septum when it is known as nose picker's carcinoma.

It is managed by a combination of surgery and radiotherapy.

Esthesioneuroblastoma/Olfactory Neuroblastoma

It is a rare malignancy constituting only 1–5% of nasal tumours.

It arises from **olfactory epithelium** lining upper 1/3rd of nose. It has bimodal age occurrence with first peak at 11–20 yrs and second at 55–60 yrs. It commonly spreads to orbits laterally and brain superiorly. MC cranial nerve involved here is olfactory nerve.

It is a neuroendocrine tumour and can secrete hormones. So before excision serum and urinary catecholamines should be tested.

Metastasis to neck is seen in 10–20% cases. It is managed by combined modality treatment with surgical resection which may involve local resection or craniofacial resection with postoperative radiotherapy.

Para-nasal Sinus Carcinoma

- The MC carcinoma of the PNS is **squamous cell carcinoma**.
- It is seen most commonly in **maxillary sinus** followed by ethmoid, frontal and sphenoid sinuses.
- There is a specific history of exposure to, nickel, chromium, leather, etc.
- The squamous cell carcinoma of the maxilla presents with blood tinged nasal discharge, nasal obstruction, widening of upper alveolus leading to poor fitting of dentures, pain and loosening of teeth, epiphora (watering from eye), facial paraesthesia.
- **Submandibular** and upper deep cervical lymph nodes are the most commonly involved.

**Note:**

In people working in hard **wood furniture** industries the **MC carcinoma is Adenocarcinoma** which is more common in the **ethmoids**. Soft wood exposure is associated with squamous cell carcinoma of the maxillary sinus.

Classification

Ohngren's Classification

An imaginary line is drawn from the medial canthus to the angle of mandible dividing the maxillary antrum into a supra and an infrastructure. This classification states that the carcinoma of supra structure has poorer prognosis than the infrastructure (this is because the carcinoma of the supra structure can easily spread to the orbit and base of skull).

TNM Classification

Carcinoma Maxilla

$T_1 \rightarrow$ Tumour confined to antral mucosa with no bony destruction.

$T_2 \rightarrow$ Bony destruction involving medial wall (middle meatus) and inferior walls (hard palate)

$T_3 \rightarrow$ Bony destruction of posterior wall of maxillary sinus, pterygoid plates, superior wall, i.e. floor of orbit, ethmoid sinuses, laterally, i.e. infratemporal fossa, anteriorly subcutaneous tissue and skin of cheek.

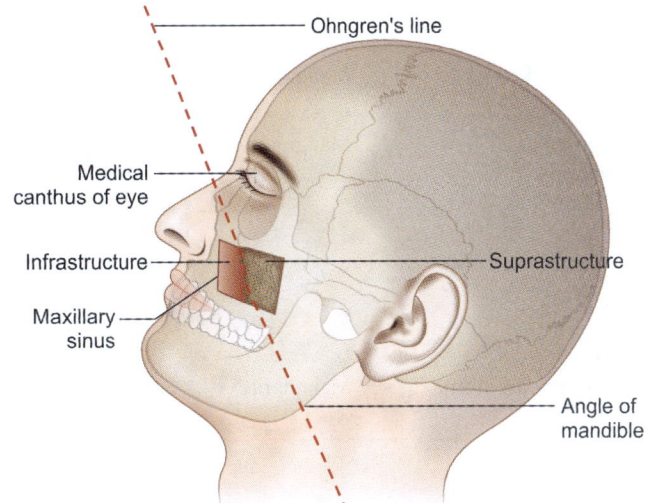

Fig. 25.1

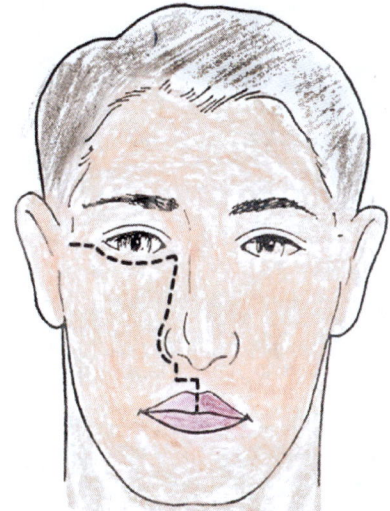

Fig. 25.2: Weber Fergusson incision

Nose

Section II

$T_4 \rightarrow$ Tumour invades orbital contents, orbital apex, cribriform plate, base of skull, nasopharynx, frontal and sphenoid sinus.

Treatment

For nearly all patients of maxillary carcinoma the treatment is surgical resection followed by radiation therapy. The surgical resection can be a partial or total maxillectomy. The incision used here is the **Weber Fergusson incision** (*see* Fig. 25.2) or a midfacial degloving approach (after giving a sub-labial incision from one molar to the other, the skin flap is raised over the face and then the procedure is carried out). Only small T1 mucosal carcinomas can be treated by surgical resection alone.

"Points to Ponder/Points for Quick revision"

Tumour/condition	Nature	Involvement/MC site	Clinical features	Treatment	Remarks
Inverted papilloma/ **Schneiderian papilloma/ Ringertz tumour.** MC benign tumour of the nasal cavity	Benign (premalignant)	Lateral wall of nose	U/L nasal obstruction and epistaxis	Wide excision	Seen in males (40–70 yrs), high recurrence
Osteoma (**MC benign tumour of the paranasal sinuses**)	Benign	Frontal sinus	Chronic sinusitis/ mucocele	External fronto-ethmoidectomy (Lynch Howarth approach)	MC histological type—Ivory osteoma. 2nd MC site—ethmoid
Fibrous dysplasia	Benign	Maxillary sinus	U/L asymmetric enlargement of maxilla	Surgical re-sculpturing	Young age. Ground glass appearance on CT
Esthesioneuroblastoma	Malignant	Olfactory epithelium	Neuro-endocrine manifestations	Surgery + radiotherapy	Rare. Bimodal age
Squamous cell carcinoma PNS 1. Squamous (MC)	Malignant	Maxillary sinus	Blood tinged nasal discharge, nasal obstruction, sub-mandibular lymphadenopathy	Surgery + radiotherapy (Weber Fergusson incision)	Ohngren's classification (line drawn from the medial canthus to the angle of mandible)—suprastructure poor prognosis. Ni, Cr and leather industry.
2. Adenocarcinoma	Malignant	Ethmoid sinus	Blood tinged nasal discharge	Surgery + radiotherapy	Hard Wood workers

PREVIOUSLY ASKED QUESTIONS

1. **Inverted papilloma arises from:**
   (AI 2006, Exam 2017)
   a. Roof of nasal cavity b. Medial wall of nose
   c. Lateral wall of nose d. None

2. **Inverted papilloma is characterised by all except:**
   (MP 2006, Exam 2017)
   a. Also called as Schneiderian papilloma
   b. Seen more often in females
   c. Presents with epistaxis and nasal obstruction
   d. Originates from lateral wall of nose

3. **True about inverted papilloma:** *(PGI 2008, 2013)*
   a. Arises mainly from nasal septum
   b. Common in children
   c. Risk of malignancy
   d. Postoperative radiotherapy useful
   e. Also known as Schneiderian papilloma

4. **All of the following are true about inverted papilloma except:** *(Delhi 2008, Exam 2017)*
   a. More common in males
   b. Arises from lateral wall of orbit
   c. Can cause epistaxis
   d. Recurrent in nature even after removal

5. **True about inverted papilloma:** *(PGI Nov 2009)*
   a. Predisposition in childhood
   b. May present with epistaxis
   c. Recurrence rare
   d. Benign in nature
   e. Arise from lateral wall of nose

6. **Most common site for osteoma is:**
   (MP 2008, Exam 2012)
   a. Maxillary sinus   b. Ethmoid sinus
   c. Frontal sinus   d. Sphenoid sinus

7. **Commonest site of Ivory osteoma:**
   (DPG 2006, Exam 2017)
   a. Frontal-ethmoidal region
   b. Mandible
   c. Maxilla
   d. Sphenoid

8. **Ground glass appearance of maxillary sinus on CT scan is seen in:** *(DPG 2007, Exam 2017)*
   a. Maxillary sinusitis
   b. Maxillary carcinoma
   c. Maxillary polyp
   d. Maxillary fibrous dysplasia

9. **Ohngren's line that divides maxillary sinus into superolateral and inferomedial zone is related to:**
   (Exam 2012)
   a. Maxillary sinusitis b. Maxillary carcinoma
   c. Maxillary osteoma d. Infratemporal carcinoma

10. **Ohngren's classification of maxillary sinus carcinoma is based on:** *(Exam 2013)*
    a. Imaginary plane between medical canthus of eye and angle of mandible
    b. Imaginary plane between lateral canthus of eye and angle of mandible
    c. Two horizontal lines, one passing through floor of orbit and other through floor of antrum
    d. None

11. **True about tumours of nose and PNS:**
    (PGI Dec 2006, Exam 2017)
    a. Squamous cell carcinoma is the most common type
    b. Adenocarcinoma can occur
    c. Melanoma is most common
    d. Adenoid cystic carcinoma is the most common
    e. Esthesioneuroblastoma is the most common type

12. **Most common malignancy in maxillary antrum is:**
    (PGI 2006, 2011)
    a. Muco-epidermoid carcinoma
    b. Adenocystic carcinoma
    c. Adenocarcinoma
    d. Squamous cell carcinoma

13. **First lymph node involved in maxillary carcinoma:**
    (RJ 2000, Exam 2017)
    a. Submental   b. Submandibular
    c. Clavicular   d. Lower Jugular

14. **Wood workers associated sinus carcinoma:**
    (PGI Dec 2006, Exam 2014)
    a. Adenocarcinoma
    b. Squamous cell carcinoma
    c. Anaplastic carcinoma
    d. Melanoma

15. **Adenocarcinoma of ethmoid sinus occurs commonly in:** *(PGI Dec 2006, 2015)*
    a. Fire workers   b. Chimney workers
    c. Watch makers   d. Wood workers

16. **Early maxillary carcinoma presents as:**
    (PGI 2000, 2014)
    a. Blood tinged nasal discharge
    b. Supraclavicular lymph node
    c. Proptosis
    d. Nasal obstruction
    e. Cheek swelling

17. **Carcinoma maxillary sinus stage III (T3 M0 N0), treatment of choice is:**
    (TN 2006, AP 2005, Exam 2017)
    a. Radiotherapy
    b. Surgery + Radiotherapy
    c. Chemotherapy
    d. Chemotherapy + Surgery

Nose

Section II

18. Tumour arising from olfactory nasal mucosa is:
    (AI 2012)

    a. Nasal Glioma
    b. Adenoid cystic carcinoma
    c. Nasopharyngeal carcinoma
    d. Esthesioneuroblastoma

19. Mucocele commonly involves: (Kerala PGMEE 2015)

    a. Maxillary sinus
    b. Sphenoid sinus
    c. Fronto-ethmoidal region
    d. Inferior turbinate

20. All are malignant tumours of nasal cavity except:
    (APPG 2015)

    a. Olfactory neuroblastoma
    b. Stewart's granuloma
    c. Malignant melanoma
    d. Ringertz tumour

21. Which is not true in fibrous dysplasia?
    (COMED 2015)

    a. Benign neoplasm of nasofacial region
    b. Presents in the first or second decade of life

    c. Classical X-ray finding of ground glass appearance
    d. Mandible is commonly affected

22. Identify the line in the given picture: (Exam 2017)

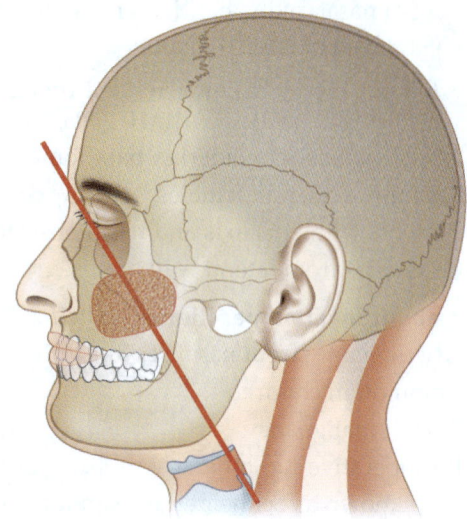

    a. Donaldson's line   b. Frankfurt's line
    c. Sebileau's line   d. Ohngren's line

ANSWERS AND EXPLANATIONS

1. **(c) Lateral wall of nose** (*Ref. Cummings, 6th ed., 741*)
2. **(b) Seen more often in females** (*Ref. Cummings, 6th ed., 741*)
3. **(c) and (e) risk of malignancy and Also known as Schneiderian papilloma** (*Ref. Cummings, 6th ed., 741*)
4. **(b) Arises from lateral wall of orbit** (*Ref. Cummings, 6th ed., 741*)
5. **(b), (d), and (e) May present with Epistaxis, benign in nature, arises from lateral wall of nose** (*Ref. Cummings, 6th ed., 741*)
6. **(c) Frontal sinus** (*Ref. Cummings, 6th ed., 746*)
7. **(a) Frontal-ethmoidal region** (*Ref. Cummings, 6th ed., 746*)
8. **(d) Maxillary fibrous dysplasia** (*Ref. Cummings, 6th ed., 749*)
9. **(b) Maxillary carcinoma** (*Ref. Cummings, 6th ed., 1180*)
10. **(a) Imaginary plane between medical canthus of eye and angle of mandible** (*Ref. Cummings, 6th ed., 1180*)
11. **(a) and (b)** (*Ref. Cummings, 6th ed., 1177*)
    - The MC carcinoma of the PNS is squamous cell carcinoma.
    - In people working in hardwood furniture industries the MC carcinoma is adenocarcinoma
    - Melanomas of the paranasal sinuses are very rare.

- Adenoid cystic carcinoma arises from the minor salivary and mucosal glands and show perineural spread.

12. **(d) Squamous cell carcinoma** (*Ref. Cummings, 6th ed., 1177*)
13. **(b) Submandibular** (*Ref. Scott Brown, Vol 3; 75*) (refer to text)
14. **(a) Adenocarcinoma** (*Ref. Cummings, 6th ed., 1177*)
15. **(d) Wood workers** (*Ref. Cummings, 6th ed., 1177*)
16. **(a) and (d) Blood tinged nasal discharge and nasal obstruction** (*Ref. Cummings, 6th ed., 1178*)
    - Nodal metastasis is uncommon, occurs late and involves submandibular and upper deep cervical lymph nodes.
    - Orbital involvement occurs late.
17. **(b) Surgery + Radiotherapy** (*Ref. Cummings, 6th ed., 1184*)
    - For all patients of carcinoma maxillary sinus (except small T1 lesions), the treatment is surgical resection (maxillectomy) followed by radiation therapy.
18. **(d) Esthesioneuroblastoma** (*Ref. Cummings, 6th ed., 1177*)
19. **(c) Fronto-ethmoidal region** (*Ref. Cummings, 6th ed., 761*)
20. **(d) Ringertz tumour** (*Ref. Cummings, 6th ed., 1177*)
21. **(d) Mandible is commonly affected** (*Ref. Cummings, 6th ed., 749*)
22. **(d) Ohngren's line** (*Ref. Scott Brown, Vol 3; 74*)

Oral Cavity and Pharynx

Anatomy and Embryology of Oral Cavity and Pharynx

DEVELOPMENT OF TONGUE

From the mesoderm of 1st branchial arch develop three thickenings. These are the two lingual swellings and one, the tuberculum impar, *see* Fig. 26.1a and b. These three fuse to form the anterior 2/3rds of tongue. So the anterior 2/3rds of tongue develops from 1st arch, *see* Figs 26.1c and 26.2b.

From the mesoderm of 3rd and 4th branchial arches develops another midline thickening known as hypobranchial eminence (Fig. 26.1a).

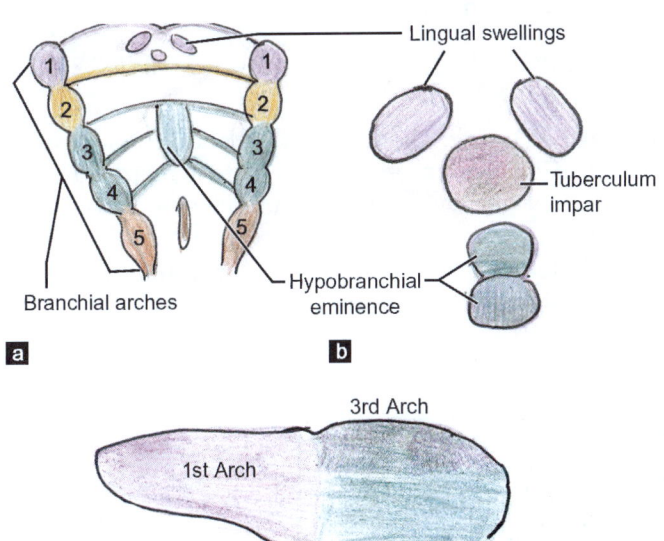

Fig. 26.1a to c

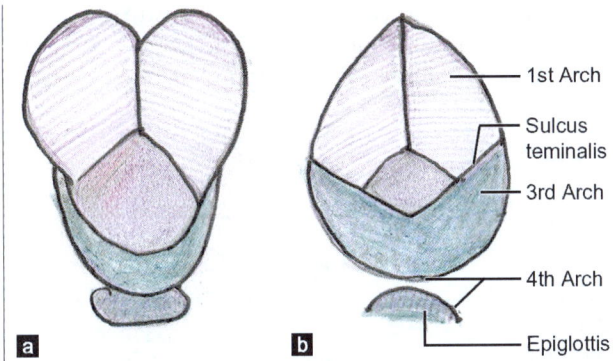

Fig. 26.2a and b

Hypobranchial eminence then divides into a cranial (from 3rd arch) and caudal (from 4th arch) part (Fig. 26.1b).

The cranial part (3rd arch) leads to the formation of the posterior 1/3rd of tongue except the posterior most part. The posterior most part of the tongue is formed by the caudal part (4th arch) of the hypobranchial eminence, *see* Figs 26.1c and 26.2b.

The rest of the caudal part leads to the formation of epiglottis.

During the formation of posterior 1/3rd of tongue the 3rd arch overgrows the 2nd arch so the 2nd arch does not contribute to the formation of tongue.

The muscles of the tongue are derived from occipital somites (myotomes) and hence are supplied by hypoglossal nerve except for palatoglossus which is supplied by pharyngeal plexus (formed by vagus along with cranial part of accessory nerve).

Arch	Part of the tongue derived	Sensory nerve supply	Taste sensation
1st	Anterior 2/3rds of tongue	Lingual nerve (a branch of mandibular which is 1st arch nerve)	Chorda tympani (the pretrematic** nerve of 1st arch)
3rd	Posterior 1/3rd of tongue	Glossopharyngeal nerve (3rd arch nerve)	Glossopharyngeal nerve
4th	Posterior most part of tongue and epiglottis	Internal laryngeal branch of Superior laryngeal nerve which is a branch of Vagus (4th arch nerve)	Internal laryngeal nerve

** The pretrematic nerve is the nerve to a particular arch given by the next arch nerve. For example, here the nerve of the 2nd arch, i.e. the facial nerve gives a pretrematic nerve to the 1st arch. This pretrematic nerve is the Chorda tympani which is responsible for taste sensation from anterior 2/3rds of tongue.

ANATOMY OF ORAL CAVITY

The external surface of lips is not included in the oral cavity. The oral cavity extends from the mucosal surface of lips anteriorly to the anterior pillar of tonsils.

Hence, the soft palate with uvula, tonsils and posterior 1/3rd of tongue (also called base of tongue) are not components of oral cavity. They are parts of oropharynx.

The oral part of tongue is separated from its oro-pharyngeal part by a V-shaped groove known as sulcus terminalis. Just anterior to sulcus terminalis are large papillae known as circumvallate papillae arranged in V-shaped.

The circumvallate papillae get special afferent taste innervation from cranial nerve IX, the Glossopharyngeal nerve even though they are anterior to the sulcus terminalis, i.e. part of the anterior 2/3rds of tongue. The rest of the anterior two-thirds of tongue get taste innervation from the chorda tympani. The sensory and taste innervation of rest of the tongue has been given in the table above.

Lymphatic Drainage of Tongue

Part of the tongue	Lymph node
Tip	Submental (level 1)
Anterior 2/3rds (lateral borders)	Submandibular (ipsilateral) (level 1)
Anterior 2/3rds (remaining middle part)	Submandibular (ipsilateral and contralateral) (level 1)
Posterior 1/3rd	Upper (also called jugulo-digastric) (level 2)and middle (jugulo-omohyoid) deep cervical (ipsilateral) (level 3)

Ultimately all the above lymph nodes drain into jugulo-omohyoid lymph nodes (middle deep cervical) which are also known as **lymph nodes of tongue**.

ANATOMY OF PHARYNX

The pharynx extends from the base of skull above to the lower border of cricoid cartilage below.

From the lower end of pharynx starts the oesophagus. This cricopharyngeal-esophageal junction is the narrowest part of the pharynx.

The pharynx is divided into three parts (Fig. 26.3):

1. **Nasopharynx or Epipharynx:** This is the upper most part of pharynx lying posterior to the nasal cavity, hence the term nasopharynx. It lies above the oropharynx (please read below) and therefore called Epipharynx. It extends from the base of skull above to the hard/soft palate below. It lies opposite the 1st cervical vertebra (C1).

2. **Oropharynx:** Below the nasopharynx is the oropharynx lying just posterior to the oral cavity. It extends from hard palate above to the hyoid below.

    The oropharynx lies opposite C2 and upper part of C3.

3. **Laryngopharynx:** It is so called it lies just behind the larynx. It lies below the oropharynx and therefore also known as hypopharynx. It extends from the hyoid above till the lower border of cricoid below. The Laryngopharynx lies opposite C3, 4, 5 and 6 cervical vertebrae.

The posterior and posterolateral pharyngeal wall is common to all the parts of pharynx.

POSTERIOR AND POSTEROLATERAL PHARYNGEAL WALL

1. **Mucosal lining:** The whole of the pharynx is lined by stratified squamous epithelium except for the nasopharynx which is lined by pseudostratified ciliated columnar epithelium.

    Hence, all the structures in the nasopharynx (adenoids, Eustachian tube opening) will be lined by

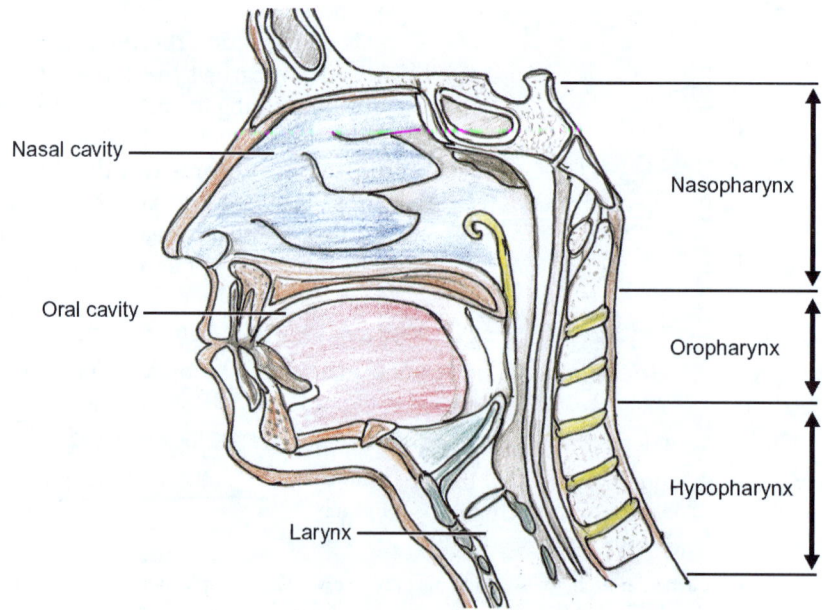

Nasal cavity

Oral cavity

Larynx

Nasopharynx

Oropharynx

Hypopharynx

Fig. 26.3: Different parts and boundaries of pharynx

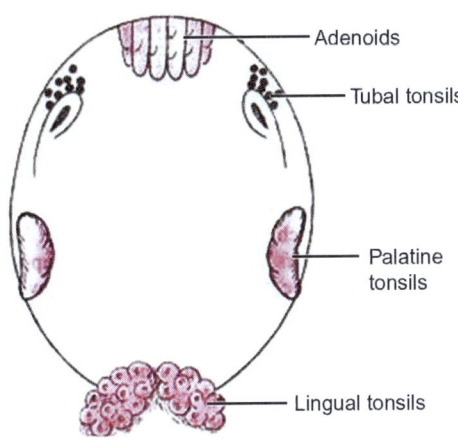

Fig. 26.4: Waldeyer's ring

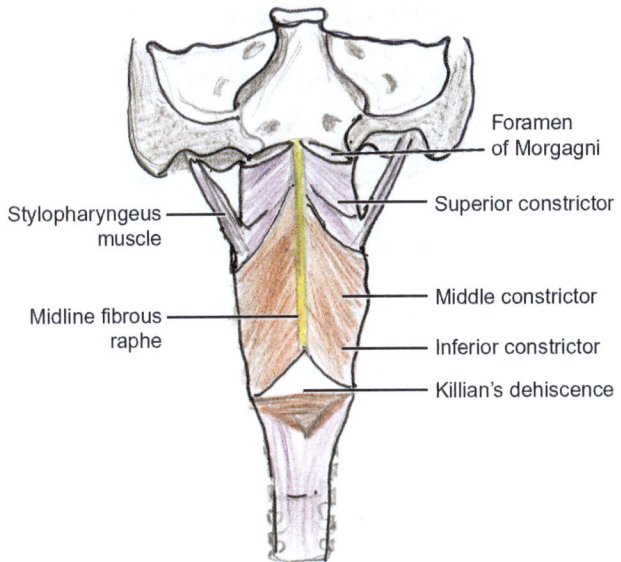

Fig. 26.5: Circular muscle layer of pharynx

ciliated columnar and elsewhere (e.g. tonsils) the structures will be lined by stratified squamous epithelium.

Since the soft palate has both nasopharyngeal and oropharyngeal surfaces, it is lined by ciliated columnar above and stratified squamous epithelium below.

2. **Waldeyer's ring:** Just beneath the epithelium is the subepithelial layer of lymphoid tissue present in the form of a ring in the nasopharynx and oropharynx. The components of this ring are:

Waldeyer's ring components	Also called	Location
Adenoids	**Lushka's or nasopharyngeal tonsil**	**Nasopharynx** (in the midline at the junction of the roof and posterior wall)
Tubal tonsils	**Gerlach's tonsils**	**Nasopharynx** (on the lateral wall behind the Eustachian tube opening)
Palatine	**Faucial tonsils**	**Oropharynx** (in between the anterior and posterior pillars)
Lingual tonsils	—	**Posterior 1/3rd, i.e. base of tongue**
Lateral pharyngeal bands and nodules	—	Posterior pharyngeal wall

3. **Pharyngobasilar fascia:** This fascia is present behind the epithelium and subepithelial lymphoid tissue, and lines the muscle layer of the pharynx anteriorly. The pharyngobasilar fascia forms the capsule of tonsil.

4. **Muscle layer:** It consists of two layers of muscles:
   a. *Inner longitudinal layer*: It contains the 3 pharyngeal muscles, stylopharyngeus, salpingopharyngeus and palatopharyngeus. They are attached above to the styloid process, Eustachian tube and palate respectively and below they all are attached to the posterior border of the thyroid cartilage. They

elevate and dilate the pharynx and help in swallowing.

   b. *Outer circular layer*: It contains the 3 constrictors (since they constrict the pharynx), superior, middle and inferior constrictor starting from base of skull above.

The uppermost constrictor muscle of the pharynx is the superior constrictor.

The upper border of the superior constrictor muscle is not attached to the base of skull. Hence, in between the base of skull and the upper border of superior constrictor is a gap which is filled by just pharyngobasilar fascia.

This gap is known as **sinus of Morgagni**. The structures that pass through the sinus of Morgagni are as follows:

Mnemonic: → **TAALA:**
   i. **T**ensor veli palatini
   ii. **A**scending palatine artery
   iii. **A**scending pharyngeal artery's palatine branch
   iv. **L**evator veli palatini
   v. **A**uditory tube (Eustachian tube)

Below the superior constrictor muscle is the middle constrictor.

The structures that pass in between **superior constrictor and middle constrictor** *are*:
   i. Glossopharyngeal nerve
   ii. Stylopharyngeus muscle

The lowermost circular muscle of the pharynx is the inferior constrictor.

In between **middle and inferior constrictor**, *passes the:*
   i. Internal laryngeal nerve (it should be remembered as Superior branch of vagus, i.e. the superior laryngeal nerve's internal laryngeal branch)
   ii. Superior laryngeal vessels.

Mnemonic: Structures passing superior to inferior constrictor are the superior nerve and vessels.

In between **inferior constrictor and oesophagus** passes the:

i. Inferior branch of vagus, i.e. the recurrent laryngeal nerve

ii. Inferior laryngeal vessels

Mnemonic: Structures passing inferior to inferior constrictor are the inferior nerve and vessels.

The **inferior constrictor** consists of two parts:

a. **Thyropharyngeus:** It arises from the oblique line of thyroid anteriorly and runs obliquely up posteriorly to attach to the midline raphe (raphe means a ridge between two halves of an organ) on the posterior wall of pharynx.

b. **Cricopharyngeus:** It arises from the cricoid anteriorly and runs horizontally backwards to attach to the midline raphe on the posterior wall of pharynx.

In between the two parts of inferior constrictor (the Thyropharyngeus running obliquely up posteriorly and Cricopharyngeus running horizontally backwards), is a gap known as **Killian's dehiscence,** also known as gateway of tears (please note tears here does not mean the natural saline drops from emotional eyes. It means tear, i.e. the pharynx lacerates or gets pulled apart from here leading to Zenker's diverticulum, *see* below).

This is the most common site for the development of the pharyngeal pouch. The pharyngeal pouch that forms from here is known as Zenker's diverticulum.

5. **Buccopharyngeal fascia:** It lines the outer surface of the constrictor muscles.

The pharyngeal wall ends at the bucco pharyngeal fascia. Behind the buccopharyngeal fascia is another fascia which is the alar fascia. Behind the alar fascia is the pre-vertebral fascia behind which are the cervical vertebrae.

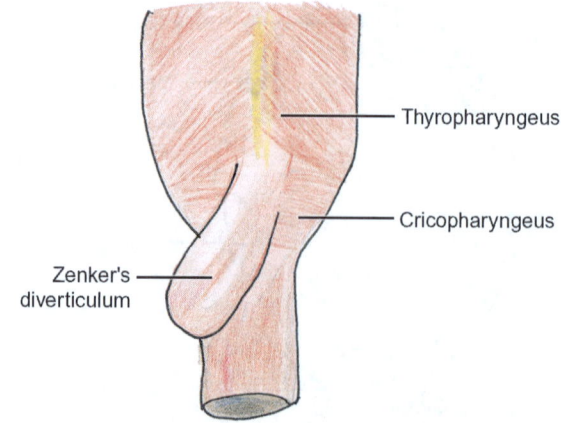

Fig. 26.6: Zenker's diverticulum (a posterior pouch)

The space in between the buccopharyngeal fascia anteriorly and the alar fascia posteriorly is known as retropharyngeal space.

The space in between the alar fascia anteriorly and prevertebral fascia posteriorly is known as Danger space or Alar space, please *see* below.

The space in between the prevertebral fascia anteriorly and vertebrae posteriorly is known as prevertebral space.

6. **Retropharyngeal space:** The retropharyngeal (behind the pharynx) space lies in between the buccopharyngeal fascia anteriorly and the alar fascia posteriorly. It starts superiorly at the base of skull and ends inferiorly at the bifurcation of trachea, i.e. T_4.

This space is divided in the midline by a fibrous raphe into two lateral spaces. These two spaces are known as **space of Gillette**. They contain lymph nodes known as **"nodes of Rouvier"**. Since this space is divided in the midline in two lateral spaces, an abscess of this space presents as a **unilateral paramedian bulge of the**

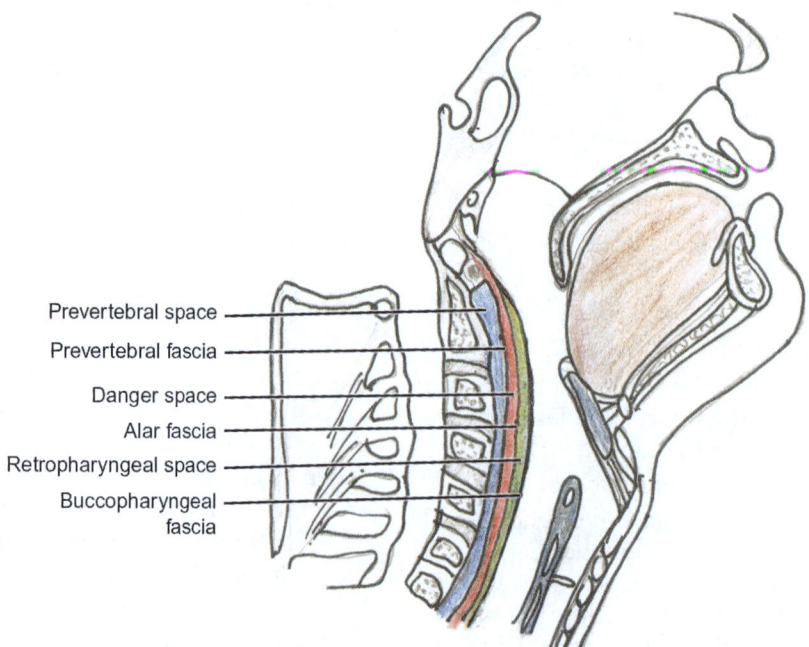

Fig. 26.7: The spaces in relation to pharynx

posterior pharyngeal wall on one side (either right or left) of the midline.

7. **Danger space:** The space in between the alar fascia anteriorly and prevertebral fascia posteriorly is known as Danger space or Alar space. It extends from the base of skull superiorly and extends through the posterior mediastinum to end inferiorly at the level of the diaphragm. It is a median space without a midline raphe and hence infection can spread easily to either side. **The danger space connects the deep cervical spaces to the mediastinum**.

It is dangerous because it is a potential path for spread of infections from the pharynx to the mediastinum. Abscess here can reach the mediastinum leading to mediastinitis, purulent pericarditis and cardiac tamponade, pleuritis, pyopneumothorax, empyema, or bronchial erosion.

8. **Prevertebral space:** The prevertebral space lies in between the prevertebral fascia anteriorly and vertebral bodies posteriorly. This space starts at the base of skull superiorly and extends down till the superior mediastinum where the prevertebral fascia is fused to the 4th thoracic vertebra.

Since this space is not divided in the midline so any abscess of prevertebral space is a **midline diffuse bulge of the posterior pharyngeal wall**.

9. **Parapharyngeal space (also called lateral pharyngeal or pharyngomaxillary space):** Just lateral to the pharyngeal wall is another space known as the parapharyngeal space. It communicates postero-medially with the retropharyngeal space of the same side.

The parapharyngeal space lies in between the lateral pharyngeal wall medially and the mandible (along with its attachments, i.e. medial pterygoid muscle on its medial surface and masseter muscle on its lateral surface) and parotid laterally. This space is in the form of inverted pyramid with base at the base of skull and apex below at the level of hyoid.

It is the smallest space of the pharynx but the most commonly infected.

The parapharyngeal space is divided into two compartments by the styloid process and the muscles attached to the styloid process:

a. Anterior compartment or **pre-styloid compartment:** It lies lateral to that part of lateral pharyngeal wall which contains tonsil. Hence any mass/abscess of this space will **push the tonsil medially** (by pushing lateral pharyngeal wall medially) and can be confused with peritonsillar abscess (also called Quinsy). *See* Chapters on Tonsils and Abscesses of pharynx.

The prestyloid compartment contains the maxillary artery and branches of the mandibular nerve (auriculotemporal, lingual and inferior alveolar).

b. Posterior compartment or **post-styloid compartment:** Through the posterior/poststyloid compartment pass very important structures from base of skull to neck or vice versa. They are internal carotid artery, internal jugular vein and the last 4 cranial nerves (9th, 10th, 11th and 12th) along with cervical sympathetic trunk (Fig. 26.8).

Any mass of post-styloid compartment will push the lateral pharyngeal wall medially producing a bulge of lateral pharyngeal wall behind the posterior pillar and also may lead to involvement of the above written important structures.

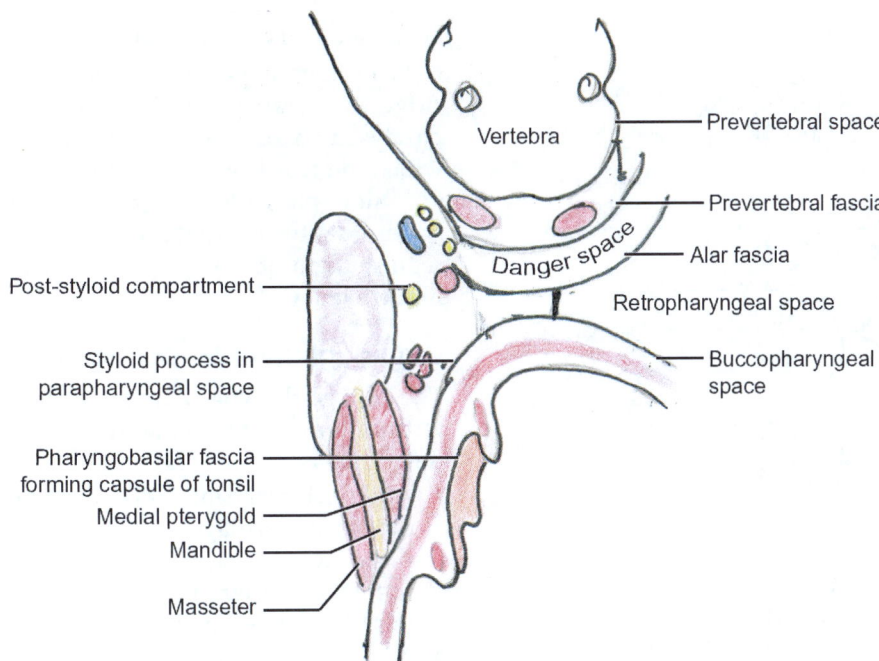

Fig. 26.8: Spaces of pharynx

Labels: Vertebra; Prevertebral space; Prevertebral fascia; Danger space; Alar fascia; Retropharyngeal space; Buccopharyngeal space; Post-styloid compartment; Styloid process in parapharyngeal space; Pharyngobasilar fascia forming capsule of tonsil; Medial pterygoid; Mandible; Masseter

CAVITY OF PHARYNX

Nasopharynx

Posterior Wall of Nasopharyngeal Cavity

In the posterior wall of nasopharynx at the junction of roof and posterior wall in the midline, is a collection of lymphoid tissue known as adenoids.

At the same site as adenoids, at the junction of roof and posterior wall, is a remnant of notochord present known as nasopharyngeal bursa or Thornwaldt's bursa.

Lateral Wall of Nasopharynx

The lateral wall of nasopharynx is the posterior continuation of the lateral wall of nose (the lateral wall of nose ends at the posterior ends of turbinates). In the lateral wall of nasopharynx from below upwards are the following structures (Fig. 26.9):

a. The **opening of Eustachian tube** is present in the lateral wall about 1.25 cm behind the posterior end of inferior turbinate.

    The cartilage of Eustachian tube produces a bulge above the Eustachian tube opening. This bulge is known as **Torus tubaris**.

b. Behind and above the bulge of Torus tubaris is a depression/fossa/recess also known as **fossa of Rosenmuller** or lateral pharyngeal recess. This is the most common site of origin of nasopharyngeal carcinoma.

c. In the lateral wall around 1 cm behind the posterior end of middle turbinate is the **sphenopalatine foramen**. This is the most common site for origin of angiofibroma. The sphenopalatine foramen connects the nasopharynx with the sphenopalatine fossa. The major vessels and nerves that supply the nose enter the nose through the sphenopalatine foramen from the sphenopalatine fossa.

The **sphenopalatine fossa** is a small pyramidal space lying posterior to the maxillary antrum. It is bounded anteriorly by the posterior wall of maxillary antrum and posteriorly by the anterior border of the pterygoid plates. Medially is the lateral wall of the nasopharynx (perpendicular plate of palatine bone), on which is the opening of sphenopalatine foramen. Laterally the fossa opens into the infratemporal fossa through the pterygomaxillary fissure (*see* Fig. 16.11, Chapter 16).

The contents of the sphenopalatine fossa are maxillary artery, maxillary nerve and the sphenopalatine (pterygopalatine) ganglion (the largest parasympathetic ganglion). Also *see* sphenopalatine foramen and fossa in Chapter 16.

Oropharynx

The oropharynx is bounded antero-superiorly by the soft palate and postero-superiorly it communicates with the nasopharynx through the nasopharyngeal isthmus (velopharyngeal isthmus).

In the **lateral wall** of the oropharynx is the palatine/faucial tonsil in between the anterior and the posterior pillars. The anterior pillar extends from the palate to the tongue and contains the palatoglossus muscle (this is the only muscle of the tongue which is supplied by pharyngeal plexus).

The posterior pillar extends from the palate to the pharyngeal wall and contains the longitudinal muscle of the pharynx, the palatopharyngeus muscle. The palatopharyngeus muscle also has circular fibres which go posteriorly in the posterior pharyngeal wall and along with the lower fibres of superior constrictor muscle forms a ridge known as **Passavant's ridge**.

When we eat or speak the words which do not have to pass through the nose, the soft palate moves posteriorly and meets the Passavant's ridge to close the nasopharyngeal/velopharyngeal isthmus.

When the soft palate is not able to meet the Passavant's ridge (e.g. cleft palate, bifid uvula, submucous cleft, paralysed palate) a gap is produced posteriorly through which the words which usually do not pass through the nose now pass and acquire nasal resonance (known as hypernasality or **rhinolalia aperta**) and also there is nasal regurgitation of food. This is known as **velopharyngeal insufficiency**.

Laryngopharynx/Hypopharynx

The laryngopharyngeal cavity can be visualised as a space with anterior, anterolateral and posterior limitations described as:

1. Anteriorly is the mucosa covering the posterior surface of cricoid cartilage, known as **postcricoid area**. The postcricoid area is the most common site of carcinoma in females suffering from Plummer-Vinson syndrome (also known as Paterson-Kelly-Brown syndrome).

2. Anterolaterally on both the sides a mucosal fold comes from the thyroid anteriorly to the cricoid posteriorly.

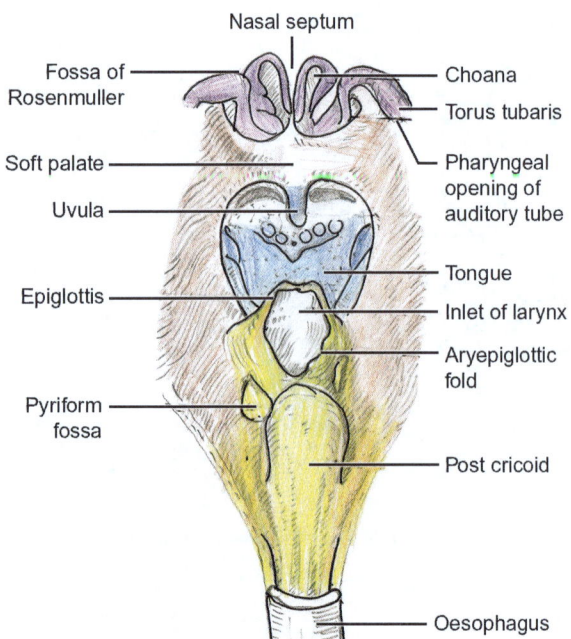

Nasal septum
Fossa of Rosenmuller
Choana
Torus tubaris
Soft palate
Pharyngeal opening of auditory tube
Uvula
Tongue
Epiglottis
Inlet of larynx
Aryepiglottic fold
Pyriform fossa
Post cricoid
Oesophagus

Fig. 26.9: The components of pharynx

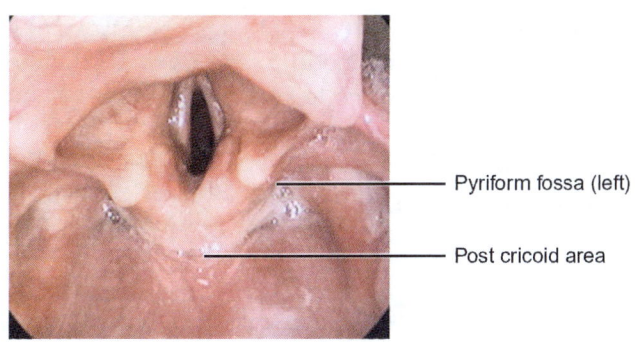

Pyriform fossa (left)

Post cricoid area

Fig. 26.10

These mucosal folds form what is known as the **pyriform fossae**.

The following are the significances of pyriform fossae:

a. The two pyriform fossae act as lateral channels for the passage of food from oropharynx down to the oesophagus.

b. They are also the site of lodgement of foreign body in the laryngopharynx.

c. The internal laryngeal nerve that passes in between the middle and inferior constrictor muscles lies very superficially (submucosally) in the pyriform fossa. This nerve gives sensory nerve supply to the larynx and hypopharynx above the level of true vocal cords.

So if we have to take a biopsy from any of these areas we will have to anaesthetise this nerve which can be done by putting anaesthetic packs in the pyriform fossa.

d. Pyriform fossae are the richest in lymphatics in the hypopharynx. So a carcinoma of the pyriform fossa metastasises very commonly to lymph nodes. This fossa drains into upper deep cervical lymph nodes.

3. **Posterior pharyngeal wall;** it is the posterior boundary of the hypopharynx.

Nerve Supply of Pharynx

• Sensory nerve supply of the nasopharynx is by maxillary nerve.

• Sensory supply of the oropharynx is mainly through glossopharyngeal and partly through maxillary nerve (lesser palatine nerve) except for the posterior most part of the base of tongue and vallecula where the sensations are given by the Vagus (internal laryngeal branch).

• Sensory supply of the hypopharynx is by Vagus (in the upper part by internal laryngeal and in the lower part by recurrent laryngeal).

• All the muscles of the pharynx are supplied by cranial part of accessory nerve through the branches of vagus (pharyngeal plexus) except for stylopharyngeus which is supplied by glossopharyngeal nerve.

• In addition to the pharyngeal plexus, the inferior constrictor also receives supply from recurrent laryngeal nerve.

"Points to Ponder/Points for Quick revision"

Cavity	Superior boundary	Inferior boundary	Anterior	Posterior	Lateral wall structures
Nasopharynx	Base of skull	Hard palate	Nose	Adenoids, Thornwaldt's bursa C1 vertebra	ET, Torus tubaris, fossa of Rosenmuller (Nasoph. Ca), spheno-palatine foramen (angiofibroma)
Oropharynx	Soft palate	Hyoid	Oral cavity	C2, C3	Faucial tonsils btw ant. & post pillars
Hypopharynx	Hyoid	Cricoid lower border	Larynx Post cricoid	C3, C4, C5, C6	Pyriform fossa

Spaces	Superior	Inferior	Anterior	Posterior	Contents
Retropharyngeal	Base of skull	T4	Bucco-pharyngeal fascia	Alar fascia	Space of Gillette, Nodes of Rouvier
Danger	Base of skull	Diaphragm	Alar fascia	Prevertebral fascia	—
Prevertebral	Base of skull	T4	Prevertebral fascia	Vertebrae	—

Space	Superior	Inferior	Medial	Lateral	Contents
Parapharyngeal (Smallest, MC—Infected)	Base of skull	Hyoid	Bucco-pharyngeal fascia/lateral pharyngeal wall	Medial pterygoid, Mandible, Masseter, parotid	Anterior compartment-branches of maxillary A & N; Post styloid compartment-ICA, IJV, CN - 9, 10 , 11, 12, cervical sympathetic chain

PREVIOUSLY ASKED QUESTIONS

1. **Not included in oral cavity cancers:** (*PGI May 2010*)
   a. Base of tongue   b. Gingivobuccal sulcus
   c. Soft palate   d. Hard palate
   e. Buccal mucosa

2. **The capsule of tonsil is formed by:** (*AI 2013*)
   a. Pharyngobasilar fascia
   b. Buccopharyngeal fascia
   c. Prevertebral fascia
   d. Mucosa

3. **Which is not a part of hypopharynx?**
   (*SRMC 2002, Exam 2016*)
   a. Posterior cricoid region
   b. Ary epiglottic folds
   c. Posterior pharyngeal wall
   d. Pyriform fossa

4. **Killian's dehiscence is seen in:**
   (*MH 2000, Exam 2017*)
   a. Oropharynx
   b. Nasopharynx
   c. Hypopharynx
   d. Vocal cords

5. **The Eustachian tube opens into nasopharynx approximately 1 cm behind the:** (*Exam 2013*)
   a. Tonsil
   b. Posterior end of superior turbinate
   c. Posterior end of middle turbinate
   d. Posterior end of inferior turbinate

6. **Which of the following structures is seen in oropharynx?** (*TN 2006, Exam 2017*)
   a. Pharyngotympanic tube
   b. Fossa of Rosenmüller
   c. Palatine tonsil
   d. Pyriform fossa

7. **Which of the following is not included in hypopharynx?** (*UP 2001, Exam 2017*)
   a. Pyriform fossa
   b. Post cricoid region
   c. Anterior pharyngeal wall
   d. Posterior pharyngeal wall

8. **Lower limit of hypopharynx is:** (*Exam 2013*)
   a. Lower border of cricoid cartilage
   b. Upper border of cricoid cartilage
   c. Upper border of thyroid cartilage
   d. Lower border of thyroid cartilage

9. **The lymphatic drainage of pyriform fossa is to:**
   (*Delhi 96, Exam 2013*)
   a. Upper deep cervical nodes
   b. Prelaryngeal node
   c. Parapharyngeal nodes
   d. Mediastinal nodes

10. **Nodes of Rouviere:** (*Exam 2013*)
    a. Retropharyngeal node
    b. Parapharyngeal node
    c. Adenoids
    d. None

11. **Gillette's space is:** (*Exam 2013*)
    a. Retropharyngeal space
    b. Peritonsillar space
    c. Parapharyngeal space
    d. None

12. **Danger space is located between:** (*AI 2013*)
    a. Buccopharyngeal and alar fascia
    b. Alar fascia and prevertebral fascia
    c. Buccopharyngeal and mandible
    d. Capsule of tonsil and superior constrictor muscle

13. **The nasopharynx is visualised in OPD by:**
    (*Exam 2013*)
    a. PNS mirror
    b. Tongue depressor
    c. Both PNS mirror and tongue depressor
    d. None

14. **The Waldeyer's group of lymph nodes do not include:** (*TN 2000, Exam 2017*)
    a. Submandibular lymph nodes
    b. Tonsils
    c. Lingual tonsils
    d. Adenoids

15. **Parapharyngeal space is also known as:**
    (*PGI June 2005, 2015*)
    a. Retropharyngeal space
    b. Pyriform sinus
    c. Lateral pharyngeal space
    d. Pharyngomaxillary space

16. **The medial bulging of pharynx is seen in:**
    (*AI 91, Exam 2016*)
    a. Parapharyngeal abscess
    b. Retropharyngeal abscess
    c. Peritonsillar abscess
    d. Paratonsillar abscess

17. **Trismus in parapharyngeal abscess is due to spasm of:** (*Exam 2015*)
    a. Masseter muscle
    b. Medial pterygoid
    c. Lateral pterygoid
    d. Temporalis

18. **True regarding nasopharynx:** (*PGI 2007, 2015*)
    a. Passavant's ridge is formed by stylopharyngeus
    b. Fossa of Rosenmüller corresponds to internal carotid artery
    c. Lower border of nasopharynx corresponds to faucial pillar
    d. Lower border lies at the level of soft palate

19. **Sinus of Morgagni lies in:** (*Exam 2016*)
    a. Between Superior and Middle constrictor
    b. Between Middle and Inferior constrictor
    c. Between Inferior constrictor and esophagus
    d. Between Base of skull and superior constrictor

20. **Adenoids are also called as:** (*Exam 2013*)
    a. Nasopharyngeal tonsils
    b. Palatine tonsils
    c. Faucial tonsil
    d. Lingual tonsil

21. **Gerlach's tonsil is:** (*Exam 2014*)
    a. Tubal tonsil   b. Palatine tonsil
    c. Pharyngeal tonsil   d. Lingual tonsil

22. **Space of Gillette is:** (*Exam 2015*)
    a. Retropharyngeal space
    b. Peritonsillar space
    c. Parapharyngeal space
    d. Pre laryngeal space

23. **The nerve carrying taste sensation from the circumvallate papillae is _____.**
    (*MH CET 2016, Exam 2016*)
    a. Lingual
    b. Chorda tympani
    c. Glossopharyngeal
    d. Hypoglossal

24. **What is the type of epithelium of the adenoid?**
    (*Exam 2015*)
    a. Pseudostratified ciliated columnar epithelium
    b. Non keratinized squamous epithelium
    c. Cuboidal epithelium
    d. Keratinized squamous epithelium

25. **Epipharynx is also called:** (*Exam 2015*)
    a. Nasopharynx   b. Oropharynx
    c. Laryngopharynx   d. Hypopharynx

26. **Passavant's ridge is formed by:** (*Exam 2015*)
    a. Cricopharyngeus and superior constrictor
    b. Palatopharyngeus and superior constrictor
    c. Palatoglossus and superior constrictor
    d. Thyropharyngeus and superior constrictor

27. **Lower limit of retropharyngeal space is at:**
    (*Exam 2015*)
    a. C7
    b. Bifurcation of trachea
    c. 4th esophageal constriction
    d. None

28. **In carcinoma base of tongue pain is referred to the ear through:** (*Exam 2016*)
    a. Hypoglossal nerve
    b. Vagus nerve
    c. Glossopharyngeal nerve
    d. Lingual nerve

IMAGE BASED PRACTICE QUESTIONS BY THE AUTHOR

29. **The marked structure in the Waldeyer's ring is:**

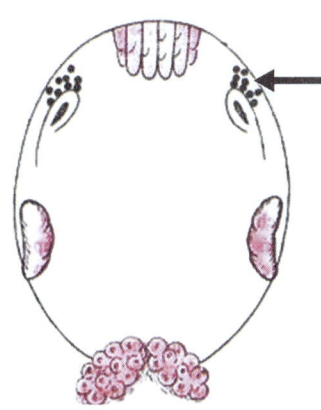

    a. Nasopharyngeal tonsil
    b. Lingual tonsil
    c. Faucial tonsil
    d. Tubal tonsil

30. **The structures passing through the area marked 1 in the figure below showing the pharyngeal musculature are all except:**

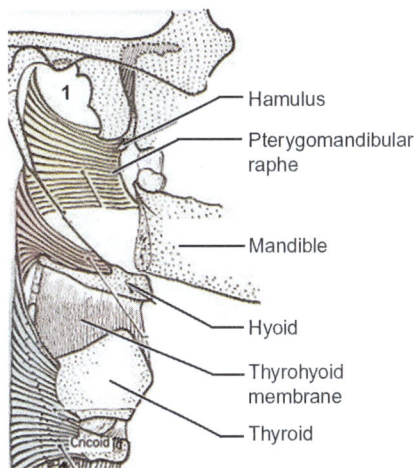

    a. Tensor tympani
    b. Eustachian tube
    c. Ascending palatine artery
    d. Levator palati

31. **The most common site of origin of the diverticulum of the pharynx seen in the barium swallow given below is:**

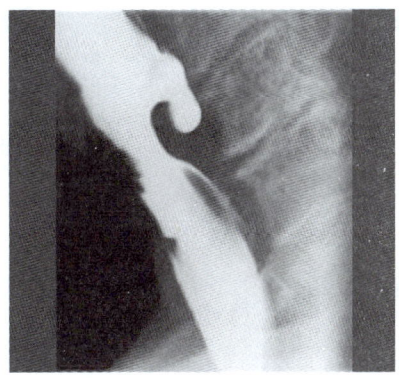

Oral Cavity and Pharynx

Section III

a. Between stylopharyngeus and palatopharyngeus
b. Between middle and inferior constrictor
c. Between inferior constrictor and esophagus
d. Between thyropharyngeus and cricopharyngeus

32. **The space through which the arrow in the picture is passing is:**

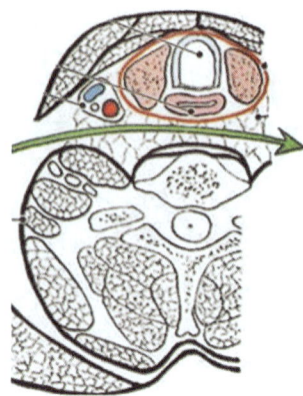

a. Retropharyngeal space
b. Peritonsillar space
c. Prevertebral space
d. Pre laryngeal space

33. **The nerves and vessels shown in the figure below are passing through:**

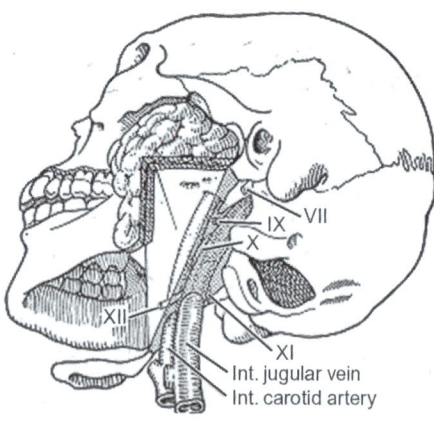

a. Retropharyngeal space
b. Parapharyngeal space
c. Prevertebral space
d. Sphenopalatine fossa

34. **Not true about the area marked in the given figure is:**

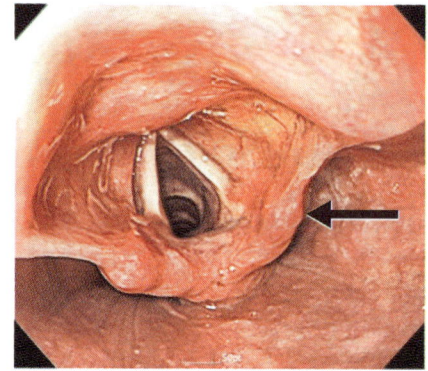

a. It is the lateral channel for passage of food
b. It is the most common site for carcinoma in Plummer-Vinson syndrome
c. It is the site of foreign body lodgement
d. It is a part of hypopharynx

35. **The area marked in the given picture is supplied by:**

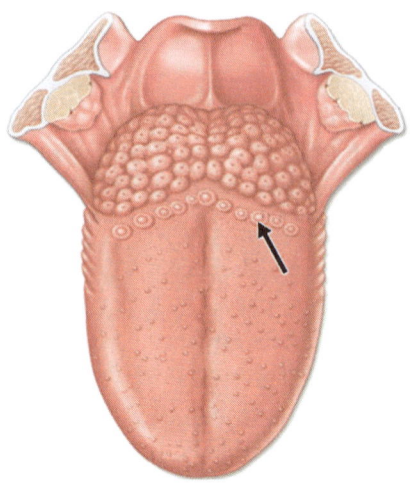

a. Lingual nerve
b. Glossopharyngeal nerve
c. Vagus nerve
d. Vidian nerve

36. **Pain from the given part of tongue is referred to the ear by:**

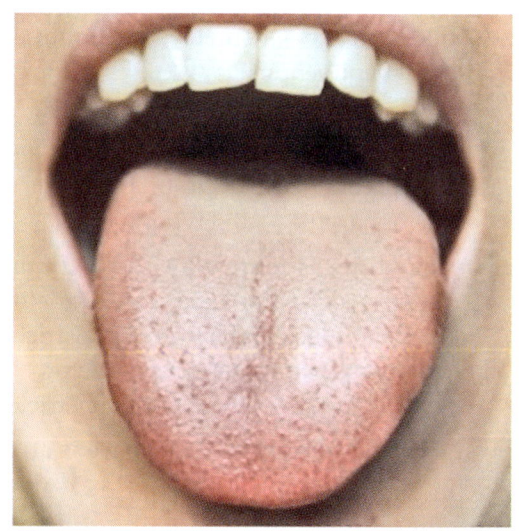

a. Lingual nerve
b. Glossopharyngeal nerve
c. Chorda tympani
d. Greater auricular nerve

37. **Tongue muscles are derived from:**   (*Exam 2018*)
a. 1st arch
b. 2nd arch
c. Occipital myotomes
d. Ultimo-branchial body

ANSWERS AND EXPLANATIONS

1. **(a), (c) Base of tongue, Soft palate** (*Ref. Scott Brown, Vol 3; 633*)
   - Base of tongue and soft palate are parts of oropharynx.

2. **(a) Pharyngobasilar fascia** (*Ref. Scott Brown, Vol 3; 741*)

3. **(b) Ary epiglottic folds** (*Ref. Scott Brown, Vol 3; 743*)
   - Aryepiglottic folds are the upper border of the quadrangular membrane which is the intrinsic membrane of larynx (please read Chapter on anatomy of larynx)
   - The 3 Ps, i.e. post cricoid region, pyriform fossa and posterior pharyngeal wall constitutes hypo- or laryngopharynx.

4. **(c) Hypopharynx** (*Ref. Scott Brown, Vol 3; 745*)
   - In between the two parts of inferior constrictor, i.e. the thyropharyngeus and cricopharyngeus is a gap which is known as Killian's dehiscence. This is the most common site for the development of pharyngeal pouch. The pharyngeal pouch that forms from here is known as Zenker's diverticulum. It lies in the hypopharynx/laryngopharynx. This area of the hypopharynx in relation to the cricoid is also known as cricopharynx.

5. **(d) Posterior end of inferior turbinate** (*Ref. Scott Brown, Vol 3; 738*)
   - Eustachian tube opens in the lateral wall of nasopharynx about 1.25 cm behind the posterior end of inferior turbinate.
   - Around 1 cm behind the posterior end of middle turbinate is the sphenopalatine foramen. This is the most common site for origin of angiofibroma.
   - There is no opening behind the superior turbinate.
   - Tonsils are present in the oropharynx.

6. **(c) Palatine tonsil** (*Ref. Scott Brown, Vol 3; 739*)
   - Palatine tonsil lies in the lateral wall of oropharynx.
   - Pharyngotympanic tube or Eustachian tube and Fossa of Rosenmüller is present in the lateral wall of nasopharynx .
   - Pyriform fossa is a component of the hypo- or laryngopharynx.

7. **(c) Anterior pharyngeal wall** (*Ref. Scott Brown, Vol 3; 743*)
   - Anterior pharyngeal wall is no entity. Anterior to the hypopharynx is the larynx. Anterior to the nasopharynx and oropharynx are nasal and oral cavities respectively.

8. **(a) Lower border of cricoid cartilage** (*Ref. Scott Brown, Vol 3; 742*)
   - Hypopharynx extends from the hyoid to the lower border of cricoid cartilage

9. **(a) Upper deep cervical nodes** (*Ref. Scott Brown, Vol 3; 751*)
   - Pyriform fossa is the richest in lymphatics in the hypopharynx.
   - It drains into upper deep cervical lymph nodes.

10. **(a) Retropharyngeal node** (*Ref. Scott Brown, Vol 3; 94*)
    - Nodes of Rouvier are the lymph nodes present in the retropharyngeal space of Gillette.
    - Adenoids is known as Lushka or nasopharyngeal tonsil.

11. **(a) Retropharyngeal space** (*Ref. Dhingra, 6th ed., 265*)
    - The retropharyngeal space is divided by a midline fibrous raphe into two spaces known as space of Gillette.
    - Parapharyngeal space is known as pharyngo-maxillary space or lateral pharyngeal space.
    - Peritonsillar space is the space between the capsule of tonsil and the circular muscles of pharynx. This contains a loose areolar tissue. Infection of this space is known as quinsy.

12. **(b) Alar fascia and prevertebral fascia** (*Ref. Scott Brown, Vol 3; 551*)
    - In between buccopharyngeal and alar fascia is the retropharyngeal space.
    - In between buccopharyngeal and mandible is the parapharyngeal space.
    - In between capsule of tonsil and superior constrictor muscle is peritonsillar space.

13. **(c) Both PNS (postnasal space) mirror and tongue depressor** (*Ref. Scott Brown, Vol 3; 98*)
    - To examine nasopharynx or post nasal space in OPD, posterior rhinoscopy is done.
    - Here the tongue is depressed using a tongue depressor and then the PNS mirror is passed behind the uvula. The glass surface of the PNS mirror is pre warmed so as to avoid mist formation, due to patient's breath, during examination.

14. **(a) Submandibular lymph nodes** (*Ref. Scott Brown, Vol 3; 741*)
    Please refer to the text for the components of the Waldeyer's group of lymphatics.

15. **(c) and (d)** (*Ref. Scott Brown, Vol 3; 624*)
    - Parapharyngeal space is also known as lateral pharyngeal space or pharyngomaxillary space.

16. **(a) Parapharyngeal abscess** (*Ref. Scott Brown, Vol 3; 551*)
    - Just lateral to the pharyngeal wall is the space known as the parapharyngeal space or pharyngomaxillary space.
    - Any mass/abscess of this space will push the lateral pharyngeal wall medially ultimately also leading to the tonsils being pushed medially.
    - It can be confused with peritonsillar abscess where also the tonsils are pushed medially.
    - Peritonsillar abscess or Quinsy is the collection of pus in the loose areolar space lateral to the capsule of the tonsil. So here only the tonsil is pushed medially in contrast to whole of the lateral pharyngeal wall in parapharyngeal abscess.
    - Retropharyngeal abscess presents with U/L paramedian bulge of the posterior pharyngeal wall.
    - There is no entity called paratonsillar abscess.

17. **(b) Medial pterygoid** (*Ref. Scott Brown, Vol 3; 551*)
   - Trismus can be because of the involvement of any of the given masseteric muscles (i.e. medial and lateral pterygoid, masseter and temporalis) but in parapharyngeal space abscess, trismus is mainly because of spasm of medial pterygoid muscle which lies just opposed to the parapharyngeal space laterally (it being attached to the medial aspect of mandible).

18. **(b) and (d)** (*Ref. Scott Brown, Vol 3; 738*)
   - Fossa of Rosenmüller lies in the lateral wall of nasopharynx. Lateral to the lateral pharyngeal wall of nasopharynx and oropharynx is the parapharyngeal space through which passes the internal carotid artery.
   - Passavant's ridge is formed by palatopharyngeus.
   - Lower border of nasopharynx extends till the hard palate/soft palate.

19. **(d) Between base of skull and superior constrictor** (*Ref. Scott Brown, Vol 3; 747, Chaurasia, 6th ed., Vol 3, 234*)

20. **(a) Nasopharyngeal tonsils** (*Ref. Scott Brown, Vol 3; 738*)

21. **(a) Tubal tonsil** (*Ref. Scott Brown, Vol 1; 285*)

22. **(a) Retropharyngeal space** (*Ref. Dhingra, 6th ed., 265*)

23. **(c) Glossopharyngeal** (*Ref. Scott Brown, Vol 3; 643*)

24. **(a) Pseudostratified ciliated columnar epithelium** (*Ref. Scott Brown, Vol 3; 739*)

25. **(a) Nasopharynx** (*Ref. Dhingra, 6th ed., 238*)

26. **(b) Palatopharyngeus and superior constrictor** (*Ref. Scott Brown, Vol 3; 746*)

27. **(b) Bifurcation of trachea** (*Ref. Scott Brown, Vol 3; 551*)

28. **(c) Glossopharyngeal nerve** (*Ref. Cummings, 6th ed., 1364, Scott Brown, Vol 3; 643*)
   - The base of tongue is mainly supplied by the glossopharyngeal nerve which also supplies the ear.

 Note: _____

- Anterior 2/3rds of tongue is supplied by lingual nerve (a branch of mandibular). Auriculotemporal nerve also a branch of mandibular nerve supplies the ear so in carcinoma anterior 2/3rds of tongue pain is referred to ear through mandibular nerve.
- Posterior 1/3rd, i.e. the base of the tongue is mainly supplied by glossopharyngeal nerve and the posterior most part of this posterior 1/3rd tongue is supplied by vagus, both of which also supply the ear, so in carcinoma of this part of tongue, pain will be referred to ear through both glossopharyngeal and vagus.
- But since glossopharyngeal supplies most of the base of the tongue so in pathologies of base of tongue the pain is referred to the ear mainly through the glossopharyngeal nerve.

29. **(d) Tubal tonsil** (*Ref. Scott Brown, Vol 3; 741*)

30. **(a) Tensor tympani** (*Ref. Scott Brown, Vol 3; 747*)
   The sinus of Morgagni is being shown

31. **(d) Between thyropharyngeus and cricopharyngeus** (*Ref. Scott Brown, Vol 3; 746*)
   - The given picture is the barium swallow showing Zenker's diverticulum

32. **(a) Retropharyngeal space** (*Ref. Scott Brown, Vol 3; 549*)

33. **(b) Parapharyngeal space** (*Ref. Scott Brown, Vol 3; 550*)

34. **(b) It is the most common site for carcinoma in Plummer-Vinson syndrome** (*Ref. Scott Brown, Vol 3; 742*)
   - Left sided pyriform fossa is being shown
   - Most common site for carcinoma in Plummer-Vinson syndrome is the postcricoid area

35. **(b) Glossopharyngeal nerve** (*Ref. Scott Brown, Vol 3; 643*)

36. **(a) Lingual nerve** (*Ref. Scott Brown, Vol 3; 643*)

37. **(c) Occipital myotomes** (*Ref. Human Embryology I, B Singh, 10th ed., 176*)

Adenoid Hypertrophy and Thornwaldt's Bursitis

In any disease of the nasopharynx the patient will have three main complaints:

1. Nasal obstruction
2. Eustachian tube obstruction leading to serous otitis media
3. Rhinolalia clausa (denasal/hyponasal voice due to nasal obstruction).

THORNWALDT'S BURSITIS/NASOPHARYNGEAL BURSITIS

Thornwaldt's bursitis is infection of the Thornwaldt's bursa. Thornwaldt's bursa or pharyngeal bursa is an inconstant blind sac located in the midline. It is present as a median recess at the junction of the roof and posterior wall of nasopharynx (in the same area as the adenoid). It extends from the mucosa of the nasopharynx to the occiput. It represents persistence of an embryonic communication between the roof of the primitive pharynx and the notochord. The opening of the bursa might get closed due to infection leading to cyst or abscess formation.

Clinical Features

Besides the above 3 common features of nasopharyngeal disease, the other symptoms, here are:

a. Persistent post nasal drip (due to bursitis)
b. Occipital headache
c. Sore throat and fever

Treatment

Antibiotics covering gram-positive and anaerobic organisms.

If cyst or abscess formation occurs then marsupialisation or cyst excision by transpalatal route is done.

ADENOID HYPERTROPHY

Adenoid or **Nasopharyngeal tonsil** is a collection of lymphoid tissue present at the junction of roof and posterior wall of nasopharynx.

Adenoid tissue is present at birth but it is not completely developed. Its hypertrophy starts at 2 years and continues till 6 years of age, after which its growth plateaus. The adenoids start to atrophy by puberty and usually disappear by 20 years of age.

There are vertical ridges on the surface of adenoid making it appear multiple, hence called adenoids.

Unlike tonsils, adenoids do not have any crypts or capsule.

Clinical Features

Any child with significant adenoid hypertrophy will present with the following:

a. **Nasal obstruction:** Because of nasal obstruction the nose is not being used for breathing leading to disuse atrophy of the nose. This leads to **absence of alar prominence** and also loss of nasolabial crease, giving the nose a pinched up appearance.

The child now respires through mouth leading to **open mouth, crowding and prominence of anterior upper teeth and high arched palate**. All these lead to dental malocclusion.

Because of nasal obstruction the child can have recurrent sinusitis. Because of repeated infections there may be **failure to thrive** (i.e. inadequate weight gain according to age).

b. **Eustachian tube obstruction:** Since adenoid is a midline mass it leads to obstruction of Eustachian tube of both sides leading to **bilateral serous otitis media** and conductive hearing loss which gives the child a **dull look** on the face (this is because of the hearing defect). The child seems lost during normal conversations.

The child can also have recurrent attacks of acute otitis media (here infection spreads to the middle ear through the Eustachian tube).

This appearance of the face with pinched up nose, absent nasolabial crease, open mouth, crowded and prominent upper teeth along with a dull look on face is known as **adenoid facies**.

c. **Rhinolalia clausa:** Due to obstruction in the nasopharynx the child has denasal/hyponasal voice.

d. **Sleep apnoea:** Chronic adenoid hypertrophy is frequently associated with tonsillar hypertrophy. This leads to sleep apnoea leading to day time somnolence.

More than 30 apnoeas (an episode of apnoea means cessation of respiration for more than 10 sec) in 7 hrs of sleep is known as sleep apnoea.

Long standing sleep apnoea causes hypoxemia leading to pulmonary vasoconstriction (please note that hypoxemia leads to vasodilatation everywhere except in pulmonary arteries where it causes vasoconstriction). This leads to pulmonary hypertension and cor pulmonale (right-sided heart failure due to pulmonary pathology).

Diagnosis

Adenoid size assessment is done by direct visualisation by **endoscopy** and **X-ray nose and nasopharynx lateral view**. See the X-ray soft tissue neck lateral view given below, the arrow pointing towards the hypertrophied adenoid mass in the nasopharynx.

Management

Acute adenoiditis should be treated by antibiotics, antihistaminics and decongestants.

If the patient does not benefit by medical management of at least 6 weeks and results in the following complications, due to now chronic significant adenoid hypertrophy, then he should be taken up for adenoidectomy. The following are the **indications for adenoidectomy**:

1. **Recurrent sinusitis** due to nasal obstruction.
2. Recurrent ear infections/chronic serous otitis media and recurrent ear discharge in a patient of safe CSOM due to Eustachian tube obstruction.
3. **Sleep apnoea**.
4. **Dental malocclusion**—following adenoidectomy the dental malocclusion, if has already occurred, does not regress but it also does not progress.

The **contraindications for adenoidectomy** are:

a. **In Velopharyngeal insufficiency** (e.g. cleft palate, submucous cleft, bifid uvula and palatal paralysis) the soft palate is not able to move posteriorly and meet the Passavant's ridge to close the nasopharyngeal (or Velopharyngeal) isthmus. So a gap is present posteriorly because of which the child has hypernasality and nasal regurgitation of food. If such a child has hypertrophied adenoids, the soft palate touches the hypertrophied adenoids and closes the nasopharyngeal isthmus and the above features are not seen.

    Following adenoidectomy such a child will present with features of Velopharyngeal insufficiency. In such a child with cleft palate and features of adenoid hypertrophy, cleft palate repair is done first and adenoidectomy is planned on a later date.

b. **Acute adenoiditis** (chances of haemorrhage and septicaemia are high in acute infection).

c. Bleeding disorders

Complications of adenoidectomy

1. Haemorrhage: The most common complication of adenoidectomy is haemorrhage. It can be managed by postnasal pack.
2. Hypernasality: This can be caused by unrecognised pre-existing velopharyngeal insufficiency.
3. Eustachian tube injury leading to its stenosis.

4. A rare complication of adenoidectomy is Grisel's syndrome. Grisel's syndrome is inflammatory subluxation of the atlanto-axial joint and can result following local postoperative inflammation or infection. The child presents with postoperative neck pain, neck stiffness and fever. It usually recovers by cervical immobilization and antibiotics.

Surgical technique used for adenoidectomy

- This is nowadays done under endoscopic visualisation by cold or hot method in Roses position (*see* Chapter 30). Previously it used to be done blindly.
- Cold method is removal of adenoids by adenoid curette or microdebrider.
- Hot method is by electrocautery.

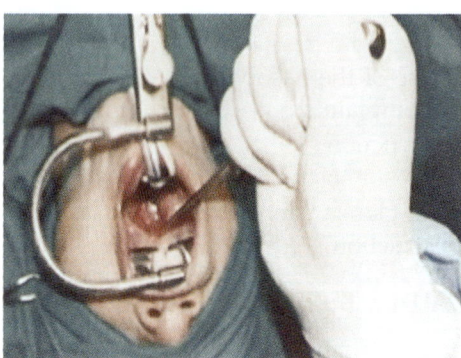

Fig. 27.1: Adenoidectomy being done by blind curettage in Roses position

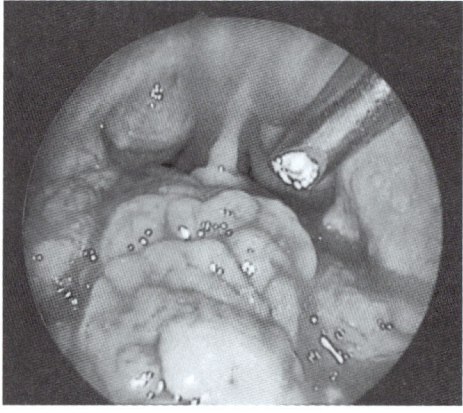

Fig. 27.2: Adenoidectomy being done by microdebrider under endoscopic visualisation

"Points to Ponder/Points for Quick revision"

- Thornwaldt's bursitis/nasopharyngeal bursitis: T/t antibiotics, Marsupialisation, Excision.
- Adenoids (nasopharyngeal tonsils): Physiological hypertrophy (2 yrs till puberty) → Regression.
- Adenoiditis CFs: 1. Adenoid Facies 2. Recurrent Sinusitis → AOM 3. B/L SOM → CHL 4. Rhinolalia Clausa 5. Sleep apnoea.
- Size assessment: Endoscopy, X-ray Nose & PNS lateral view
- Indications for adenoidectomy: Chronic CFs 2 to 5.
- Contraindications: Velopharyngeal insufficiency, acute infection, bleeding disorders.
- Complications: Haemorrhage (MC), Unveiling of Velopharyngeal insufficiency (if done in cleft palate).

PREVIOUSLY ASKED QUESTIONS

1. Thornwaldt's cyst: *(Exam 2013)*
   a. Laryngeal cyst
   b. Nasopharyngeal cyst
   c. Ear cyst
   d. None

2. Thornwaldt's abscess false is: *(Exam 2013)*
   a. Antibiotics
   b. Marsupialisation
   c. Removal of cyst
   d. Anti-tubercular treatment

3. Adenoids are also called: *(Exam 2013)*
   a. Nasopharyngeal tonsils
   b. Palatine tonsils
   c. Faucial tonsils
   d. Lingual tonsils

4. A 5-year-old child with recurrent sinusitis, cause is: *(Exam 2013)*
   a. Adenoids
   b. Angiofibroma
   c. Nasal carcinoma
   d. All of the above

5. Regarding adenoids true is/are: *(PGI 2002, 2015)*
   a. There is failure to thrive
   b. Mouth breathing is seen
   c. CT scan should be done to assess size
   d. High arched palate is present
   e. Immediate surgery even for minor symptoms

6. True about enlarged adenoids: *(Exam 2013)*
   a. Mouth breathing
   b. Failure to thrive
   c. High arched palate
   d. All

7. Adenoidectomy is contraindicated in: *(Exam 2013)*
   a. Large adenoids
   b. Large tonsils
   c. Cleft lip
   d. Cleft palate

8. Adenoidectomy contraindicated in: *(Exam 2013)*
   a. SOM
   b. CSOM
   c. Bleeding disorder
   d. None

9. Adenoids hypertrophy with symptoms treatment is all except: *(Exam 2013)*
   a. Nasal decongestants
   b. Antibiotics
   c. β_2 agonists
   d. adenoidectomy

10. Indication for adenoidectomy in children includes all except: *(AP 2000, Exam 2017)*
    a. Recurrent upper respiratory tract infections
    b. Recurrent middle ear infection with deafness
    c. Chronic serous otitis media
    d. Multiple adenoids

11. Adenoidectomy with grommet insertion is treatment of choice for: *(Exam 2013)*
    a. Serous otitis media in children
    b. Serous otitis media in adults
    c. Adenoiditis in children
    d. All of the above

12. Management of a 6-year-old child with recurrent URTI with mouth breathing and failure to thrive with high arched palate and impaired hearing is: *(AI 2010)*
    a. Tonsillectomy
    b. Grommet insertion
    c. Myringotomy with grommet insertion
    d. Adenoidectomy with grommet insertion

13. Rhinolalia clausa is associated with the following except: *(AI 2007, Exam 2017)*
    a. Adenoids
    b. Allergic rhinitis
    c. Palatal paralysis
    d. Nasal polyps

14. In a patient with hypertrophied adenoids the voice abnormality that is seen is: *(JIPMER 2000/Exam 2017)*
    a. Rhinolalia clausa
    b. Rhinolalia aperta
    c. Hot potato voice
    d. Staccato voice

15. Complications of adenoidectomy are all except: *(Exam 2015)*
    a. Hyponasality of speech
    b. Velopharyngeal insufficiency
    c. Hemorrhage
    d. Grisel's syndrome

16. Child with adenoids hypertrophy and blockage of Eustachian tube has future risk for: *(JIPMER 2015)*
    a. Primary acquired cholesteatoma
    b. Secondary acquired cholesteatoma
    c. Congenital cholesteatoma
    d. Otosclerosis

17. Dodd sign is seen in: *(Exam 2015)*
    a. Antrochoanal polyp
    b. Angiofibroma
    c. Nasopharyngeal carcinoma
    d. Adenoid hypertrophy

18. What is the type of epithelium of the adenoid: *(Exam 2016)*
    a. Pseudostratified ciliated columnar epithelium
    b. Non-keratinized squamous epithelium
    c. Cuboidal epithelium
    d. Keratinized squamous epithelium

19. All of the following are features of enlarged adenoids except: *(Exam 2016)*
    a. Serous otitis media
    b. Nasal obstruction
    c. Failure to thrive of child
    d. Odynophagia

20. Speech problem after adenoidectomy is due to: *(Exam 2016)*
    a. Trauma to larynx
    b. Velopharyngeal insufficiency
    c. Trauma to vocal cord
    d. Trauma to superior constrictor

Oral Cavity and Pharynx

Section III

21. **A 5-year-old child after adenoidectomy developed hypernasality and nasal regurgitation of food. What could be the cause?** *(Exam 2016)*
    a. Velopharyngeal insufficiency
    b. Glossopharyngeal nerve injury
    c. Reactionary hemorrhage
    d. Trauma to soft palate

IMAGE BASED PRACTICE QUESTIONS BY THE AUTHOR

22. **This 6-year-old child presents with recurrent URTI, with mouth breathing, with high arched palate and impaired hearing. This appearance is known as:**

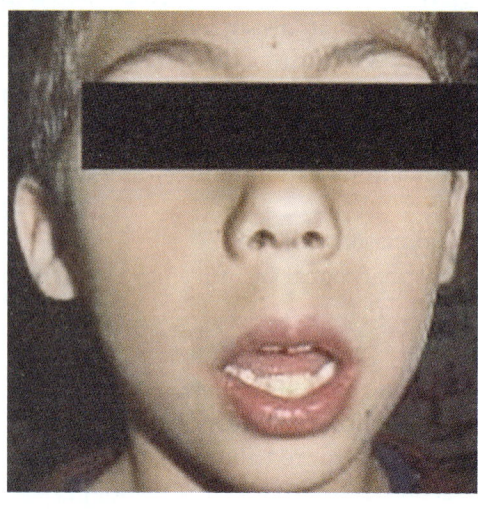

    a. Fish mouth appearance
    b. Frog facies

    c. Adenoid facies
    d. Leonine facies

23. **A 5-year-old child presents with recurrent URTI with mouth breathing and snoring. His X-ray STN is given below. This child should be advised for adenoidectomy if the following are present except:**

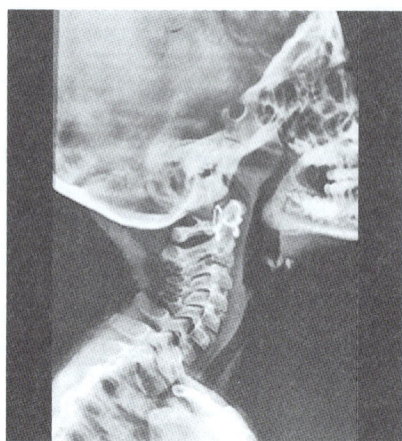

    a. Recurrent upper respiratory tract infections and sinusitis
    b. Recurrent middle ear infection with deafness
    c. Sleep apnoea
    d. Hypernasality

24. **Pharyngeal bursa gives origin to:** *(Exam 2017)*
    a. Thornwaldt's cyst
    b. Chordoma
    c. Craniopharyngioma
    d. Tubal tonsils

ANSWERS AND EXPLANATIONS

1. **(b) Nasopharyngeal cyst** (*Ref. Cummings, 6th ed., 1420*)

2. **(d) Anti-tubercular treatment** (*Ref. Cummings, 6th ed., 1421*)

3. **(a) Nasopharyngeal tonsils** (*Ref. Scott Brown Vol 3; 738*)
   - Palatine tonsils are also known as faucial tonsils Lingual tonsils are present in the base of tongue.

4. **(a) Adenoids** (*Ref. Scott Brown, Vol 2; 286*)
   - Because of nasal obstruction the child can have recurrent sinusitis. Angiofibroma and nasopharyngeal carcinoma are not seen at this age.

5. **(a) (b) and (d) options are true** (*Ref. Scott Brown, Vol 2; 286*)
   - Endoscopy and X-ray nose and nasopharynx (lateral view) are done for assessing the size.
   - Indications for doing adenoidectomy are various complications arising out of clinically significant adenoid hypertrophy (please refer to the text).

6. **(d) all** (*Ref. Scott Brown, Vol 2; 286*)

7. **(d) Cleft palate** (*Ref. Scott Brown, 6th ed., 6/18/12*)
   - Adenoidectomy in a child with cleft palate will lead to nasopharyngeal/velopharyngeal insufficiency so it is a contraindication.
   - Large adenoids causing complications as discussed in the text is an indication of adenoidectomy.
   - In a child who is simultaneously suffering due to large tonsils, tonsillectomy is done along with adenoidectomy in the same sitting.
   - Cleft lip does not lead to nasopharyngeal/velopharyngeal insufficiency after adenoidectomy.

8. **(c) Bleeding disorder** (*Ref. Scott Brown, 6th ed., 6/18/12*)

9. **(c) β_2 agonists** (*Ref. Scott Brown, Vol 2; 288*)
   - β_2 agonists (salbutamol/terbutaline) have no role in respiratory obstruction due to adenoids. They are used in lower airway obstruction diseases, e.g. asthma, etc.

10. **(d) Multiple adenoids** (*Ref. Scott Brown, Vol 2; 286*)
    - Multiple adenoids are no term. Adenoid tissues normally have vertical ridges on its surface which makes it appear multiple that is why the term adenoids instead of adenoid.

11. **(a) Serous otitis media in children** (*Ref. Scott Brown, Vol 2; 286*)
    - Adenoids start to atrophy by puberty so will not lead to SOM in an adult.

- Adenoidectomy with grommet insertion is done for Serous otitis media due to persistently hypertrophied adenoids in children.

12. **(d) Adenoidectomy with grommet insertion** (*Ref. Scott Brown, Vol 2; 288*)
    - Recurrent URTI with mouth breathing and failure to thrive in the given 6-year-old child with high arched palate is due to persistently hypertrophied adenoids.
    - The impaired hearing is due to serous otitis media which in turn is because of hypertrophied adenoids blocking the Eustachian tubes.
    - So treatment will be adenoidectomy with grommet insertion.

13. **(c) Palatal paralysis** (*Ref. Scott Brown, Vol 2; 181*)
    - Palatal paralysis leads to Rhinolalia aperta.

14. **(a) Rhinolalia clausa** (*Ref. Scott Brown, Vol 2; 181*)
    - Rhinolalia clausa means denasal or hyponasal voice. It is seen in conditions causing obstruction of nose and nasopharynx, e.g. adenoids, nasal polyps, allergic rhinitis and any nasal or nasopharyngeal mass.
    - Rhinolalia aperta means hypernasality seen in conditions causing velopharyngeal insufficiency, e.g. cleft palate, submucous cleft, bifid palate and palatal palsy.
    - Hot potato voice or muffled speech is seen in painful oropharyngeal conditions, e.g. quinsy.
    - Staccato voice along with scanning speech is seen in multiple sclerosis and Friedreich's and other ataxias. They occur due to cerebellar dysfunction. In these the articulation is slow, ataxic, and jerky or explosive owing to asynergy of the muscles of phonation.

15. **(a) Hyponasality of speech** (*Ref. Scott Brown, Vol 2; 289*)

16. **(a) Primary acquired cholesteatoma** (*Ref. Cummings 6th ed., 2143*)
    - Adenoid hypertrophy leading to prolonged blockage of Eustachian tube can result in retraction pocket formation and primary acquired cholesteatoma.

17. **(a) Antrochoanal polyp** (*Ref. Dhingra, 6th ed., 175; https://pinterest.com*)
    Refer to Chapter 21

18. **(a) Pseudostratified ciliated columnar epithelium** (*Ref. Scott Brown, Vol 3; 739*)

19. **(d) Odynophagia** (*Ref. Scott Brown, Vol 3; 739*)

20. **(b) Velopharyngeal insufficiency** (*Ref. Cummings, 6th ed., 2935*)

21. **(a) Velopharyngeal insufficiency** (*Ref. Cummings, 6th ed., 2935; Ref. Scott Brown, Vol 2; 181*)

22. **(c) Adenoid facies** (*Ref. Cummings, 6th ed., 2881*)

23. **(d) Hypernasality** (*Ref. Scott Brown, Vol 2; 289*)

24. **(a) Thornwaldt's cyst** (*Ref. Cummings, 6th ed., 1420*)

Section III   Oral Cavity and Pharynx

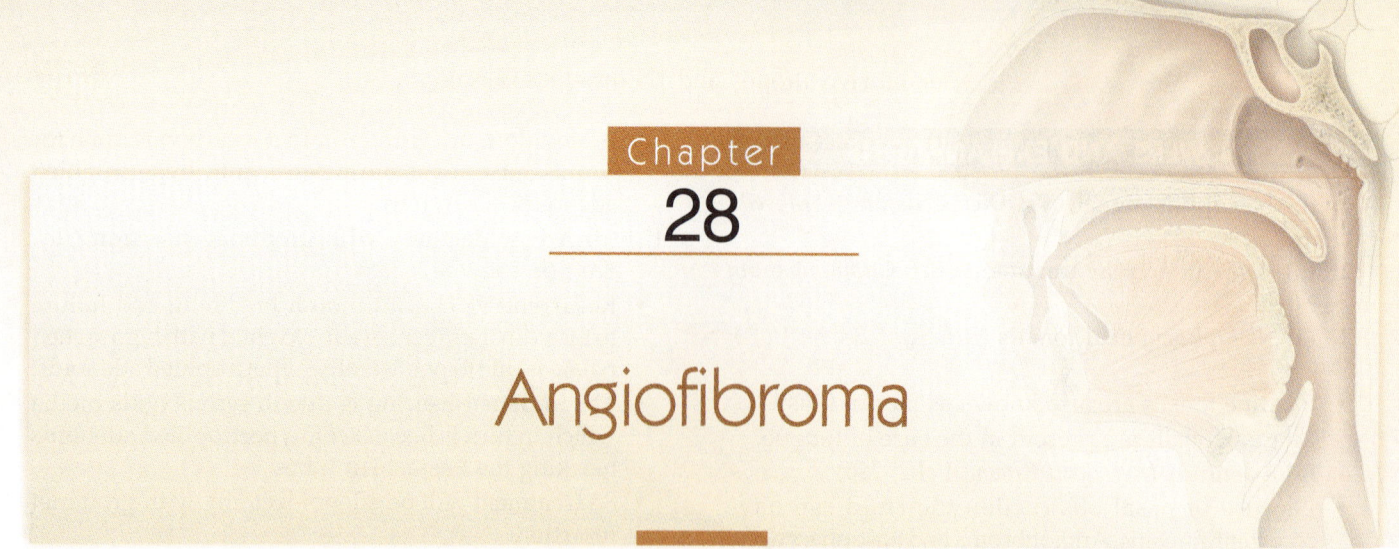

Angiofibroma

Angiofibroma is the **most common benign tumour** of the nasopharynx. It is a benign but locally invasive tumour. It is also known as nasopharyngeal fibroma.

It is typically seen in **young adolescent males**, i.e. occur near puberty, hence also called juvenile nasopharyngeal angiofibroma (exclusive occurrence in males near puberty indicates the possibility of an underlying hormonal etiology). Recently it has been proposed that angiofibroma are vascular malformations arising from vascular remnants of 1st branchial arch.

It arises from the **sphenopalatine foramen** which connects the nasopharynx with the sphenopalatine fossa. Please also see anatomy of sphenopalatine fossa and sphenopalatine foramen in anatomy of lateral wall of nose.

Clinical Features

1. From the sphenopalatine foramen it grows into the nasopharynx and adjoining nasal cavity. As the name angiofibroma contains only blood vessels (angio) and fibrous tissue (fibroma) with no muscular coat. The patient here presents most commonly with **recurrent episodes of profuse epistaxis** and **unilateral nasal obstruction**. Because of its growth in the nasal cavity there occurs splaying (falling apart, widening) of nasal bones leading to broadening of nasal bridge.

   On anterior rhinoscopy, a **red fleshy mass** can be seen in the nasal cavity.

2. Due to obstruction of the Eustachian tube opening, which is present in the lateral wall of nasopharynx the patient has U/L serous otitis media and conductive hearing loss. Later on with spread to the opposite side, in the nasopharynx there can occur B/L serous otitis media.

3. The tumour then grows laterally from the sphenopalatine foramen into the sphenopalatine fossa. It fills the fossa completely. It derives its main blood supply from the maxillary artery and its sphenopalatine branch which are also present here (*see* Chapter 16). On further expansion in the sphenopalatine fossa it pushes the posterior wall of maxillary antrum (the anterior boundary of sphenopalatine fossa) anteriorly (*see*

Holman Miller sign below) and pterygoid plates (its posterior boundary) posteriorly.

4. It can enter the orbit through the inferior orbital fissure leading to **proptosis**.

5. It can grow out of the sphenopalatine fossa through its lateral boundary, i.e. the pterygomaxillary fissure into the infratemporal fossa and cheek leading to **swelling in the cheek**.

   The nasal bridge broadening along with proptosis and swelling in the cheek gives rise to **frog face deformity**.

6. It can also go intracranially through floor of middle cranial fossa or sphenoid sinus or through cribriform plate or through the orbit via the superior orbital fissure.

Investigations

The **best** investigation for the diagnosis of angiofibroma is **CECT** where the pathognomonic finding is widening of the sphenopalatine foramen and the anterior bowing of posterior wall of maxillary antrum by a hyper vascular enhancing mass, known as **antral sign/Holman Miller sign**. Also the pterygoid plates are pushed posteriorly which on CT appears as floating pterygoids.

To see the intracranial extension or extension into orbits or infratemporal fossa CECT has to be augmented with MRI.

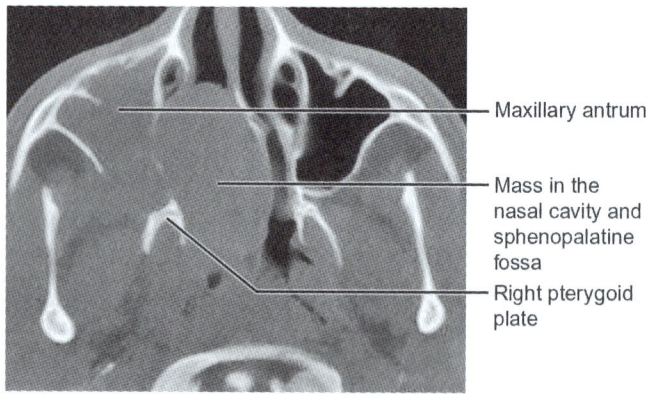

Maxillary antrum

Mass in the nasal cavity and sphenopalatine fossa

Right pterygoid plate

Fig. 28.1: CT showing mass in the sphenopalatine fossa and right nasal cavity

Since it contains only blood vessels (angio) and fibrous tissue (fibroma) with no muscular coat (hence retraction does not occur), biopsy can lead to profuse bleeding and is contraindicated here.

Carotid angiography is done so as to know the feeding vessel to angiofibroma so that preoperative embolisation of this vessel can be done.

STAGING OF ANGIOFIBROMA

The staging system proposed by Sessions et al divides tumours into three stages:

- **Stage I**
  - **Ia:** Limited to nasal cavity/nasopharynx
  - **Ib:** Extension into one or more paranasal sinuses
- **Stage II**
  - **IIa:** Minimal extension through sphenopalatine foramen into sphenopalatine/pterygomaxillary fossa
  - **IIb:** Fills sphenopalatine fossa bowing the posterior wall of the maxillary antrum anteriorly or extending into the orbit via the inferior orbital fissure
  - **IIc:** Extends beyond sphenopalatine fossa into the cheek and infratemporal fossa.
- **Stage III:** Intracranial extension.

A modification of sessions system has been proposed by Radowski. It is the most recent classification system of Juvenile nasopharyngeal angiofibroma (JNA). Here stages Ia, Ib, IIa, IIb and IIc are same as sessions. Stage III is divided into IIIa and IIIb as:

Stage IIIa: Erosion of skull base (middle cranial fossa or pterygoids) with minimal intracranial spread.

Stage IIIb: Erosion of skull base with significant intracranial spread.

Treatment

The main management of angiofibroma is surgical excision.

Since it is a very vascular tumour preoperative embolisation of feeding vessel is done.

The **surgical approaches** depend upon the extent of the tumour. The following approaches can be used:

a. Endoscopic approach: Nowadays, endoscopic resection is preferred over external approaches for most of the juvenile angiofibromas except for the ones with extensive skull base infiltration, intracranial extension and in tumours deriving extensive blood supply from internal carotid artery.

b. Transpalatine: Here incision is given in between the hard and soft palate to approach the nasopharynx when the tumour is confined to the nasopharynx.

c. Transpalatine + sub-labial (Sardana's approach): When the tumour from the nasopharynx has also extended into the cheek, it can be approached additionally through the sub-labial incision.

d. Medial maxillectomy by lateral rhinotomy approach: Here incision is given in the nasofacial crease (lateral rhinotomy), and the medial wall of maxilla (i.e. lateral wall of nose) is removed, to approach the sphenopalatine foramen and sphenopalatine fossa posterior to it. It can also be done by midfacial degloving approach (here a sub-labial incision is given from one molar to another and the skin flap is raised). The benefit of degloving approach is that there is no external scar of incision on the face.

e. Transmaxillary approach (by lateral rhinotomy/ midfacial degloving)

f. Infratemporal fossa approach

Since the patient here is young and radiotherapy is not preferred in young as it can induce second tumours (e.g. papillary carcinoma thyroid, leukaemia, etc.), main treatment of angiofibroma is surgical excision.

Radiotherapy is indicated in stage III when the tumour has **intracranial extension** where complete excision will not be possible and the tumour has become unresectable because of deriving its blood supply from intracranial vessels.

The **recurrence** rate of this tumour is high.

 "Points to Ponder/Points for Quick revision"

- JNA: MC benign tumour of nasopharynx.
- Young M: Recurrent epistaxis & U/L nasal obstruction; Frog facies.
- Bx: C/I; CECT (Hollman Miller sign) → diagnosis.
- T/t: Preop-embolization, surgical excision (till stage IIb/IIIa)
- Recurrence rate—high.

PREVIOUSLY ASKED QUESTIONS

1. **Most common site of origin of nasopharyngeal angiofibroma:** *(JIPMER 2004, Exam 2017)*
   a. Roof of nasopharynx
   b. At sphenopalatine foramen
   c. Vault of skull
   d. Lateral wall of nose

2. **Nasopharyngeal angiofibroma is:** *(TN 91, Exam 2014)*
   a. Benign
   b. Malignant
   c. Benign but potentially malignant
   d. None of the above

3. **A 10-year-old boy has U/L nasal obstruction, recurrent profuse epistaxis, swelling over cheek, the diagnosis is:** *(AIIMS 99, AI 2001, UP 2008, Exam 2013)*
   a. Nasal polyp
   b. Nasopharyngeal carcinoma
   c. Angiofibroma
   d. Inverted papilloma
   e. Foreign body

4. **In angiofibroma of nasopharynx all are correct except:** *(Kolkata 2000, Exam 2017)*
   a. Common in females
   b. Most common presentation is epistaxis
   c. Arises from the lateral wall of nasopharynx at the sphenopalatine foramen
   d. In late cases frog face deformity occurs

5. **Angiofibroma bleeds excessively because:** *(Exam 2001, Exam 2017)*
   a. It lacks a capsule
   b. Vessels lack a contractile component
   c. It has multiple sites of origin
   d. All of the above

6. **Clinical features of nasopharyngeal angiofibroma are:** *(PGI 2002, 2013)*
   a. Present in 3rd to 4th decade
   b. Adolescent male
   c. Epistaxis and nasal obstruction are the cardinal symptoms
   d. Radiotherapy is the treatment of choice
   e. Arises from posterior nasal cavity

7. **A 14-year-old boy presented with repeated torrential epistaxis, and a swelling in cheek. Which of these statements may be correct?** *(PGI 2003, 2012)*
   a. Diagnosis is nasopharyngeal angiofibroma
   b. CECT should be done to see the extent
   c. High propensity to spread via lymphatics
   d. Arises from roof of nose
   e. Surgery is therapy of choice

8. **True about juvenile nasopharyngeal angiofibroma:** *(PGI June 2006, 2014)*
   a. Surgery is treatment of choice
   b. It is malignant tumour

   c. Increased incidence in females
   d. Biopsy is done for the diagnosis
   e. Holman Miller's sign positive

9. **True about nasopharyngeal angiofibroma:** *(PGI Dec 2003, 2013)*
   a. Commonly seen in girls
   b. Hormonal etiology
   c. Surgery is treatment of choice
   d. Radiotherapy can be given
   e. Recurrence is common

10. **Most appropriate investigation for angiofibroma is:** *(AIIMS 97, Exam 2011)*
    a. Angiography
    b. CECT scan
    c. MRI
    d. Plain X-ray

11. **A 10-year-old boy presents with nasal obstruction and intermittent profuse epistaxis. He has a firm pinkish mass in the nasopharynx. All of the following investigations are done in this case except:** *(AI 97, Exam 2012)*
    a. MRI
    b. Carotid angiography
    c. CECT scan
    d. Biopsy

12. **An 18-year-old boy presented with repeated epistaxis and there was a mass extending into the nose and nasopharynx. It was decided to operate him. All of the following are true regarding his management except:** *(AIIMS 2002, Exam 2017)*
    a. Requires radiotherapy before surgery
    b. A lateral rhinotomy approach may be used
    c. Transpalatal approach is used
    d. Transmaxillary approach

13. **Treatment of choice for angiofibroma:** *(RJ 2002, Exam 2017)*
    a. Surgery
    b. Radiotherapy
    c. Both
    d. Chemotherapy

14. **Frog face deformity of nose caused by:** *(DPG 2008, Exam 2017)*
    a. Rhinoscleroma
    b. Angiofibroma
    c. Antral polyp
    d. Ethmoidal polyp

15. **A 12-year-old child presents with U/L pink nasal mass. Most important investigation prior to undertaking surgery is:** *(AI 97, Exam 2013)*
    a. Ultrasound
    b. FNAC
    c. Biopsy
    d. Contrast CT scan

16. **Antral sign is seen in:** *(Exam 2013)*
    a. Juvenile angiofibroma
    b. Otosclerosis
    c. CSOM
    d. Sinusitis

17. **Radiotherapy is used in treatment of angiofibroma when it involves:** *(MP 2004, Exam 2017)*
    a. Cheek
    b. Orbit
    c. Middle cranial fossa
    d. Pterygopalatine fossa

18. **Which of the following is not true for juvenile angiofibroma?** *(Exam 2013, Exam 2018)*
    a. Biopsy for diagnosis
    b. Benign tumour
    c. Surgical excision
    d. Typically occurs in second decade

19. **Stage 2B nasopharyngeal angiofibroma best treated with:** *(Exam 2013)*
    a. Surgery
    b. Chemotherapy
    c. Radiotherapy
    d. None

20. **Antral sign is seen in:** *(WB PG 2015)*
    a. Nasopharyngeal carcinoma
    b. Antrochoanal polyp
    c. Angiofibroma
    d. Chronic maxillary sinusitis

21. **True about nasopharyngeal fibroma:** *(Exam 2015)*
    a. Arises from fossa of Rosenmuller
    b. Benign but locally invasive
    c. Radiotherapy is the treatment of choice
    d. Caused by EBV

22. **Juvenile nasopharyngeal angiofibroma is supplied by:** *(AIIMS 2015)*
    a. Internal maxillary artery
    b. Ascending pharyngeal artery
    c. Facial artery
    d. Lingual artery

IMAGE BASED PRACTICE QUESTION BY THE AUTHOR

23. Given below is a CECT (showing an enhancing mass in the nose, sphenopalatine fossa and infratemporal fossa) of an 18-year-old male presenting with recurrent epistaxis, nasal obstruction and swelling of cheek. He should be managed by the following except:

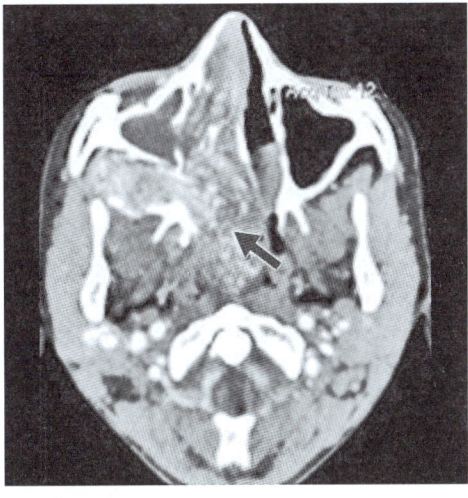

    a. Surgical excision
    b. Preoperative radiotherapy
    c. Preoperative embolisation
    d. Biopsy is contraindicated here

24. A 13-year-old boy with U/L nasal obstruction and recurrent epistaxis. CECT shows enhancing lesion in the nose with minimal extension to sphenoid sinus and no lateral extension. Radowski stage: *(AIIMS 2018)*
    a. Ia
    b. Ib
    c. IIa
    d. IIb

Oral Cavity and Pharynx

Section III

ANSWERS AND EXPLANATIONS

1. **(b) At sphenopalatine foramen** (*Ref. Cummings, 6th ed., 1421; Scott Brown, 8th ed., Vol1; 1265*)
   - Most common site of origin of nasopharyngeal angiofibroma is from the sphenopalatine foramen which is present around 1 cm behind the posterior border of the middle turbinate in the lateral wall of nasopharynx.
   - The lateral wall of the nose ends at the posterior end of turbinates. So it is not the answer
   - Angiofibroma spreads to the roof of nasopharynx from where it can go intracranially.
   - Vault of skull is not valid.

2. **(a) Benign** (*Ref. Cummings, 6th ed., 1421*)
   - Nasopharyngeal angiofibroma is benign but locally invasive tumour.
   - It is not considered malignant or the one with malignant potential because it does not show metastasis.

3. **(c) Angiofibroma** (*Ref. Cummings, 6th ed., 1421*)
   - Any child of pubertal age with these complaints should be investigated for angiofibroma.
   - The nasal polyp (Antrochoanal polyp/Killian's polyp) presents with unilateral nasal obstruction but they, having very poor blood supply, do not present with epistaxis. They do not cause swelling over the cheek.
   - Though nasopharyngeal carcinoma can also occur in young age it presents with upper deep cervical lymphadenopathy in most of the cases. Here the complaints regarding nasopharyngeal obstruction by the tumour and cheek swelling occur late.
   - Considering the age it cannot be foreign body. Also a foreign body will not lead to recurrent profuse epistaxis and swelling over the cheek. The swelling over the cheek is because of the angiofibroma coming from the sphenopalatine fossa into the infratemporal fossa through the pterygomaxillary fissure.
   - Inverted papilloma is the most common benign tumour of the nasal cavity. It arises from the lateral wall of the nose so it causes U/L nasal obstruction but epistaxis is not profuse here. It can also lead to swelling in the cheek because it is also a locally invasive tumour but inverted papilloma is seen in the age group of 40–70 yrs and not in a 10-year-old child.

4. **(a) Common in females** (*Ref. Cummings, 6th ed., 1421*)

5. **(b) Vessels lack a contractile component** (*Ref. Cummings, 6th ed., 1421; Scott Brown, 8th ed., Vol1; 1266*)

6. **(b) and (c)** (*Ref. Cummings, 6th ed., 1423*)

7. **(a), (b) and (e)** (*Ref. Cummings, 6th ed., 1422*)

8. **(a) and (e) are true** (*Ref. Scott Brown, 8th ed., Vol 1; 1266*)

9. **(b), (c), (d) and (e)** (*Ref. Cummings, 6th ed., 1423; 744*)

10. **(b) CECT scan** (*Ref. Cummings, 6th ed., 1422; 744*)

11. **(d) Biopsy** (*Ref. Cummings, 6th ed., 1421*)
    This is most likely a case of angiofibroma.
    - Biopsy is contraindicated in a case of suspected angiofibroma, as it will result into profuse bleeding because here the blood vessels lack the muscular component so contraction does not occur.
    - The most appropriate investigation for the diagnosis of angiofibroma is CECT.
    - Carotid angiography is done so as to know the feeding vessel to angiofibroma so that preoperative embolisation of this vessel can be done.
    - To see the intracranial extension or extension into orbits or infratemporal fossa CECT has to be augmented with MRI.

12. **(a) Requires radiotherapy before surgery** (*Ref. Cummings, 6th ed., 745*)

13. **(a) Surgery (best option)** (*Ref. Cummings, 6th ed., 1422*)
    - Radiotherapy is indicated in angiofibroma only when the tumour has intracranial extension.

14. **(b) Angiofibroma** (*Ref. Dhingra, 6th ed., 246*)
    - The appearance of nose in Rhinoscleroma is known as woody nose or Hebra nose.
    In antrochoanal and ethmoidal polyp no external deformity of nose is seen.

15. **(d) Contrast CT scan** (*Ref. Cummings, 6th ed., 1422*)
    - An adolescent male with U/L pink nasal mass has to be investigated to rule out angiofibroma. So the next best investigation prior to undertaking surgery is a Contrast enhanced CT scan.
    - FNAC and biopsy are contraindicated here for the fear of profuse bleeding.

16. **(a) Juvenile angiofibroma** (*Ref. Dhingra, 6th ed., 248*)

17. **(c) Middle cranial fossa** (*Ref. Cummings, 6th ed., 1423; 744*)

18. **(a) Biopsy for diagnosis** (*Ref. Cummings, 6th ed., 1421*)

19. **(a) Surgery** (*Ref. Cummings, 6th ed., 1423*)

20. **(c) Angiofibroma** (*Ref. Scott Brown, 8th ed., Vol 1; 1266*)

21. **(b) Benign but locally invasive** (*Ref. Cummings, 6th ed., 1421*)

22. **(a) Internal maxillary artery** (*Ref. Scott Brown, 8th ed., Vol 1; 1266*)

23. **(b) Preoperative radiotherapy** (*Ref. Cummings, 6th ed., 1422*)

24. **(b) Ib** (*Ref. Scott Brown, 8th ed., Vol 1; 1266*)

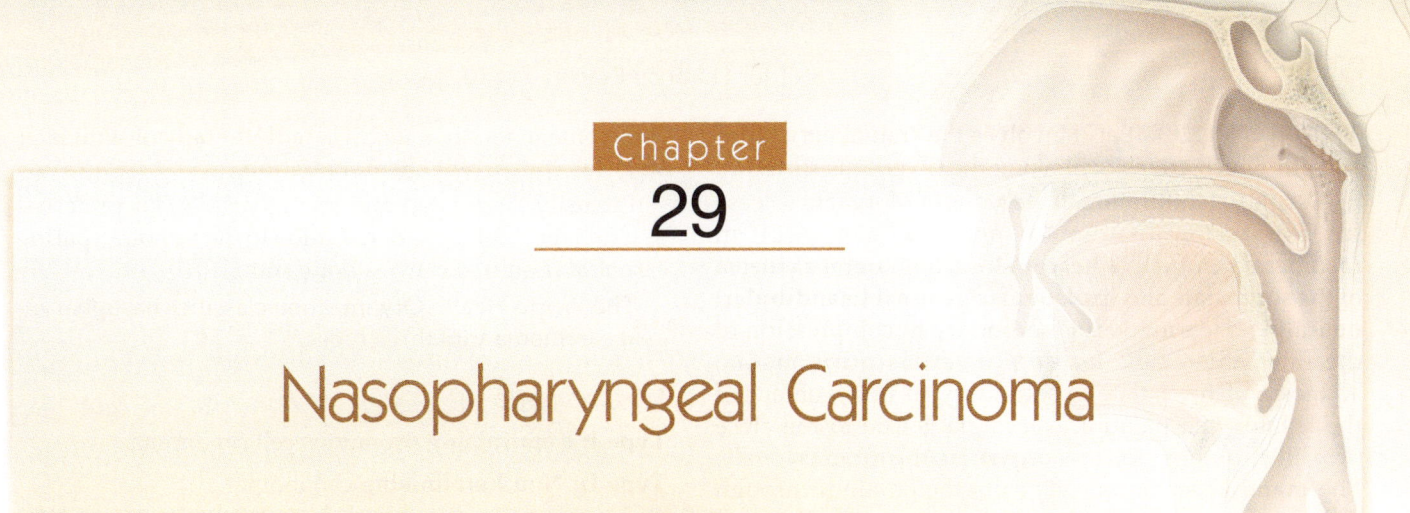

Nasopharyngeal Carcinoma

The most common carcinoma of the nasopharynx is nasopharyngeal carcinoma.

It is a **squamous cell carcinoma** (please note that the lining of nasopharynx is similar to the lining of paranasal sinuses, nose, larynx and bronchi, being pseudo-stratified ciliated columnar and most commonly the carcinomas in these locations are of squamous cell variety).

The most common site of origin of nasopharyngeal carcinoma is **fossa of Rosenmüller** (lateral pharyngeal recess) in the lateral wall of nasopharynx just behind the bulge of Eustachian tube cartilage, i.e. torus tubaris, *see* Chapter on anatomy of oral cavity and pharynx.

The exact etiology of this tumour is not known. There are 3 main postulations:

1. **Genetic etiology:** People living in south East Asian countries like **Southern China, Hong Kong, Indonesia and Taiwan (Mongolians)** have high genetic susceptibility. The highest incidence is seen in southern China among the Cantonese population of **Guangdong** province. An association with the HLA allele located on the chromosome no. 6 has been found. Therefore, all the family members of the patient should be screened.

2. **Environmental etiology:** Exposure to nitrosamines used in food preservatives (salted fish), polycyclic hydrocarbons (in burning of wood and incense) and smoking can predispose to this tumour.

3. **Viral etiology:** Infection with **Epstein-Barr virus (EBV)** is associated with this tumour. Immuno-globulin A against the viral capsid antigen (**IgA VCA**) of EBV has been used as the **serological marker** for screening of nasopharyngeal carcinoma in endemic regions of this tumour. More than 90% patients have elevated antibody titres of IgA class to EBV antigens. The titres of IgA VCA is also useful in follow up of patients after treatment to see recurrence. IgA against nuclear core early antigen (EA) is also raised in these individuals. IgA VCA is more sensitive and IgA EA is more specific.

Clinical Features

Nasopharyngeal carcinoma has bi-modal age occurrence with two peaks, the 1st at 15–25 yrs and the 2nd at 55–65 yrs of age.

Nearly **75% of patients** of nasopharyngeal carcinoma present with **painless cervical lymphadenopathy** of mainly the upper deep cervical lymph node (level II) and posterior triangle (level V). The nasopharynx drains into the retropharyngeal lymph node of Rouvier but this is inaccessible to inspection as well as palpation. From here the 2nd echelon nodes are the jugulo-digastric (upper deep cervical) and posterior triangle lymph nodes which are the first palpable nodes.

The other symptoms of any mass in the nasopharynx as mentioned below come later on.

Nasal: Nasal obstruction, denasal or hyponasal voice, i.e. Rhinolalia clausa, blood tinged nasal discharge.

Ear: U/L serous Otitis media due to obstruction of the same side Eustachian tube. Any adult with U/L serous Otitis media should be investigated for nasopharyngeal carcinoma.

Inferiorly it may spread to the soft palate and oropharynx.

Posteriorly it may spread to retropharyngeal space

Laterally it may spread to the parapharyngeal space (post styloid compartment) where it involves the 9th, 10th, 11th cranial nerves (known as jugular foramen syndrome), 12th cranial nerve, cervical sympathetic chain (causing **Horner's syndrome**).

Orbital: Tumours may directly invade the orbit leading to exophthalmos and blindness. Here it can also lead to diplopia and ophthalmoplegia due to involvement of cranial nerves 3rd, 4th and 6th.

Superiorly it extends intracranially by direct invasion through foramen lacerum and foramen ovale, sphenoid bone and sphenoid sinus causing multiple cranial nerve palsies. The most common nerves affected in descending order of frequency are 5th (V2 involved in the pterygopalatine fossa and V3 in the foramen ovale), 6th,

9th, 10th and 12th. It also involves the cranial nerves 3rd and 4th which are present along the cavernous sinus.

Neoplastic infiltration of the sinus of Morgagni (please *see* Chapter on anatomy of pharynx) can result in **ipsilateral conductive hearing loss, ipsilateral akinesia of the soft palate and ipsilateral trigeminal (mandibular) neuralgia**. Hearing loss is secondary to compression of the Eustachian tube leading to **serous otitis media**. Akinesia of the palate is secondary to involvement of the levator veli palatini. Neuralgia is due to the close proximity of the sinus of Morgagni to the foramen ovale. The **mandibular nerve**, V3, exits the cranium through the foramen ovale, and is responsible for pain in the lower jaw, ear and lateral side of the face. This is known as **Trotter's Triad** or **sinus of Morgagni syndrome**.

Mnemonic: Nasopharyngeal carcinoma **NPC** (**N**euralgia ipsilateral side of head, **P**alatal palsy, **C**onductive hearing loss).

As the neoplasm grows, the maxillary nerve, V2, which passes through the foramen rotundum into the nearby pterygopalatine fossa, may also be affected.

Distant metastasis: Skeletal metastasis to most commonly the thoracolumbar spine is seen followed by lung and liver.

Diagnosis: Nasopharyngeal carcinoma is diagnosed by transnasal endoscopic biopsy. CT and MRI are done to see the extent of the tumour.

Treatment

Because of difficulty in obtaining adequate surgical margins, the definitive treatment for nasopharyngeal carcinoma in its early stages is **radiotherapy** or with later stages is **concurrent chemoradiation**.

Intensity modulated radiotherapy (IMRT) is preferred as it delivers high dose of radiation to the tumour, sparing essential tissues, e.g. eyes, brainstem.

The World Health Organization classifies nasopharyngeal carcinoma into three types.

WHO Criteria

Type I: Keratinising squamous cell carcinoma.

Type II: Non-keratinising carcinoma.

Type IIa: Non-keratinising differentiated carcinoma.

Type IIb: Non-keratinising undifferentiated carcinoma.

Usually well differentiated keratinizing squamous cell carcinomas are relatively radio resistant but the non-keratinising **undifferentiated** nasopharyngeal carcinoma (II b) which is the **most common subtype** in endemic areas, is **very radiosensitive** though it is very aggressive.

The **prognosis** of this tumour is **very poor**.

 "Points to Ponder/Points for Quick revision"

- NPC: Squamous cell carcinoma
- Southern China (Guandong); Bimodal age; Genetic/Viral (EBV)/Nitrosamines
- Upper neck mass (MC presentation)
- Multiple cranial N, Trotter's triad (NPC)
- Screening: IgA VCA, IgA EA; Diagnosis—Bx
- T/t: Radiotherapy—early stages; Concurrent Chemoradiation—late stages.

PREVIOUSLY ASKED QUESTIONS

1. **Nasopharyngeal carcinoma is caused by:**
   (MAHE 2005, Exam 2017)
   a. EBV
   b. Papilloma virus
   c. Herpes virus
   d. Adeno virus

2. **Nasopharyngeal carcinoma involve:**
   (PGI 2002, 2011)
   a. Nasal cavity
   b. Oropharynx
   c. Pyriform fossa
   d. Tympanic cavity
   e. Orbit

3. **Most common site for origin of nasopharyngeal carcinoma:** *(AIIMS 97, MP 2002, Exam 2013)*
   a. Nasal septum
   b. Fossa of Rosenmüller
   c. Vault of nasopharynx
   d. Antero-superior wall

4. **Nasopharyngeal carcinoma presents as:**
   (Exam 2013, 2018)
   a. Epistaxis
   b. Mass in neck
   c. Headache
   d. Nasal stuffiness
   e. Hoarseness of voice

5. **A 70-year-old male presents with neck nodes and right sided deafness. Examination reveals a dull tympanic membrane. Tympanometry shows curve B. The most probable diagnosis is:**
   (AI 2008, Exam 2013, AIIMS 2013)
   a. Nasopharyngeal carcinoma
   b. Pyriform fossa carcinoma
   c. Tumour in inner ear
   d. Adenoid hypertrophy

6. **Nasopharyngeal carcinoma causes deafness by:**
   (Exam 2014)
   a. Temporal bone metastasis
   b. Middle ear infiltration
   c. Serous effusion
   d. Radiation therapy

7. **Trotter's triad is seen in carcinoma of:**
   (Comed 2008, Exam 2013)
   a. Maxilla
   b. Larynx
   c. Nasopharynx
   d. Ethmoid sinus

8. **True about Trotter's triad:** *(PGI Dec 2008, 2012)*
   a. Conductive deafness
   b. Involvement of 6th cranial nerve
   c. Involvement of 5th cranial nerve
   d. Palatal paralysis
   e. Associated with nasopharyngeal angiofibroma

9. **Trotter's triad includes all of the following except:**
   (AI 2009, Exam 2013)
   a. Mandibular neuralgia
   b. Deafness
   c. Palatal palsy
   d. Seizures

10. **Horner's syndrome is caused by:** *(Exam 2011)*
    a. Nasopharyngeal carcinoma metastasis
    b. Facial bone injury
    c. Maxillary sinusitis
    d. Ethmoid polyp

11. **Nasopharyngeal carcinoma:** *(PGI 2002, 2014)*
    a. MC nerve involved upon intracranial spread is vagus
    b. U/L serous Otitis media is seen
    c. Treatment of choice—radiotherapy
    d. Metastasised to cervical lymph nodes
    e. EBV is responsible

12. **Which among the following is not true regarding nasopharyngeal carcinoma:** *(PGI 2002, 2013)*
    a. Associated with EBV infection
    b. Starts in the fossa of Rosenmüller
    c. Radiotherapy is the treatment of choice
    d. Adenocarcinoma is usual
    e. If elderly patients present with unilateral otitis media it is highly suggestive

13. **Treatment of choice in advanced nasopharyngeal carcinoma:** *(Exam 2016)*
    a. Concurrent chemoradiation
    b. Chemotherapy
    c. Surgery
    d. Surgery and radiotherapy

14. **Treatment of nasopharyngeal carcinoma T1, and T2:** *(Karnataka 2005, Exam 2017)*
    a. Radiation therapy
    b. Surgery
    c. Local resection
    d. Chemotherapy

15. **Most radiosensitive tumour of the following is:**
    (AI 2001, Exam 2017)
    a. Supraglottic carcinoma
    b. Carcinoma glottis
    c. Carcinoma nasopharynx
    d. Subglottic carcinoma

16. **All of the following statements about nasopharyngeal carcinoma are true, except:** *(AI 2010)*
    a. Bimodal age distribution
    b. Nasopharyngectomy with radical neck dissection is the treatment of choice
    c. IgA antibody to EBV is observed
    d. Squamous cell carcinoma is the most common histological subtype

17. **Type of speech seen in nasopharyngeal carcinoma:**
    (Manipal 2008, Exam 2017)
    a. Rhinolalia clausa
    b. Rhinolalia aperta
    c. Hot potato voice
    d. Hoarse voice

18. **Nasopharyngeal carcinoma is most common in:**
    (Exam 2013)
    a. India
    b. Pakistan
    c. China
    d. Japan

Oral Cavity and Pharynx

Section III

19. **Category of non-keratinized squamous cancer of nasopharynx according to WHO is:** (*Exam 2011*)
    a. Type 1   b. Type 2
    c. Type 3   d. Type 4

20. **Branch of trigeminal nerve involved in Trotter's triad:** (*Exam 2014*)
    a. Ophthalmic   b. Mandibular
    c. Maxillary   d. Greater auricular

21. **Which one of the following statements is TRUE regarding nasopharyngeal carcinoma:** (*APPG 2016*)
    a. Anti-EBV therapy + chemotherapy is the treatment of choice
    b. Eighth cranial nerve is the most commonly involved nerve
    c. It most often arises from fossa of Rosenmüller in the lateral wall of the nasopharynx
    d. It is the commonest head and neck malignancy among males in India

22. **Nasopharyngeal carcinoma is most common in which race?** (*Exam 2015*)
    a. Mongoloids   b. Caucasians
    c. Aryans   d. Dravidians

23. **Trotter's triad is seen in:** (*Exam 2015*)
    a. Juvenile nasal angiofibroma
    b. Acoustic neuroma
    c. Nasopharyngeal carcinoma
    d. Glomus tumour

24. **Most common presentation of nasopharyngeal carcinoma is:** (*Exam 2015*)
    a. Neck mass   b. Trotter's triad
    c. Ophthalmoplegia d. Glue ear

25. **Which cancer has maximum propensity to spread to cervical lymph nodes?** (*Exam 2016*)
    a. Nasopharyngeal carcinoma
    b. Carcinoma of hard palate
    c. Carcinoma of soft palate
    d. Carcinoma of mandible

IMAGE BASED PRACTICE QUESTIONS BY THE AUTHOR

26. **This patient presents with right neck mass not benefitting by medical management. Biopsy shows nonkeratinising undifferentiated carcinoma. CT shows a soft tissue mass arising from the lateral wall of nasopharynx**

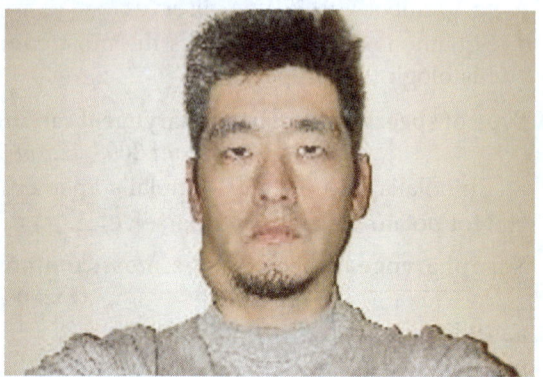

Not true about this tumour is:
    a. Level 4 cervical lymph node is earliest to be involved
    b. Radiotherapy is treatment of choice
    c. May be associated with U/L serous otitis media
    d. Associated with EBV

27. **The marked area is the site of origin of:**

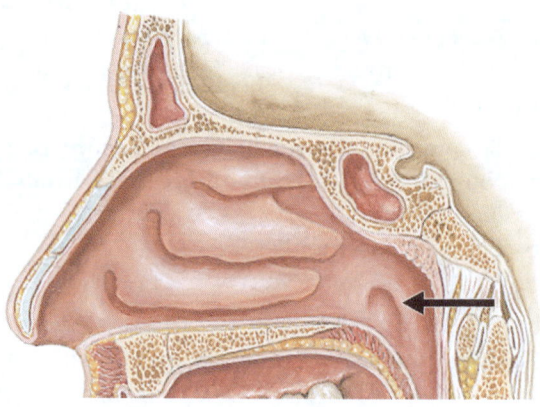

    a. Angiofibroma
    b. Nasopharyngeal carcinoma
    c. Antrochoanal polyp
    d. Inverted papilloma

28. **A 25-year-old male presents with right upper deep cervical lymphadenopathy, nasal obstruction and decreased hearing in right ear. CT shows a soft tissue mass arising from the lateral wall of nasopharynx. His audiogram shows a 40 dB conductive hearing loss in the right ear. His tympanogram of right ear is given below. True about this condition is all except:**

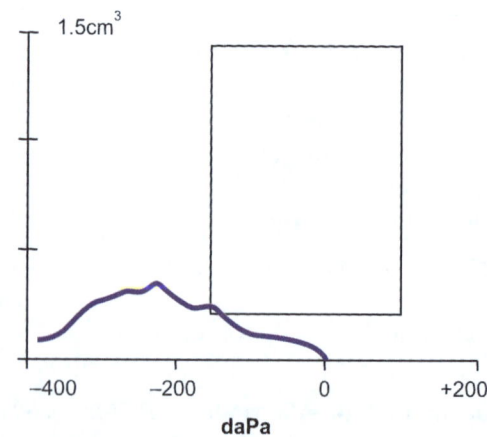

    a. He has serous otitis media in the right ear
    b. Biopsy should be taken for diagnosis
    c. He is a patient of angiofibroma
    d. Other siblings of this patient should also be screened for the same

29. **Guandong carcinoma is:** (*Exam 2018*)
    a. Nasopharyngeal carcinoma
    b. Glottic carcinoma
    c. Pyriform fossa carcinoma
    d. Glomus tympanicum

ANSWERS AND EXPLANATIONS

1. **(a) EBV** (*Ref. Cummings, 6th ed., 1424; Scott Brown, 8th ed., Vol 3; 95*)
2. **(a) (b) (d) and (e)** (*Ref. Scott Brown, 8th ed., Vol 3; 94*)
   - Nasopharyngeal carcinoma does not involve the pyriform fossa.
   - The rest of the structures mentioned are involved. Please refer to the text.
3. **(b) Fossa of Rosenmüller** (*Ref. Scott Brown, 8th ed., Vol 3; 93*)
4. **(b) Mass in neck** (*Ref. Cummings, 6th ed., 1425; Scott Brown, 8th ed., Vol 3; 97*)
   Nearly 75% of patients of nasopharyngeal carcinoma present with painless cervical lymphadenopathy of mainly the upper deep cervical lymph node.
5. **(a) Nasopharyngeal carcinoma** (*Ref. Cummings, 6th ed., 1425*)
   - The dull tympanic membrane, deafness and B type tympanogram all suggest serous otitis media. Any adult with unilateral serous otitis media, nasopharyngeal carcinoma should be ruled out.
   - Since this tumour arises from fossa of Rosenmüller just behind the Eustachian tube, it leads to unilateral Eustachian tube compression and unilateral serous otitis media.
   - Also the patient here is presenting with neck nodes which is the presentation in nearly 75% of patients of nasopharyngeal carcinoma.
   - Adenoid disappears by 20 years and leads to bilateral serous otitis media.
   - In pyriform fossa carcinoma neck nodes are present but it presents with dysphagia and not deafness.
   - Tumour in the inner ear presents with sensorineural deafness.
6. **(c) Serous effusion** (*Ref. Scott Brown, 8th ed., Vol 3; 97*)
7. **(c) Nasopharynx** (*Ref. Dhingra, 6th ed., 251*)
8. **(a), (c), and (d)** (*Ref. Dhingra, 6th ed., 251*)
   Involvement of 6th cranial nerve occurs upon intracranial spread in nasopharyngeal carcinoma but it is not a part of the Trotter's triad.
9. **(d) Seizures** (*Ref. Dhingra, 6th ed., 251*)
10. **(a) Nasopharyngeal carcinoma metastasis** (*Ref. Scott Brown, 8th ed., Vol 3; 98*)
    Nasopharyngeal carcinoma metastasis or direct extension laterally to the parapharyngeal space post styloid compartment leads to the involvement of cervical sympathetic chain which is known as Horner's syndrome. Signs of Horner's syndrome: (*Mnemonic:* **AMPLE**)
    1. **A**nhidrosis (decreased sweating on the affected side of the face)
    2. **M**iosis (small pupils)
    3. **P**tosis (drooping of the upper eyelid from loss of sympathetic innervation to the superior tarsal muscle, also known as Müller's muscle)
    4. **L**oss of ciliospinal reflex (i.e. no dilation of the ipsilateral pupil in response to pain stimuli applied to the neck).

5. **E**nophthalmos (the impression that the eye is sunk in)
11. **(b), (c), (d) and (e)** (*Ref. Cummings, 6th ed., 1426*)
12. **(d) Adenocarcinoma is usual** (*Ref. Cummings, 6th ed., 1424; Scott Brown, 8th ed., Vol 3; 101*)
    The nasopharyngeal carcinoma is most commonly squamous cell carcinoma.
13. **(a) Concurrent chemoradiation** (*Ref. Cummings, 6th ed., 1427*)
14. **(a) Radiation therapy** (*Ref. Cummings, 6th ed., 1427; Scott Brown, 8th ed., Vol 3; 102*)
15. **(c) Carcinoma nasopharynx** (*Ref. Stell & Maran, 5th ed., 596*)
    - The more undifferentiated a tumour, the more radiosensitive it is.
    - Hence the undifferentiated nasopharyngeal carcinoma (it being the most common subtype in endemic areas) is very radiosensitive. But despite its high radio sensitivity since it is undifferentiated so it is very aggressive and prognosis is very poor
    - The remaining 3 options of carcinoma of the larynx can be undifferentiated but are mostly well or moderately differentiated.
16. **(b) Nasopharyngectomy with radical neck dissection is the treatment of choice** (*Ref. Scott Brown, 8th ed., Vol 3; 101*)
    - The definitive treatment for nasopharyngeal carcinoma and its regional node metastasis is radiotherapy.
17. **(a) Rhinolalia clausa** (*Ref. Scott Brown, 8th ed., Vol 1; 181*)
    - Rhinolalia aperta is caused by conditions leading to velopharyngeal insufficiency, e.g. cleft palate, bifid uvula, paralysed palate.
    - Hot potato voice is produced by painful mass lesions of the oropharynx.
    - Hoarse voice is produced by pathologies of vocal cord.
18. **(c) China** (*Ref. Cummings, 6th ed., 1423; Scott Brown, 8th ed., Vol 3; 94*)
    The incidence of nasopharyngeal carcinoma is highest in southern China. It is rare in India, Pakistan or Japan.
19. **(b) Type 2** (*Ref. Cummings, 6th ed., 1426*)
20. **(b) Mandibular** (*Ref. Stell & Maran, 5th ed., 63*)
21. **(c) It most often arises from fossa of Rosenmüller in the lateral wall of the nasopharynx** (*Ref. Cummings, 6th ed., 1426*)
22. **(a) Mongoloids** (*Ref. Scott Brown, 8th ed., Vol 3; 94*)
23. **(c) Nasopharyngeal carcinoma** (*Ref. Dhingra, 6th ed., 251*)
24. **(a) Neck mass** (*Ref. Cummings, 6th ed., 1425*)
25. **(a) Nasopharyngeal carcinoma** (*Ref. Cummings, 6th ed., 1425; Scott Brown, 8th ed., Vol 3; 97*)
26. **(a) Level 4 cervical lymph node is the earliest to be involved** (*Ref. Stell & Maran, 5th ed. 592*)
27. **(b) Nasopharyngeal carcinoma** (*Ref. Cummings, 6th ed., 1426*)
    The marked area is fossa of Rosenmüller
28. **(c) He is a patient of angiofibroma** (*Ref. Cummings, 6th ed., 1426*)
29. **(a) Nasopharyngeal carcinoma** (*Ref. Scott Brown, 8th ed., Vol 3; 94*)

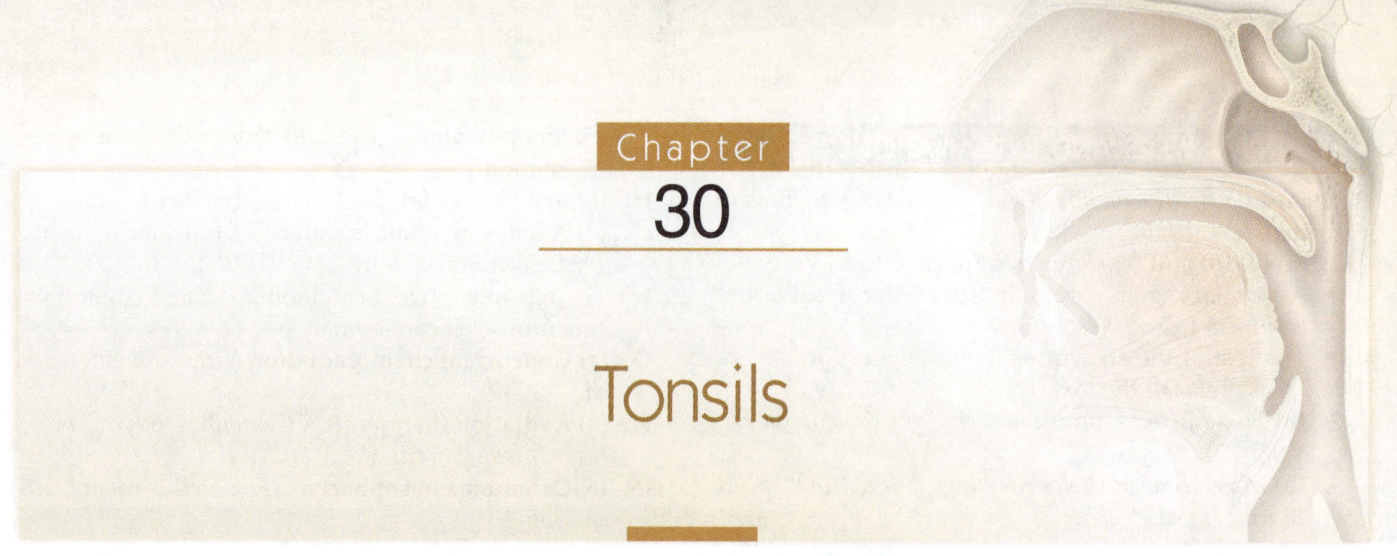

Chapter

30

Tonsils

Embryology and Anatomy

The tonsils are present in the lateral wall of oropharynx in between the anterior and posterior pillars. The tonsils are composed of lymphoid tissue (predominantly B) and have a role in providing local and systemic immunity. The tonsils are present at birth and achieve their maximum size by puberty. They regress after puberty.

The tonsils develop from the **2nd pharyngeal pouch**.

The tonsil is lined by non-keratinizing stratified squamous epithelium. This epithelium dips in the tonsillar tissue forming crypts.

There are around 12–15 crypts on the medial surface of tonsil.

The remnant of the ventral portion of 2nd pharyngeal pouch in the tonsil is the largest crypt of tonsil known as **crypta magna** or intratonsillar cleft.

The tonsil is bounded by a **capsule** on its lateral surface. The capsule is formed by pharyngobasilar fascia.

Only the medial surface of tonsil is visible, the upper and lower poles being covered by mucosal folds.

The upper pole of tonsil is covered by a semilunar fold of mucosa known as **plica semilunaris** and the lower pole is covered by a triangular fold of mucosa known as **plica triangularis**.

Everything lateral to the tonsil constitutes what is known as the bed of tonsil.

Lateral to the capsule of tonsil is the circular muscle layer (superior constrictor) of pharynx in the lateral pharyngeal wall.

In between the capsule and circular muscle layer called **peritonsillar space** is a loose areolar tissue in which runs the paratonsillar vein also known as **external palatine vein** responsible for draining the tonsil.

Clinical Importance of Peritonsillar Space

a. Injury to paratonsillar or external palatine vein is the most common cause of haemorrhage following tonsillectomy.

b. The infection of the loose areolar tissue in the peritonsillar space is what is known as Quinsy or peritonsillar abscess.

The other structures in the bed of the tonsil are the Glossopharyngeal nerve entering the pharynx in between the superior and middle constrictor, and the buccopharyngeal fascia (lining the outer surface of circular constrictor muscles).

Still more laterally is the facial artery along with its branches (tonsillar and ascending palatine) and internal carotid and styloid process in the parapharyngeal space.

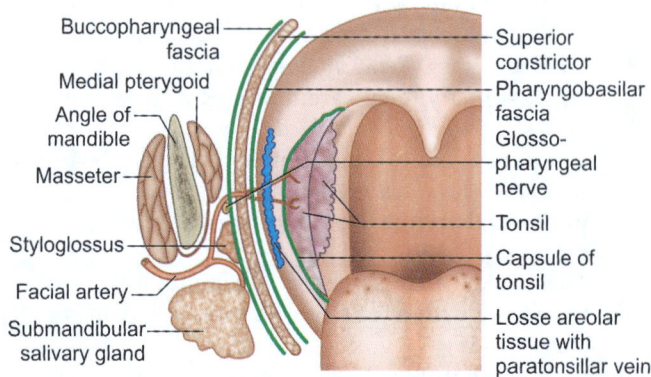

Fig. 30.1: Bed of tonsil

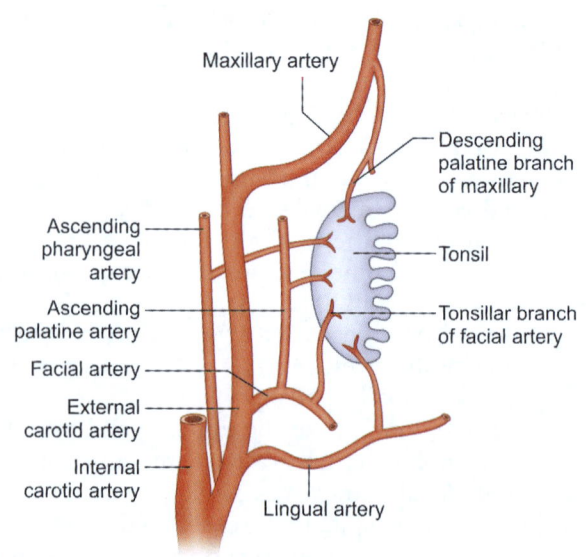

Fig. 30.2: Arterial supply of tonsil

Oral Cavity and Pharynx

Note:

The enlarged styloid process in **Styalgia/eagle's syndrome** (odynophagia & foreign body sensation in the throat due to enlarged styloid process) and the glossopharyngeal nerve in **Glossopharyngeal neuralgia** (stabbing pain in the oropharyngeal region because of compression/irritation of glossopharyngeal nerve) are approached through the tonsillar bed by a preliminary tonsillectomy.

Blood Supply

The whole of the **arterial supply** of tonsil is by external carotid. The branches of external carotid supplying the tonsil are as follows:

1. Facial gives 2 branches:
   a. Tonsillar artery: This is the main artery supplying the tonsil.
   b. Ascending palatine
2. Tonsillar branch of ascending pharyngeal
3. Dorsal linguae branches of lingual artery
4. Descending palatine branch of maxillary

The **venous drainage** of tonsil is by paratonsillar vein also known as external palatine vein.

Lymphatic drainage of tonsil is to upper deep cervical lymph node i.e. jugulo-digastric lymph node.

The most common cause of enlargement of these lymph nodes is the tonsillar infection because of which they are also known as tonsillar nodes.

Nerve supply of tonsil is by glossopharyngeal nerve and lesser palatine branch of maxillary nerve.

ACUTE TONSILLITIS

Like rhinitis, sinusitis and pharyngitis most common causes to acute tonsillitis are viral infections.

Among bacterial infections the most common organism causing acute tonsillitis is group A beta hemolytic streptococcus (GABHS).

Presentation

The patient presents with fever, sore throat, difficulty in swallowing and earache (referred pain via glossopharyngeal).

On Examination there may be

a. Yellowish spots on the tonsils due to purulent material in the crypts (called **follicular tonsillitis**) (Fig. 30.3).
b. Exudation from crypts may coalesce to form a membrane over the tonsil (known as **membranous tonsillitis**). This is actually a pseudomembrane formed by the **exudate**. Any bacterial infection involving the tonsil (these are mainly the gram + bacteria here) can lead to the formation of such pseudomembrane. Other than these infections a patient of membranous or more appropriately pseudomembranous tonsillitis, if not responding to antibiotics, should also be investigated for some other important conditions, read below, which can also lead to membrane formation over tonsils (Fig. 30.4).

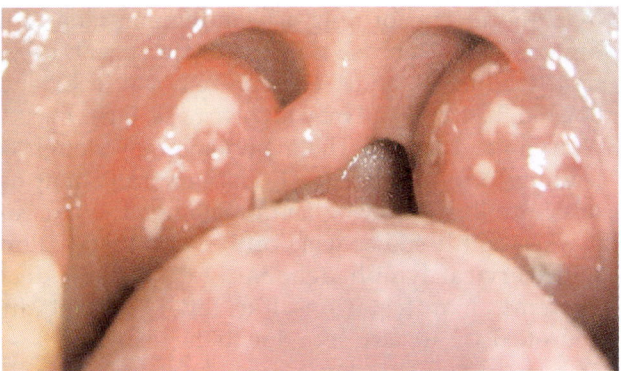

Fig. 30.3

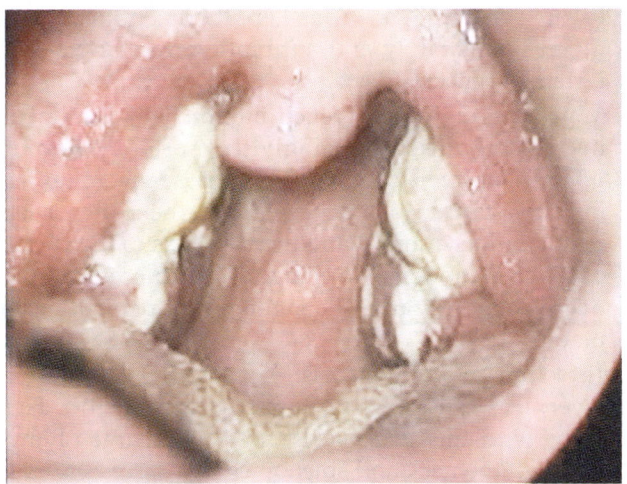

Fig. 30.4

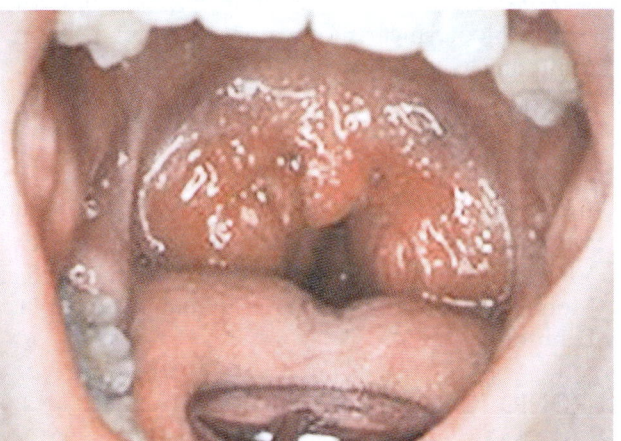

Fig. 30.5

c. The tonsil is uniformly enlarged and red (called **parenchymatous tonsillitis**) (Fig. 30.5).

Differential Diagnosis of Membranous or Pseudomembranous Tonsillitis

1. **Moniliasis (candidiasis)**
2. **Diphtheria:** Diphtheria is a bacterial infection of the pharynx caused by *Corynebacterium diphtheriae* that mainly occurs in the unimmunised population. It is an airborne infection with an incubation period of 2–5 days. It releases a toxin which leads to necrosis resulting in mucosal ulcers. Fibrino-suppurative exudates form

Oral Cavity and Pharynx

Section III

over the ulcers forming a pseudomembrane. This diphtheritic membrane is dirty grey in appearance, is tightly adherent and bleeds on removal. It extends beyond the tonsil and may involve nose, other parts of pharynx and larynx. The membrane may slough off leading to respiratory tract obstruction. Patient has difficulty in swallowing and breathing. There occurs marked soft tissue oedema of the neck tissues along with cervical lymphadenopathy called bull neck. Systemic manifestations like fever, cardiac and neurotoxicity are also seen due to the toxin.

Diagnosis: Throat swab (Chinese letter characters).

Management: Aims to neutralise the toxin and prevent its further formation. Thus Diphtheria antitoxin to be given immediately and antibiotics are started (Beta lactams or macrolides).

3. **Vincent's angina or Trench mouth:** This is an acute **necrotizing ulcerative gingivitis** caused by *Borrelia vincenti* **(spirochete)** and *F. fusiformis* **(anaerobe).** The infection starts in inter dental papillae (hence never seen in edentulous mouth) and then spreads to the surface of gingiva and tonsil forming ulcer and greyish **black necrotic membrane**. Management is penicillin and metronidazole.

4. **Infectious mononucleosis:** Also known as glandular fever, it is caused by Epstein-Barr virus (EBV). Here along with enlarged tonsils there are enlarged lymph nodes in the neck and splenomegaly.
   - Diagnosis is by the Paul Bunnel or monospot test which shows high titres of heterophile antibodies.
   - The blood smear shows atypical lymphocytosis.

5. **Malignancy of tonsil**
6. **Trauma**
7. **Aphthous ulcers**
8. **Leukaemia**
9. **Agranulocytosis** (by predisposing to above infections)
   Mnemonic: **AL VITAMIN D**–**A**granulocytosis, **L**eukaemia, **V**incent's, **I**nfectious mononucleosis, **A**phthous ulcers, **M**oniliasis, **I**nfections of throat (Gram +), **N**eoplasia, **D**iphtheria.

CHRONIC TONSILLITIS

Recurrent attacks of acute tonsillitis can lead to chronic tonsillitis where the patient complains of chronic throat irritation and halitosis. The cardinal signs of chronic tonsillitis are the following:

a. Flushing of anterior pillars as compared to rest of the pharynx.
b. **Irwin Moore sign:** On pressure of anterior pillar there is expression of cheesy material from the tonsil.
c. Enlarged jugulo-digastric lymph node.

Complications of Acute/Chronic Tonsillitis

a. **Local:**
   1. Acute otitis media (infection involving middle ear via Eustachian tube)

2. Peritonsillar abscess
3. Parapharyngeal abscess
4. Cervical abscess (due to the suppurative lymphadenitis of cervical lymph node)
5. Tonsillolith (it is formed by the inspissated secretions of the blocked crypt) and tonsillar cyst

b. **Systemic:**
   1. Acute glomerulonephritis (post-streptococcal)
   2. Rheumatic fever
   3. Subacute bacterial endocarditis
   4. Cor pulmonale: Chronic tonsillitis can lead to hypertrophied tonsils leading to sleep apnoea which can lead to pulmonary hypertension and Cor pulmonale, also *see* Chapter on adenoid hypertrophy.

INDICATIONS OF TONSILLECTOMY

Absolute Indication

1. Recurrent episodes of acute tonsillitis
   a. 3 episodes/year for 3 consecutive years
   b. 5 episodes/year for 2 consecutive years
   c. 7 episodes in a single year
2. Febrile seizures due to fever in tonsillitis
3. Chronic tonsillitis
4. Peritonsillar abscess (after 2 episodes in adults and single episode in a child)
5. Obstructive sleep apnoea and dysphagia due to hypertrophied tonsils.
6. Unilateral enlargement of tonsils with suspected malignancy

Relative indication: Streptococcal and diphtherial carrier Tonsillectomy **as an approach to other surgeries**:

a. **Styalgia (Eagle's syndrome):** The styloid process in the parapharyngeal space is enlarged and calcified. This leads to pain in the tonsillar area during swallowing.
b. **Glossopharyngeal neuralgia:** In this condition the glossopharyngeal nerve is transected where it enters the pharynx in between the superior and middle constrictor.
c. **UPPP (Uvulo-palato-pharyngoplasty):** In cases of sleep apnoea due to hypertrophied tonsil and bulky oropharynx, both the tonsils are removed along with the uvula and the anterior and posterior pillars are sutured together to increase the oropharyngeal airway.

While doing tonsillectomy the patient is made to lie down on the O T table in **Rose's position**.

In this position both the head and neck are extended. This is done by keeping a sand bag under the patient's shoulder blade in supine position. Tonsils are removed by dissection and snare method or by LASER (*see* Fig. 30.6).

Besides tonsillectomy, adenoidectomy and tracheostomy procedures are also done in Rose's position (*Mnemonic:* **A** (**A**denoidectomy) **Ton** (**Ton**sillectomy) of **Roses position**ed in the **Tray** (**Tra**cheostomy). In this position the larynx lies at a higher level than the oral cavity hence the risk of aspiration is reduced greatly.

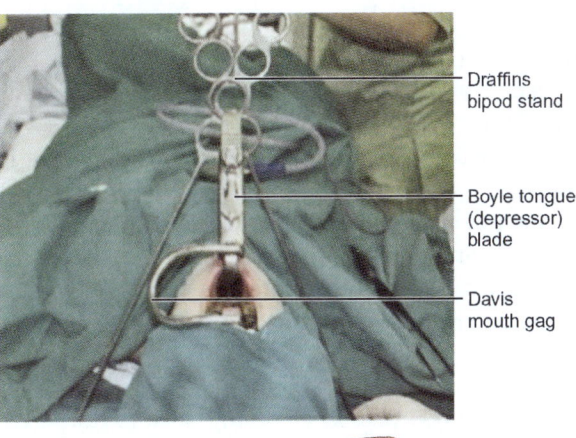

Draffins bipod stand

Boyle tongue (depressor) blade

Davis mouth gag

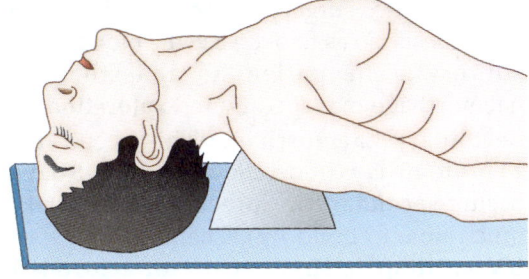

Fig. 30.6: Above; Patient ready for tonsillectomy. Below; Roses position (a sand bag has been inserted below the shoulder so that the head and neck got extended)

TYPES OF TONSILLECTOMY

Tonsillectomy is of two types:

1. **Extra-capsular (total tonsillectomy):** Here the whole of the tonsil along with its capsule is removed as a single unit.

2. **Intra-capsular (subtotal/partial tonsillectomy/tonsillotomy):** In partial tonsillectomy/tonsillotomy, most of the tonsil is removed, preserving a rim of lymphoid tissue and tonsillar capsule which acts as a biologic dressing and promotes faster recovery. It is preferred in children with obstructive sleep apnoea for debulking the tonsils.

TECHNIQUES OF TONSILLECTOMY

Cold Methods: These methods do not use heat. They are **employed in extra-capsular approach** to tonsillectomy.

- **Cold knife:** Dissection and snare method. It is sharp dissection technique using scissors, knife, dissector and the tonsil snare.

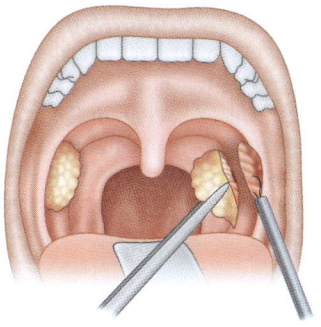

Fig. 30.7: Dissection and Snare method

- **Microdebrider tonsillectomy:** The microdebrider is a powered rotatory shaving device with continuous suction, made up of a tube, and connected to a hand piece.

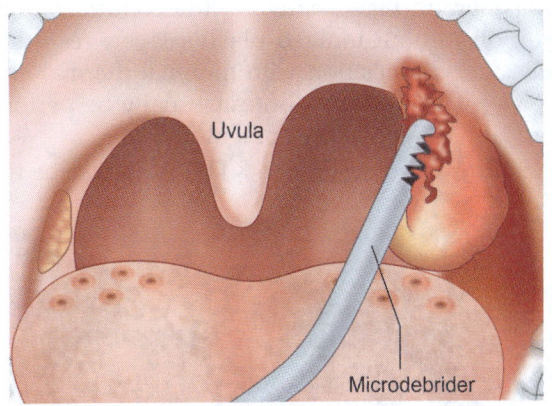

Uvula

Microdebrider

Fig. 30.8: Tonsillectomy by microdebrider

- **Harmonic scalpel:** It uses ultrasonic energy to vibrate its blade at 55,000 cycles per second. The vibration transfers energy to the tissue, providing simultaneous cutting and coagulation.

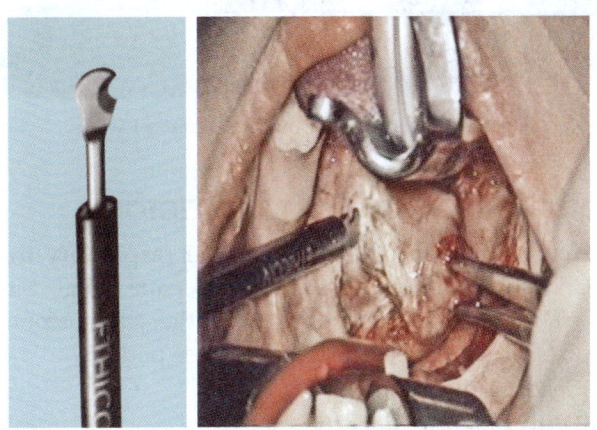

Fig. 30.9: Harmonic scalpel and tonsillectomy using it

- **Cryosurgery:** This is a process in which very cold instrument or substance is applied to tonsil. The tonsil here is removed by the process of repeated freezing and thawing. This procedure requires a lot of operating time. It is used only in patients with known bleeding diathesis.

Hot methods: These methods use heat

- **Cautery:** Both unipolar and bipolar cautery can be used.

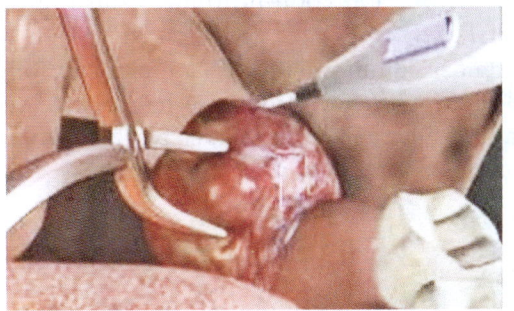

Fig. 30.10: Tonsillectomy by unipolar electo-cautery

Oral Cavity and Pharynx

Section III

- **Bipolar radiofrequency ablation with coblation wand**
  The equipment includes a radiofrequency generator, foot control, saline irrigation and the coblation wand. During a bipolar radiofrequency ablation tonsillectomy, the coblation wand converts the conductive saline solution into an ionized plasma layer, resulting in molecular dissociation with minimal thermal energy transfer. Haemostasis also can usually be performed here with the coblation wand alone.
- **LASER:** A CO_2 LASER or a KTP LASER can be used.

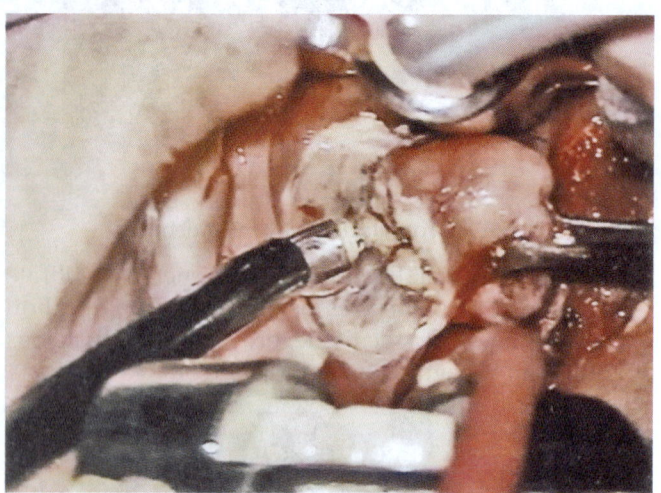

Fig. 30.11: Tonsillectomy by Coblation wand

CONTRAINDICATIONS OF TONSILLECTOMY

1. **Acute infection of tonsil or upper respiratory tract:** Chances of haemorrhage and septicaemia is high. Since it is not an emergency surgery, surgery is postponed till after three weeks of infection free period.
2. **Bleeding disorders**
3. **Polio epidemic:** Since the polio virus gets concentrated in the lymphoid tissues of tonsil and adenoid, tonsillectomy can lead to entry of virus into the blood stream triggering paralytic polio.
4. **Cleft palate, submucous cleft:** These are relative contraindications as these patients are at risk for velopharyngeal insufficiency getting unmasked post-surgery.

COMPLICATIONS OF TONSILLECTOMY

The most common complication of tonsillectomy is **haemorrhage**.

The most common site of haemorrhage following tonsillectomy is venous from external palatine vein, i.e. the paratonsillar vein. This venous bleed slowly fills the tonsillar fossa.

Torrential haemorrhage following tonsillectomy can occur due to injury to aberrantly large or aberrantly placed main artery of the tonsil, i.e. tonsillar artery, a branch of facial artery.

Haemorrhage during/following tonsillectomy is of 3 types:

1. **Primary haemorrhage:** This is the haemorrhage occurring **during surgery** secondary to injury to blood vessels while operating.
2. **Reactionary haemorrhage:** This occurs **after surgery to within 24 hours**. This occurs because of dislodgement of clot or slippage of ligature because of the blood pressure coming back to normal after surgery (since surgery is done here in hypotensive anaesthesia, so as to decrease the blood loss during surgery). The patient is anaesthetised and haemorrhage managed by **re-exploration**.
3. **Secondary haemorrhage:** This occurs between 24 hrs to 10 days (most commonly at **5–8 days**). This occurs **secondary to infection** (which takes this much time to build up). The patient is started on **I/V antibiotics first** and if not controlled he is anaesthetised and haemorrhage managed.

Management of Haemorrhage Following Tonsillectomy

The haemorrhage following tonsillectomy can be managed by the following steps:

1. Removal of clots: This is the 1st step for management of haemorrhage following tonsillectomy. Removal of clots allows retraction to occur and bleeding to stop.
2. Pressure with vasoconstrictors
3. Cauterisation or ligation of the local bleeding vessel
4. Putting a pressure pack in the tonsillar fossa and suture the anterior and posterior pillars together.

"Points to Ponder/Points for Quick revision"

- Physiological hypertrophy (till puberty) → Regression (like adenoids).
- Tonsils develop from 2nd pouch (remnant-crypta magna).
- Pharyngobasilar fascia → Capsule.
- Peritonsillar space between the Capsule and Superior constrictor–Infection → Quinsy.
- Main arterial supply—Facial.
- Sensory N—glossopharyngeal (referred-earache).
- Draining LN—upper deep cervical.
- Venous drainage—paratonsillar/external palatinevein (MC cause of haemorrhage following tonsillectomy).
- GABHS (MC) → Acute tonsillitis.
- Membrane over tonsil—AL Vitamin D.
- Tonsillectomy—extracapsular/intracapsular; cold/hot; MC complication—haemorrhage (1°/Reactionary/Secondary).

PREVIOUSLY ASKED QUESTIONS

1. **Tonsils reach their maximum size by:** (*Exam 2010*)
   a. 1 year
   b. 3 years
   c. 5 years
   d. 12 years

2. **Most common cause of acute tonsillitis:**
   (*AI 98, Exam 2014*)
   a. *Streptococcus pneumonia*
   b. *H. influenza*
   c. β hemolytic streptococci
   d. *Staphylococcus aureus*

3. **Commonest organism causing acute tonsillitis in children:** (*JIPMER 92, Exam 2014*)
   a. Streptococcus
   b. Hemophilus
   c. Staphylococcus
   d. *Treponema vincenti*

4. **Referred pain from tonsils to the middle ear is along the:** (*Kolkata 2001, Exam 2017*)
   a. Vagus nerve
   b. Glossopharyngeal nerve
   c. Auriculotemporal nerve
   d. Greater auricular nerve

5. **Arterial supply of tonsil is mainly:**
   (*AI 97, Exam 2015*)
   a. Tonsillar branch of facial artery
   b. Maxillary artery
   c. Middle meningeal artery
   d. Internal carotid artery

6. **The palatine tonsil receives its arterial supply from all of the following, except:**
   (*AIIMS May 2005, Exam 2017*)
   a. Facial
   b. Ascending palatine
   c. Sphenopalatine
   d. Dorsal lingual

7. **All of the following vessels supply blood to the tonsils except:** (*Exam 2013*)
   a. Ascending pharyngeal artery
   b. Tonsillar branch of facial artery
   c. Superior labial artery
   d. Dorsal lingual artery

8. **The commonest lymph node to enlarge in acute tonsillitis is:** (*TN 95, Exam 2015*)
   a. Jugulo-omohyoid
   b. Jugulo-digastric
   c. Posterior cervical
   d. Submandibular

9. **All of the following cause a grey white membrane on the tonsil, except:**
   (*AIIMS 2004, SGPGI 2005, Exam 2017*)
   a. Infectious mononucleosis
   b. Ludwig's angina
   c. Streptococcal tonsillitis
   d. Diphtheria

10. **Patch on tonsil is not caused by:**
    (*Exam 2010, 2017*)
    a. Vincent's angina
    b. Candida
    c. Staphylococcus
    d. Ludwig's angina

11. **All can cause white membrane over tonsils, except:**
    (*DPG 2009*)
    a. Streptococcus
    b. Candida
    c. Diphtheria
    d. *Borrelia vincenti*

12. **Black coloured patch in the mouth is seen in:**
    (*AI 91, Exam 2011*)
    a. Acute tonsillitis
    b. Peritonsillar abscess
    c. Vincent's angina
    d. Leukaemia

13. **Trench mouth is:** (*UP 2007, Exam 2017*)
    a. Sub mucosal fibrosis
    b. Tumour at uveal angle
    c. Ulcerative lesion of the gingiva
    d. Retention cyst of the tonsil

14. **The typical characteristic of diphtheritic membrane is:** (*Exam 2008, Exam 2017*)
    a. Loosely attached and does not bleed on removal
    b. Pearly white in colour
    c. Firmly attached and bleeds on removal
    d. Membrane is confined to the tonsil

15. **Vincent's angina is caused by:**
    (*Exam 2007, Exam 2017*)
    a. Borrelia and F. fusiformis
    b. Beta-hemolytic streptococci
    c. Microaerophilic streptococci
    d. *Treponema pallidum*

16. **Vincent's angina affect:** (*Exam 2011, Exam 2017*)
    a. Sub-mandibular space
    b. Heart
    c. Gums
    d. Larynx

17. **All of the following are indications for tonsillectomy except:** (*Exam 2009, Exam 2017*)
    a. Foreign body in tonsils
    b. Unilateral enlargement of tonsils with suspected malignancy
    c. Chronic tonsillitis
    d. Recurrent quinsy

18. **Tonsillectomy is indicated in:**
    (*Exam 2006, Exam 2017*)
    a. Acute tonsillitis
    b. Aphthous ulcers in the pharynx
    c. Tonsillitis causing rheumatic fever
    d. Physiological enlargement

19. **Contraindications to tonsillectomy are all, except:**
    (*MH 2002, Exam 2017*)
    a. Submucous fibrosis
    b. Bleeding disorders
    c. Epidemic of polio
    d. Acute tonsillitis

20. **Not a contraindication of routine tonsillectomy:**
    (*MP 2003, Exam 2016*)
    a. Upper respiratory tract infections
    b. Bleeding disorders
    c. Diphtheria carriers
    d. Cleft palate

21. Contraindication of tonsillectomy: (*PGI 2007, 2015*)
    a. URTI   b. Age less than 4 years
    c. Epidemic of polio d. Bleeding disorders
    e. Chronic tonsillitis

22. Tonsillectomy is contraindicated in which of the following situation: (*MP 2004, Exam 2017*)
    a. Peritonsillar abscess
    b. Acute tonsillitis
    c. For avulsion of glossopharyngeal nerve
    d. Suspected tonsillar malignancy

23. A 5-year-old child is scheduled for tonsillectomy. On the day of surgery he had running nose, temperature 37.5°C and dry cough. Which of the following should be the most appropriate decision for surgery: (*AI 2006, Exam 2017*)
    a. Surgery should be done next day and child should be put on I/V antibiotics and paracetamol
    b. Can proceed for surgery on the same day after starting I/V antibiotics and paracetamol
    c. Get X-ray chest done and if normal proceed for surgery
    d. Cancel surgery for 3 weeks and put the patient on antibiotics

24. The position adopted for tonsillectomy is also adopted for this procedure: (*JIPMER 2003, Exam 2016*)
    a. Direct laryngoscopy b. Bronchoscopy
    c. Tracheostomy   d. Indirect laryngoscopy

25. Commonest postoperative complication of tonsillectomy is: (*Exam 2016*)
    a. Palatal palsy   b. Hemorrhage
    c. Injury to uvula   d. Infection

26. Haemorrhage during tonsillectomy is usually from: (*Exam 2013*)
    a. Maxillary artery   b. Paratonsillar vein
    c. Lingual artery   d. Middle meningeal artery

27. Torrential bleed during tonsillectomy is due to: (*AI 2000, Exam 2013*)
    a. Lingual artery   b. Tonsillar artery
    c. Paratonsillar vein   d. None

28. Ramu 15-year-old male presents with haemorrhage 5 hours after tonsillectomy. Best treatment for this patient is: (*AIIMS 2003, Exam 2017*)
    a. External gauze packing
    b. Antibiotics and mouth wash
    c. Irrigation with cold saline
    d. Re explore immediately

29. Secondary haemorrhage after tonsillectomy usually presents at: (*AI 2011*)
    a. 12 hours   b. 24 hours
    c. 6 days   d. 12 days

30. Haemorrhage occurring 6 hours after tonsillectomy is called: (*TN 2000, Exam 2017*)
    a. Primary haemorrhage
    b. Secondary haemorrhage

    c. Reactionary haemorrhage
    d. None of the above

31. After tonsillectomy, secondary haemorrhage occurs: (*JIPMER 2003, Exam 2013*)
    a. Within 24 hours
    b. After 2 weeks
    c. 5–10 postoperative days
    d. After 1 month

32. Which of the following can cause secondary haemorrhage after tonsillectomy?   (*AI 2002, Exam 2017*)
    a. Injury to blood vessels
    b. Patient not taking antibiotics
    c. Slipping of surgical knot
    d. None of these

33. Laser uvulopalatoplasty is done for: (*AIIMS Nov 2012*)
    a. Snoring   b. Pharyngotonsillitis
    c. Cleft palate   d. Stammering

34. Palatine tonsil not seen is: (*Exam 2014*)
    a. Develops from second pharyngeal pouch
    b. Branch of facial artery is main blood supply
    c. Covered by fibrous capsule
    d. Leads to ear pain due to Xth nerve

35. Pseudomembrane over tonsil and pharynx is caused by: (*AIIMS MAY 2014*)
    a. Gram +ve bacteria   b. Gram -ve bacteria
    c. SSRNA virus   d. None of the above

36. Palatine tonsil is covered with which epithelium: (*NIMHANS 2015*)
    a. Ciliated columnar
    b. Stratified squamous non-keratinized
    c. Stratified squamous keratinized
    d. Simple cuboidal

37. Palatine tonsil seen is: (*Exam 2015*)
    a. Develops from 2nd pharyngeal arch
    b. Branch of maxillary is the main blood supply
    c. Covered by fibrous capsule
    d. Leads to ear pain due to transmission by Xth nerve

38. All of the following instruments are commonly used in tonsillectomy, except: (*Exam 2016*)
    a. Bipolar cautery   b. Conduction wand
    c. Harmonic scalpel   d. Microdebrider

39. Crypta magna is the remnant of: (*Exam 2012*)
    a. First pharyngeal pouch
    b. Second pharyngeal pouch
    c. Third pharyngeal pouch
    d. Fourth pharyngeal pouch

40. Tonsil develops from: (*Exam 2016*)
    a. First pharyngeal pouch
    b. Second pharyngeal pouch
    c. Third pharyngeal pouch
    d. Fourth pharyngeal pouch

41. Anterior tonsillar pillar is formed by: (*Exam 2016*)
a. Palatopharyngeal fold
b. Palatoglossal fold
c. Pterygopalatine arch
d. Valleculae

42. All of the following are true regarding tonsillectomy in children, except: (*Exam 2016*)
a. Extra capsular approach is best for cold approach
b. Sleep apnoea is an indication
c. Adenoids should also be removed along with tonsils if significantly enlarged
d. Hemorrhage following tonsillectomy is usually arterial

IMAGE BASED PRACTICE QUESTIONS BY THE AUTHOR

43. A patient presents with sore throat, fever and pain in the ear. Examination of throat shows the following finding. He can be treated by the following except:

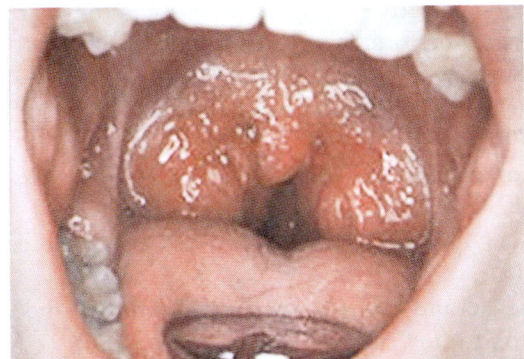

a. Penicillin
b. 2nd generation cephalosporin
c. Macrolides
d. Ciprofloxacin

44. A 25-years-old male presents with fever, sore throat and odynophagia. He was diagnosed as acute tonsillitis and was started on amoxyclav. Inspite of the management his condition worsened and examination of the throat shows the following. He should be investigated for the following except:

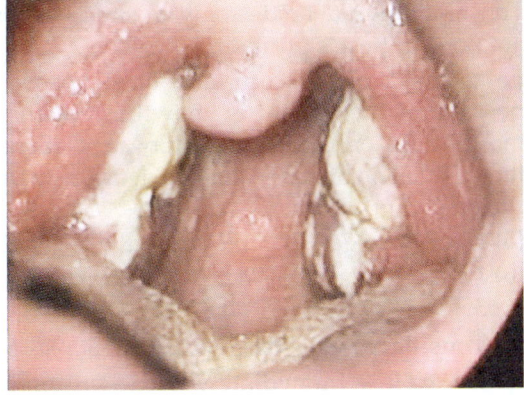

a. Diphtheria
b. Infectious mononucleosis
c. Submucous fibrosis
d. Candidiasis

45. Not true about the marked structure in the given figure is:

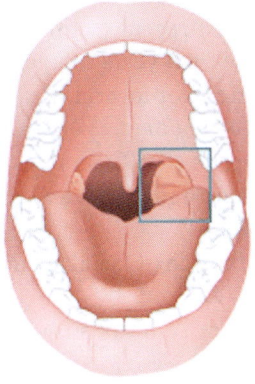

a. Its capsule is formed by buccopharyngeal fascia
b. Pain can be referred from here through glosso-pharyngeal nerve
c. While its removal haemorrhage is usually venous
d. Its largest crypt is crypta magna

46. Tonsillectomy is being done in the given patient. This position is:

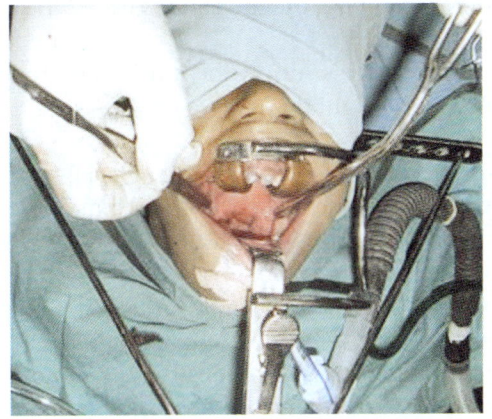

a. Rose's position   b. Trendelenburg position
c. Barking dog position d. Boyce position

47. A 12-year-old unimmunised girl presents with sore throat, fever and pain in the throat. Throat examination reveal membrane over the tonsil which bleed on removal as shown in the picture below. Most probable diagnosis is: (*Exam 2019*)

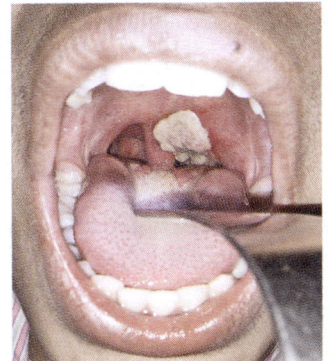

a. Ludwig's angina   b. Diphtheria
c. Peritonsillar abscess d. Pertussis

Oral Cavity and Pharynx

Section III

Oral Cavity and Pharynx *(Section III)*

ANSWERS AND EXPLANATIONS

1. **(d) 12 years** (*Ref. Scott Brown, 8th ed., Vol 3; 635*)
   - The tonsils are present at birth and achieve their maximum size by 5 years of age.
2. **(c) β hemolytic streptococci** (*Ref. Cummings, 6th ed., 3046; Scott Brown, 8th ed., Vol 2; 436*)
3. **(a) Streptococcus** (*Ref. Cummings, 6th ed., 3046*)
4. **(b) Glossopharyngeal nerve** (*Ref. Scott Brown, 8th ed., Vol 3; 558; 742*)
5. **(a) Tonsillar branch of facial artery** (*Ref. Scott Brown, 8th ed., Vol 3; 742*)
   - The arterial supply to tonsil is by external carotid artery branches.
   - Maxillary artery also supplies the tonsil but the main artery supplying is the tonsillar branch of facial (please refer to text).
   - Middle meningeal artery, a branch of maxillary artery, does not supply the tonsil.
6. **(c) Sphenopalatine** (*Ref. Chaurasia, 6th ed., Vol 3; 230*)
   - The Sphenopalatine artery which is a branch of maxillary does not supply the tonsil. It is the main artery supplying the nose and is called the artery of epistaxis.
     The rest arteries supply the tonsil (refer to text).
7. **(c) Superior labial artery** (*Ref. Chaurasia, 6th ed., Vol 3; 230*)
   - Superior labial artery a branch of facial supplies the upper lip, ala of nose and nasal septum (Little's area). It does not supply the tonsils.
     Rest supply the tonsil.
8. **(b) Jugulo-digastric lymph node** (*Ref. Scott Brown, 8th ed., Vol 3; 742*)
   - Lymphatic drainage of tonsil is to jugulo-digastric lymph node (upper deep cervical lymph node). The most common cause of enlargement of these lymph nodes is the tonsillar infection because of which they are also known as tonsillar nodes.
   - Jugulo-omohyoid lymph nodes (middle deep cervical lymph nodes) are known as lymph nodes of tongue as the lymphatics from all over the tongue ultimately drain here.
9. **(b) Ludwig's angina** (*Ref. Scott Brown, 8th ed., Vol 3; 550*)
   - Ludwig's angina is cellulitis of the sub-mandibular space.
   - The rest of the options can cause membrane over tonsils (*refer* to text).
10. **(d) Ludwig's angina** (*Ref. Scott Brown, 8th ed., Vol 3; 550*)
    - Ludwig's angina does not involve tonsil. The other options can lead to patch/pseudomembrane on the tonsil.
11. **(d)** *Borrelia vincenti* (*Ref. Scott Brown, 6th ed., 5/4/14*)
    - In Vincent's angina greyish black necrotic patch is formed over the gingiva and tonsil. Rest of the options cause grey white membrane over tonsil.

12. **(c) Vincent's angina** (*Ref. Scott Brown, 6th ed., 5/4/14*)
13. **(c) Ulcerative lesion of the gingiva** (*Ref. Scott Brown, 6th ed., 5/4/14*)
    - Trench mouth also known as Vincent's angina is acute necrotizing ulcerative gingivitis.
14. **(c) Firmly attached and bleeds on removal** (*Ref. Scott Brown, 8th ed., Vol 3; 799*)
15. **(a) Borrelia and F. fusiformis** (*Ref. Scott Brown, 6th ed., 5/4/14*)
16. **(c) Gums** (*Ref. Scott Brown, 6th ed., 5/4/14*)
    - Vincent's angina is acute necrotizing ulcerative gingivitis spreading over to the tonsil.
    - Ludwig's angina involves submandibular space.
17. **(a) Foreign body in tonsils** (*Ref. Scott Brown, 8th ed., Vol 2; 438*)
    - Rest are indications
    - The most common site of lodgement of a sharp foreign body (e.g. fish bone) is the tonsillar fossa. Here the foreign body is removed and there is no need to do tonsillectomy.
18. **(c) Tonsillitis causing rheumatic fever** (*Ref. Scott Brown, 6th ed., 5/4/18*)
19. **(a) Submucous fibrosis** (*Ref. Scott Brown, 6th ed., 5/4/18*)
20. **(c) Diphtheria carriers** (*Ref. Scott Brown, 6th ed., 5/4/18*)
21. **(a), (c) and (d) are the contraindications.** Kindly refer to text (*Ref. Scott Brown, 6th ed., 5/4/18*).
22. **(b) Acute tonsillitis** (*Ref. Cummings, 6th ed., 3047*)
23. **(d) Cancel surgery for 3 weeks and put the patient on antibiotics** (*Ref. Scott Brown, 6th ed., 5/4/17*)
    - Tonsillectomy is an elective surgery done under GA. Intubation during upper respiratory tract infection carries a high risk of laryngospasm and lung complications. Also a chance of haemorrhage is increased during respiratory tract infections. Here antibiotics are given and the surgery postponed for 3 weeks.
24. **(c) Tracheostomy** (*Ref. Stell & Maran, 5th ed., 275*)
    - Tonsillectomy, adenoidectomy and tracheostomy all are done in Rose's position.
    - For direct laryngoscopy and bronchoscopy the position of the patient is known as "sniffing the morning air" or barking dog or Boyce position. Here there is flexion at cervical and extension at atlanto-occipital joint
25. **(b) Haemorrhage** (*Ref. Scott Brown, 8th ed., Vol 2; 440*)
26. **(b) Paratonsillar vein** (*Ref. Scott Brown, 8th ed., Vol 3; 635*)
27. **(b) Tonsillar artery** (*Ref. Scott Brown, 6th ed., 5/4/20*)
28. **(d) Re explore immediately** (*Ref. Scott Brown, 8th ed., Vol 2; 288*)
    - Hemorrhage following tonsillectomy till within 24 hours is called reactionary hemorrhage and requires re-exploration.

29. **(c) 6 days** (*Ref. Scott Brown, 8th ed., Vol 2; 440*)

30. **(c) Reactionary haemorrhage** (*Ref. Scott Brown, 8th ed., Vol 2; 288*)

31. **(c) 5–10 postoperative days** (*Ref. Scott Brown, 8th ed., Vol 2; 440*)

32. **(b) Patient not taking antibiotics** (*Ref. Scott Brown, 8th ed., Vol 2; 440*)
   - Injury to blood vessels at the time of surgery leads to primary haemorrhage.
   - Slipping of surgical knot leads to reactionary haemorrhage.

33. **(a) Snoring** (*Ref. Cummings, 6th ed., 2863*)
   - Uvulopalatoplasty also known as Uvulopalato-pharyngoplasty (UPPP) is done in obstructive sleep apnoea due to hypertrophied tonsils and bulky oropharynx which usually presents with excessive snoring during sleep and day time somnolence. Kindly refer to text.

34. **(d) Leads to ear pain due to Xth nerve** (*Ref. Scott Brown, 8th ed., Vol 3; 742*)
   - Referred pain from tonsils is through the IXth i.e. Glossopharyngeal nerve.

35. **(a) Gram +ve bacteria** (*Ref. Scott Brown, 8th ed., Vol 3; 799*)

36. **(b) Stratified squamous non-keratinized** (*Ref. Scott Brown, 8th ed., Vol 3; 743*)

37. **(c) Covered by fibrous capsule** (*Ref. Scott Brown, 8th ed., Vol 3; 743; 542*)

38. **(b) Conduction wand** (*Ref. Cummings, 6th ed., 2861*)
   - Coblation wand is used here

39. **(b) Second pharyngeal pouch** (*Ref. Scott Brown, 8th ed., Vol 3; 208; Chaurasia, 6th ed., Vol 3; 230*)

40. **(b) Second pharyngeal pouch** (*Ref. Scott Brown, 8th ed., Vol 3; 542*)

41. **(b) Palatoglossal fold**, *see* Chapter 26 (*Ref. Scott Brown, 8th ed., Vol 3; 742*).

42. **(d) Hemorrhage following tonsillectomy is usually arterial** (*Ref. Cummings, 6th ed., 2861*)

43. **(d) Ciprofloxacin** (*Ref. Cummings, 6th ed., 3047*)

44. **(c) Submucous fibrosis** (*Ref. Scott Brown, 8th ed., Vol 3; 799; 805*)

45. **(a) Its capsule is formed by buccopharyngeal fascia**, *see* Chapter 26 (*Ref. Scott Brown, 8th ed., Vol 3; 742*)
   - Its capsule is formed by pharyngobasilar fascia

46. **(a) Rose's position** (refer to text) (*Ref. Stell & Maran 5th ed., 275*)
   - Trendelenburg position: Here the body is laid flat on the table with head lower the pevis. It is used for abdominal or gynaecological procedures.
   - For direct laryngoscopy the patient is made to lie supine with flexion at his cervical spine and extension at atlanto-occipital joint. This is known as sniffing the morning air, or barking dog position or Boyce position.

47. **(b) Diphtheria** (*Ref. Harrison's, 20th ed., Chapter 145*)

Abscesses of Pharynx

PERITONSILLAR ABSCESS/QUINSY

The peritonsillar space is the space just lateral to the capsule of tonsil, i.e. **between the capsule of tonsil and superior constrictor muscle**.

Any infection of the oropharynx can affect the tonsil and through its crypts (usually **crypta magna**, it being the deepest) can reach the peritonsillar space, leading to peritonsillar abscess. Since the tonsil becomes atrophic in adults, the crypta magna easily reaches up to the capsule, transmitting oropharyngeal infection easily to peritonsillar space. Hence it is seen more commonly in adults.

Peritonsillar abscess is a **unilateral** condition.

It is caused by **mixed aerobic (Group A beta haemolytic strept, GABHS-MC) and anaerobic** bacteria.

Clinical Presentation

The patient presents with
a. Odynophagia: Painful swallowing
b. Muffled or plummy speech known as **hot potato voice** (any painful oropharyngeal mass can lead to a voice which resembles as if there is a hot potato in the mouth) and drooling of saliva.
c. Pain in the ear (referred pain via glossopharyngeal nerve).
d. **Trismus** (limited mouth opening) due to spasm of muscles.
e. Constitutional symptoms (fever)

On Examination

Because of the pus collection lateral to the capsule of tonsil the **tonsil is pushed medially** pushing the uvula to the opposite side. Also there is a bulge of the soft palate (this bulge is due to the collection of pus in the peritonsillar space in relation to the upper pole of the tonsil).

Management

1. **Incision and drainage:** The incision is given either at the maximum bulge or just lateral to where a vertical line drawn at the anterior border of anterior pillar meets a horizontal line passing at the base of uvula.
2. **Antibiotics** (beta lactum group along with metronidazole, to cover aerobes and anaerobes respectively).

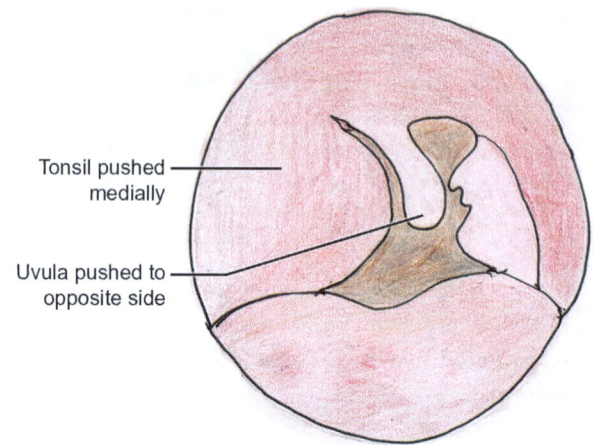

Tonsil pushed medially

Uvula pushed to opposite side

Fig. 31.1: Peritonsillar abscess

3. **Interval tonsillectomy:** This means tonsillectomy is done here after an interval of **6 weeks** after the very 1st episode of quinsy in children. Interval tonsillectomy is done after 6 weeks after the 2nd episode of quinsy in adults.

The rationale of doing interval tonsillectomy despite initial incision and drainage is that repeated infections and repeated incision and drainage will lead to fibrosis making an ultimate tonsillectomy difficult.

Hot tonsillectomy, i.e. tonsillectomy at the time of acute episode is not done because of increased chances of haemorrhage and septicaemia during acute infection, *see* chapter on tonsils.

PARAPHARYNGEAL ABSCESS

In parapharyngeal abscess the abscess is in the parapharyngeal or pharyngo-maxillary space just lateral to the lateral pharyngeal wall.

In spite of it being the smallest space in relation to the pharynx it is the **most commonly infected** space of the pharynx as infections from tonsil (most commonly), dental, parotid, retropharyngeal, prevertebral and submandibular space can all lead to parapharyngeal abscess.

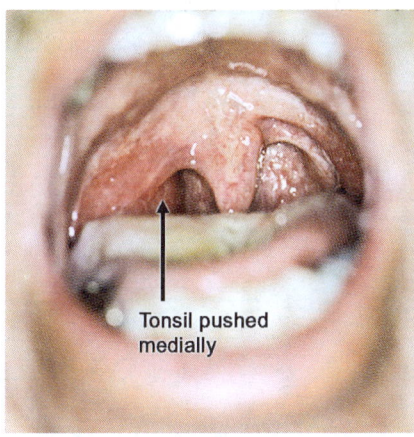

Fig. 31.2

It can involve the anterior compartment, i.e. the pre-styloid compartment or posterior (post-styloid) compartment (please refer to chapter on anatomy of pharynx).

If the **pre-styloid compartment** is involved a **triad of** following **features** are seen:

1. **Tonsils pushed medially** (here the tonsils are pushed medially because of the lateral pharyngeal wall being pushed medially). The patient below is having a parapharyngeal mass/abscess on the right side pushing the tonsil medially.
2. **Trismus** (due to the spasm of medial pterygoid muscle).
3. **Bulge in the neck at the angle of jaw**, i.e. at the upper 1/3rd of sternocleidomastoid.

The parapharyngeal space extends below till the level of hyoid bone causing bulge at the angle of jaw or the upper 1/3rd of sternocleidomastoid.

This is the differentiating feature of an anterior compartment parapharyngeal abscess from a peritonsillar abscess. In peritonsillar abscess only the 1st two signs, i.e. the tonsils being pushed medially and trismus are present.

In posterior compartment parapharyngeal space abscess, there is torticollis due to spasm of prevertebral muscles and also the symptoms because of involvement of the nerves of post-styloid compartment (9th, 10th, 11th, and 12th cranial) and cervical sympathetic chain. There can also be complications involving the major vessels in this space (internal jugular vein thrombosis and rupture of internal carotid).

Treatment

Incision and drainage is done by a horizontal incision 2–3 cm below the lower border of mandible along with I/V antibiotics.

Note:

Any incision in the neck is always given 2 fingers below the lower border of mandible to avoid injury to the marginal mandibular branch of facial nerve. This nerve curves to ascend up from the neck crossing the mandible to supply the corner of mouth and lower lip. Its injury gives rise to inability of that corner of the mouth and lower lip to move down while speaking and smiling giving rise to a cosmetic deformity.

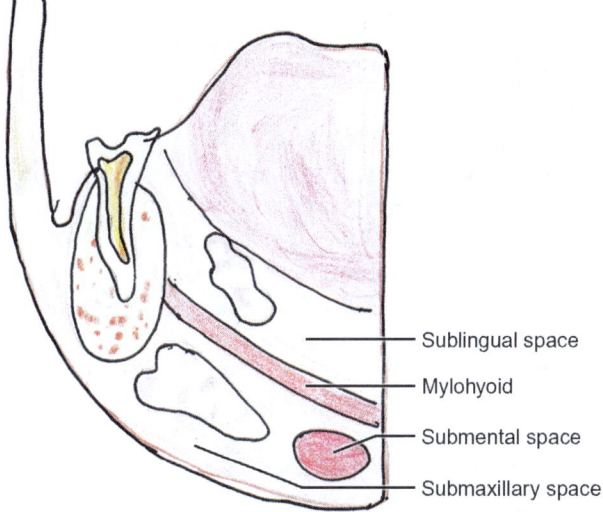

Fig. 31.3: Submandibular space

LUDWIG'S ANGINA

This is infection of the **submandibular space**, i.e. **floor of mouth**.

The most common cause of Ludwig's angina is dental caries.

The organisms responsible are **mixed aerobic** (alpha haemolytic streptococcus, staphylococcus) and **anaerobic** (bacteroides).

The submandibular space is divided into 2 spaces by the mylohyoid muscle (also known as **oral diaphragm**).

The space above the mylohyoid is known as sublingual space. Here the infection spreads from premolar tooth.

The space below the mylohyoid is known as submaxillary space laterally and submental space in the centre. Infection to this space follows carious molars.

Presentation

Infection of the **sublingual space** leads to raised floor of mouth, difficulty in eating and speaking.

The infection of the **submaxillary and submental space** presents with a very tense swelling (brawny oedema) with **woody** feel of the skin of neck below the chin and mandible (as this is a very tense space) and trismus (trismus here is due to the tense mass below the mandible).

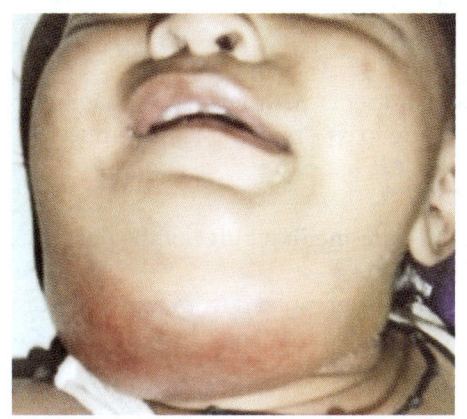

Fig. 31.4

Ultimately both these spaces get involved as they communicate with each other behind the medial border of mylohyoid.

There are four Goldring's criteria to diagnose Ludwig's angina.

1. It is always a **cellulitis** and not an abscess. If an abscess is present it is known as submandibular abscess and not Ludwig's angina.
2. It is always **bilateral**
3. It **spreads through tissue spaces** and not through lymphatics.
4. It does not involve the submandibular and sublingual salivary glands.

Management

1. **Incision and drainage:** In spite of Ludwig's angina being a cellulitis and not an abscess, a horizontal incision is given 2–3 cm below the lower border of mandible extending from one angle of mandible to the other. This is given to relieve the tissue pressure and accelerate healing as this is a very tense space.
2. Antibiotics are given covering aerobes as well as anaerobes.

RETROPHARYNGEAL ABSCESS

The retropharyngeal space lies in between the buccopharyngeal fascia anteriorly and the alar fascia posteriorly, *see* chapter on anatomy of pharynx.

It is divided longitudinally by a midline fibrous raphe into two paramedian spaces known as space of Gillette which contains lymph nodes known as nodes of Rouviere.

The nasopharynx and the oropharynx drains into these lymph nodes.

Acute Retropharyngeal Abscess

Acute suppurative lymphadenitis of these lymph nodes (of Rouviere) leads to acute retropharyngeal abscess.

Since nasopharyngeal (adenoiditis) and oropharyngeal infections (tonsillitis) are **more common in children**, acute retropharyngeal abscess is also more common in children than adults. In adults it occurs more commonly due to penetrating injuries (e.g. fish bone, etc.) of the posterior pharyngeal wall.

Presentation

The patient presents with fever, dysphagia, stridor and torticollis (due to spasm of paraspinal muscles).

On Examination

A **unilateral para-median bulge** of the **posterior pharyngeal wall** is seen.

It has to be differentiated from a prevertebral abscess in which a midline diffuse bulge of the posterior pharyngeal wall is present.

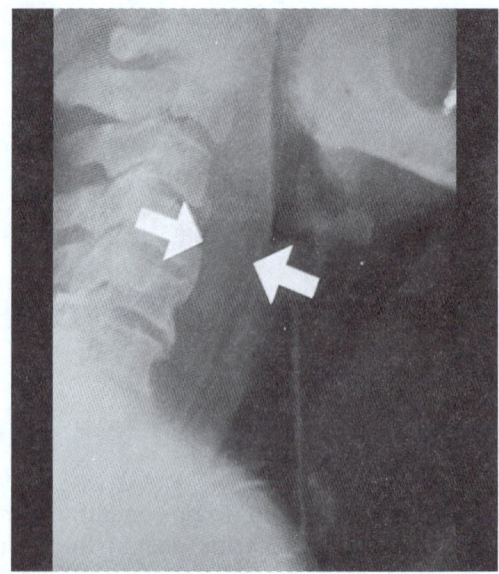

Fig. 31.5

X-ray soft tissue neck (STN) lateral view in both retropharyngeal and prevertebral abscesses will show increased prevertebral shadow.

So an X-ray cannot differentiate the two.

Features on X-ray (STN) Suggestive of Retropharyngeal Abscess

1. Widened retropharyngeal space:
   Normal thickness of retropharyngeal space:
   - Children: At C 2–7 mm and at C 6–14 mm
   - Adults: At C 6–22 mm
2. Reversal of normal cervical lordosis
3. Air-fluid level
4. Gas

Management

Incision and drainage: The incision is given intra-orally at the site of maximum bulge.

Chronic Retropharyngeal Abscess

This is seen most commonly in **adults**. The most common cause of chronic retropharyngeal abscess is **tuberculous infection** of these lymph nodes (of Rouviere) following Pott's spine or caries spine.

Management

1. ATT: It is the mainstay of treatment.
2. If nerve compression symptoms or stridor is present antigravity aspiration is done (the aspiration is antigravity in a TB abscess so as to reduce the chances of a sinus formation).
3. If no relief despite antigravity aspiration, drainage can be done by an external incision either at the anterior border (for low abscess) or at the posterior border (for high abscess) of sternocleidomastoid.

"Points to Ponder/Points for Quick revision"

- **Peritonsillar abscess/quinsy (MC–adults):** Oropharyngeal infection → Crypta magna → peritonsillar space.
- Odynophagia, hot potato voice, trismus, referred earache (glossopharyngeal N); Tonsils pushed medially.
- T/t: Intraoral I & D, antibiotics → interval tonsillectomy (after 6 weeks; 1st episode–children; 2nd episode–adults).
- **Parapharyngeal abscess:**
- Trismus, tonsils pushed medially, bulge at the angle of jaw (differentiates quinsy).
- T/t—I & D, antibiotics.
- **Ludwig's angina:** Cellulitis of B/L sub-mandibular space (MC—following odontogenic infection).
- Raised floor of mouth, brawny oedema, woody feel.
- I & D, antibiotics.
- **Retropharyngeal abscess:** Acute (MC—children); chronic (adults).
- U/L Bulge in posterior pharyngeal wall—one side of midline (differentiates prevertebral abscess—midline diffuse bulge).
- X-ray—↑ prevertebral shadow.
- T/t—I & D, antibiotics (acute); ATT (chronic).

Features	Quinsy	Parapharyngeal abscess	Ludwig's angina
Trismus	+	+	+
Tonsils pushed medially	+	+	−
U/L bulge at angle of jaw	−	+	−
Raised floor of mouth	−	−	+
B/L woody brawny oedema of skin below mandible	−	−	+

Features	Retropharyngeal abscess	Prevertebral abscess
Dysphagia	+	+
Stridor	+	+
Torticollis	+	+
Prevertebral shadow ↑ on X-ray	+	+
Bulge of posterior pharyngeal wall	U/L paramedian bulge	Midline diffuse bulge

Oral Cavity and Pharynx

Section III

Section III — Oral Cavity and Pharynx

PREVIOUSLY ASKED QUESTIONS

1. In which of the following locations there is collection of pus in the quinsy: *(AIIMS 2004, Exam 2016)*
   a. Peritonsillar space
   b. Parapharyngeal space
   c. Retropharyngeal space
   d. Within the tonsil

2. Abscess between tonsillar area and superior constrictor muscle is known as: *(MH 2000, Exam 2016)*
   a. Quinsy
   b. Dental abscess
   c. Parapharyngeal abscess
   d. Retropharyngeal abscess

3. Quinsy is synonymous with: *(AI 99, Exam 2013)*
   a. Parapharyngeal abscess
   b. Retropharyngeal abscess
   c. Peritonsillar abscess
   d. Paratonsillar abscess

4. True about quinsy is: *(PGI 2002, 2016)*
   a. Penicillin is used in treatment
   b. Abscess is located in capsule
   c. Commonly occurs bilaterally
   d. Immediate tonsillectomy should be done
   e. Patient presents with odynophagia and drooling of saliva

5. All of the following are true about peritonsillar abscess, except: *(AP 2006, Exam 2013)*
   a. Bulge in soft palate
   b. Does not involve floor of mouth
   c. Abscess is collected lateral to the superior constrictor
   d. Trismus is commonly associated

6. Treatment for peritonsillar abscess is: *(AP 2005, Exam 2016)*
   a. Immediate tonsillectomy
   b. Incision and drainage
   c. Antibiotics alone
   d. I and D plus antibiotics

7. A 7-year-old child presents with peritonsillar abscess with trismus. The best treatment is: *(AIIMS 2003, Exam 2016)*
   a. Immediate abscess drain orally
   b. Drainage externally
   c. Systemic antibiotics up to 48 hours then drainage
   d. Tracheostomy

8. The ideal time for tonsillectomy after an attack of quinsy is: *(Exam 2015)*
   a. 2 weeks   b. 4 weeks
   c. 6 weeks   d. 12 weeks

9. Infection of submandibular space is seen in: *(Manipal 2008, Exam 2013)*
   a. Ludwig angina   b. Vincent angina
   c. Prinzmetal angina d. Unstable angina

10. True about Ludwig's angina: *(PGI 2007, 2013)*
    a. Involves both submandibular and sublingual spaces
    b. Most common cause is dental infection
    c. Bilateral
    d. Spreads by lymphatics

11. True about Ludwig's angina: *(PGI 2003, 2014)*
    a. Rapidly spreading cellulitis of left sided chest wall
    b. *H. influenzae* is the most common cause
    c. Oedema of floor of mouth
    d. Sub lingual and sub maxillary spaces are involved

12. Ludwig's angina is characterised by all the following, except: *(AI 94, Exam 2014)*
    a. Cellulitis of the floor of the mouth
    b. Caused by anaerobic organisms
    c. Aphthous ulcers in the pharynx
    d. Infection spreads to parapharyngeal space

13. Which of the following is not true about acute retropharyngeal abscess? *(Exam 2013)*
    a. Dysphagia
    b. Swelling on posterolateral wall of pharynx
    c. Torticollis
    d. Caries of cervical spine is usually a common cause

14. All of the following are true about retropharyngeal abscess except: *(AIIMS Nov 2010)*
    a. Confined to one side of the midline
    b. Can be palpable per orally by pressing the finger on posterior pharyngeal wall
    c. Lies behind the prevertebral fascia
    d. Presents with dysphagia and difficulty in breathing

15. Commonest cause of chronic retropharyngeal abscess: *(Kolkata 2001, Exam 2016)*
    a. Suppuration of retropharyngeal lymph node
    b. Caries of cervical spine
    c. Infective foreign body
    d. Caries teeth

16. True statement about chronic retropharyngeal abscess: *(PGI 2003, 2015)*
    a. Association with tuberculosis of spine
    b. Causes psoas spasm
    c. Suppuration of Rouviere lymph node
    d. Treatment by surgery

17. A 30-year-old male underwent tooth extraction for dental caries. Now he presents with fever and trismus. Oropharyngeal examination is revealing that the tonsils are pushed medially. There is also a swelling in the neck at the upper border of sternocleidomastoid muscle. Most likely diagnosis is: *(AIIMS 2001, Exam 2016)*
    a. Retropharyngeal abscess
    b. Ludwig's angina
    c. Peritonsillar abscess
    d. Parapharyngeal abscess

18. Middle age diabetic with tooth extraction with ipsilateral swelling over upper one third of sterno-cleidomastoid and displacement of ipsilateral tonsil towards contralateral side: *(Exam 2013)*
    a. Parapharyngeal abscess
    b. Retropharyngeal abscess
    c. Ludwig's angina
    d. None

19. The medial bulging of pharynx is seen in: *(AI 91, Exam 2012)*
    a. Pharyngomaxillary abscess
    b. Retropharyngeal abscess
    c. Peritonsillar abscess
    d. Prevertebral abscess

20. Parapharyngeal abscess—all true except: *(Exam 2013)*
    a. Midline swelling
    b. Abscess in pharyngo maxillary space
    c. Trismus
    d. Torticollis

21. True about peritonsillar abscess except: *(Exam 2014)*
    a. Follows sore throat
    b. Hot potato voice
    c. Shifting of uvula to same side
    d. Odynophagia

22. Most common cause of parapharyngeal abscess is: *(Exam 2015)*
    a. TB   b. Adenoiditis
    c. Tonsillitis   d. Lymphadenitis

23. HOT potato voice is characteristic of: *(Exam 2015)*
    a. Nasopharyngeal   b. Glottic mass
    c. Subglottic mass   d. Oropharyngeal mass

24. Trismus can be seen in all except: *(Exam 2015)*
    a. Ludwig angina   b. Quinsy
    c. Prevertebral abscess d. Parapharyngeal abscess

25. In quinsy, the part of tonsil to be affected first is: *(Exam 2016)*
    a. Inferior pole   b. Capsule of tonsil
    c. Crypta magna   d. Posterior pillar area

26. This young boy came with history of fever and severe throat pain and odynophagia. His voice is

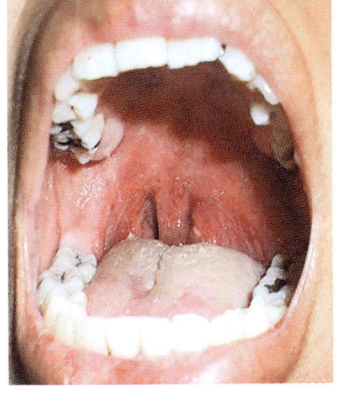

muffled (hot potato voice). This is his picture. Which one of the following is the most likely cause of his complaints: *(APPG 2015)*
    a. Candidial infection
    b. Glossitis
    c. Chronic fibrotic tonsillitis
    d. Quinsy

IMAGE BASED PRACTICE QUESTIONS BY THE AUTHOR

27. This patient gives the history of toothache since one week. What is the diagnosis:

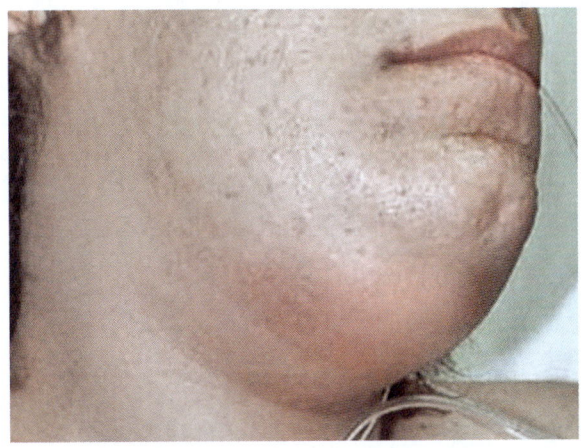

    a. Acute parotitis   b. Angioneurotic edema
    c. Ludwig's angina   e. Parapharyngeal abscess

28. A 35-year-old male presents with dysphagia and difficulty in breathing. On examination there is a bulge of posterior pharyngeal wall confined to right side of the midline. His X-ray STN is given. True about the above is:

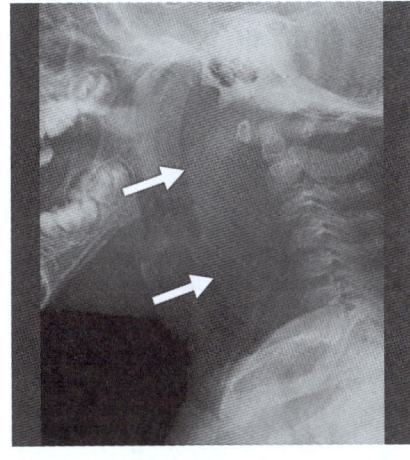

    a. Abscess Lies behind the prevertebral fascia
    b. Suppuration of retropharyngeal lymph node
    c. Involves both submandibular and sublingual spaces
    d. Abscess in pharyngo maxillary space

29. Given below is the picture of a 30-year-old male who underwent tooth extraction for dental caries. Now he presents with fever, difficulty in swallowing and trismus. Oropharyngeal examination is

revealing that the tonsils are pushed medially. Most likely diagnosis is:

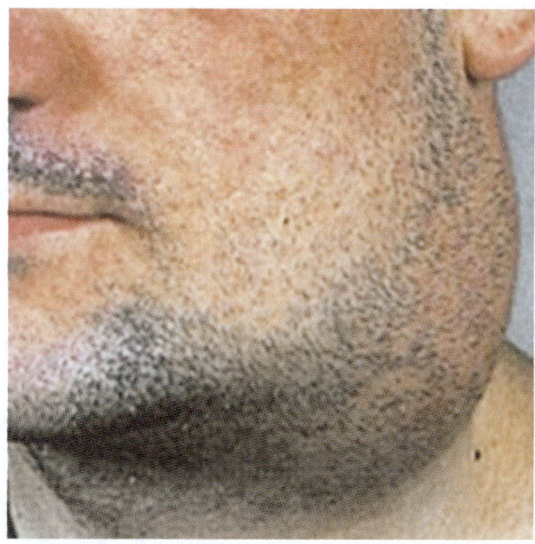

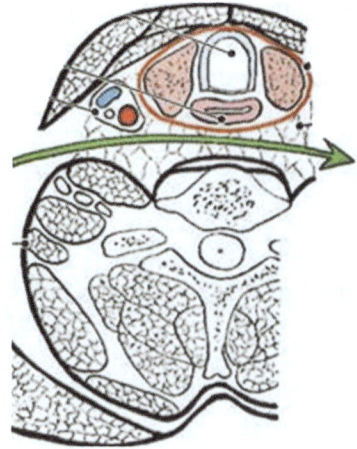

a. Retropharyngeal abscess
b. Ludwig's angina
c. Peritonsillar abscess
d. Parapharyngeal abscess

30. **Not true about the space through which arrow in the picture is passing is:**

a. It contains nodes of Rouviere
b. Acute abscess of this space more common in children
c. Abscess presents as a unilateral paramedian bulge of posterior pharyngeal wall
d. It is prevertebral space

31. **Ludwig's angina arises from:**   (*AIIMS 2018*)
a. Peritonsillar space
b. Parapharyngeal space
c. Submandibular space
d. Sublingual space

ANSWERS AND EXPLANATIONS

1. **(a) Peritonsillar space** (*Ref. Scott Brown, 8th ed., Vol 3; 626*)
2. **(a) Quinsy** (*Ref. Scott Brown, 8th ed., Vol 3; 626*)
3. **(c) Peritonsillar abscess** (*Ref. Scott Brown, 8th ed., Vol 3; 626*)

   There is no entity called Paratonsillar abscess.
4. **(a) and (e) are true** (*Ref. Scott Brown, 8th ed., Vol 3; 797*)
   - Penicillin along with metronidazole (since the flora is mixed aerobic and anaerobic) is given intravenously during treatment.
   - Quinsy is a unilateral condition.
   - In Quinsy the abscess forms in the loose areolar tissue just lateral to the capsule of tonsil and not in the capsule.
   - Here tonsillectomy is done after an interval of 6 weeks. This is known as Interval tonsillectomy.
5. **(c) Abscess is collected lateral to the superior constrictor** (*Ref. Scott Brown, 8th ed., Vol 3; 626*)
   - The abscess is collected in the peritonsillar space medial to the superior constrictor.
   - Rest all are true (kindly refer to the text)
6. **(d) I and D plus antibiotics** (*Ref. Scott Brown, 8th ed., Vol 3; 797*)
   - The treatment of peritonsillar abscess is incision and drainage along with antibiotics followed by interval tonsillectomy.
7. **(a) Immediate abscess drain orally** (*Ref. Scott Brown, 8th ed., Vol 3; 797*)
   - In peritonsillar abscess immediate Incision and drainage is done by an intraoral incision.
   - The trismus here is never so much that mouth cannot be opened for Incision and drainage.
   - Systemic antibiotics are started along with drainage.
8. **(c) 6 weeks** (*Ref. Scott Brown, 6th ed., 5/4/4*)
   - This is known as interval tonsillectomy.
9. **(a) Ludwig angina** (*Ref. Scott Brown, 8th ed., Vol 3; 628; Stell & Maran, 5th ed., 229*)
   - Ludwig angina is infection of the submandibular space, i.e. floor of mouth.
   - Vincent angina is ulcerative gingivitis along with involvement of the tonsils.
   - Prinzmetal angina and unstable angina are the acute coronary syndromes.
10. **(a) (b) and (c)** (*Ref. Scott Brown, 8th ed., Vol 3; 550; Stell & Maran, 5th ed., 229*)
    - In Ludwig's angina infection spreads through tissue spaces and not through lymphatics.
11. **(c) and (d)** (*Ref. Stell & Maran, 5th ed., 229*)
12. **(c) Aphthous ulcers in the pharynx** (*Ref. Stell & Maran, 5th ed., 229*)
13. **(d) Caries of cervical spine is usually a common cause** (*Ref. Scott Brown, 8th ed., Vol 3; 628*)

14. **(c) Lies behind the prevertebral fascia** (*Ref. Scott Brown, 8th ed., Vol 3; 628*)
    - Retropharyngeal abscess lies retro to the pharynx, i.e. behind its last lining the buccopharyngeal fascia. It lies in front of the prevertebral fascia. Behind the prevertebral fascia is the prevertebral space, hence the abscess here is known as prevertebral abscess.
15. **(b) Caries of cervical spine** (*Ref. Scott Brown, 6th ed., 5/4/5*)
16. **(a) and (c)** (*Ref. Scott Brown, 6th ed., 5/4/5*)
    - Chronic retropharyngeal abscess is the tuberculous suppuration of lymph nodes of Rouviere following TB spine.
    - Since retropharyngeal space ends at the level of tracheal bifurcation, i.e. T4 it does not cause psoas spasm.
    - Treatment is mainly by ATT.
17. **(d) Parapharyngeal abscess** (*Ref. Scott Brown, 8th ed., Vol 3; 550*)
    - Ludwig's angina is cellulitis of the submandibular space. Its most common underlying cause is dental caries. The patient has fever and trismus. Here the floor of mouth is raised pushing the tongue up and also there is swelling in the neck below the mandible on both sides. The tonsils are not pushed medially here.
    - Peritonsillar abscess or Quinsy can also follow dental caries. The patient here presents with fever and trismus. On examination, the tonsils are pushed medially but external swelling at the upper border of sternocleidomastoid is not seen here.
    - Parapharyngeal abscess can also follow dental infection. The patient presents with fever and trismus.
    - On examination, the tonsils are pushed medially, because of the lateral pharyngeal wall being pushed medially.
    - Since the lower boundary of the parapharyngeal space is hyoid, here external swelling at the upper border of sternocleidomastoid will also be seen.
    - In retropharyngeal abscess a unilateral para-median bulge of the posterior pharyngeal wall is seen, the tonsil is not displaced here.
18. **(a) Parapharyngeal abscess** (*Ref. Scott Brown, 8th ed., Vol 3; 796*)
    - Please *see* the explanation to the above question.
19. **(a) Pharyngomaxillary abscess** (*Ref. Stell & Maran 5th ed., 229*)
    - In pharyngomaxillary/parapharyngeal abscess, the lateral pharyngeal wall is pushed medially.
    - In retropharyngeal and prevertebral abscess, the posterior pharyngeal wall is pushed anteriorly.
    - In peritonsillar abscess there is no bulging of the pharyngeal wall, only the tonsil is pushed medially.

Oral Cavity and Pharynx

Section III

20. **(a) Midline swelling** (*Ref. Scott Brown, 8th ed., Vol 3; 550*)
- Midline swelling is seen in prevertebral abscess.

21. **(c) Shifting of uvula to same side** (*Ref. Scott Brown, 8th ed., Vol 3; 796*)

22. **(c) Tonsillitis** (*Ref. Scott Brown, 8th ed., Vol 3; 551*)

23. **(d) Oropharyngeal mass** (*Ref. Dhingra, 6th ed., 264; Scott Brown, 8th ed., Vol 3; 796*)

24. **(c) Prevertebral abscess** (*Ref. Scott Brown, 8th ed., Vol 3; 628*)

25. **(c) Crypta magna** (*Ref. Scott Brown, 8th ed., Vol 3; 796*)

26. **(d) Quinsy** (*Ref. Scott Brown, 8th ed., Vol 3; 797*)

27. **(c) Ludwig's angina** (*Ref. Scott Brown, 8th ed., Vol 3; 628*)

28. **(b) Suppuration of retropharyngeal lymph node** (*Ref. Scott Brown, 8th ed., Vol 3; 551*)
- Though X-ray cannot differentiate between the options a and b but since on examination there is a bulge of posterior pharyngeal wall confined to right side of the midline therefore answer is (b).

29. **(d) Parapharyngeal abscess** (*Ref. Scott Brown, 8th ed., Vol 3; 551*)

30. **(d) It is prevertebral space** (*Ref. Scott Brown 8th ed. Vol 3; 549*)

31. **(c) Submandibular space** (*Ref. Scott Brown 8th ed. Vol 3; 550*)
- It is a better answer since sublingual space is a part of submandibular space.

Section III   Oral Cavity and Pharynx

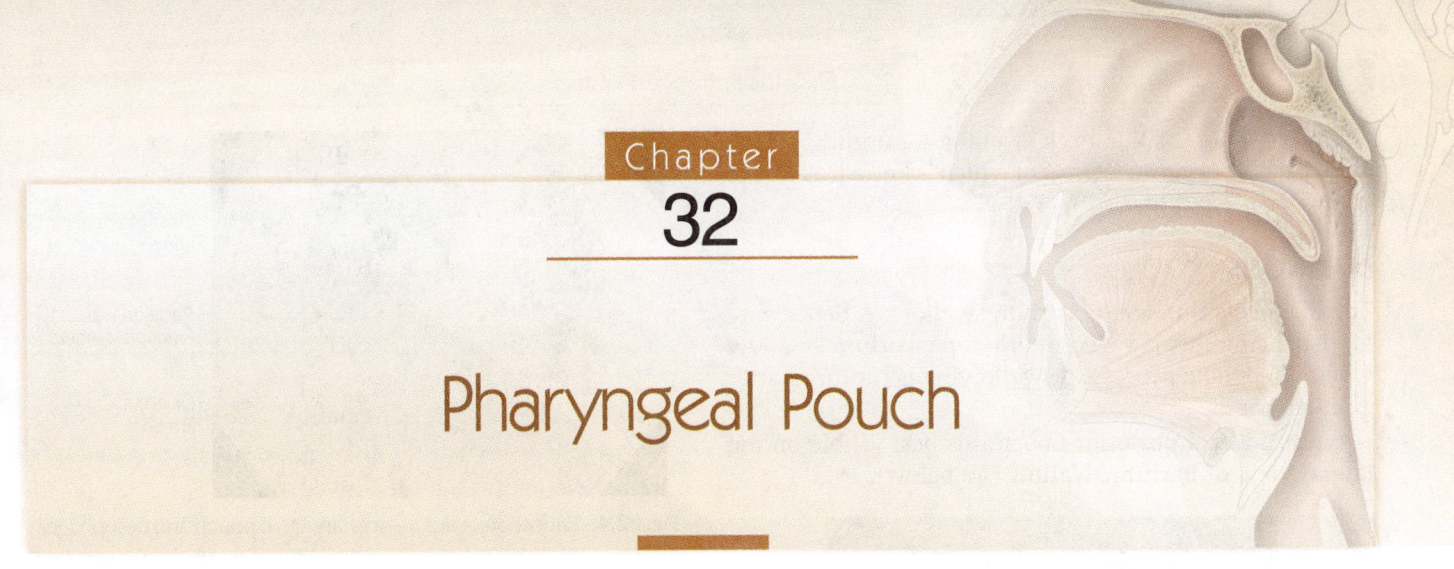

Pharyngeal Pouch

Pharyngeal pouch or diverticulum (a diverticulum is defined as an out pouching from a tubular structure) forms when there is a neuromuscular in coordination while swallowing as a result of which the muscles above the cricopharyngeal sphincter contract to push the food down but the cricopharyngeal sphincter does not open. The pressure is now applied on the walls of the pharynx above the cricopharyngeal sphincter and where there is a site of weakness of pharyngeal wall, pharyngeal out pouching results.

The most common such area of weakness and, therefore, pharyngeal out pouching or diverticulum formation is the **Killian's dehiscence (gateway of tears)** which lies in between the thyropharyngeus (going obliquely upwards and backwards) and Cricopharyngeus (going horizontally backwards, forming the cricopharyngeal sphincter) parts of inferior constrictor muscle, in the hypopharynx.

Killian's dehiscence is present in the posterior wall of hypopharynx so the pharyngeal pouch or diverticulum from here is a **posterior pouch** (lying posterior to the cervical oesophagus initially). This is also known as **Zenker's diverticulum or hypopharyngeal diverticulum**. Zenker's diverticulum is a **pulsion diverticulum** (as it occurs due to increased intraluminal pressure).

A true diverticulum contains all the layers of the tubular structure. Zenker's diverticulum is a **false diverticulum** as it does not involve all the layers of the pharyngeal wall. It contains only mucosa, lined with stratified squamous epithelium with a thin lamina propria. No muscular layer is present here.

PRESENTATION

This is seen usually in **elderly** above 60 years.

The patient presents mainly with **dysphagia** (once the pouch gets filled with food, it starts compressing the cervical oesophagus), **halitosis** (foul breath, due to retained food in the pouch), gurgling sounds in the neck and regurgitation of undigested food (this occurs particularly while lying down).

The regurgitation can cause **aspiration**, cough, recurrent laryngitis, hoarseness, pneumonia and even lung abscess.

Since we do not have much space for the expansion of this pouch posteriorly, when this pouch further enlarges, it comes most commonly on the left side of oesophagus and now becomes visible in the neck. This may be due to the slight convexity of the cervical esophagus to the left side and to the more laterally positioned carotid artery on the left side, creating a potential space for the sac on the left side.

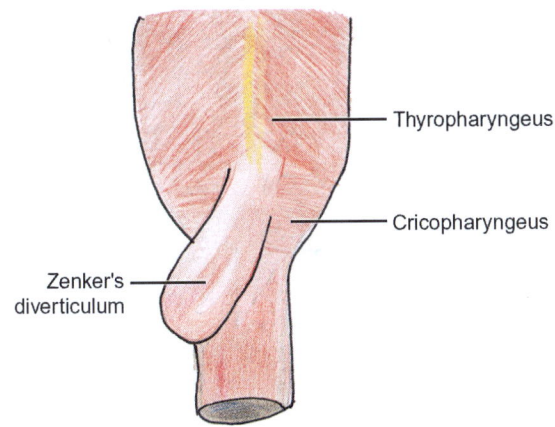

Fig. 32.1: Zenker's diverticulum (a posterior pouch)

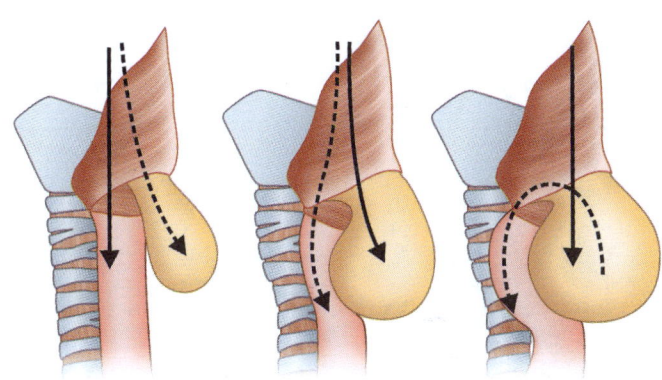

Fig. 32.2: The progressive stages in the development of Zenker's diverticulum. With progressive dilatation of the pouch the oesophageal lumen gets compressed leading to dysphagia and regurgitation of food into the oesophagus and larynx

On palpation of this neck swelling a gurgling sound (cervical borborygmi) is present which is known as **Boyce sign**.

DIAGNOSIS

The diagnosis is made by barium swallow. A better way of visualising this is video fluoroscopic barium swallow where the whole process of swallowing is captured after giving barium.

Since this is a posterior pouch it is best visible on the **lateral view of barium swallow** (*see* below).

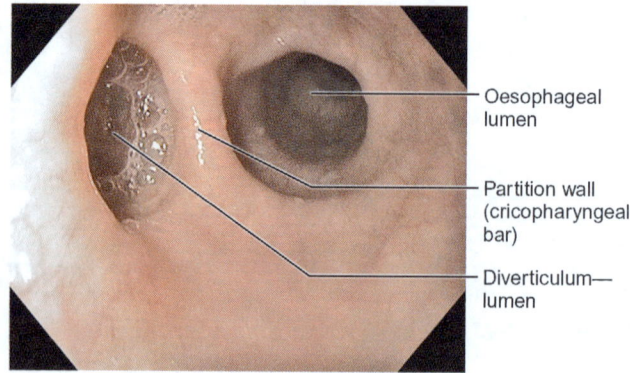

Fig. 32.4: Endoscopic picture of pharyngeal pouch and oesophageal lumen

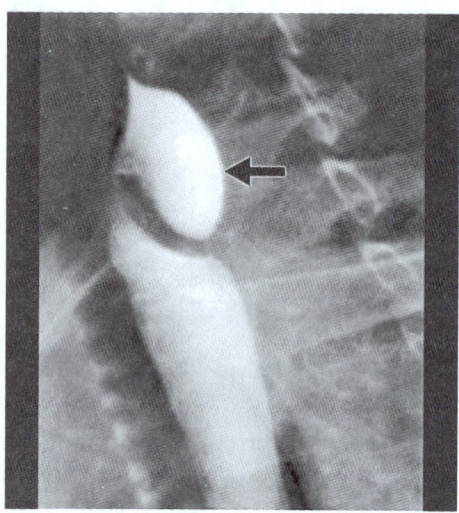

Fig. 32.3

MANAGEMENT

Excision of pouch: The pouch is excised and cricopharyngeal myotomy is done to relax the cricopharyngeal sphincter.

Endoscopic stapling diverticulotomy: This is presently the preferred modality. The endoscopic surgery aims at converting the oesophageal and pouch lumen into a common cavity to avoid collection of food. This is done by cutting the cricopharyngeal bar, i.e. the partition wall between the oesophageal lumen and pouch (diverticulotomy), *see* the endoscopic picture above. The raw mucosal edges arising as a result of cutting of the partition wall are stapled.

Division of the cricopharyngeal partition wall can also be done by CO_2 LASER. Historically this concept of creating a common cavity was successfully practiced by Dohlman who used diathermy to first coagulate the common wall before cutting it (**Dohlman's procedure**).

 "Points to Ponder/Points for Quick revision"

- Elderly: Neuromuscular incoordination—pulsion diverticulum, false diverticulum.
- Killians dehiscence, posterior gap, posterolateral pouch, Zenker's (MC left side of neck)—Boyce sign.
- Halitosis, regurgitation of undigested food, laryngeal and lung symptoms.
- Diagnosis: Barium swallow.
- Management: Endoscopic stapling.

PREVIOUSLY ASKED QUESTIONS

1. Which of the following is known as "Gateway of tears"? *(DPG 2008, Exam 2016)*
   a. Killian's dehiscence
   b. Rathke's pouch
   c. Waldeyer's ring
   d. Sinus of Morgagni

2. One of the following is true regarding Zenker's diverticulum: *(AI 95, Exam 2015)*
   a. It is mostly asymptomatic
   b. Occurs in the mid oesophagus
   c. Treatment is simple excision
   d. It occurs in children

3. Dohlman's operation is related to:
   (DPG 2009, Exam 2016)
   a. Carcinoma esophagus
   b. Carcinoma larynx
   c. Zenker's diverticulum
   d. Nasal carcinoma

4. An elderly male presents with history of dysphagia, regurgitation, foul breath, hoarseness and cough. Right sided lung crepts are noted on examination. The most likely diagnosis is: *(AI 2012)*
   a. Schatzki ring
   b. Zenker's diverticulum
   c. Corkscrew esophagus
   d. Plummer-Vinson syndrome

5. All of the following are true about Zenker's Diverticulum except: *(AI 2011)*
   a. It is an acquired condition
   b. It is a false diverticulum
   c. Barium swallow, lateral view is the IOC
   d. Out pouching of anterior pharyngeal wall above cricopharyngeus muscles

6. Zenker's diverticulum is a: *(Exam 2016)*
   a. Prepharyngeal diverticulum
   b. Parapharyngeal diverticulum
   c. Pharyngotympanic diverticulum
   d. Hypopharyngeal diverticulum

7. One of the following is true regarding Zenker's diverticulum: *(Exam 2016)*
   a. It is a pulsion diverticulum
   b. It projects anteriorly
   c. Commonly seen in young males
   d. It is between superior and middle constrictor

8. Killian dehiscence is seen in: *(Exam 2016)*
   a. Superior constrictor
   b. Inferior constrictor
   c. Middle constrictor
   d. None

IMAGE BASED PRACTICE QUESTION BY THE AUTHOR

9. An elderly male presents with history of dysphagia, halitosis, regurgitation, hoarseness and cough. His barium swallow is given below. Following is true about this condition except:

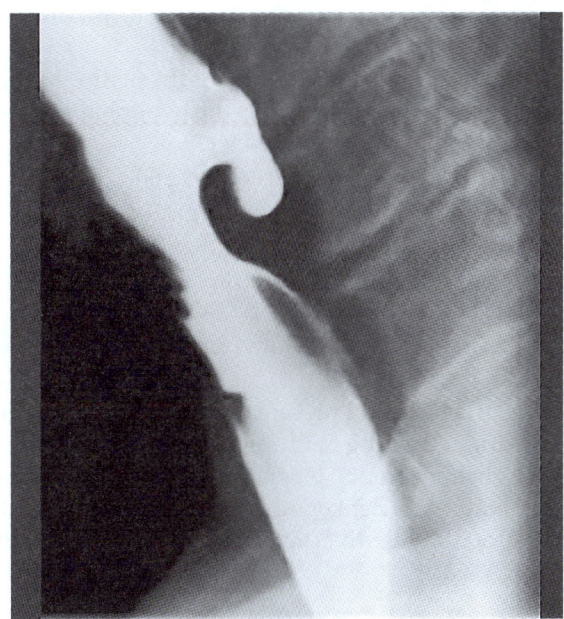

   a. It is a posterior pouch
   b. It is a false diverticulum
   c. Should be managed by excision
   d. Due to traction from outside the oesophagus

ANSWERS AND EXPLANATIONS

1. **(a) Killian's dehiscence** (*Ref. Scott Brown, 8th ed., Vol 3; 811*)
   - The most common site of pharyngeal pouch formation is Killian's dehiscence hence known as Gateway of tears.
   - **Rathke's pouch** is a depression in the roof of the developing pharynx. This pouch eventually loses its connection with the pharynx giving rise to the anterior pituitary (adenohypophysis).
   - Waldeyer's ring which is the ring of lymphatics in the naso and oropharynx and sinus of Morgagni which is the gap between the upper border of superior constrictor and base of skull are not the sites for pharyngeal pouch formation.

2. **(c) Treatment is simple excision** (*Ref. Stell & Maran, 5th ed., 231*)
   - It usually presents with dysphagia and symptoms due to regurgitation of food into the respiratory tract (refer the text).
   - Zenker's diverticulum occurs from the Killian's dehiscence that is present in the hypopharynx above the cricopharyngeal sphincter.
   - It occurs usually in elderly above 60 years.
     Simple excision and other surgical procedures are mentioned in the text.

3. **(c) Zenker's diverticulum** (*Ref. Scott Brown, 8th ed., Vol 3; 816*)

4. **(b) Zenker's diverticulum** (*Ref. Scott Brown, 8th ed., Vol 3; 812*)
   - The given clinical presentation, where dysphagia is mentioned along with regurgitation (hoarseness, cough, lung crepts) is consistent with an oropharyngeal cause, i.e. Zenker's diverticulum. Here the collected food in the diverticulum leads to foul breath.

- Schatzki ring and Corkscrew oesophagus can also lead to dysphagia but they being distal oesophageal conditions are characterised by associated symptoms like retrosternal chest pain and heart burn. In these oesophageal pathologies the chances of regurgitation are far less.
- Schatzki ring is a narrowing of the lower part of the esophagus that can cause intermittent dysphagia especially during hurried ingestion of solid food.
- Corkscrew esophagus also known as nutcracker esophagus, is a spastic motility disorder in which uncoordinated contractions of the esophagus occur because of which food cannot be effectively propelled to the stomach.
- Plummer-Vinson syndrome (PVS), also called Paterson-Brown-Kelly syndrome, however is a proximal oesophageal condition and presents as a triad of postcricoid dysphagia, upper esophageal web and iron deficiency anemia. Regurgitation can occur due to the proximal location of oesophageal web. However, it usually occurs in postmenopausal women.

5. **(d) Out pouching of anterior pharyngeal wall above cricopharyngeus muscles** (*Ref. Scott Brown, 8th ed., Vol 3; 813*)
   - In Zenker's diverticulum there is out pouching of posterior hypopharyngeal wall above cricopharyngeus sphincter.

6. **(d) Hypopharyngeal diverticulum** (*Ref. Scott Brown, 8th ed., Vol 3; 811*)

7. **(a) It is a pulsion diverticulum** (*Ref. Stell & Maran, 5th ed., 231*)

8. **(b) Inferior constrictor** (*Ref. Stell & Maran, 5th ed., 231*)

9. **(d) Due to traction from outside the oesophagus** (*Ref. Scott Brown, 8th ed., Vol 3; 812*)

Section III | **Oral Cavity and Pharynx**

Oral Cancers and Miscellaneous Conditions

RANULA

Ranulas are **extravasation cysts**, originating from the **sublingual gland** in the floor of the mouth.

The development of ranulas depends on the disruption of the flow of saliva from the secretory apparatus of the sublingual salivary glands (due to trauma, sialolith, stenosis, etc.).

Experimentally ligation of the sublingual duct leads to ranula formation, whereas ligation of the submandibular duct and parotid duct does not (they tend to atrophy). The difference lies in the fact that the sublingual glands secrete continuously in inter-digestive period, whereas the other two major salivary glands secrete only in response to stimuli, such as eating.

Therefore, with trauma, if a sublingual salivary duct is obstructed, secretory back pressure builds and leads to extravasation and ranula formation.

Ranulas are divided into 2 types:

1. **Oral ranulas**
2. **Cervical or plunging ranulas**

Oral ranulas as the name lie in the oral cavity below the tongue superior to the mylohyoid muscle.

The mylohyoid muscle which is regarded as the diaphragm of the floor of the mouth can be dehiscent. The sites of dehiscence provide a route of egress for the cyst leading to the formation of cervical or plunging ranulas.

Presentation

A ranula is most commonly observed as a **translucent bluish soft cystic fluctuant** swelling (remotely resembling the belly of a frog (*Rana* species), hence the name) located below the tongue (easy to remember RANULA–sub Lingual gland).

The mass may interfere with speech, mastication, respiration, and swallowing because of the upward and medial displacement of the tongue.

Plunging ranula usually manifests as asymptomatic, enlarging neck mass.

Management

i. **Marsupialisation:** It involves unroofing the cyst and tacking the edges of the cyst to adjacent tissue.
ii. **Sclerosing agents:** Bleomycin, OK-432, etc.
iii. **Sublingual gland excision along with excision of ranula:** here the advantage is that the recurrence rate is very low. The recurrence is high with the above two procedures.

APHTHOUS ULCERS

Aphthous ulcers (canker sores) are painful, shallow ulcers often covered with white/yellow exudates surrounded by an erythematous margin.

They are seen exclusively on **soft oral mucosal surfaces**, e.g. lip, buccal mucosa, floor of mouth, lateral part of tongue and soft palate (in sharp contrast ulcers following

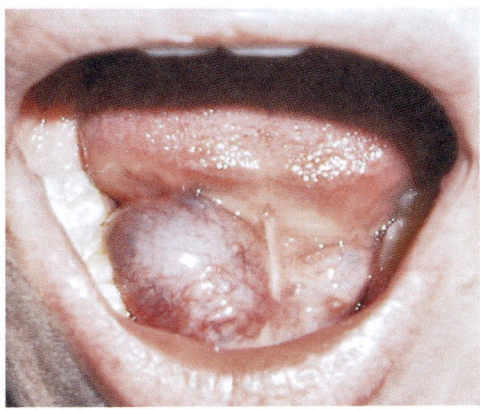

Fig. 33.1: Ranula

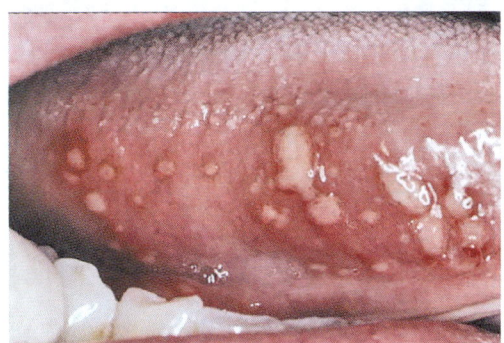

Fig. 33.2: Aphthous ulcers

HSV are vesicular and involve hard mucosal surfaces in the mouth, e.g. gingival, hard palate and dorsal surface of tongue).

The underlying cause of aphthous ulcer is **multifactorial**, e.g. vitamin deficiencies, iron and other mineral deficiencies, stress, allergies, chronic trauma due to ill-fitting dentures, immunologic abnormalities such as celiac disease and genetic predisposition.

They **frequently recur** at irregular intervals. They do not have malignant potential.

Treatment

Multivitamins and minerals, topical anaesthetics and **steroids**.

FORDYCE SPOTS

Fordyce spots or granules are yellowish white spots present on the buccal mucosa and lips in large majority of people. They are **normal sebaceous glands**.

PLUMMER–VINSON SYNDROME

Plummer-Vinson syndrome (PVS), also called Paterson-Brown-Kelly syndrome, presents as a **triad of** postcricoid dysphagia, **Hypopharyngeal/upper** esophageal webs, **and** iron deficiency anaemia (IDA).

Clinical Features

It is seen largely in women over 40–50 years of age.

Dysphagia is typically limited to solids initially and can later on be to liquids also. Here obstruction to food is usually felt in the throat in contrast to conditions affecting lower oesophagus, e.g. Schatzki ring where the obstruction is felt in the epigastric region.

Choking spells and aspiration may occur because of the proximal location of the web.

Weakness, fatigue, and dyspnoea are secondary to iron deficiency anaemia. Other manifestations of tissue iron deficiency, e.g. angular cheilitis, glossitis and koilonychia (spoon nails) may be evident.

Iron deficiency leads to mucosal atrophy and web formation in the postcricoid region of the hypopharynx. There is also atrophy of the gastric mucosa leading to achlorhydria (with achlorhydria there will be interference

with the absorption of iron itself and also vitamin B_{12} and calcium). Therefore, frequently patients with PV syndrome are found to be deficient in vitamin B_{12} also.

If these alterations are of long duration this may lead to carcinoma. In fact in females suffering from Plummer-Vinson syndrome, **postcricoid carcinoma** is the most common carcinoma of hypopharynx otherwise the commonest site for carcinoma in the hypopharynx is pyriform fossa. Approximately **5–15%** of women with PV syndrome develop post-cricoid carcinoma. There is also an increased incidence of carcinomas of tongue, oesophagus and stomach in patients of PV syndrome.

Diagnosis

Blood tests show a microcytic hypochromic anemia that is consistent with the iron-deficiency anemia. Serum ferritin, % transferrin saturation and serum iron are low and TIBC is raised.

Barium swallow or upper gastrointestinal endoscopy (UGIE) may reveal the web in the esophagus. UGIE will also help in taking biopsy to differentiate it from malignancy.

Biopsy of involved mucosa typically reveals epithelial atrophy (shrinking) and varying amounts of submucosal chronic inflammation and submucosal fibrosis. Epithelial atypia or dysplasia may be present (it being a premalignant condition).

Treatment

Treatment is primarily aimed at correcting the iron-deficiency anemia. This may improve dysphagia and pain.

If there is no relief, the web can be dilated during upper endoscopy to allow normal swallowing and passage of food.

PREMALIGNANT CONDITIONS OF ORAL CAVITY AND OROPHARYNX

1. Leukoplakia

It is a white patch in the mucosa that cannot be rubbed off, and cannot be characterised clinically or histopathologically as any other disease or lesion. Leucoplakia is often associated with tobacco smoking though it can be idiopathic. This is the **most common premalignant condition** of the oral cavity. It is managed by **cessation of smoking** and close follow up or **excision** of the leukoplakic patch.

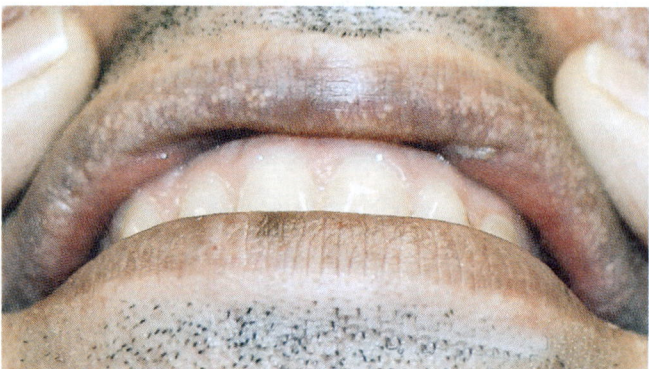

Fig. 33.3: Fordyce spots

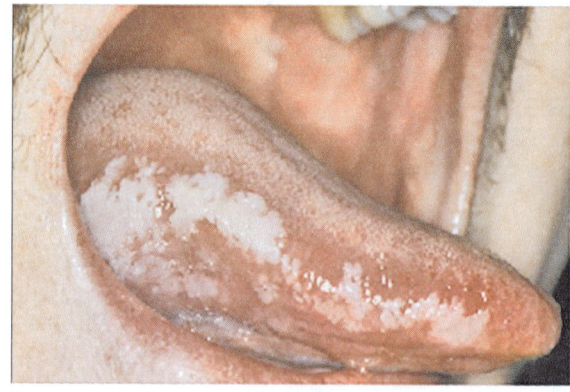

Fig. 33.4: Leukoplakia

2. Erythroplakia

As its name it is a red plaque on the mucosa. It is rare. It carries **higher risk** of carcinoma than leukoplakia. Management is **excision** and close follow up.

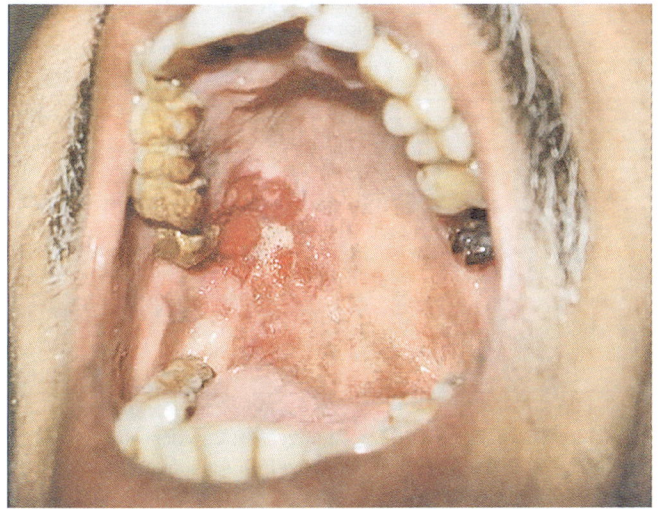

Fig. 33.5: Erythroplakia

3. Sub-mucous Fibrosis (SMF)

It is an uncommon premalignant disorder characterised by inflammation and progressive fibrosis of the sub-mucosal tissues (lamina propria and deeper connective tissues) inside the mouth.

Sub-mucous fibrosis is often associated with chewing betel nuts. It is due to chronic exposure to **arecoline** present in the betel nuts.

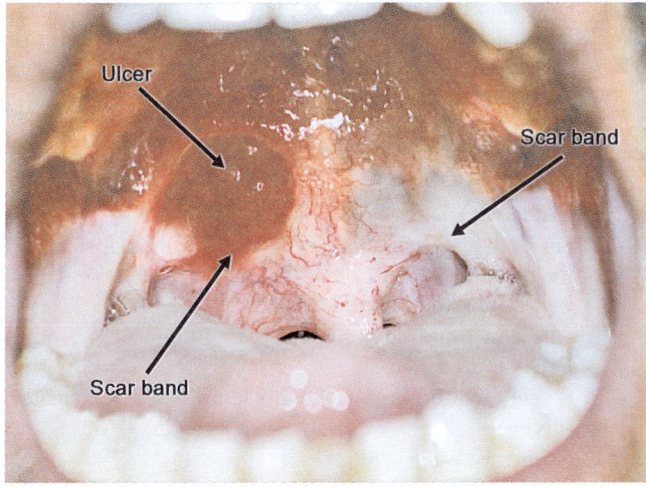

Fig. 33.6: Sub-mucous fibrosis

Presenting features: The condition starts with redness, blistering and ulceration inside the mouth that is eventually replaced with stiff fibrous tissue as it heals. In the advanced stage the oral mucosa loses its resiliency and becomes blanched (white) and stiff. There is progressive inability to open mouth.

Treatment: If the disease is detected at a very early stage, cessation of chewing of betel nuts is sufficient.

Steroids: Weekly submucosal intra-lesional injections of steroids with hyaluronidase may help prevent further damage.

Placental extracts have anti-inflammatory effect hence, useful in preventing or inhibiting mucosal damage.

4. Lichen Planus

These appear as white lacy striae (Wickham's striae) in the oral cavity. Patients often complain of increased sensitivity of the oral mucosa to hot or spicy food and a roughness in the lining of the mouth. The erosive variety of lichen planus is very painful.

It is often associated with skin lichen planus lesions on the flexor surfaces of the wrists, forearm and thigh which are described as 5Ps—**p**urple, **p**ruritic, **p**lanar, **p**olygonal, **p**apules.

Treatment: Steroids.

Rare cases of malignant transformation have been reported.

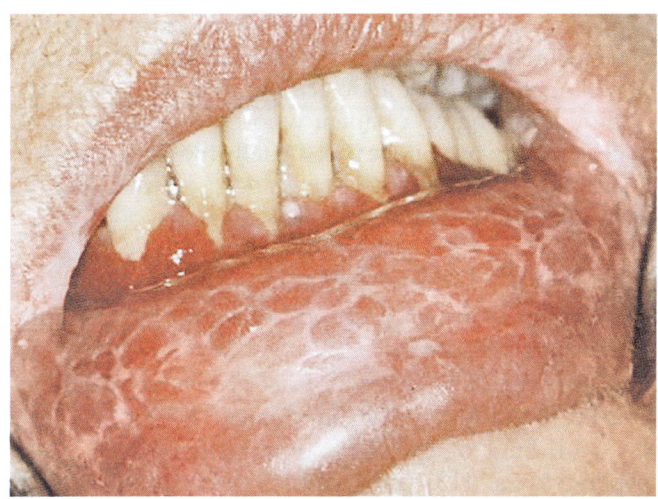

Fig. 33.7: Lichen planus

ORAL CANCERS

Important Learning Facts

- Carcinoma of the oral cavity is overall the **most common carcinoma in males** in India, lung cancer being the 2nd most common here. Oral cavity extends from mucosal surface of lips up to the level of anterior pillar of tonsil. The most important predisposing factors are tobacco (chewing and smoking) and alcohol.
- Most common carcinoma of the oral cavity **worldwide** is carcinoma of the tongue. The carcinoma of the **lateral border of tongue** constitutes 85% of the carcinomas of the tongue.
- **In India,** however the most common carcinoma of the oral cavity is carcinoma of the **gingivo-buccal/bucco-alveolar sulcus**.
- Most common carcinoma of the mouth (oral cavity + external surface of lips) and oropharynx is the **squamous cell carcinoma**.
- An uncommon variant of squamous cell carcinoma called Verrucous carcinoma, is a slow growing and

Oral Cavity and Pharynx

Section III

very well differentiated carcinoma of low metastatic potential. It presents with **fungating/warty** soft **papillary lesion** in the oral cavity. Superficial biopsy in Verrucous carcinoma shows **hyperkeratosis and acanthosis**. Deep biopsy shows dysplasia. Verrucous carcinoma has good prognosis.

- Among lip cancers, 98% carcinomas occur in the **lower lip** (squamous cell Ca). Only 2% of the carcinomas occur in the upper lip (most common carcinoma of the upper lip is basal cell carcinoma).
- Prolonged exposure to sunlight is an important predisposing factor in carcinoma of lip.
- Most common carcinoma of the oropharynx is carcinoma of tonsil.
- The prevalence of **HPV** (16 and 18) positive tumours in head and neck squamous cell carcinoma has increased tremendously. HPV related head and neck cancers most commonly arise from the oropharynx specifically the tonsils and base of tongue.
- Second primary tumour means a new, unrelated primary cancer in a person with a history of cancer at some other site in the past. It should not be confused with metastasis of the first cancer. For example, in the clinical setting of a patient who has had a head and neck malignancy in the past, usually the oral cavity and oropharyngeal squamous cell cancers may occur as the second primary tumours.

Prognosis of Oral Cancers

- Carcinoma of the lip carries **best prognosis** among carcinoma of mouth.
- Carcinoma of mouth with least lymphatic metastasis is lip cancer followed by hard palate.
- Carcinoma of the floor of mouth carries worst prognosis. However, the highest incidence of lymph node metastasis is seen in carcinoma of the tongue followed by carcinoma of the floor of mouth because tongue is the richest in lymphatics in the oral cavity.

Nodal Spread of Oral Cancers

- Nodal spread from carcinoma lip involves submental and submandibular lymph nodes (level 1). Upper lip also drains into preauricular and parotid nodes.
- The lateral border of tongue, floor of mouth and Buccal mucosa drain into ipsilateral submandibular (**level I**) as well as to jugulo-digastric or upper deep cervical (**level II**), jugulo-omohyoid or middle deep cervical (**level III**) and lower jugular or lower deep cervical (**level IV**) lymph nodes. Midline tumours drain bilaterally.
- Oropharyngeal tumours drain into jugulo-digastric or upper deep cervical (level II), jugulo-omohyoid or middle deep cervical (level III) and lower jugular or lower deep cervical (level IV) lymph nodes.

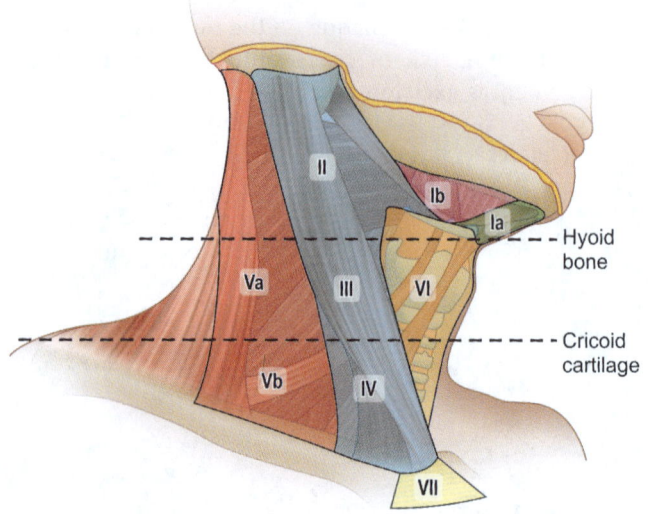

Level Ia: Submental	**Level Va:** Posterior triangle
Level Ib: Submandibular	**Level Vb:** Supraclavicular
Level II: Upper deep cervical	**Level VI:** Anterior compartment lymph nodes
Level III: Middle deep cervical	
Level IV: Lower deep cervical	**Level VII:** Superior mediastinal

Levels of lymph node in the neck

AJC Staging of Oral Cavity Carcinoma

T_1	Tumours ≤ 2 cm and ≤ 5 mm depth of invasion
T_2	Tumours > 2 cm and up till 4 cm and < 10 mm depth or Tumours ≤ 2 cm and > 5, < 10 mm depth of invasion
T_3	Tumours > 4 cm or > 10 mm depth of invasion
T_{4a}	Locally advanced disease (tumour may involve mandible, hard palate, muscles of tongue, maxillary sinus, skin of face, **medial pterygoid** muscle)
T_{4b}	Very advanced disease, tumour invades **lateral pterygoid** muscle, **pterygoid plates,** masticator space, skull base and/or internal carotid artery.

N_0	No cervical lymph nodes
N_1	Single ipsilateral node ≤3 cm without Extra Nodal Extension (ENE-ve)
N_2	Single ipsilateral node 3–6 cm (N_{2a}), multiple ipsilateral (N_{2b}), contralateral or bilateral nodes (N_{2c}) ≤ 6 cm. All without Extra Nodal Extension
N_{3a}	Single or multiple nodes > 6 cm without Extra Nodal Extension
N_{3b}	Single or multiple nodes with Extra Nodal Extension (ENE +)
M_0	No metastasis
M_1	Distant metastasis

Management

1. **Carcinoma Lip, Oral tongue, Buccal mucosa and Floor of mouth:**

A. T1, T2:

   i. Excision and repair or

   ii. Radiotherapy: The early tumours also do well with radiotherapy. The radiotherapy here can be brachytherapy (i.e. implantation of radioactive sources most commonly iridium within the tumour) or external beam which is usually intensity modulated radiotherapy (IMRT). Brachytherapy delivers radiation dose mainly to the tumour sparing normal tissue hence decreasing toxicity.

Lip reconstruction following excision:

Defect arising after excision	Intervention
Less than 1/3rd of the length of lip	Primary closure
1/3rd to 2/3rd of the length of the lip	Abbe flap (*see* below)
More than 2/3rd of the length of the lip	Gillies fan flap

Abbe flap is based on the main artery of the orbicularis oris, the labial artery. A portion of the uninvolved lip (either upper or lower) is rotated across the mouth and placed into the surgical defect of the involved lip while maintaining the blood supply from the labial artery.

After 10–14 days, the blood supply of the flap would have been established to the point where the artery could be divided. The defect of the uninvolved lip from which the flap has been taken is sutured primarily.

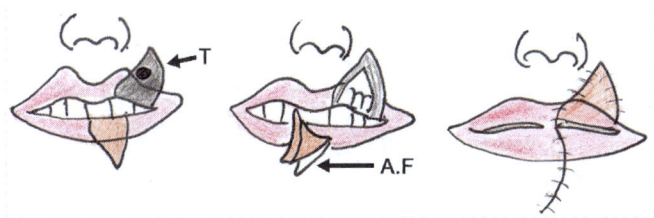

Fig. 33.8: ABBE Flap

Gillies fan flap borrow tissue from the cheek and adjacent sites.

- In tumours of the lateral border of tongue which are less than 2 cm in size, i.e. T_1 interstitial irradiation (brachytherapy) or excision i.e. partial glossectomy is the choice. If the tumour is more than 2 cm in size, i.e. T_2 then hemiglossectomy or external beam radiotherapy (IMRT) is preferred.

*Note:*

As stated above since tongue and floor of mouth have very rich lymphatics therefore in these sites in T_1 T_2 tumours with no palpable neck nodes, the **treatment of neck** should also be done because of high incidence of occult neck metastasis. If the primary tumour is treated with radiotherapy, the neck should receive prophylactic irradiation. Where the primary tumour is treated surgically **selective supra-omohyoid (level I to III) or extended supra-omohyoid neck dissection (level I to IV)** (for neck dissection *see* Chapter 39, carcinoma larynx) should be done.

B. T_3, T_4: Excision + ipsilateral/contralateral neck dissection + radiotherapy ± chemotherapy.

2. **Carcinoma Base of tongue:** T_1, T_2, T_3, and T_4: Concurrent chemoradiation.

3. **Carcinoma lower Gingivo-buccal/lower bucco-alveolus:** Since radiation to the mandible carries risk of **osteoradionecrosis**, carcinoma lower alveolus/gingivo-buccal is dealt **surgically in all the stages**.

The surgical excision can be:

a. Rim resection/marginal mandibulectomy or
b. Segmental resection of the mandible

Marginal mandibulectomy involves excising a rim of mandible but with maintenance of the mandibular arch. These defects should be made in a curvilinear manner, and at least 1 cm of mandibular height should be retained.

The advantage of the rim/marginal mandibulectomy is that it encompasses only a rim or margin of the mandible (from inner/outer surface or upper/lower border) while leaving the mandibular arch intact largely.

Indications for rim/marginal resection of the mandible are:

i. Tumour involving mucosa of the mandible.
ii. Tumour involving mandibular periosteum.
iii. Tumour involving mandibular periosteum and superficial cortex only.

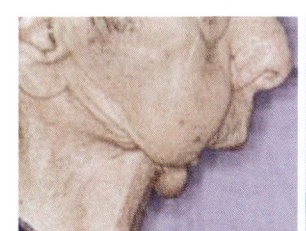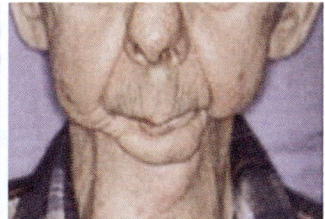

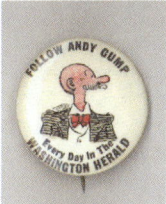

Fig. 33.9

Segmental mandibulectomy involves resection of a full-thickness segment of bone, which creates a discontinuity defect. Lack of reconstruction causes significant functional and cosmetic morbidity.

In carcinomas of anterior floor of mouth leading to extensive invasion of mandible the complete anterior segment of mandible must be resected. After resection, segmental anterior defects should be corrected by reconstruction with osseous free tissue transfer. If this reconstruction is not done, loss of anterior arch of mandible results in a disabling cosmetic deformity known as **"Andy Gump" deformity** (absent chin and severely retrognathic lower jaw) after the character in American strip cartoon.

Indications for segmental (a portion of mandible with periosteum on both its inner and outer surfaces) resection of the mandible are:

i. Invasion of the medullary space of the mandible.
ii. Tumour fixation to the occlusal surface (i.e. the surface which comes in contact with the maxilla

during mouth closure) of the mandible in the edentulous patient (Edentulous mandible is generally hypoplastic, i.e. the vertical height of the mandible is decreased making rim resection difficult).

iii. Invasion of tumour into the mandible via the mandibular or mental foramen.

COMMANDO (COMbined **MA**ndibulectomy and **N**eck **D**issection with **O**ropharyngeal resection) operation: This is radical resection of the tumour in the oral cavity/oropharynx with mandibulectomy (marginal/segmental/hemi) and neck dissection. This is done for T_3 and T_4 tumours of the oral cavity/oropharynx involving the mandible.

"Points to Ponder/Points for Quick revision"

- **Ranula:** Extravasation cyst of sublingual gland.
- Cystic fluctuant swelling—floor of mouth; can be plunging
- T/t: Excision of cyst with sublingual gland.
- **Plummer Vinson syndrome:** MC–F (Fe deficiency); IDA + Post-cricoid dysphagia + hypopharyngeal web; ↑-post cricoid Ca.
- T/t: Iron supplements, dilatation of web.
- **Premalignant conditions:** Leukoplakia, Erythroplakia, SMF (arecoline → progressive trismus).
- MC Ca—oral cavity–lateral border tongue; Oropharynx—tonsil; Hypopharynx—Pyriform fossa.
- T/t (preferred modality)—oral cavity—surgical excision; Oro- and Hypo-pharynx—chemoradiation.

PREVIOUSLY ASKED QUESTIONS

1. **Ranula is:** *(JIPMER 95, Exam 2015)*
   a. Hypertrophied lymphoid tissue
   b. Arises from floor of mouth
   c. Hard and haemorrhagic
   d. An abscess

2. **Regarding ranula all are true except:**
   (MAHE 2005, Exam 2014)
   a. Extravasation cyst
   b. Arises from submandibular gland
   c. Translucent
   d. Plunging may be a feature

3. **Ranula is:** *(Exam 2013)*
   a. Leukoplakia
   b. Extravasation cyst
   c. Premalignant
   d. Arise from submandibular gland

4. **Ranula is a:** *(AP 2003, Exam 2014)*
   a. Extravasation cyst
   b. Tumour
   c. Submandibular gland swelling
   d. Swelling on dorsum of tongue

5. **True about aphthous ulcer:** *(PGI June 2005, 2013)*
   a. Viral predisposition
   b. Recurrent ulcer
   c. Deep ulcers
   d. Involves the mucosa of the hard palate
   e. Steroids given as treatment

6. **Fordyce spots in oral cavity arise from:**
   (AIIMS 2004, Exam 2015)
   a. Mucous glands   b. Sebaceous glands
   c. Taste buds   d. Minor salivary glands

7. **All statement about Plummer-Vinson syndrome are true except:** *(PGI 96, Exam 2013)*
   a. Commonly leads to carcinoma in lower third of oesophagus
   b. Common with iron deficiency
   c. Common in females
   d. Premalignant

8. **Which of the following region is involved in Plummer-Vinson syndrome?** *(UP 2001, Exam 2013)*
   a. Pyriform sinus
   b. Post-cricoid region
   c. Valleculae
   d. Posterior pharyngeal wall

9. **Women with vitamin B$_{12}$ deficiency presents with dysphagia and anemia. What is the syndrome mentioned in the presentation?** *(Exam 2012)*
   a. Plummer-Vinson syndrome
   b. Eagle syndrome
   c. Job's syndrome
   d. Treacher Collin syndrome

10. **In Plummer-Vinson syndrome what is the percentage of post-cricoid carcinoma:**
    (JIPMER 2002, Exam 2014)
    a. 10%   b. 30%
    c. 50%   d. 75%

11. **All are precancerous lesions of oral cavity except:**
    (MP 2009, Exam 2014)
    a. Leukoplakia
    b. Erythroplakia
    c. Diffuse oral submucous fibrosis
    d. Diffuse aphthous ulcers

12. **The most common pre-malignant condition of oral carcinoma is:** *(AI 95, Exam 2014)*
    a. Leukoplakia   b. Erythroplakia
    c. Lichen planus   d. Submucous Fibrosis

13. **Premalignant lesion of oral cavity includes:**
    (PGI Nov 2010)
    a. Erythroplakia   b. Fordyce's spot
    c. Leukoplakia   d. Keratoacanthoma
    e. Aphthous ulcer

14. **Premalignant lesions are:** *(Kolkata 2000, Exam 2014)*
    a. Submucous fibrosis b. Leukoplakia
    c. Erythroplakia   d. All of the above

15. **Treatment of leukoplakia:** *(Exam 2013)*
    a. Local excision
    b. Excision and radiotherapy
    c. Topical chemotherapy
    d. Repositioning of ill fitting dentures

16. **The most common malignant tumour of adult males in India is:** *(AI 2004, UPSC 2015)*
    a. Oropharyngeal carcinoma
    b. Gastric carcinoma
    c. Colo-rectal carcinoma
    d. Lung cancer

17. **Which carcinoma has best prognosis?**
    (AIIMS 98, Exam 2014)
    a. Carcinoma lip   b. Carcinoma cheek
    c. Carcinoma tongue d. Carcinoma palate

18. **The commonest site of oral cancer among Indian population is:** *(AI 2004, Exam 2013)*
    a. Tongue
    b. Floor of mouth
    c. Alveolo buccal complex
    d. Lip

19. **Carcinoma tongue most frequently develops from:**
    (AI 2002, Exam 2014)
    a. Tip   b. Lateral border
    c. Dorsal portion   d. All portions equally

20. **Carcinoma of buccal mucosa commonly drain to the following lymph node sites:**
    (AI 97, AIIMS 96, Exam 2011)
    a. Lower deep cervical b. Submandibular
    c. Supraclavicular   d. Mediastinal

Section III | **Oral Cavity and Pharynx**

21. In carcinoma of lower lip secondaries are seen in: *(AI 2001, Exam 2015)*
   a. Submandibular LN
   b. Preauricular LN
   c. Mediastinal LN
   d. Supraclavicular LN

22. True about AJC staging of oral cavity carcinoma: *(PGI June 2009, 2014)*
   a. Involvement of pterygoid plate in T_3
   b. Involvement of pterygoid plate in T_4
   c. Involvement of lateral pterygoid muscle in stage T_4
   d. Involvement of medial pterygoid muscle T_3

23. A patient has carcinoma of tongue on its right lateral border (anterior 2/3rd), with lymph node of size 4 cm in level 3 on left side of the neck, stage of disease is: *(AIIMS May 2007, AI 2010)*
   a. N_0 b. N_1
   c. N_2 d. N_3

24. Tumour in cheek with 3 cm size with contralateral mobile lymph nodes comes under: *(Exam 2015)*
   a. $T_3N_2M_0$ b. $T_2N_2M_0$
   c. $T_4N_2M_0$ d. $T_3N_3M_0$

25. True statement about oral cancer is/are: *(PGI 2004, 2015)*
   a. Most common in buccal mucosa
   b. Lymphatic metastasis uncommon
   c. Responds to radiotherapy
   d. Surgery is treatment of choice
   e. Smoking predisposes

26. The most common site for squamous cell carcinoma in oral cavity is: *(DPG 2009, Exam 2014)*
   a. Tongue
   b. Floor of mouth
   c. Upper and lower alveolus
   d. Buccal mucosa

27. The highest frequency of palpable metastasis in neck on presentation is: *(DPG 2009, Exam 2013)*
   a. Carcinoma tongue   b. Buccal mucosa
   c. Alveolus   d. Lip

28. What is N3 in TNM staging of head and neck malignancy: *(Exam 2018)*
   a. Contralateral nodes of 3–6 cm
   b. B/L nodes of 3–6 cm
   c. Contralateral nodes of > 6 cm
   d. Single ipsilateral node 3–6 cm

29. A patient presented with 1–1.5 cm growth on the lateral border of tongue. The treatment indicated would be: *(AIIMS 2002, Exam 2014)*
   a. Tongue shaving
   b. Interstitial brachytherapy
   c. External beam radiotherapy
   d. Chemotherapy

30. An edentulous patient had carcinoma of the oral cavity infiltrating into the lower alveolar margin. All the following are possible treatment options except: *(AI 2002, Exam 2012)*
   a. Segmental mandibulectomy
   b. Marginal mandibulectomy with removal of outer table
   c. Radiotherapy
   d. Commando

31. A 70-year-old male who had been chewing Tobacco for the past 50 years, presents with a 6 months history of fungating soft papillary lesion in the oral cavity. Lymph nodes are not palpable. 2 biopsies from the lesion show benign appearing papillomas with hyperkeratosis and acanthosis. Most likely diagnosis is: *(AIIMS 2005, Exam 2014)*
   a. Verrucous carcinoma
   b. Squamous cell carcinoma
   c. Malignant mixed tumour
   d. Basal cell carcinoma

32. A 50-year-male came with an ulcero-proliferative growth measuring 3 cm in the left buccal mucosa with a 5 cm right submandibular lymph node and clinically no evidence of distant metastasis. What is the TNM staging: *(Exam 2015)*
   a. $T_2 N_3 M_0$
   b. $T_2 N_2b M_0$
   c. $T_2 N_2c M_0$
   d. $T_3 N_2c M_0$

33. True about Andy Gump deformity: *(PGI May 2015)*
   a. Occurs due to defects of the anterior mandibular arch
   b. Hemimandibulectomy can cause it
   c. Marginal mandibulectomy can cause it
   d. Treatment is adequate reconstruction of anterior mandibular arch with bone and graft

34. Which one of these four images is most likely to be a premalignant condition: *(APPG 2016)*

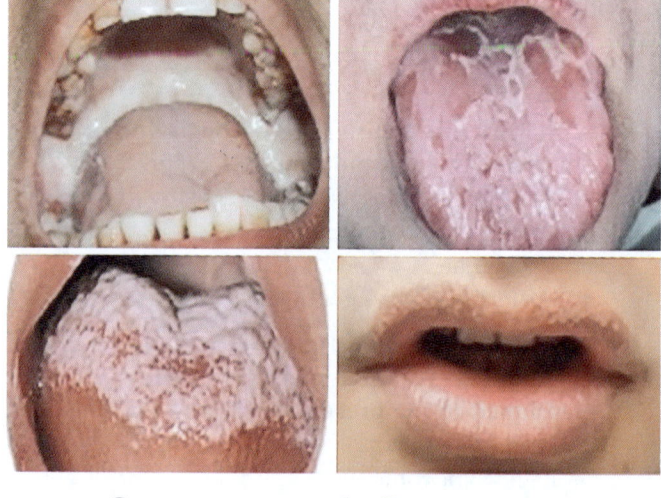

   a. C   b. D
   c. A   d. B

35. HPV do not cause: *(AIIMS 2015)*
   a. Base of tongue carcinoma
   b. Carcinoma tonsil
   c. Nasopharyngeal carcinoma
   d. Cervical cancer

36. A 70-year-old man has h/o smoking since 25 years. He presented with an ulcer on vermillion, i.e. upper border of upper lip. Most probable diagnosis is: *(UPSC 2015)*

   a. BCC   b. SCC
   c. Melanoma   d. Melanocytic nevus

IMAGE BASED PRACTICE QUESTIONS BY THE AUTHOR

37. A patient presents with a mass on the lateral border of anterior 2/3 of tongue. Biopsy shows squamous cell carcinoma. This will tend to metastasize to the lymph nodes at which levels:

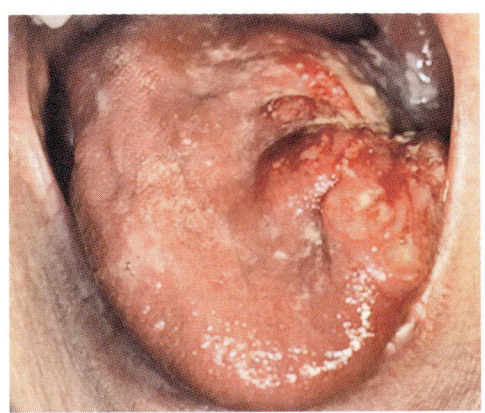

   a. I, II, III
   b. II, IV, V
   c. III, IV, V
   d. I, II, VI

38. A 30-year-old gentleman but a pan masala addict, presents with inability to open the mouth fully, along with restriction of tongue movement. Examination of the oral cavity reveals the following. What is the most likely diagnosis:

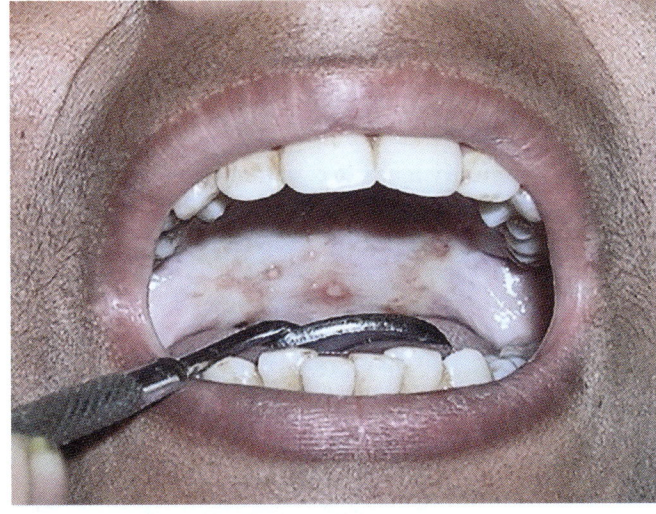

   a. Leukoplakia
   b. Submucous fibrosis
   c. Carcinoma in situ
   d. Lichen planus

Section III | **Oral Cavity and Pharynx**

ANSWERS AND EXPLANATIONS

1. **(b) Arises from floor of mouth** (*Ref. Scott Brown, 8th ed., Vol 2; 444*)

2. **(b) Arises from submandibular gland** (*Ref. Scott Brown, 8th ed., Vol 2; 444*)

3. **(b) Extravasation cyst** (*Ref. Scott Brown, 8th ed., Vol 2; 444*)
   - They are mucous retention cysts of sublingual glands. They are not premalignant.

4. **(a) Extravasation cyst** (*Ref. Scott Brown, 8th ed., Vol 2; 444*)

5. **(b) and (e) are true, please refer the text** (*Ref. Cummings, 6th ed., 1314*)

6. **(b) Sebaceous glands** (*Ref. Scott Brown, 8th ed., Vol 3; 634*)

7. **(a) Commonly leads to carcinoma in lower third of oesophagus** (*Ref. Sleisenger Gastrointestinal & Liver Disease, 8th ed.,; 851*)
   - Plummer-Vinson syndrome affects the postcricoid area and upper part of oesophagus.

8. **(b) Post-cricoid region** (*Ref. Sleisenger Gastrointestinal & Liver Disease, 8th ed.,; 851*)

9. **(a) Plummer-Vinson syndrome** (*Ref. Sleisenger Gastrointestinal & Liver Disease, 8th ed.,; 851*)
   - Triad of postcricoid dysphagia, oesophageal webs, and iron deficiency anemia constitutes Plummer Vinson syndrome. Due to iron deficiency there occurs atrophy of the gastric mucosa leading to achlorhydria.
   - Intrinsic factor (IF) is needed for the absorption of dietary cobalamin, i.e. vitamin B_{12}. This binding of IF with B_{12} prevents the proteolytic digestion of B_{12}. Intrinsic factor is secreted by the parietal cells of the cardiac and fundic mucosa of the stomach, which also secrete hydrochloric acid (HCl). The IF-cobalamin complex then reaches terminal ileum where cobalamin gets absorbed.
   - In PV syndrome due to atrophy of gastric mucosa therefore there is no IF available leading to poor absorption of vitamin B_{12}.
   - Eagle syndrome is pain in the tonsillar fossa area due to enlarged calcified styloid process.
   - Job's syndrome is hyperimmunoglobulin E syndrome.
   - Treacher Collin syndrome is 1st arch hypoplasia causing maxillo-mandibular hypoplasia.

10. **(a) 10%** (*Ref. Sleisenger Gastrointestinal & Liver Disease, 8th ed.,; 951*)

11. **(d) diffuse aphthous ulcers** (*Ref. Cummings, 6th ed., 1435*)

12. **(a) Leukoplakia** (*Ref. Cummings, 6th ed., 1299*)
    - All the other choices also are pre-malignant but leukoplakia is the most common premalignant condition.

13. **(a), (c) Erythroplakia, Leukoplakia** (*Ref. Cummings, 6th ed., 1435*)
    - Keratoacanthoma (KA) is a low-grade (unlikely to metastasize or invade) skin tumour that is believed to originate from the neck of the hair follicle.

14. **(d) All of the above** (*Ref. Cummings, 6th ed., 1366*)

15. **(a) Local excision** (*Ref. Cummings, 6th ed., 1302*)

16. **(d) Lung cancer** (*Ref. Stell & Maran, 5th ed., 558*)
    - In India, in males, **Oral cavity Cancer (buccoalveolar sulcus)** is the most common registered **Cancer**, followed by **Lung cancer**.
    - To create confusion oropharyngeal carcinoma has been put in the options, so one should carefully read all the options!

17. **(a) Carcinoma lip** (*Ref. Cummings, 6th ed., 1372*)

18. **(c) Alveolo buccal complex** (*Ref. Stell & Maran, 5th ed., 558*)

19. **(b) Lateral border** (*Ref. Stell & Maran, 5th ed., 563*)
    - 85% carcinomas of tongue arise from the lateral border.

20. **(b) Submandibular** (*Ref. Cummings, 6th ed., 1365*)
    - Buccal mucosa drains into ipsilateral submandibular (level I) as well as to upper deep cervical (level II), middle deep cervical (level III) and lower deep cervical (level IV).

21. **(a) submandibular LN** (*Ref. Cummings, 6th ed., 1364*)
    - Nodal spread from carcinoma lower lip involves submental and submandibular lymph nodes (level 1).

22. **(b) and (c)** (*Ref. Cummings, 6th ed., 1369*)
    - Involvement of pterygoid plate or pterygoid muscles is T_4.

23. **(c) N_2** (*Ref. Cummings, 6th ed., 1369*)

24. **(b) $T_2N_2M_0$** (*Ref. Cummings, 6th ed., 1369*)
    - Refer to staging of oral cancers in the text.

25. **(c), (d) and (e) are true** (*Ref. Cummings, 6th ed., 1375*)
    - Worldwide most common site of oral cancer is lateral border of tongue.
    - Lymphatic metastasis in oral cancers except carcinoma hard palate is very common.

26. **(a) Tongue** (*Ref. Cummings, 6th ed., 1375*)

27. **(a) Carcinoma tongue** (*Ref. Cummings, 6th ed., 1375*)

28. **(c) Contralateral nodes of > 6 cm** (*Ref. Scott Brown, 8th ed., Vol 3; 39*)

29. **(b) Interstitial brachytherapy** (*Ref. Cummings, 6th ed., 1373*)

30. **(c) Radiotherapy** (*Ref. Cummings, 6th ed., 1372*)
    - Since radiation to the mandible carries risk of osteoradionecrosis, carcinoma lower alveolus/mandible is dealt with surgically in all the stages.
    - Chemotherapy may be given in T_3, T_4 tumours.

31. **(a) Verrucous carcinoma** (*Ref. Cummings, 6th ed., 1366*)

32. **(c) $T_2 N_2 c M_0$** (*Ref. Cummings, 6th ed., 1369*)

33. **(a) and (d)** (*Ref. Cummings, 6th ed., 1390*)

34. **(c) A** (*Ref. Cummings, 6th ed., 1307*)
    A: Sub-mucous fibrosis
    B: Geographic tongue
    C: Candidiasis
    D: Fordyce spots

35. **(c) Nasopharyngeal carcinoma is caused by EBV** (*Ref. Cummings, 6th ed., 1439*)

36. **(a) BCC** (*Ref. Cummings, 6th ed., 1370*)

37. **(a) I, II, III** (*Ref. Cummings, 6th ed., 1364*)

38. **(b) Submucous fibrosis** (*Ref. Cummings, 6th ed., 1306*)

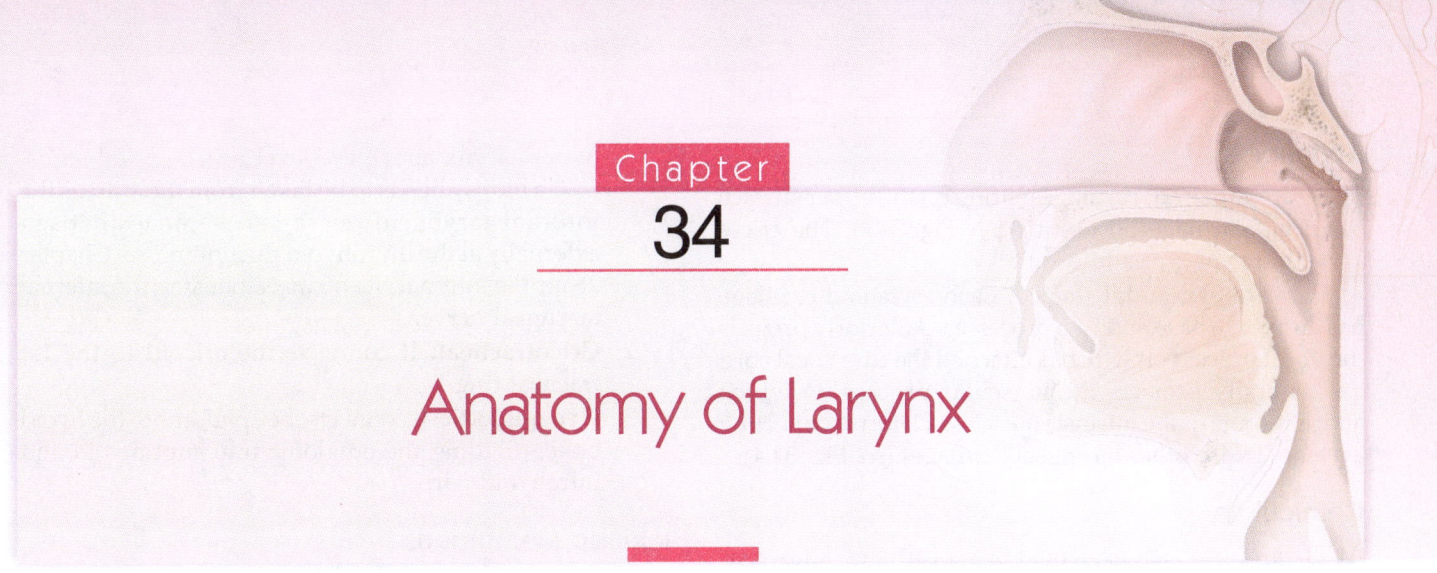

Anatomy of Larynx

EMBRYOLOGY

Larynx develops from the **4th and 6th branchial arches**.

The part of the larynx above the true vocal cords is supraglottis which develops from the 4th arch and hence is supplied by **superior laryngeal nerve (the 4th arch nerve)**.

The part of the larynx at the level of true vocal cords (called glottis) and below it, i.e. subglottis develops from the 6th arch, and hence is supplied by recurrent laryngeal nerve (the 6th arch nerve).

So the **epiglottis** (present in supraglottis) develop from **4th arch** and cricoid (present in subglottis) develops from 6th arch (*see* the anatomy of larynx below). However, the entire thyroid cartilage develops from 4th arch.

ANATOMY

The larynx in an adult person lies opposite the **C3, 4, 5, and 6 cervical vertebrae**. The length of the larynx is 44 mm and 36 mm in adult male and female respectively. When we push the larynx posteriorly and move it from side to side, we can feel a **laryngeal crepitus**.

This crepitus is produced because of rubbing of two bony surfaces with each other (anteriorly cricoid and posteriorly vertebral bodies).

The absence of this crepitus means that these two surfaces are not able to meet with each other i.e. either there is something behind the cricoid say post cricoid carcinoma or something in front of vertebrae say retropharyngeal or prevertebral abscess. This absence of laryngeal crepitus is known as **Moure's sign**.

The larynx consists of **3 unpaired and 3 paired cartilages:**

Unpaired cartilages	Paired cartilages
1. Thyroid	Arytenoids
2. Cricoid	Corniculate
3. Epiglottis	Cuneiform

The **thyroid**, cricoid and the arytenoids are hyaline hence they calcify with age (therefore visible on X-rays and prone to fractures). The rest of the cartilages, i.e. epiglottis, corniculate, and cuneiform are elastic and remain the same throughout life. *Mnemonic*—of the above

6 cartilages, 4 important ones are Epiglottis, Arytenoids, Cricoid and Thyroid so **E** for **E** (**E**piglottis–**E**lastic) and **ACTH** (**A**rytenoid, **C**ricoid, **T**hyroid–**H**yaline).

Thyroid

This is the largest cartilage of the larynx. It has two alae, which meet in the midline at an angle of **90°** in **males**. Due to this males have the laryngeal prominence known as Adam's apple. In **females** the angle is **120°**.

The thyroid ala on each side on their lateral aspect, projects superiorly and inferiorly to form superior and inferior cornu of thyroid. The inferior cornu of thyroid articulates with the cricoid, this crico-thyroid joint is a pivot joint.

On the external surface of each thyroid ala runs a line obliquely from the base of superior cornu to the midpoint of inferior border. It is known as **oblique line of thyroid** (Fig. 34.1). **Three muscles attach** to the oblique line of thyroid. They are:

1. Sternothyroid
2. Thyrohyoid
3. Thyropharyngeus part of inferior constrictor

On the midpoint of laryngeal surface of thyroid angle attaches the epiglottis just above the attachment of the true vocal cords.

Epiglottis

It is a **leaf shaped** cartilage. Its upper surface near the tongue is called the lingual surface and its lower surface facing the laryngeal cavity is known as the laryngeal surface. The epiglottis is attached above to the hyoid bone by hyoepiglottic ligament and below, it is attached to the midpoint of thyroid angle (Fig. 34.2). So as per the attachment, epiglottis is divided into suprahyoid and infrahyoid parts.

Cricoid

Cricoid is the only complete ring cartilage of the larynx, hence it is also known as **signet ring** cartilage (Fig. 34.2). The significance of it being the only complete ring cartilage is that any injury of cricoid leading to necrosis and fibrosis will ultimately lead to **laryngeal stenosis** here (also called subglottic stenosis).

Arytenoids

These are 2 (paired) cartilages sitting on the upper surface of cricoid cartilage posteriorly (*see* Fig. 34.2). The crico-arytenoid joint is a saddle joint.

They are **pyramidal** shaped. Each arytenoid cartilage has an apex, a base and two processes. Anteriorly projects the vocal process on which is attached the true vocal cord and laterally projects the muscular process on which attaches some of the intrinsic muscles of larynx connecting arytenoid with other laryngeal cartilages (*see* Fig. 34.4).

Corniculate

At the apex of each arytenoid sits a cartilage known as corniculate cartilage. It is also known as **cartilage of Santorini**.

Cuneiform Cartilage

Just lateral to the corniculate cartilage on each side is the rod shaped cartilage known as cuneiform cartilage. These are also known as **cartilage of Wrisberg**.

The above six laryngeal cartilages are attached to each other by membranes and muscles known as intrinsic membranes and intrinsic muscles of larynx. They are also connected to the external surrounding structures superiorly and inferiorly by extrinsic membranes and extrinsic muscles.

Extrinsic Membranes

They connect the laryngeal framework externally, superiorly and inferiorly to the surrounding structures (*see* Fig. 34.1.). These membranes and ligaments of larynx act as barriers for the spread of laryngeal tumours.

The extrinsic membranes are:

1. **Thyrohyoid:** It connects the thyroid to the hyoid above. The **internal laryngeal nerve** (a branch of superior laryngeal nerve, the 4th arch nerve) and **superior laryngeal vessels enter the larynx after piercing this membrane**. The internal laryngeal nerve gives sensory supply to the larynx and

hypopharynx above the level of true vocal cords. So if a biopsy needs to be taken from these areas the internal laryngeal nerve can be anaesthetised externally at the thyrohyoid membrane, *see* Chapter 26 for the internal site of anaesthetising the internal laryngeal nerve.

2. **Cricotracheal:** It connects the cricoid to the 1st tracheal ring.
3. **Hyoepiglottic:** It connects the epiglottis to the hyoid bone, dividing the epiglottis into suprahyoid and infrahyoid parts.

Intrinsic Membranes

The membranes which connect the laryngeal cartilages with each other are known as intrinsic membranes.

The two intrinsic membranes are (both named according to their shape):

1. **Quadrangular membrane:** This membrane extends from both the sides of epiglottis to the arytenoids. The upper border of quadrangular membrane on each side is known as **Ary-Epiglottic fold (AE fold)**. The lower border of quadrangular membrane forms the **false vocal cord/fold**. The false vocal cords attach anteriorly to the thyroid cartilage just below the epiglottis and posteriorly to the arytenoids. The false vocal cords are also known as ventricular folds or vestibular folds, as they form the upper border of ventricle and lower border of vestibule respectively (*see* Fig. 34.5).

2. **Conus elasticus (cricovocal membrane):** Conus elasticus or cricovocal membrane is a cone-shaped membrane.

The lower border of the cricovocal membrane attaches to the entire upper border of cricoid on each side. The upper border of the cricovocal membrane on each side is free and forms the **true vocal cord/fold** which attaches anteriorly to the laryngeal

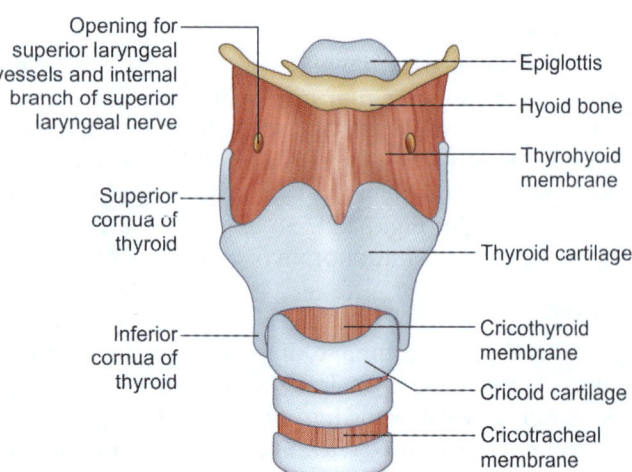

Fig. 34.1: External laryngeal frame work

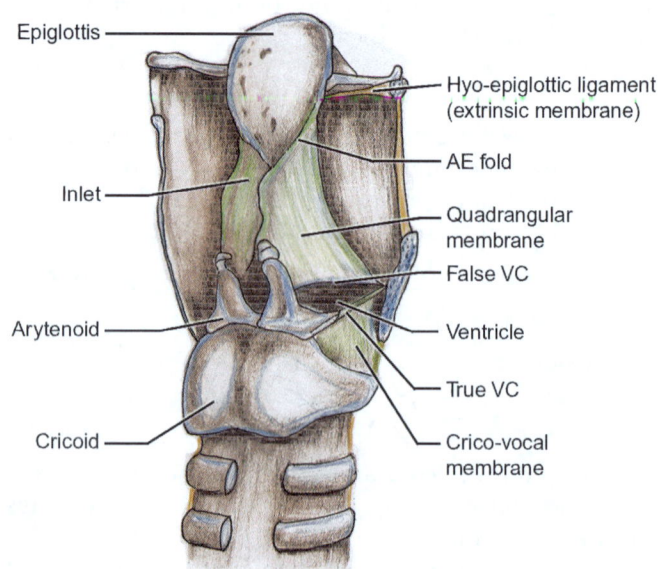

Fig. 34.2: Larynx

surface of thyroid angle just below the false vocal cords by a thick fibrous tissue known as Broyle's ligament or anterior commissure tendon. It is attached posteriorly to the vocal process of arytenoids.

From the upper border of cricoid the two cricovocal membranes go medially upwards in the form of a cone (the tip of the cone being the true vocal cords) hence known as conus elasticus.

In between the cricoid and thyroid anteriorly the cricovocal membrane is thickened to form cricothyroid membrane.

The **cricothyroid membrane**, which is the anterior thickening of cricovocal membrane, lies externally connecting cricoid and thyroid. In spite of lying externally, it is not considered as an extrinsic membrane (because by definition an extrinsic membrane is the one which connects the larynx to the surrounding external structures but the cricothyroid membrane connects the cricoid with thyroid, i.e. the two laryngeal cartilages and hence is considered as an intrinsic membrane).

The cricothyroid membrane is the site for **Cricothyrotomy** which is an emergency procedure to restore airway when the obstruction is at or above the level of vocal cords.

Similarly the cricothyroid muscle lies externally but is an intrinsic muscle, read below.

PARTS OF LARYNX

Supraglottis

Everything **above the true vocal cords is known as supraglottis**. The components of supraglottis are (*see* Fig. 34.2):
- Epiglottis (both lingual and laryngeal surfaces)
- Arytenoids
- Quadrangular membrane with its upper borders, i.e. the aryepiglottic folds and lower borders, i.e. the false vocal cords
- Ventricle
  - (Please note that the suprahyoid epiglottis, aryepiglottic folds and the arytenoid and interarytenoid area (all forming the inlet of larynx) are together known as **epilarynx**).
- **Ventricle** is the space in between the false vocal cords above and true vocal cords below.

The ventricle goes laterally to form a sac like structure known as **saccule**. Whenever there is a growth at the ventricle which allows the air to enter the saccule but does not allow its exit or whenever there is increased transglottic air pressure as in trumpet players or in glass blowers, it leads to enlargement of the saccule which is known as **laryngocele** (*see* Fig. 34.3).

A laryngocele can remain intrinsic when it lies inside the larynx only or can become extrinsic when it pierces the thyrohyoid membrane and presents as a swelling in the antero-superior part of neck. This swelling increases on Valsalva.

Glottis

This is the **narrowest part** of the larynx in **adults.** In **children** the narrowest part of larynx is **subglottis**, see below. Glottis lies **at the level of true vocal cords** and extends till 1 cm below it.

The components of glottis are:
1. **Anterior commissure:** This is where the two true vocal cords meet anteriorly on the medial surface of thyroid cartilage.
2. **The true vocal cords:** The true vocal cord (VC) is formed in its anterior 2/3rd by the upper free border of cricovocal membrane and in its posterior 1/3rd by the vocal process of arytenoids.

   So only the **anterior 2/3rd** of the true vocal cords is **membranous**. The **posterior 1/3rd** of true vocal cords is **cartilaginous** formed by the vocal process of arytenoids. The average length of VC in males is approx. 23 mm and in females is 17 mm.
3. **Posterior commissure/Posterior Glottis:** The vocal process of arytenoids along with the interarytenoid area is known as posterior commissure.

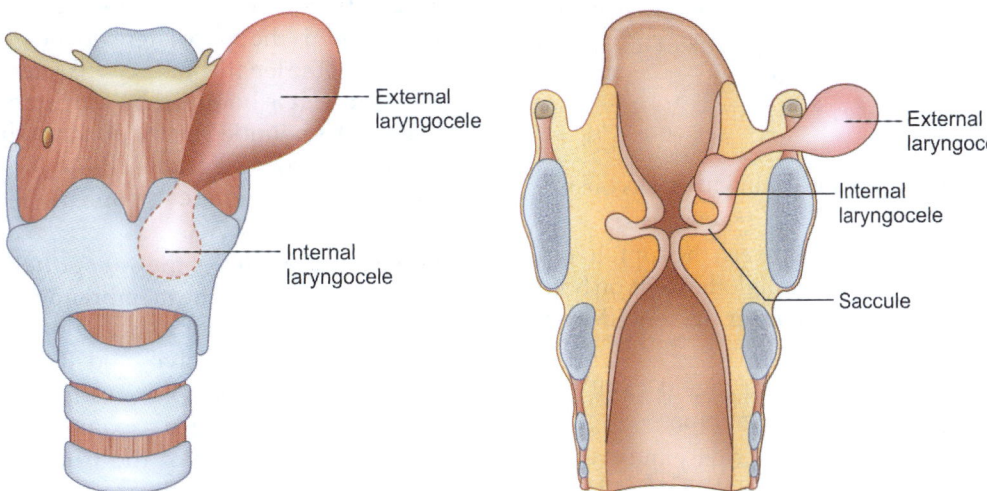

Fig. 34.3: Laryngocele

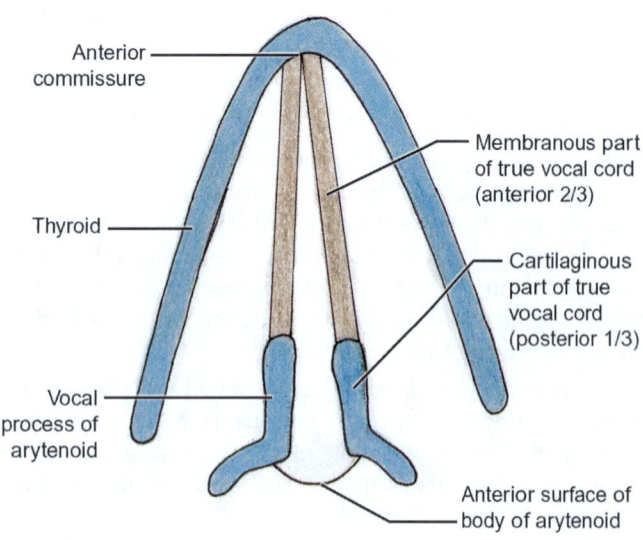

Fig. 34.4: Parts of glottis of larynx

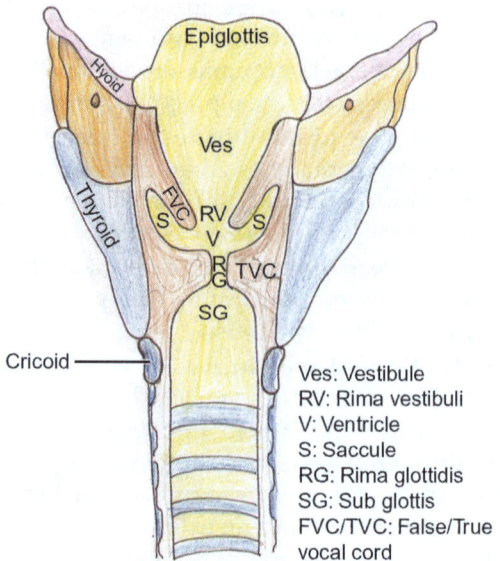

Ves: Vestibule
RV: Rima vestibuli
V: Ventricle
S: Saccule
RG: Rima glottidis
SG: Sub glottis
FVC/TVC: False/True vocal cord

Fig. 34.5: Cavity of larynx

Epithelial Lining

The whole of the larynx is lined by pseudostratified ciliated columnar epithelium except for the following three structures which are lined by stratified squamous epithelium:

- True vocal cords
- Lingual and upper part of laryngeal surface of epiglottis
- Upper part of AE folds which are lined by stratified squamous epithelium.

Lymphatic Drainage

The true vocal cords, i.e. glottis acts as a watershed for lymphatics. Above it, i.e. the **supraglottis** drains into **upper and middle deep cervical lymph nodes** and below it the **subglottis** drains into **lower deep cervical** and mediastinal lymph nodes (either directly or through prelaryngeal or pretracheal lymph nodes). So the **glottis** has got literally **no lymphatics**. Hence carcinoma of glottis has least lymphatic metastasis and therefore carries the best prognosis.

Subglottis

From 1 cm **below the level of true vocal cords** till the lower border of cricoid is the subglottis. This is the narrowest part of the larynx in children.

Cavity of Larynx

The cavity of the larynx from above downwards consists of the following:

1. **Inlet of larynx:** The inlet lies in between the suprahyoid epiglottis anteriorly, the two aryepiglottic folds on both the sides and arytenoids and inter arytenoid area posteriorly (*see* Fig. 34.2).
2. **Vestibule:** This is the part of laryngeal cavity in between the two quadrangular membranes.
3. **Rima vestubuli:** This is the part of cavity in between the two false vocal cords, i.e. the lower border of quadrangular membranes.

4. **Ventricle (also known as sinus of Morgagni of larynx):** This is the part of cavity in between the false vocal cord above and true vocal cords below. This goes laterally to form sac like structure known as saccule. The saccule contains mucus glands, secretions of which lubricate the VC, hence also called "oil can of larynx".
5. **Rima glottidis:** This is the part of cavity in between the two true vocal cords (which are formed by the upper free border of conus elasticus).
6. **Sub glottis:** The part of cavity below the glottis in between the two cricovocal membranes and cricoid cartilage is known as subglottis.

Spaces in Relation to Larynx

There are 3 spaces in relation to the larynx.

1. **Pre-epiglottic space:** This is also known as **space of Boyer**. This space lies in between the thyroid and thyrohyoid membrane anteriorly and the epiglottis posteriorly. It communicates with the paraglottic space laterally.
2. **Paraglottic space:** This is also known as **space of Tucker**. This is the space lateral to the larynx. It extends throughout the length of the larynx laterally from above downwards. It is bounded by the thyroid ala laterally. Medially it is bounded by the quadrangular membrane, ventricle and conus elasticus. Posteriorly it is bounded by pyriform fossa of the hypopharynx, *see* Chapter 26 on anatomy of pharynx.
3. **Reinke's space:** This is the **subepithelial space** in the medial free border **of the membranous true vocal cords** extending from anterior to posterior commissure. The vocal nodule, vocal polyp, and Reinke's oedema all arise from this space.

Just below the stratified squamous epithelium of the medial or free border of the true vocal cord is the subepithelial connective tissue called lamina propria. The lamina propria consists of superficial, intermediate and deep layers. The superficial layer of lamina propria is known as Reinke's space. In the intermediate and deep layers of lamina propria the elastin and collagen fibres fuse to form a ligament known as vocal ligament, which forms the superior border of the conus elasticus.

Between the epithelium of vocal cord medially and the vocal ligament laterally is Rienke's space.

The vocal ligament extends throughout the length of the free margin of the membranous part of true vocal cord. The upper and lower attachments of this vocal ligament on the upper and lower surface of true vocal cords are visible as faint white lines called superior and inferior arcuate lines respectively.

Lateral to the vocal ligament are the muscles of the vocal cord (Vocalis). So while excision of the vocal nodule or polyp, the surgeon should not go lateral to the superior arcuate line.

So the **boundaries of Rienke's space** are as follows:
- Anteriorly → anterior commissure
- Posteriorly → posterior commissure
- Superiorly → superior arcuate line
- Inferiorly → inferior arcuate line
- Medially → stratified squamous epithelium along the free margin of vocal cords
- Laterally → vocal ligament

MUSCLES OF LARYNX

Intrinsic Muscles

The intrinsic muscles of larynx **connect the laryngeal cartilages with each other**. They have been named according to which two cartilages they connect.
1. Thyroarytenoid and **Vocalis** (the **medial most part of the thyroarytenoid** is called vocalis)
2. Thyroepiglottic
3. Cricothyroid
4. Lateral cricoarytenoid
5. Posterior cricoarytenoid
6. Interarytenoid (transverse arytenoid)
7. Oblique arytenoids
8. Aryepiglottic

Note:

- All the muscles are paired except **interarytenoid** which is the **only unpaired muscle** of the larynx. Because it is unpaired, interarytenoid is supplied by recurrent laryngeal nerve of both the sides. Hence **interarytenoid** is the only intrinsic muscle of larynx with **dual nerve supply**.
- The only intrinsic muscle that **lies externally** is **cricothyroid**.

Actions of the intrinsic muscles of larynx:
Muscles acting on laryngeal inlet:
- **Opener of the laryngeal inlet:** Thyroepiglottic
- **Closure of the laryngeal inlet:** Aryepiglottic, oblique arytenoids

Muscles acting on vocal cords
- **Abductor** of the vocal cords: **Posterior cricoarytenoid** (please note that this is the only muscle which abducts the vocal cord, helping in respiration hence also known as **safety muscle** of larynx).
- The remaining muscles in the above list, i.e. thyroarytenoid, vocalis, cricothyroid, lateral cricoarytenoid and interarytenoid are **adductors** of the true vocal cords.
- Of these cricothyroid and vocalis are additionally **tensors** of the vocal cords.

The tensors of the VC act on the length of the vocal cord to either increase (cricothyroid) or decrease (vocalis) the tension.

Extrinsic Muscles of Larynx

These **connect the larynx to the neighbouring structures**. These are elevators and depressors of the larynx.

1. **Elevators of larynx:**
   i. Longitudinal muscles of pharynx (stylopharyngeus, salpingopharyngeus and palatopharyngeus).
   ii. Thyrohyoid, mylohyoid, stylohyoid, geniohyoid
   iii. Digastric
2. **Depressors of larynx:**
   i. Sternothyroid
   ii. Sternohyoid and Omohyoid

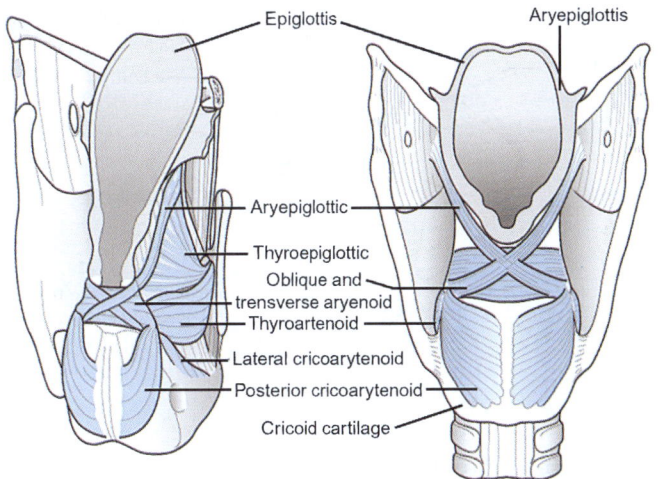

Fig. 34.6: Muscle of larynx

FUNCTIONS OF LARYNX

1. **Respiration:** Larynx is the conducting pathway for ventilation of lungs.
2. **Protection of lower airways:** Aspiration is prevented at three levels in the larynx. The first is at the inlet of larynx, next is at the false vocal cords and the last is at the true vocal cords. Larynx also helps in the generation of cough and thereby protects the lower respiratory tract by throwing out any noxious thing which has entered the airways.
3. **Speech:** Speech is produced by the vibration of the vocal cords, while they are held in adduction, by the

subglottic air coming from the lower airways during exhalation.

4. **Chest fixation:** Voluntary closure of the glottis leads to fixation of the chest, which helps in lifting heavy weights or in activities requiring increased intra-abdominal pressure, e.g. defecation, parturition, etc.

EXAMINATION OF LARYNX

Indirect Laryngoscopy

In the ENT OPD examination of the larynx is done by indirect laryngoscopy (I/L) or by rigid or flexible fibre optic endoscopy.

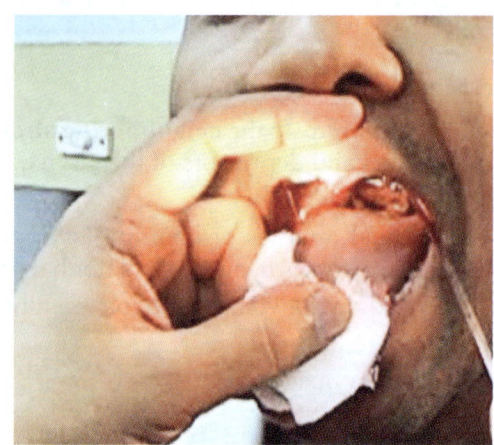

Fig. 34.7

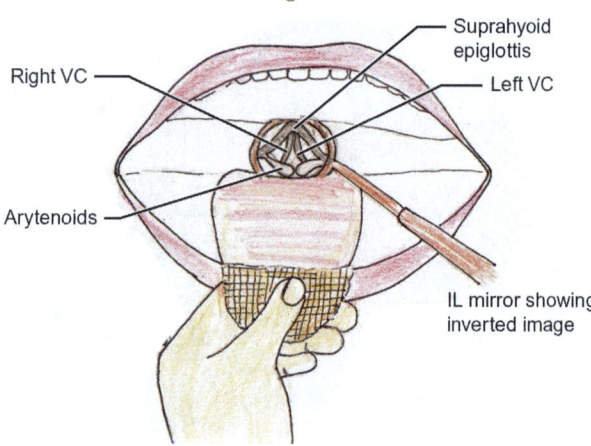

Fig. 34.8: Indirect laryngoscopy

Indirect laryngoscopy is done with the help of a laryngeal mirror which is placed in the oropharynx against the soft palate. Before using, the laryngeal mirror is **pre warmed** by placing its glass surface near the bulb of Bull's eye lamp or on flame or in warm water. This is done to **prevent fogging** caused due to breathing.

Since we are looking at the larynx in the mirror the image produced is **inverted**, i.e. the right half of the patient's larynx will be seen making the left half of the mirror image and also there will be antero-posterior reversal (epiglottis will be seen posteriorly, forming the top and arytenoids will be seen anteriorly, towards the bottom).

In indirect laryngoscopy whole of the larynx except for infrahyoid epiglottis, ventricle, anterior commissure and subglottis can be seen. These structures not seen on I/L are called **hidden areas of larynx**.

To examine these areas either rigid or flexible fiberoptic endoscopy is done.

Direct Laryngoscopy

In addition to **direct visualisation** of the larynx and hypopharynx, like the rigid or flexible fiberoptic endoscope, direct laryngoscopy which is done with the rigid laryngoscope can also be used to do **laryngeal procedures**.

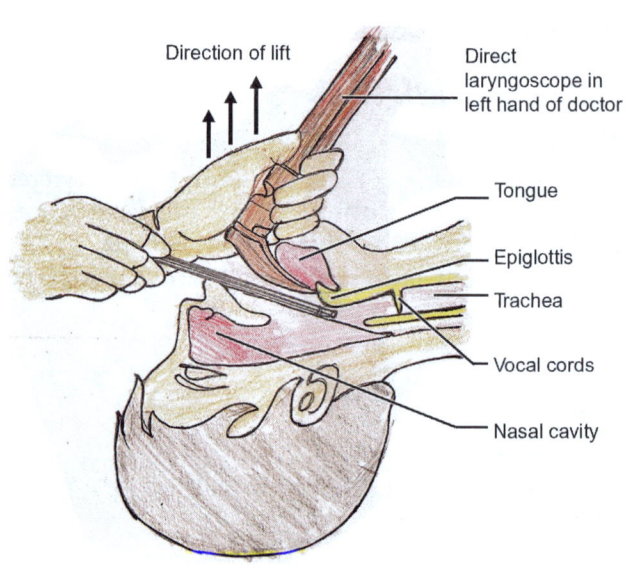

Fig. 34.9: Direct laryngoscopy

Larynx in infants	Larynx in adults
Initially it lies opposite C2–C3. Later on descends, as the child grows, to lie opposite C3 and C4	It lies opposite C3, 4, 5, and 6
Epiglottis is omega shaped	Leaf shaped
Thyroid cartilage is flat	Angulated
Larynx is inverted conical or funnel shaped	Cylindrical shaped
Narrowest part is sub-glottis	Narrowest part is glottis
Sub mucosal tissue is more and loose, hence oedema and stridor occurs following infections and trauma.	Less and dense. Infections usually do not lead to stridor.
Laryngeal cartilages are soft and collapsible so injury usually does not lead to fracture	Ossified and hard so laryngeal fractures may occur following injury.

Table 34.1: Difference of larynx in infants and adults

Here the patient is made to lie supine with flexion at his cervical spine and extension at atlanto-occipital joint. This is known as sniffing the morning air, or **barking dog position** or **Boyce position**.

The laryngoscope is held in the **left hand by a right handed** doctor, to keep his right hand free to do various procedures.

It is done to take biopsy from the larynx and hypopharynx and to remove foreign body. It is used along with the microscope to do micro-laryngeal surgeries, e.g. excision of vocal nodule, vocal polyp, papilloma, Reinke's oedema, etc.

It is also useful to see the larynx in children where indirect laryngoscopy or fiberoptic endoscopy is not possible.

During swallowing, the already **higher situated**, infant's larynx reaches C1–C2 and the epiglottis meets the soft palate. This makes a separate nasopharyngeal channel for nasal breathing while at the same time, the milk passes from the sides of the epiglottis into the hypopharynx (through the pyriform fossa on each side) thus allowing **simultaneous nasal breathing and swallowing during suckling,** whereas in adults nasal respiration and swallowing is not possible simultaneously.

Larynx

Section IV

Larynx

Section IV

PREVIOUSLY ASKED QUESTIONS

1. **Epiglottis develops from:**   *(Exam 2013)*
   a. 2nd arch   b. 3rd arch
   c. 4th arch   d. 6th arch

2. **The larynx consists of:**   *(MH 2003, Exam 2016)*
   a. 3 paired; 3 unpaired cartilage
   b. 2 paired; 3 unpaired cartilage
   c. 3 paired; 2 unpaired cartilage
   d. 2 paired; 2 unpaired cartilage

3. **All are paired cartilage of larynx except:**
                                (RJ 2001, Exam 2016)
   a. Arytenoid   b. Corniculate
   c. Cuneiform   d. Cricoid

4. **The following are unpaired:** *(PGI Nov. 2005, 2013)*
   a. Interarytenoid   b. Corniculate
   c. Vocal cord   d. Cricothyroid
   e. Thyroid

5. **Which of the following cartilage has signet ring shape?**   *(TN 2008, AIIMS 2013)*
   a. Thyroid   b. Cricoid
   c. Cuneiform   d. Arytenoid

6. **Elastic cartilage is present in:**   *(Exam 2013)*
   a. Thyroid cartilage   b. Epiglottis
   c. Cricoid   d. Arytenoid cartilage

7. **Laryngeal crepitus is absent in the following conditions except:**   *(AIIMS 2001, Exam 2016)*
   a. Postcricoid malignancy
   b. Retropharyngeal abscess
   c. Parapharyngeal abscess
   d. Prevertebral abscess

8. **Which of the following is extrinsic membrane of larynx?**   *(AIIMS 2005, Exam 2016)*
   a. Quadrangular   b. Conus elasticus
   c. Thyrohyoid   d. None

9. **All of the following are extrinsic laryngeal membranes/ligaments, except:**
                                (AI 2010, Exam 2016)
   a. Hyoepiglottic   b. Cricothyroid
   c. Cricotracheal   d. Thyrohyoid

10. **Inlet of larynx is formed by:**
                                (Kolkata 2003, Exam 2016)
    a. Ventricular fold
    b. Aryepiglottic fold
    c. Glossoepiglottic fold
    d. Vocal cord

11. **Supraglottis includes all of the following except:**
                                (PGI 2003, 2016)
    a. Aryepiglottic fold
    b. False cord
    c. Lingual surface of epiglottis
    d. Vocal cord

12. **Epilarynx includes:**   *(PGI Nov 2010, Exam 2016)*
    a. Suprahyoid epiglottis
    b. Infrahyoid epiglottis
    c. Arytenoids
    d. False cords
    e. Aryepiglottic folds

13. **Saccules in the larynx are present in:**
                                (UP 2007, Exam 2016)
    a. Paraglottic space   b. Pyriform fossa
    c. Reinke's space   d. Laryngeal ventricles

14. **Vocal cord is lined by:**   *(Delhi 96, Exam 2015)*
    a. Stratified columnar epithelium
    b. Ciliated columnar epithelium
    c. Stratified squamous epithelium
    d. Cuboidal epithelium

15. **Landmark for superior laryngeal nerve block:**
                                (JIPMER 2018)
    a. Cricothyroid membrane
    b. Greater cornu of hyoid
    c. C7 transverse process
    d. Cricotracheal membrane

16. **True about Reinke's space is:**   *(AI 99, Exam 2014)*
    a. Located in true cord
    b. Oedema of this space can be seen in smokers
    c. Associated with vocal polyps
    d. All of the above

17. **Space of Tucker is seen in:**   *(Exam 2013)*
    a. Larynx
    b. Oesophagus
    c. Femoral canal
    d. Laparoscopic approach to hernia

18. **Abductor of vocal cord is:**
                      (AI 95, Exam 2013, PGM-CET 2015)
    a. Posterior cricoarytenoid
    b. Lateral cricoarytenoid
    c. Cricothyroid
    d. Thyroarytenoid

19. **Tensor of vocal cord is:**   *(TN 2006, Exam 2016)*
    a. Posterior cricoarytenoid
    b. Lateral cricoarytenoid
    c. Cricothyroid
    d. Thyroarytenoids-external part

20. **Which of the following is the only intrinsic muscle of larynx that lies outside the laryngeal framework?**   *(Exam 2013)*
    a. Cricothyroid   b. Superior constrictor
    c. Cricopharyngeus   d. Lateral cricothyroid

21. **Closure of glottis is by all except:**
                                (TN 2008, Exam 2016)
    a. Posterior cricoarytenoids
    b. Lateral cricoarytenoids
    c. Cricothyroid
    d. Thyroarytenoids

22. Which of the following open the inlet of larynx?
    (TN 2006, Exam 2016)
    a. Thyroepiglotticus   b. Vocalis
    c. Cricoarytenoid   d. Thyroarytenoid

23. Tensors of vocal cord are: *(TN 2007, Exam 2016)*
    a. Posterior cricothyroid, internal interarytenoid
    b. Lateral cricothyroid, internal interarytenoid
    c. Thyroarytenoid, internal interarytenoid
    d. Cricothyroid and internal thyroarytenoid

24. All are elevators of larynx except:
    (AP 2004, Exam 2016)
    a. Thyrohyoid   b. Digastric
    c. Stylohyoid   d. Sternohyoid

25. Which of the following is a depressor of larynx?
    (Bihar 2002, Exam 2016)
    a. Mylohyoid   b. Stylopharyngeus
    c. Sternohyoid   d. Digastric

26. Superior margin of the infant's larynx is at the level of: *(AIIMS 2000, Exam 2016)*
    a. Cervical spine C1   b. Cervical spine C2
    c. Cervical spine C4   d. Cervical spine C6

27. A neonate while suckling milk can respire without difficulty due to: *(AIIMS Nov 2010, MH CET 2016)*
    a. Small soft palate   b. Small tongue
    c. High larynx   d. Small arytenoids

28. True about larynx in an infant: *(PGI 2003, 2015)*
    a. Epiglottis is large and omega shaped
    b. Cricoid narrowest part
    c. It extends C4, 5, 6 vertebrae
    d. Breathing and swallowing at the same time
    e. Funnel shaped

29. Narrowest part in infant's respiratory tract is:
    (RJ 2005, Exam 2016)
    a. Subglottis   b. Glottis
    c. Carina   d. None of these

30. Which of the following are functions of larynx?
    (PGI 2002, 2014)
    a. Respiration   b. Phonation
    c. Fixation of chest   d. Protection of lower airway
    e. All of the above

31. Laryngeal mirror is warmed before use by placing:
    (2001, Exam 2016)
    a. Glass surface on flame
    b. Back of mirror on flame
    c. Whole mirror into flame
    d. Mirror in boiling water

32. Which of the following is difficult to visualize or examine on Indirect Laryngoscopy?
    (MH 2008, Exam 2016)
    a. True vocal cord   b. Anterior commissure
    c. Epiglottis   d. False vocal cord

33. In indirect laryngoscopy not seen is:
    (CUPGEE 2002, Exam 2016)
    a. Base of tongue   b. Pyriform fossa
    c. Glottis   d. Subglottis

34. In right handed person, direct laryngoscope is held by which hand?   *(AIIMS May 2012)*
    a. Left   b. Right
    c. Both   d. Either of these

35. In direct laryngoscopy which of the following cannot be visualized: *(PGI Dec 2001, 2015)*
    a. Cricothyroid
    b. Lingual surface of epiglottis
    c. Arytenoids
    d. Pyriform fossa
    e. Tracheal cartilage

36. Safety muscle of the larynx is: *(Exam 2013)*
    a. Posterior cricoarytenoid
    b. Thyroarytenoid
    c. Cricothyroid
    d. Interarytenoid

37. Which one of the following is an intrinsic laryngeal membrane?   *(APPG 2016)*
    a. Cricotracheal   b. Thyrohyoid
    c. Cricothyroid   d. Cricovocal

38. Which of the following statements is true regarding vocal cords?   *(APPG 2015)*
    a. Two muscles adduct (close) the vocal cords
    b. One muscle abducts (opens) the vocal cords
    c. One muscle adjusts the length of the vocal cords
    d. One muscle adjusts the tension of the vocal cords

39. How many muscles are the tensors of vocal cords:
    (MH CET 2015)
    a. 1   b. 2
    c. 3   d. 4

40. Pre-epiglottic space is also called: *(MH CET 2015)*
    a. Reinke's space   b. Sinus of larynx
    c. Rima glottidis   d. Space of boyer

41. Moure's sign can be detected in: *(Exam 2016)*
    a. Nasopharyngeal carcinoma
    b. Oropharyngeal carcinoma
    c. Postcricoid carcinoma
    d. Supraglottic carcinoma

42. Supraglottic part of larynx drains into: *(Exam 2016)*
    a. Upper and middle deep cervical LN
    b. Middle and lower deep cervical LN
    c. Submandibular and submental group of LN
    d. Posterior triangle LN

43. Indirect laryngoscopy is primarily used to visualize:
    (Exam 2016)
    a. Vocal cords   b. Fossa incudis
    c. Bronchi   d. Trachea

Larynx

Section IV

IMAGE BASED PRACTICE QUESTIONS BY THE AUTHOR

44. The marked structures in the figure are:

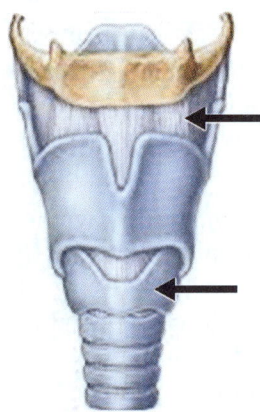

a. Thyrohyoid membrane and cricoid cartilage
b. Cricothyroid membrane and cricoid cartilage
c. Quadrangular membrane and thyroid cartilage
d. Thyrohyoid membrane and first tracheal ring

45. The marked muscle is:

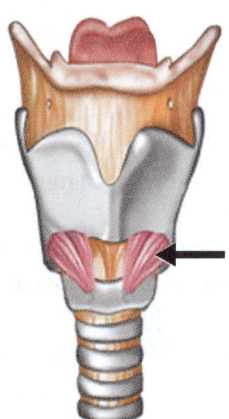

a. Thyroarytenoid   b. Thyroepiglottic
c. Cricoepiglottic   d. Cricothyroid

46. The function of the marked muscle is:

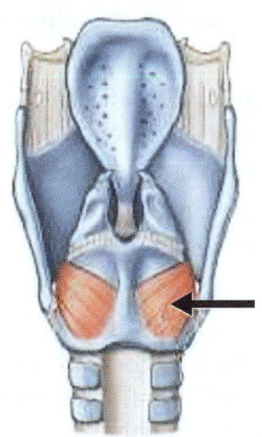

a. Adductor
b. Abductor
c. Tensor
d. Relaxer

47. The black highlighted area is:

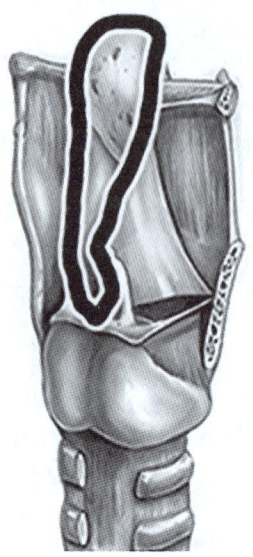

a. Vestibule
b. Ventricle
c. Inlet
d. Subglottis

48. The lymphatic drainage of the marked area is:

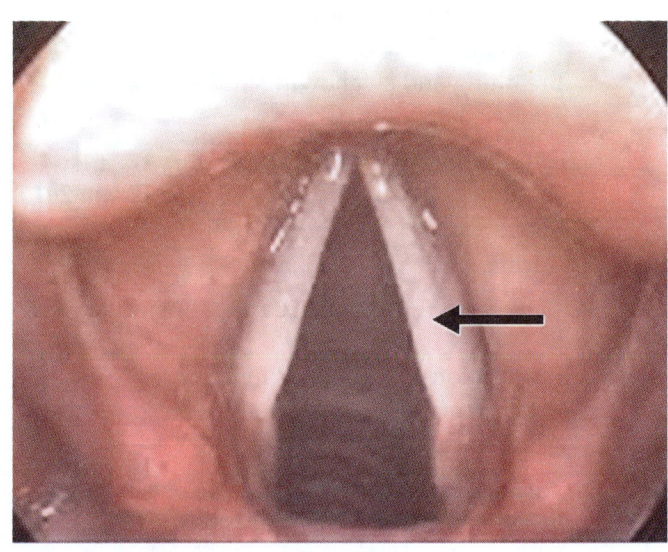

a. Upper deep cervical
b. Lower deep cervical
c. No lymphatics
d. Mediastinal lymph nodes

ANSWERS AND EXPLANATIONS

1. **(c) 4th arch** (*Ref. Scott Brown, 8th ed., Vol 3; 883*)
   Please refer to text

2. **(a) 3 paired; 3 unpaired cartilage** (*Ref. Chaurasia, 6th ed., Vol 3; 253*)
   Please refer to text

3. **(d) Cricoid** (*Ref. Cummings, 6th ed., 826; Scott Brown, 8th ed., Vol 3; 886*)

4. **(a) and (e)** (*Ref. Scott Brown, 8th ed., Vol 3; 889*)

5. **(b) Cricoid** (*Ref. Cummings, 6th ed., 826; Scott Brown, 8th ed., Vol 3; 543*)

6. **(b) Epiglottis** (*Ref. Scott Brown, 8th ed., Vol 3; 886*)
   Please refer to the text

7. **(c) Parapharyngeal abscess** (*Ref. CDT-Otolaryngology. Lalwani, 3th ed.; 460*)

8. **(c) Thyrohyoid** (*Ref. Scott Brown, 8th ed., Vol 3; 887*)

9. **(b) Cricothyroid** (*Ref. Scott Brown, 8th ed., Vol 3; 887*)
   Please *see* text.

10. **(b) Aryepiglottic fold** (*Ref. Scott Brown, 8th ed., Vol 3; 885*)

11. **(d) Vocal cord** (*Ref. Cummings, 6th ed., 1602; Scott Brown, 8th ed., Vol 3; 885*)

12. **(a), (c) and (e)** (*Ref. Cummings, 6th ed., 1602*)

13. **(d) Laryngeal ventricles** (*Ref. Scott Brown, 8th ed., Vol 3; 888*)

14. **(c) Stratified squamous epithelium** (*Ref. Scott Brown, 8th ed., Vol 3; 891*)

15. **(b) Greater cornu of hyoid** (*Ref. Scott Brown, 8th ed., Vol 3; 891*)

16. **(d) All of the above** (*Ref. Cummings, 6th ed., 913*)

17. **(a) Larynx** (*Ref. CDT-Otolaryngology. Lalwani, 3th ed.; 459*)

18. **(a) Posterior cricoarytenoid** (*Ref. Cummings, 6th ed., 826*)

19. **(c) Cricothyroid** (*Ref. Scott Brown, 8th ed., Vol 3; 888*)

20. **(a) Cricothyroid** (*Ref. Scott Brown, 8th ed., Vol 3; 889*)

21. **(a) Posterior cricoarytenoid** (*Ref. Scott Brown, 8th ed., Vol 3; 888*)
   - The Posterior cricoarytenoid is the only abductor of the true vocal cord, i.e. it opens the glottis.

22. **(a) Thyroepiglotticus** (*Ref. Scott Brown, 8th ed., Vol 3; 889*)
   Rest of the muscles act on the vocal cords.

23. **(d) Cricothyroid and internal thyroarytenoid** (*Ref. Scott Brown, 8th ed., Vol 3; 888*)

24. **(d) Sternohyoid** (*Ref. Scott Brown, 8th ed., Vol 3; 888*)

25. **(c) Sternohyoid** (*Ref. Scott Brown, 8th ed., Vol 3; 888*)
   - The muscles that attach to the thyroid or hyoid from below the larynx depress it and are known as depressors of larynx.
   - The depressors of larynx are sternothyroid, sternohyoid and omohyoid.

26. **(b) Cervical spine C2** (*Ref. Dhingra, 6th ed., 285*)
   Refer to the text

27. **(c) High larynx** (*Ref. Cummings, 6th ed., 825*)

28. **(a) (b) (d) and (e)** (*Ref. Scott Brown, 6th ed., 1/12/3; Dhingra, 6th ed., 285*)

29. **(a) Subglottis** (*Ref. Scott Brown, 8th ed., Vol1; 326*)
   - In infant's larynx the diameter of cricoid cartilage is smaller than the glottis, making subglottis the narrowest part, whereas in adults the narrowest part is the glottis.

30. **(e) All of the above** (*Ref. Cummings, 6th ed., 828*)
   Please refer to text.

31. **(a) Glass surface on flame** (*Ref. Dhingra, 6th ed., 384*)
   - Laryngeal mirror is warmed before use by placing the glass surface on flame to prevent fogging caused due to breathing.
   - Putting back of mirror on flame or will heat its back surface also which when held against the soft palate of the patient, while doing I/L, will cause burn injury.

32. **(b) Anterior commissure** (*Ref. Scott Brown, 6th ed., 1/12/15*)

33. **(d) Subglottis** (*Ref. Scott Brown, 6th ed., 1/12/15*)

34. **(a) Left** (*Ref. Dhingra, 6th ed., 422*)
   - In right handed person, direct laryngoscope is held by left hand so that the right hand is free to take biopsy or remove foreign body.

35. **(a) Cricothyroid** (*Ref. Dhingra, 6th ed., 422*)
   - In Direct laryngoscopy we are visualising the cavity of the larynx from within so cricothyroid muscle or membrane which lie externally cannot be seen.

36. **(a) Posterior Cricoarytenoid** (*Ref. Cummings, 6th ed., 826*)

37. **(c), (d)** (*Ref. Scott Brown, 8th ed., Vol 3; 887*) (the choices were wrongly set in this question, so two answers)
   - Cricothyroid membrane is the anterior thickening of Cricovocal membrane which is an intrinsic membrane.

38. **(b) One muscle abducts (opens) the vocal cords** (*ref. Scott Brown, 8th ed., Vol 3; 889*)
   - All muscles of VC are adductors
   - The tensors alter the length, hence tension of vocal cords. There are two tensors of VC.

39. **(b) 2** (*Ref. Scott Brown, 8th ed., Vol 3; 888; 889*)

40. **(d) Space of Boyer** (*Ref. Dhingra, 6th ed., 285*)

41. **(c) Postcricoid carcinoma** (*Ref. CDT- Otolaryngology. Lalwani, 3th ed.; 460; Matary Textbook of Differential Diagnosis, 4th ed.*)

42. **(a) Upper and middle deep cervical LN** (*Ref. Scott Brown, 8th ed., Vol 3; 893*)

43. **(a) Vocal cords** (*Ref. Dhingra, 6th ed., 384*)

44. **(a) Thyrohyoid membrane and cricoid cartilage** (*Ref. Cummings, 6th ed., 826; Scott Brown, 8th ed., Vol 3; 885*)

45. **(d) cricothyroid** (*Ref. Cummings, 6th ed., 827*) (the only intrinsic muscle lying outside the larynx)

46. **(b) Abductor** (*Ref. Cummings, 6th ed., 827*)
   The marked muscle is posterior cricoarytenoid

47. **(c) Inlet** (*Ref. Chaurasia, 6th ed., Vol 3; 256*)

48. **(c) No lymphatics** (*Ref. Scott Brown, 8th ed., Vol 3; 893*)
   - The true vocal cords do not have lymphatics

Infections and Inflammatory States of Larynx

ACUTE EPIGLOTTITIS

Since epiglottis is a part of supraglottis, epiglottitis is also known as acute supraglottic laryngitis.

Acute epiglottitis is a **rapidly progressive** cellulitis of epiglottis that can lead to fatal airway obstruction. Previously acute epiglottitis was most commonly caused by *H. influenzae* **type b (Hib)** but because of Hib vaccination under the universal immunisation programme, the overall incidence of acute epiglottitis has gone down. Also nowadays due to the same reason it is most commonly caused by Gp A β hemolytic Streptococcus (GABHS). Acute epiglottitis may occur in all ages but is most commonly seen in children of 2–6 years of age.

 Note:

- Less commonly bacteria like, Hib (in unimmunised children) *Streptococcus pneumonae* and *Staph. aureus*, etc. cause acute epiglottitis.
- Viruses have not been implicated as causes to acute epiglottitis.

Clinical Presentation

A **child** of acute epiglottitis presents with **acute onset fever and inspiratory stridor**. The child may find it difficult to breathe unless he is sitting up, as supine position may close off airway because of the swollen epiglottis. The child usually prefers to sit leaning forwards or in the tripod position with hands against the bed and head held in sniffing position, so that the edematous tissue fall in front and obstruction decreases. The child usually also has **odynophagia** and **drooling of saliva**.

Epiglottitis/supraglottic laryngitis involves the supraglottis. Glottis (vocal cords) is not involved so the voice of the child remains normal (so the child has **normal cry** here) and the stridor is inspiratory.

 Note:

If obstruction is supraglottic or glottic, stridor is inspiratory. If obstruction is subglottic or in cervical trachea, stridor is biphasic. If obstruction is in intrathoracic trachea, main bronchus and secondary bronchi, stridor is expiratory.

An **adult** patient with acute epiglottitis presents with **sore throat** and **odynophagia**.

This is because the sub mucosal tissue in an adult larynx is less and dense as compared to child where it is more and loose, so gross oedema resulting in stridor does not occur in adults with acute epiglottitis. Whenever the patient swallows, the infected swollen epiglottis moves down to close the inlet of larynx and food passes over this infected epiglottis leading to odynophagia (painful deglutition).

On Examination

Indirect laryngoscopy (I/L) shows **congested swollen epiglottis**, though I/L is usually avoided since it may precipitate laryngospasm. Sometimes the congested epiglottis may give a "rising beam appearance" from behind the base of tongue.

X-ray soft tissue neck (lateral view) shows the epiglottis (which normally is thin leaf shaped) to be swollen appearing like a thumb (white arrow in the X-ray picture) known as **thumb sign**.

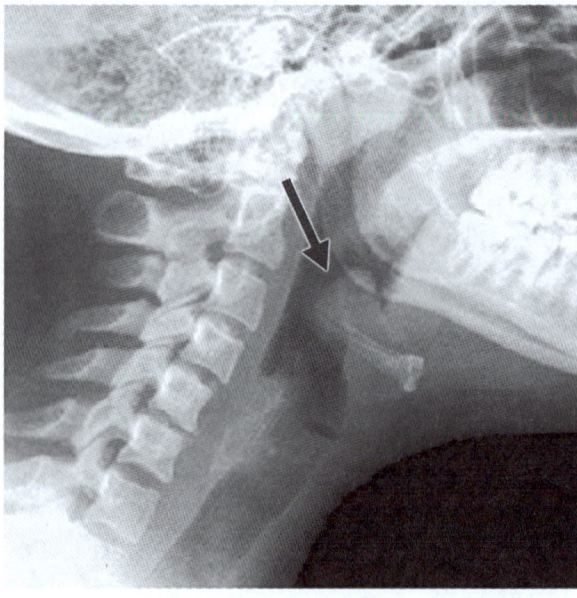

Fig. 35.1: X-ray soft tissue neck showing thumb sign

Management

The mainstay of management are:

a. Antibiotics (**beta lactum** are the drug of choice here).

b. Steroids, at times, are added for a short period to decrease the inflammation.

If in spite of the above medical management the airway obstruction due to epiglottits persists and the child goes into respiratory distress, intubation (preferably) or tracheostomy should be performed. In acute epiglottitis death due to airway obstruction may occur if appropriate treatment is not done.

LARYNGO-TRACHEO-BRONCHITIS (CROUP)

It is the most common infectious cause of airway obstruction in children. The underlying cause is viral infections, most commonly the **parainfluenza virus**.

It involves the larynx (mainly the **sub-glottis,** leading to sub-glottis oedema) and progresses to trachea and bronchi.

Clinical Features

For reasons unclear it is seen more commonly in a male than female child. Generally the age of the child is less than 3 years.

Patient presents with **gradual onset fever, barking cough (Seal like), hoarseness and stridor** (which is biphasic and has a distinct expiratory component).

Diagnosis

It is made on clinical picture.

X-ray (AP view) neck shows the sub-glottis and the upper trachea to be narrowed which appear like inverted V (^) resembling the steeple of a church. This is known as **"steeple sign"** or pencil tip appearance (*see* the X-ray film below). Other findings on X-ray are **dilatation of the hypopharynx** and normal epiglottis."

Management

i. Humidification,

ii. Nebulisation with epinephrine

iii. Decongestants

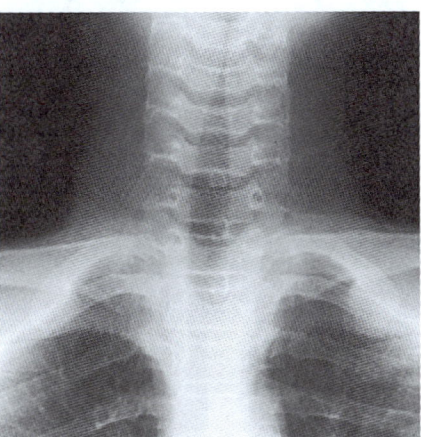

Fig. 35.2: X-ray AP view neck showing "steeple sign"

iv. Local and systemic steroids.

Inspite of the medical management, if the airway obstruction worsens:

v. Intubation (preferably) or tracheostomy can be done.

PACHYDERMIA LARYNGIS/CONTACT ULCER/KISS ULCER

Due to prolonged voice abuse when the two vocal processes of arytenoids (which form **posterior 1/3rd** of true vocal cords) forcefully rub against each other, **heaping** of epithelium, i.e. granulations at the posterior commissure area (the posterior commissure area includes, the vocal process of arytenoids along with anterior surface of body of arytenoids) occurs.

The heaping on the medial edge of one vocal process produces a saucer shaped indentation on the medial edge of other vocal process which appears like an ulcer hence known as contact ulcer.

It is **not a true ulcer** since there is no breach of the epithelium, it is just an indentation.

It is not a premalignant condition. Like a lot of other laryngeal conditions, it gets aggravated by gastroesophageal reflex, read below.

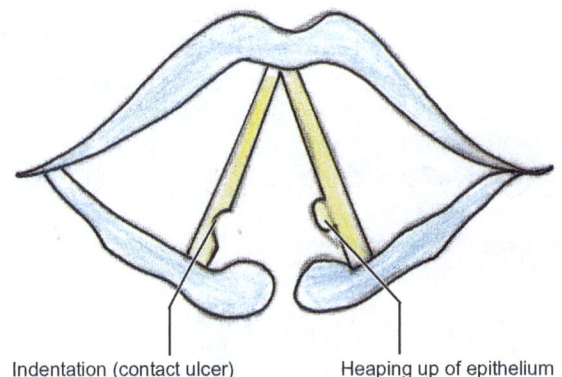

Indentation (contact ulcer)   Heaping up of epithelium

Fig. 353: Contact ulcer

Management

Micro laryngeal biopsy is done to differentiate it from tuberculosis of larynx and carcinoma larynx. The biopsy here shows hyperkeratosis.

They usually regress by voice rest and speech therapy.

If they do not regress by the above then removal of the granulations is done by micro laryngeal surgery.

REFLUX LARYNGITIS/GASTROESOPHAGEAL REFLUX DISEASE (GERD)

This is also known as pharyngolaryngeal reflux or extraesophageal reflux disease (EERD).

GERD (with or without the typical symptoms of heartburn and regurgitation) may lead to the following complications of larynx:

i. Chronic laryngitis (patient presents with pain throat, mild hoarseness, repeated throat clearing tendency and chronic cough)

ii. Posterior glottic stenosis

iii. Laryngeal pseudosulcus (refer to chapter on voice and speech disorders)
iv. A foreign body sensation in the throat (globus)
v. Aggravation of a lot of laryngeal inflammatory conditions, e.g. pachydermia laryngis, Rienke's oedema, vocal nodule, etc.

Unlike esophageal adenocarcinoma (in the background of Barrett's esophagus) a causal relationship of GERD with laryngeal cancer is still uncertain.

KERATOSIS LARYNGIS/LEUKOPLAKIA

It is hyperkeratosis of the vocal cord epithelium. It occurs due to chronic laryngeal irritation due to smoking. Unlike Pachydermia laryngis, Keratosis laryngis is a **premalignant** condition. It is managed by surgical excision by instruments or LASER. The excised specimen is sent for biopsy.

RIENKE'S OEDEMA

This is chronic and irreversible oedema of the Rienke's space, i.e. sub-mucosal space of the membranous true vocal cords along their free medial margin.

It can follow any chronic irritation of the larynx, but is most commonly due to smoking hence also known as smoker's larynx. Other chronic irritation conditions which may cause Rienke's oedema are voice abuse, pharyngolaryngeal reflux (due to gastroesophageal reflux), chronic sinusitis and postnasal drip leading to microaspiration.

Patient presents with low pitch voice, effortful speaking and hoarseness.

Diffuse symmetrical pale swelling is seen on the free edges of both the vocal cords.

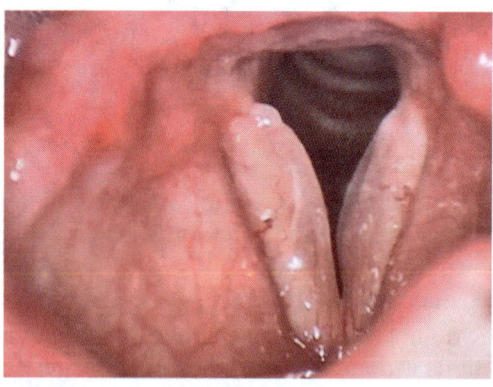

Fig. 35.4: Rienke's oedema

Management

Reduction glotto-plasty is done with instruments or LASER (KTP). Here the incision is given on the superior aspect of the vocal cord. Mucosa is elevated and the myxedematous contents are aspirated. The mucosal flap is then replaced. Voice rest and speech therapy is given in the postoperative period.

ATROPHIC LARYNGITIS/LARYNGITIS SICCA

It is the extension of atrophic rhinitis in the larynx. It is caused by *Klebsiella ozaenae*, *see* Chapter 19.

Clinical features: Hoarseness and dry irritating cough.

On laryngoscopic examination atrophy of the laryngeal mucosa with excessive crust formation is seen.

Management

Antibiotics
Laryngeal sprays containing glucose in glycerine.

GRANULOMATOUS CONDITIONS OF LARYNX

Tuberculosis of Larynx

It is usually secondary to pulmonary TB.

Clinical features: The earliest symptom is weakness of voice followed by hoarseness.

Later on the main symptom becomes odynophagia, i.e. painful deglutition due to involvement of epiglottis. Please note that whereas TB of the ear and nose are painless, TB of the larynx is an **extremely painful** condition.

Signs: TB starts in the **posterior part** of larynx.
1. The earliest sign is hyperaemia of the vocal cord and posterior commissure area and loss of complete adduction.
2. The arytenoids appear very swollen known as **mamillated arytenoids**.
3. There are multiple ulcers on the vocal cord giving it a **mouse nibbled appearance**.
4. Epiglottis which is affected late in the disease appears very swollen due to cellular infiltration (pseudoedema) and is known as **turban epiglottis**.

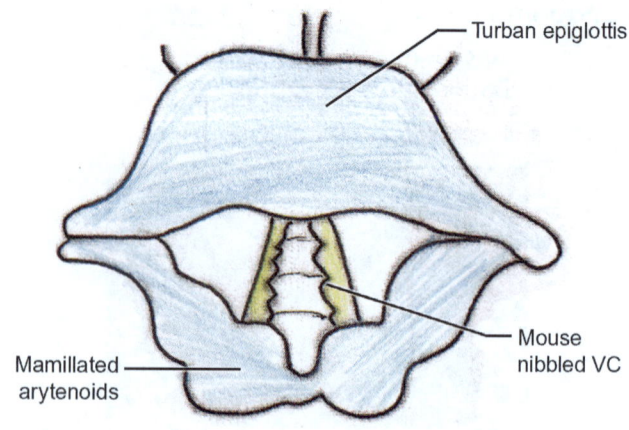

Fig. 35.5: Signs in TB larynx

Management

Anti tubercular therapy (ATT).

Differential diagnosis
- i. Pachydermia laryngis
- ii. Carcinoma of the larynx.

SCLEROMA OF LARYNX

This is the extension of Rhinoscleroma, *see* Chapter 22. It is caused by *Klebsiella rhinoscleromatis*. Here granulomas are present mainly in the subglottic region. Hoarseness and dyspnea is the presenting symptom.

Management

- i. Streptomycin, tetracycline, rifampicin
- ii. Steroids are given to ↓ fibrosis.

INTUBATION GRANULOMA

Intubation, rigid bronchoscopy or direct laryngoscopy can lead to abrasion of the arytenoid perichondrium or pressure necrosis of vocal process area (cartilaginous part of true vocal cord). Following this, a reparative granuloma forms in this area which is known as intubation granuloma. It can lead to posterior glottic incompetence or arytenoid fixation. It is managed by excision.

 "Points to Ponder/Points for Quick revision"

Symptoms	Supraglottic obstruction	Glottic obstruction	Subglottic obstruction
Stridor	Inspiratory	Inspiratory	Expiratory
Voice	Normal	Hoarse	Normal
Odynophagia	Present	Absent	Absent
Drooling of saliva	Present	Absent	Absent
Stridor ↑ supine	Present	Absent	Absent
Stridor ↓ prone	Present	Absent	Absent
Examples	Acute epiglottitis	Croup	Subglottic stenosis

Note: Laryngomalacia (*see* Chapter 37) which involves supraglottis will show all the features of supraglottic obstruction except for odynophagia and drooling of saliva which are because of painful infective oedema.

- Acute epiglottitis: Gp A Strept (MC); X-ray STN lateral view–Thumb sign
- Croup: Viral; X-ray neck AP view; Steeple sign
- Contact ulcer: Voice abuse—not true ulcer
- Keratosis laryngis: Smokers; premalignant
- Rienke's edema: Smokers larynx
- TB larynx, contact ulcer, intubation granuloma—involve posterior part of larynx.

Larynx

Section IV

PREVIOUSLY ASKED QUESTIONS

1. **Epiglottitis in a 2-year-old child occurs most commonly due to infection with:**
   (AIIMS May 2005, Exam 2016)
   a. Influenza virus
   b. Group A Streptococcus
   c. *Hemophilus influenzae*
   d. Respiratory syncytial virus

2. **Thumb sign in lateral X-ray of neck is seen in:**
   (PGI Dec 2004, 2011)
   a. Epiglottitis   b. Internal haemorrhage
   c. Saccular cyst   d. Carcinoma epiglottis
   e. Valecular cyst

3. **The antibiotic of choice in acute epiglottitis pending culture sensitivity report is:**
   (JIPMER 2001, Exam 2016)
   a. Erythromycin   b. Tetracycline
   c. Doxycycline   d. Ampicillin

4. **In acute epiglottitis common cause of death is:**
   (Delhi 96, Exam 2011)
   a. Acidosis   b. Respiratory obstruction
   c. Atelectasis   d. Aspiration

5. **Steeple sign is seen in:**
   (SGPGI 2005, UP 2005, Exam 2013)
   a. Croup   b. Acute epiglottitis
   c. Laryngomalacia   d. Quinsy

6. **The cause for contact ulcer in vocal cords is:**
   (Kerala 95, Exam 2012)
   a. Voice abuse   b. Smoking
   c. TB   d. Malignancy

7. **Site of involvement in Pachydermia laryngis:**
   (AP 2003, Exam 2016)
   a. Junction of anterior and middle 1/3rd of true vocal cords
   b. Posterior commissure
   c. Anterior commissure
   d. Vestibular fold

8. **A patient with hoarseness of voice was found to be having Pachydermia laryngis. All of the following are true except:** *(AIIMS 2002, Exam 2016)*
   a. It is a hyperkeratotic lesion present within the anterior 2/3rd of the vocal cords
   b. It is not premalignant lesion
   c. Diagnosis is made by biopsy
   d. On microscopy it shows hyperkeratosis

9. **Which of the following statements is true for contact ulcer?** *(AIIMS 2003, Exam 2016)*
   a. The commonest site is the junction of anterior 1/3rd and middle 1/3rd of vocal cord and voice abuse is the causative factor
   b. Can be caused by intubation injury

   c. The vocal process is the site and is aggravated by acid reflux
   d. Immediate surgery is the management

10. **A middle aged male comes to the OPD with complaint of hoarseness of voice for the past 2 months. He has been a chronic smoker for 30 years. On examination a reddish area of mucosal irregularity overlying a portion of both cords was seen. Management would include all except:**
    (AI 2003, Exam 2017)
    a. Cessation of smoking
    b. Radiotherapy
    c. Microlaryngeal biopsy
    d. Regular follow up

11. **Rienke's edema is seen in:**
    (Karnataka 2001, Exam 2016)
    a. Vestibular folds
    b. Vocal cords
    c. Between true and false vocal cords
    d. In pyriform fossa

12. **True about laryngitis sicca:** *(PGI June 2005, 2014)*
    a. Caused by *Klebsiella ozaenae*
    b. Caused by *Klebsiella rhinoscleromatis*
    c. Excessive crust formation is seen
    d. Antifungal are effective
    e. Microlaryngoscopic surgery is a modality of treatment

13. **Tubercular laryngitis affects primarily:**
    (TN 2001, 2016)
    a. Anterior commissure
    b. Posterior commissure of larynx
    c. Anywhere within the larynx
    d. Superior surface of larynx

14. **True about TB larynx:** *(PGI 2002, 2013)*
    a. Turban epiglottis
    b. Odynophagia
    c. Cricoarytenoid fixation
    d. Mamillated arytenoids
    e. Paralysis of vocal cords

15. **Mouse nibbled appearance of vocal cord is seen in:** *(CUPGEE 2001, Exam 2012)*
    a. TB   b. Syphilis
    c. Cancer   d. Papilloma

16. **Which one of the following conditions is considered to be definitely precancerous in the larynx?**
    (AP 2007, Exam 2016)
    a. Vocal nodules   b. Subglottic hemangiomas
    c. Leukoplakia   d. Vocal polyp

17. **Which of the following is precancerous lesion?**
    (PGI 2001, 2011)
    a. Pachydermia of larynx
    b. Laryngitis sicca

c. Keratosis of larynx

d. Scleroma larynx

e. Laryngeal papillomatosis

18. **Reflux laryngitis causes:** *(PGI Dec 2004, 2014)*
    a. Posterior glottic stenosis
    b. Carcinoma larynx
    c. Cord fixation
    d. Globus
    e. Laryngitis

19. **Treatment of Leukoplakia:** *(MH 2002, Exam 2016)*
    a. Stripping and decortication
    b. Radiotherapy
    c. Topical chemotherapy
    d. Systemic chemotherapy

20. **A child presents with biphasic stridor, barking cough and difficulty in breathing since 2–3 days. He has fever. All of the following statements about his condition are true, except:** *(AI 2010)*
    a. Subglottis stenosis and hypopharyngeal dilatation may be seen on X-rays
    b. Boys are more commonly affected than girls
    c. Symptoms are predominantly caused by involvement of the supraglottis
    d. Antibiotics do not have role in treatment

21. **Sign of acute laryngotracheobronchitis:** *(Exam 2013)*
    a. Thumb sign   b. Vallecula sign
    c. Steeple sign   d. None

22. **Regarding acute epiglottitis which of the following is/are true:** *(PGI Dec 2008, 2015)*
    a. Caused by *Haemophilus influenzae* type B
    b. Thumb sign on X-ray
    c. Ciprofloxacin is drug of choice
    d. Diagnosis is made by indirect laryngoscopy
    e. Odynophagia and drooling of saliva can occur

23. **Which of the following is seen in TB of larynx?** *(Exam 2011)*
    a. Mamillated appearance of arytenoids
    b. Mouse nibbled appearance of vocal cords
    c. Turban epiglottis
    d. All of the above

24. **A 2½ years old fully immunised child developed sore throat, dysphagia, fever and stridor in quick succession. Within 2 hours of onset of symptoms the child was very sick, pale and looked terrified. An hour later, the child became quiet and floppy. And within next one hour the child expired. The most likely diagnosis was:** *(APPG 2014)*
    a. Acute laryngotracheal bronchitis
    b. Acute epiglottitis
    c. Laryngeal diphtheria
    d. Foreign body aspiration

25. **A 4-year-old male child is brought to the paediatric outpatient department with sore Throat, fever and noisy breathing with inability to swallow for the past four hours. Examination showed a toxic, tachypnoeic child with inspiratory stridor and drooling of saliva. There is suprasternal, supraclavicular and inter costal recession during inspiration. No stridor heard during expiration. The child's clinical presentation suggests:** *(COMEDK 2013)*
    a. Intrathoracic airway obstruction
    b. Extrathoracic airway obstruction
    c. Belladonna poisoning
    d. Bronchopneumonia

26. **The appropriate next course of action is:** *(COMEDK 2013)*
    a. Arrange things for securing airway
    b. Give urgent stomach wash
    c. Immediate throat examination for a foreign body
    d. Sedate the child

27. **X-ray neck lateral view in this child is likely to reveal:** *COMEDK 2013*
    a. Steeple sign
    b. Thumb sign
    c. Scabbard trachea
    d. Normal airway

28. **The child needs to be treated with:** *(COMEDK 2013)*
    a. Neostigmine
    b. Chelating agents
    c. Urgent adenoidectomy
    d. Antibiotics

29. **Turban epiglottis is seen in:** *(Exam 2015)*
    a. Laryngeal TB
    b. Leprosy
    c. Laryngeal papilloma
    d. Epiglottis

30. **True about Reinke's oedema:** *(PGI 2014)*
    a. Usually unilateral
    b. Common in smoker
    c. Corticosteroid is mainstay of treatment
    d. Involve whole of membranous part of the vocal cords
    e. Patient has low pitch voice

31. **A 2-year-old girl is brought with acute onset of fever and breathing difficulty. Audible stridor and drooling of saliva present. No h/o cough. No vaccination. Pathogen most commonly involved:** *(Exam 2016)*
    a. *Streptococcus pneumoniae*
    b. *Legionella pneumophila*
    c. *Group A Strept*
    d. Influenza virus

32. **A 2 months old child has stridor for the past few days. The child has no other problems. The stridor is mainly during expiration. The child is taking**

feeds and is active. Which of the following is seen in the child: *(Exam 2015)*

a. Increase in the severity of stridor when the child is made to lie down in supine position
b. Indirect laryngoscopy will show omega-shaped epiglottis
c. X-ray soft tissue neck will show decreased or narrow airway in the subglottic area
d. All are seen

IMAGE BASED PRACTICE QUESTIONS BY THE AUTHOR

33. **A child is presented with h/o pain during swallowing and noisy breathing. Examination showed a toxic, tachypnoeic child with inspiratory stridor and drooling of saliva. The X-ray soft tissue neck, lateral view is shown. The most probable diagnosis is:**

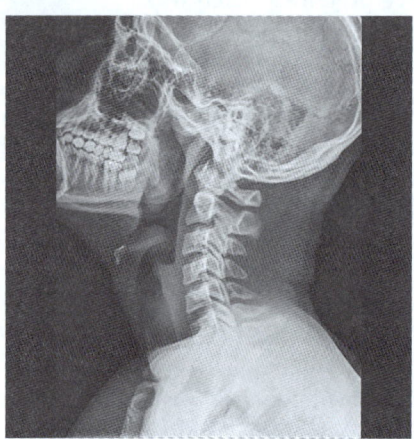

a. Acute epiglottitis
b. Croup
c. Retropharyngeal abscess
d. Prevertebral abscess

34. **A child presents with fever, stridor and barking cough. His X-ray is given below:**
Following is true about the patient:

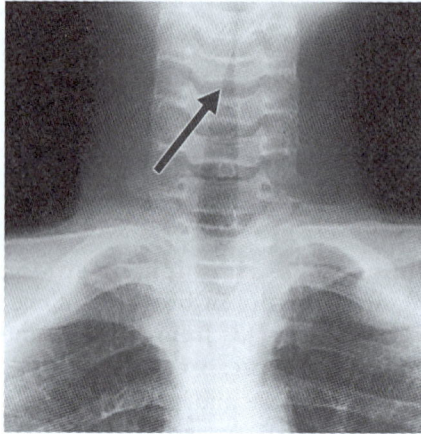

a. Symptoms are predominantly caused by involvement of subglottis
b. Antibiotics should be started immediately
c. X-ray is showing thumb sign
d. Caused by *H. influenzae b*

35. **Inspiratory stridor is seen in obstruction of:**
(Exam 2019)

a. Supraglottic   b. Subglottic
c. Tracheal   d. Bronchial

ANSWERS AND EXPLANATIONS

1. **(b) Group A Streptococcus** (*Ref. Harrison's 20th ed.; Scott Brown, 8th ed., Vol 1; 329*)
2. **(a) Epiglottitis** (*Ref. Cummings, 6th ed., 3051; Scott Brown, 8th ed., Vol 1; 329*)
3. **(d) Ampicillin** (*Ref. Cummings, 6th ed., 3052*)
   - Due to the GI side effects of ampicillin, these days' amoxicillin+ clavulanic acid, 2nd or 3rd generation cephalosporins are the preferred agents.
   - Macrolides and tetracyclines have only mild effect on Group A streptococcus.
4. **(b) Respiratory obstruction** (*Ref. Scott Brown, 8th ed., Vol 1; 330*)
5. **(a) Croup** (*Ref. Cummings, 6th ed., 3049; Scott Brown, 8th ed., Vol 1; 326*)
   Please refer the text
6. **(a) Voice abuse** (*Ref. Cummings, 6th ed., 916*)
7. **(b) Posterior commissure** (*Ref. Scott Brown, 6th ed., 5/5/10*)
   - Pachydermia laryngis involves the posterior commissure area.
   - Vocal nodule and vocal polyp arise at the junction of anterior 1/3rd and middle 1/3rd of true vocal cords.
8. **(a) It is a hyperkeratotic lesion present within the anterior 2/3rd of the vocal cords** (*Ref. Scott Brown, 6th ed., 5/5/10*)
   Rest are true, please refer the text
9. **(c) The vocal process is the site and is aggravated by acid reflux** (*Ref. Cummings, 6th ed., 916*)
   - Voice abuse causes contact ulcer in posterior commissure area. Voice abuse causes vocal nodules and polyp at the junction of anterior 1/3rd and middle 1/3rd of vocal cord.
   - Intubation leads to contact granuloma at the site of injury to perichondrium on the vocal process of arytenoids. It is unilateral.
   - Initial and mainstay management of contact ulcer is voice rest and speech therapy (refer to text).
10. **(b) Radiotherapy** (*Ref. Cummings, 6th ed., 1608*)
    - This presentation can be of a patient of contact ulcer, carcinoma or TB of the larynx. In any case the next step is to take a microlaryngeal biopsy. Cessation of smoking and regular follow up is required in all the three.
    - In case biopsy shows carcinoma, then radiotherapy will be the preferred treatment as the carcinoma is involving the vocal cords (stage II), please refer the chapter on carcinoma larynx.
11. **(b) Vocal cords** (*Ref. Cummings, 6th ed., 913; Scott Brown, 8th ed., Vol 3; 1017*)
12. **(a) and (c) Caused by *Klebsiella ozaenae*, Excessive crust formation is seen** (*Ref. Scott Brown, 8th ed., Vol 3; 1020*)
    - *Klebsiella rhinoscleromatis* leads to scleroma of larynx.
    - Antibiotics and glucose in glycerine spray is used in the management of laryngitis sicca.
13. **(b) Posterior commissure of larynx** (*Ref. Scott Brown, 8th ed., Vol 3; 1018*)
    - Mostly the granulomatous conditions of the larynx start in the anterior part of the larynx except for tuberculosis which starts and mainly involves the posterior part.
14. **(a) (b) and (d)** (*Ref. Dhingra, 6th ed., 293*)
    Please refer to text
15. **(a) TB** (*Ref. Dhingra, 6th ed., 293*)
16. **(c) Leukoplakia** (*Ref. Cummings, 6th ed., 1609*)
    Rest are not precancerous.
    - Subglottic hemangiomas are benign vascular tumours. They are rare as such but can lead to progressive stridor. They are commonly associated with cutaneous hemangiomas (the most common benign skin vascular tumours in children). Most subglottic hemangiomas spontaneously resolve by 5 years of age. If large and progressive they can be excised by CO_2 LASER or surgically.
17. **(c) and (e) are precancerous** (*Ref. Cummings, 6th ed., 1609*)
    - Malignant transformation can be seen in laryngeal papillomatosis though it is rare, *see* Chapter 39.
    - Keratosis of larynx, i.e. Leukoplakia occurs due to chronic laryngeal irritation due to smoking and is premalignant.
18. **(a), (d) and (e)** (*Ref. Cummings, 6th ed., 913*)
    Please refer to the text
19. **(a) Local excision** (*Ref. Cummings, 6th ed., 1608*)
20. **(c) Symptoms are predominantly caused by involvement of the supraglottis** (*Ref. Cummings, 6th ed., 3048; Scott Brown, 8th ed., Vol 1; 326*)
    - Fever, biphasic stridor and barking cough suggest the diagnosis to be laryngotracheobronchitis which mainly affects the subglottis along with trachea and bronchi. The underlying cause being viral (most commonly parainfluenza) so antibiotics have no role.
    - Rest of the options are true. Kindly refer to text.
21. **(c) Steeple sign** (*Ref. Cummings, 6th ed., 3048; Scott Brown, 8th ed., Vol 1; 326*)
    - Thumb sign is seen in epiglottitis.
    - Vallecula sign is the absence of air in the vallecula due to oedema of epiglottis seen on X-ray (lateral view) soft tissue neck of a patient of acute epiglottitis.
22. **(a) (b) (d) and (e) are true** (*Ref. Cummings, 6th ed., 3052; Scott Brown, 8th ed., Vol 1; 329*)
    Please remember that ciprofloxacin is not effective against group A Streptococcus, so beta lactum antibiotics covering these bacteria, are therefore the DOC here.
23. **(d) All of the above** (*Ref. Dhingra, 6th ed., 293*)
24. **(b) Acute epiglottitis** (*Ref. Cummings, 6th ed., 3051; Scott Brown, 8th ed., Vol 1; 329*)

Larynx

Section IV

- Since there is fever, foreign body is ruled out. Also since the child is immunised so practically no chances of diphtheria. Even if the child is immunised against Hib, the other mentioned bacteria in the text can lead to epiglottitis. Laryngotracheobronchitis (croup) can also present in the same fashion but it being mainly a subglottic involvement, dysphagia is not seen here. Also in croup there is a gradual development of clinical manifestations. Dysphagia and fast development of clinical symptoms point towards the acute epiglottitis.

25. **(b) Extrathoracic airway obstruction** (*Ref. Cummings, 6th ed., 3051; Scott Brown, 8th ed., Vol 1; 312*)

   It is a case of epiglottitis

26. **(a) Arrange things for securing airway** (*Ref. Cummings, 6th ed., 3052; Scott Brown 8th ed., Vol 1; 330*)

27. **(b) Thumb sign** (*Ref. Cummings, 6th ed., 3051; Scott Brown, 8th ed., Vol 1; 329*)

28. **(d) Antibiotics** (*Ref. Cummings, 6th ed., 3052*)

29. **(a) Laryngeal TB** (*Ref. Dhingra, 6th ed., 293*)

30. **(b), (d), (e) Common in smoker, Involve whole of membranous part of the vocal cords, Patient has low pitch voice** (*Ref. Cummings, 6th ed., 913*)

31. **(c) Group A *Strept*** (*Ref. Cummings, 6th ed., 3051; Scott Brown, 8th ed., Vol 1; 329*)

32. **(c) X-ray soft tissue neck will show decreased or narrow airway in the subglottic area** (*Ref. Current Diagnosis & Treatment Otolaryngology, Lalwani, 3rd ed., 481; Scott Brown, 8th ed., Vol 1; 312*)

33. **(a) Acute epiglottitis** (*Ref. Cummings, 6th ed., 3051; Scott Brown, 8th ed., Vol 1; 329*)

34. **(a) Symptoms are predominantly caused by involvement of subglottis** (*Ref. Cummings, 6th ed., 3049; Scott Brown, 8th ed., Vol 1; 326*)

35. **(a) Supraglottic** (*Ref. Scott Brown, 8th ed., Vol 3; 1038*)

Voice and Speech Disorders

VOCAL NODULE

Prolonged periods of voice abuse as seen in teachers, singers, vendors, etc. leads to sub-mucosal haemorrhage, appearing as small nodules (<3 mm) at the site of maximum vibration of the free edge of true vocal cords, i.e. the **junction of anterior 1/3rd and posterior 2/3rd** (or midpoint of membranous part of true VC).

This is known as vocal nodule, also called singer's or screamer's nodules.

They are **bilaterally symmetrical** and sessile.

It is seen more commonly in women and children. Infections, allergies and laryngopharyngeal reflux (LPR) aggravate this condition.

Clinical Features

Hoarseness and voice fatigue.

Management

Early vocal nodules (i.e. reddish in appearance as haemorrhage has just occurred) can be treated by **voice rest and speech therapy**. Infections, allergies and LPR should be treated.

Later on if hyalinisation and fibrosis occurs, then these nodules will not regress by voice reduction. They will require precise **excision** without damage of vocal ligament and muscles laterally.

Excision is done with a microscope with a lens of **400 mm** focal length known as microlaryngeal surgery **(MLS)**.

Speech therapy has to be given in the postoperative period to prevent recurrence.

VOCAL POLYPS

It is a benign solitary swelling (>3 mm) arising from the free edge of the true vocal cord. It is due to a sudden voice abuse (e.g. shouting) particularly if the vocal cords are inflamed due to infection or LPR.

It is unilateral and pedunculated and present at the site of maximum vibration of vocal cords, i.e. **junction of anterior 1/3rd and posterior 2/3rd** (*see* endoscopic photo below).

It is more commonly seen in men. Patient presents with hoarseness of voice. Since it is unilateral, the vibratory frequency of both the vocal cords is different leading to **diplophonia** (double voice).

Management

It has to be always excised by microlaryngeal surgery **(MLS),** followed by speech therapy.

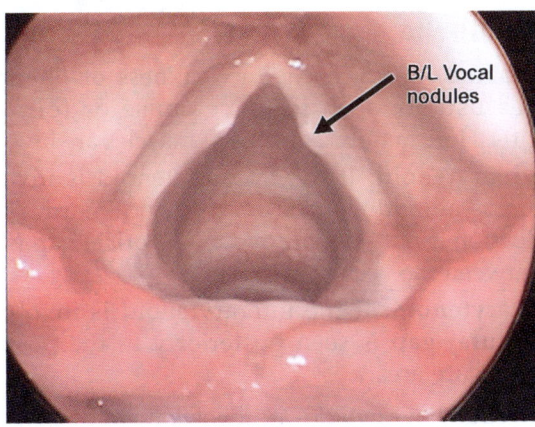

Fig. 36.1: Vocal nodules

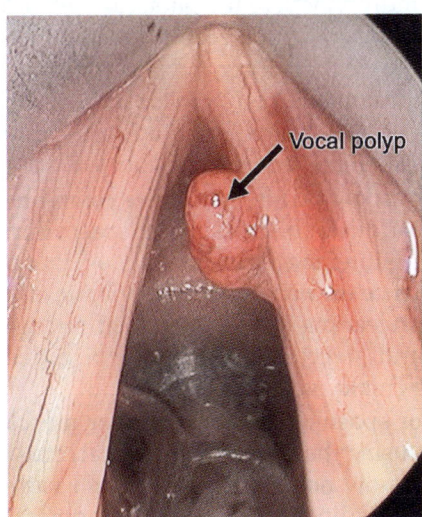

Fig. 36.2: Endoscopic view of vocal polyp

So to summarise both vocal nodule and vocal polyp occur after voice abuse and the site being the same, i.e. at the junction of anterior 1/3rd and posterior 2/3rd. The two differ from each other as given in Table 36.1.

Table 36.1	
Vocal nodule	*Vocal polyp*
Occurs after prolonged periods of voice abuse	Due to sudden voice abuse (shouting)
Bilaterally symmetrical	Unilateral
Sessile	Pedunculated
Voice fatigue and hoarseness	Diplophonia (double voice)
Initially treated with voice rest	MLS is the only option

VIDEOSTROBOSCOPY

It is an important investigation to **differentiate various lesions of the vocal cord** and in monitoring rehabilitation during speech therapy. It is based on the principle that putting light flashes on a vibrating object below the frequency at which it vibrates makes it appear vibrating in slow motion.

Hence it allows the **visualisation of mucosal wave** occurring at the medial edge of vocal fold in slow motion, making it easy to differentiate lesions and know their exact site of involvement.

SPEECH DISORDERS

Dysphonia Plica Ventriculars

Normally the **voice** is produced by the true vocal cords. If the true vocal cords are not functioning either due to organic cause (paralysis, fixation, and tumour) or non-organic cause (functional), their function is taken up by **false vocal cords, i.e. ventricular folds.** The voice then produced is a rough, low pitched voice. This is known as dysphonia plica ventricularis.

Management

Treatment of the organic cause. Functional cases are treated by psychotherapy.

Spasmodic Dysphonia/Laryngeal Dystonia

This is a condition where the phonatory muscles go into involuntary spasm during speech leading to dysphonia. It is a **neurological disorder** and is often **associated with other dystonias,** e.g. blepharospasms, oromandibular dystonias, etc. It is of three types, adductor, abductor and mixed. It is differentiated on the basis of voice of the patient:

a. **Adductor spasm:** This is the **more common** condition. Here the adductor muscles go into spasm during speech leading to stiffening and slamming together of the vocal cords. Hence they are not able to vibrate effectively on phonation leading to a very strained, strangled (full of effort) and staccato (in pieces) voice described as **scratchy croaky voice.**

b. **Abductor spasm:** Here the abductor muscles go into spasm causing the opening up of vocal cords. The vocal cords are now not able to adduct and vibrate during phonation leading to leakage of air leading to a **breathy or whispery voice.**

Management

Percutaneous botulinum toxin injection in the muscles involved, is the main treatment.

In **adductor** spasmodic dysphonia, **botulinum** toxin is given in the **thyroarytenoid** muscle (an adductor muscle) and in **abductor** dysphonia it is given in the only abductor muscle, i.e. **posterior cricoarytenoid** muscle.

For adductor spasmodic dysphonia type 2 thyroplasty can also be done.

Hysterical Aphonia/Functional (Non-organic) Aphonia/Habitual Dysphonia

It is seen mostly in **emotionally labile females** in the age group of 15–30 years.

Here in relation to stressful events sometimes the patient starts speaking in whispering voice. The quality of pitch of voice is often not constant. At times the patient complains of sudden complete loss of voice which is not accompanied by any other neurological deficit and she starts communicating through actions.

On laryngoscopic examination the vocal cords are in abducted position and fail to adduct on phonation but on coughing adduction is present, indicating that it is not vocal cord palsy but deliberate effort by the patient during phonation.

It is managed by **psychotherapy** and reassurance.

Puberophonia/Mutational Falsetto

At puberty the high pitch voice of a boy changes to the low pitch voice of an adult male due to lengthening and relaxation (i.e. decrease in tension) of the vocal cords. If low pitch voice fails to develop, the **adult male continues to have a high pitched voice.** This is known as puberophonia.

It is usually seen in introvert and emotionally insecure males.

Management

If these patients produce a low pitch voice on pressing the thyroid prominence backwards and downwards (relaxing the overstretched vocal cords), known as **Gutzmann's pressure test,** they should be treated by **type III thyroplasty** which is a procedure for relaxing the vocal cord by shortening it anteroposteriorly.

PHONASTHENIA

It is weakness of voice due to **weakness of phonatory muscles** usually seen in voice abuse or following laryngitis. Here mainly 2 groups of muscles are involved:

1. **Thyroarytenoid:** If the thyroarytenoid is involved which is an adductor of the true vocal cord, proper adduction is not possible and an **elliptical gap** is seen in between the vocal cords.

2. **Interarytenoid:** If the interarytenoid is involved a **triangular gap** is seen posteriorly in the posterior commissure area.

If both the above muscles are involved, a **key hole appearance** of the glottis is seen (*see* the endoscopic view below).

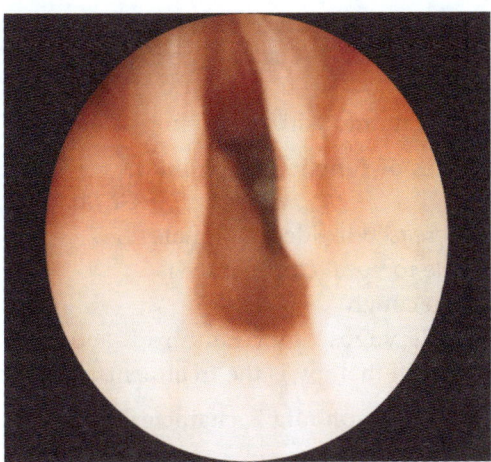

Fig. 36.3: Endoscopic view of the glottis following weakness of both thyroarytenoid and interarytenoid

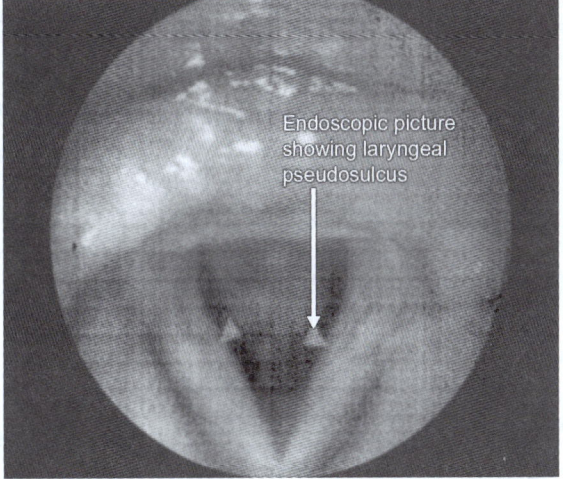

Fig. 36.4: Laryngeal pseudosulcus

Management

Voice rest.

LARYNGEAL PSEUDOSULCUS

Sulcus vocalis is an abnormal anatomical change where there is adhesion of the vocal cord epithelium to the underlying vocal ligament. This makes the vocal cords appear grooved on its medial surface.

Pharyngolaryngeal reflux, also called extraesophageal reflux disease (EERD), refers to retrograde flow of gastric contents to the upper aerodigestive tract. It leads to infraglottic oedema on the under surface of vocal cord extending throughout its length from anterior to posterior, giving it a similar appearance like sulcus vocalis, and is known as laryngeal pseudosulcus.

Management

Control of gastroesophageal reflux (GERD) and thereby pharyngolaryngeal reflux by **PPI** (to decrease acid production) and **domperidone** (which help by its prokinetic action and by increasing the tone of lower esophageal sphincter).

 "Points to Ponder/Points for Quick revision"

- Prolonged voice abuse—vocal nodule; Sudden voice abuse-vocal polyp; MC site for both is junction of anterior 1/3rd & posterior 2/3rd (*see* Table 36.1).
- Dysphonia plica ventricularis—false VC/Ventricular folds.
- Adductor spasmodic dysphonia—scratchy croaky voice.
- Abductor spasmodic dysphonia—breathy/whispery voice.
- Puberophonia: Gutzmann pressure test; type III thyroplasty.

PREVIOUSLY ASKED QUESTIONS

1. **Condition involving anterior larynx**
   (MP 2001, Exam 2017)
   a. TB
   b. Vocal nodule
   c. Contact ulcer
   d. Intubation granuloma

2. **Most common location of vocal nodule:**
   (UP 2004, Exam 2017)
   a. Anterior 1/3 and posterior 2/3 of junction
   b. Anterior commissure
   c. Posterior 1/3 and anterior 2/3 of junction
   d. Posterior commissure

3. **True about vocal nodule is/are:** *(PGI 2000, 2012)*
   a. Also known as screamer's node
   b. Occur at junction of anterior 1/3rd and posterior 2/3rd of vocal cords
   c. Most common presentation is aphonia
   d. Microlaryngoscopic surgery is not useful

4. **Treatment of choice in early vocal nodule is:**
   (AIIMS 95, Exam 2014)
   a. Radial excision
   b. Microlaryngoscopic removal
   c. Cryotherapy
   d. Voice rest and speech therapy

5. **A lady singer with singer's node with history of reflux, the best treatment is:**
   (AI 2008, Exam 2017)
   a. Voice therapy and PPI
   b. Microlaryngeal excision and PPI
   c. LASER excision and PPI
   d. Vocal cord stripping

6. **Functions of videostroboscopy include all except:**
   (AIIMS 2002, Exam 2017)
   a. Examine vocal fold mucosa for general health
   b. Vocal fold anatomical defects
   c. Differentiate vocal cord cyst from vocal nodule
   d. Vocal fold biochemical disturbances

7. **In Dysphonia plica ventricularis sound is produced by:** *(AIIMS 99, Exam 2015)*
   a. False vocal cords
   b. True vocal cords
   c. Ventricle of larynx
   d. Tongue

8. **A 26-year-old female complaining of scratchy croaky voice. Which of the following is true?**
   (AIIMS May 2009)
   a. The best treatment is botulinum in cricoarytenoid
   b. Type I thyroplasty can be used as treatment
   c. Adductor dysphonia is the cause
   d. Abductor dysphonia is the cause

9. **All are true about the spasmodic dysphonia except:**
   (AIIMS 2010)
   a. Local laryngeal disorder
   b. May be associated with other focal dystonias
   c. Adductor groups are having the strangulated voice while abductor type is having the breathy voice
   d. Botulinum toxin is used in treatment

10. **Features of functional aphonia:**
    (PGI June 2006, 2013)
    a. Increased incidence in males
    b. Due to vocal cord paralysis
    c. Can cough
    d. On laryngoscopy vocal cord is abducted
    e. Speech therapy is the treatment of choice

11. **Habitual dysphonia is characterized by:**
    (PGI Dec 2004, 2015)
    a. Seen more commonly in females
    b. Related to stressful events
    c. Treatments is psychotherapy and reassurance
    d. Whispering voice
    e. Quality of voice is constant

12. **Key knob appearance is seen in:**
    (MP 2008, Exam 2017)
    a. Functional aphonia
    b. Puberophonia
    c. Phonasthenia
    d. Vocal cord paralysis

13. **Pseudosulcus in larynx occurs due to:**
    (AIIMS Nov 2012)
    a. Vocal abuse
    b. Tuberculosis
    c. Pharyngolaryngeal reflux
    d. Chronic steroid use

14. **All of the following are true about Spasmodic Dysphonia, except:** *(Exam 2014)*
    a. It may be of adductor or abductor type
    b. Abductor type is characterized by whispering quality of voice
    c. Adductor type is characterized by breathlessness
    d. It is local laryngeal dystonia

15. **Puberophonia can be corrected by doing:**
    (Exam 2016)
    a. Type I thyroplasty
    b. Type II thyroplasty
    c. Type III thyroplasty
    d. Type IV thyroplasty

16. **Gutzmann's pressure test is done to diagnose:**
    (Exam 2016)
    a. Puberophonia
    b. Androphonia
    c. Hysterical aphonia
    d. Spasmodic dysphonia

17. **Most common cause of singer's nodule is:**
    (Exam 2016)
    a. Infection
    b. Vocal abuse
    c. Allergy
    d. Carcinoma

18. A teacher presents with tiredness of voice and hoarseness. On laryngoscopic examination, keyhole appearance of glottis is present. Which of the following is true regarding management:

(Exam 2012)

   a. Treated with voice rest and speech therapy
   b. Weakness of thyroarytenoid alone
   c. Treated with excision
   d. Muscles fail to abduct

IMAGE BASED PRACTICE QUESTIONS BY THE AUTHOR

19. The patient presented with hoarseness following a protest. Endoscopy showed the following appearance. He should be managed by:

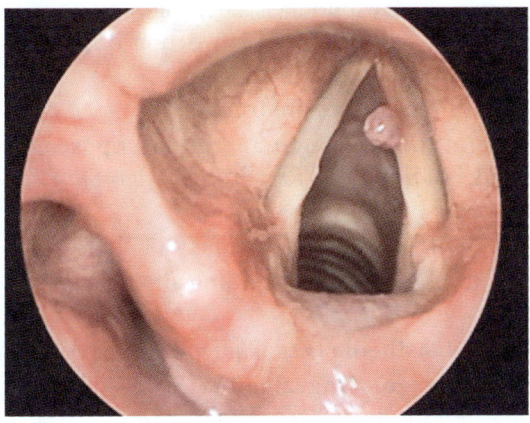

   a. Voice rest and speech therapy
   b. Microlaryngoscopic removal
   c. Radiotherapy
   d. Cryotherapy

20. A teacher presents with hoarseness. His laryngeal endoscopy is given below. True about this condition is:

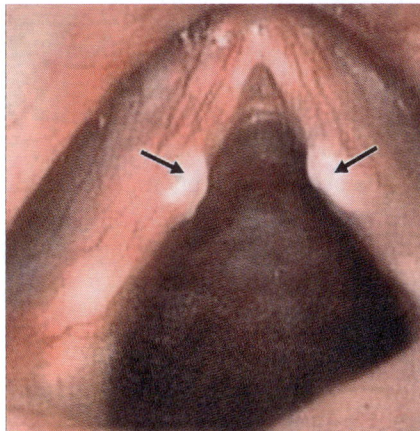

   a. Also known as screamer's nodule
   b. Occurs at the junction of anterior 2/3rd and posterior 1/3rd of vocal cords
   c. Most common presentation is aphonia
   d. Microlaryngoscopic surgery is to be done immediately

ANSWERS AND EXPLANATIONS

1. **(b) Vocal nodule** (*Ref. Cummings, 6th ed., 905; Scott Brown, 8th ed., Vol 3; 984*)
   - The commonest site for vocal nodule is the junction of anterior 1/3rd and middle 1/3rd of vocal cord (or anterior 1/3rd and posterior 2/3rd of vocal cord). Rest all involve the posterior part

2. **(a) Anterior 1/3 and posterior 2/3 of junction** (*Ref. Cummings, 6th ed., 905; Scott Brown, 8th ed., Vol 3; 951; 984*)
   - The conditions involving the posterior commissure are contact ulcer, intubation granuloma and TB.
   Rest two locations given in the options are not specific for any condition

3. **(a) and (b) are true** (*Ref. Cummings, 6th ed., 905; Scott Brown, 8th ed., Vol 3; 984*)
   Please *see* the text

4. **(d) Voice rest and speech therapy** (*Ref. Cummings, 6th ed., 905; Scott Brown, 8th ed., Vol 3; 984*)
   - Early vocal nodule is managed conservatively
   - MLS removal is done in persistent nodules despite speech therapy

5. **(a) Voice therapy and PPI** (*Ref. Cummings, 6th ed., 906; Scott Brown, 8th ed., Vol 3; 951; 984*)
   - Initial management of vocal nodule is conservative by advising voice rest and speech therapy. Pharyngo-laryngeal reflux of acid is a common aggravating cause of most of the laryngeal pathologies, so PPI also will benefit this singer.
   - Microlaryngeal excision with knife or LASER is done in persistent nodules despite speech therapy
   - Vocal cord stripping is done in keratosis laryngis/leukoplakia and Reinke's oedema.

6. **(d) Vocal fold biochemical disturbances** (*Ref. Cummings, 6th ed., 834*)
   - Videostroboscopy is a physical test to evaluate vocal cord pathologies. It does not measure biochemical parameters. Kindly *see* the text.

7. **(a) False vocal cords** (*Ref. Dhingra, 6th ed., 313*)

8. **(c) Adductor dysphonia is the cause** (*Ref. Scott Brown, 8th ed., Vol 3; 957; 997*)

- Scratchy croaky is a high pitched sound arising due to rubbing of vocal cords in adductor dysphonias. The best treatment here will be percutaneous botulinum injection in the thyroarytenoid muscle.
- Percutaneous botulinum injection in the cricoarytenoid muscle (the only abductor of VC), is done in abductor dysphonias.
- In abductor dysphonia the voice produced is low pitched breathy and whispery.
- Isshiki Type I thyroplasty is medialisation of vocal cords done in unilateral complete paralysis of vocal cords, *see* Chapter 38.

9. **(a) Local laryngeal disorder** (*Ref. Scott Brown, 8th ed., Vol 3; 957;997*)
   - Spasmodic dysphonia is a neurological disorder and is often associated with other dystonias e.g. blepharospasms
   Rest of the choices are true.

10. **(c) and (d) can cough and on laryngoscopy vocal cord is abducted** (*Ref. Scott Brown, 8th ed., Vol 3; 964*)
    Psychotherapy is the treatment of choice.

11. **(a), (b), (c), and (d)** (*Ref. Scott Brown, 8th ed., Vol 3; 964*)

12. **(c) Phonasthenia** (*Ref. Dhingra, 6th ed., 314*)

13. **(c) Pharyngolaryngeal reflux** (*Ref. Cummings, 6th ed., 912; Scott Brown, 8th ed., Vol 3; 987*)

14. **(d) It is local laryngeal dystonia** (*Ref. Scott Brown, 8th ed., Vol 3; 997*)

15. **(c) Type III thyroplasty** (*Ref. Scott Brown, 8th ed., Vol 3; 958*)

16. **(a) Puberophonia** (*Ref. Dhingra, 6th ed., 314*)

17. **(b) Vocal abuse** (*Ref. Cummings, 6th ed., 905*)

18. **(a) Treated with voice rest and speech therapy** (*Ref. Dhingra, 6th ed., 314*)

19. **(b) Microlaryngoscopic removal** (*Ref. Cummings, 6th ed., 908*)
    Endoscopy shows vocal polyp

20. **(a) Also known as screamer's nodule** (*Ref. Cummings, 6th ed., 907*)

Chapter 37

Congenital Lesions of Larynx and Laryngocele

Stridor is the abnormal high, medium or low pitched sound due to turbulent airflow through an **obstructed larynx**, trachea or large bronchi.

Any obstruction in the **nose, nasopharynx or oropharynx** leads to the abnormal sound termed as **stertor** (inspiratory snoring).

Obstruction below the secondary bronchi produce wheeze.

Obstruction	Stridor
Supraglottic, glottic	**Inspiratory**
Subglottic and cervical trachea	**Biphasic**
Intrathoracic trachea and primary and secondary bronchi	**Expiratory**

LARYNGOMALACIA (CONGENITAL LARYNGEAL STRIDOR)

This is the **most common** congenital anomaly of the larynx and also the most common cause of stridor in infants.

Clinical Features

Initially the child does not show any signs of respiratory abnormality at birth, but after few days to few weeks the child develops intermittent **inspiratory stridor** (hinting the cause to be supraglottic). This inspiratory stridor is initially mild and peaks by around 6 months.

Here in laryngomalacia the **supraglottis is bulky and floppy**. Whenever the child inspires, all the floppy and redundant tissue of supraglottis is sucked in blocking the larynx leading to stridor. This stridor worsens on crying or any exertion and while sleeping in supine position.

The stridor **disappears** on making the child lie in **prone position,** when all the redundant tissue falls in front.

Since it is a supraglottic condition the glottis, i.e. **vocal cords are normal** so the **cry** of the child remains **normal**.

Diagnosis

The diagnosis is confirmed on **direct laryngoscopy** which shows the following four important signs:
1. Elongated and large **omega shaped (Ω)** epiglottis curled upon itself.

2. Floppy aryepiglottic folds
3. Prominent arytenoids
4. Excessive redundant tissue in the supraglottis

Management

As the larynx grows all the redundant tissue is taken up and the stridor **disappears by 2 years** of age. So management is conservative by re-assurance. Rarely when the stridor is very severe leading to failure to thrive (i.e. weight gain of the child is not appropriate as per the growing age), excision of the excessive redundant tissue is done called supraglottoplasty.

VOCAL CORD PARALYSIS

This is the second most common congenital anomaly of the larynx leading to stridor.

The most common congenital CNS abnormality resulting in vocal cord paralysis is Arnold-Chiari malformation due to hydrocephalus.

Other causes of vocal cord paralysis in neonates are birth trauma following forceps delivery, intubation, CTVS surgery, repair of tracheoesophageal fistula.

Presentation has been discussed in chapter on vocal cord paralysis.

Management

Tracheostomy, if the airway is significantly compromised. Laryngeal surgery is postponed till the larynx develops fully.

SUBGLOTTIC STENOSIS

The subglottis is the narrowest part of the larynx in children. Cricoid cartilage being the only complete ring cartilage of larynx, any slight decrease in diameter of subglottis will lead to significant obstruction.

A subglottic diameter of ≤ 4 mm in a full term neonate or less than 3 mm in premature neonate is considered abnormal.

Congenital subglottic stenosis is the 3rd leading congenital anomaly of larynx causing stridor. Subglottic

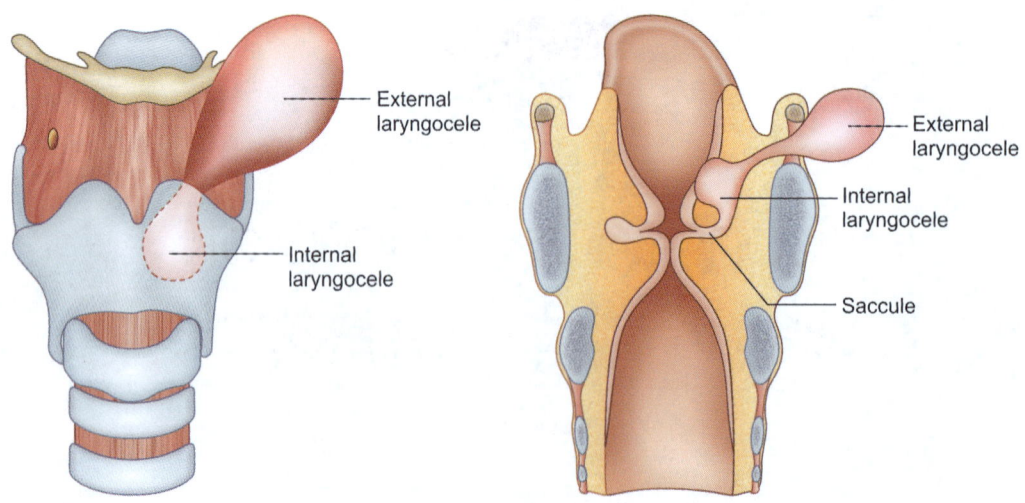

Fig. 37.1: Laryngocele

stenosis can be acquired also. The **most common cause** of acquired subglottic stenosis is **prolonged intubation** (most commonly consequent upon respiratory distress syndrome and prematurity these days) leading to pressure necrosis and fibrosis of subglottic mucosa.

Subglottic stenosis has been graded as follows by **Meyer-Cotton grading system:**

Grade	Degree of obstruction
I	0–50%
II	51–70%
III	71–99%
IV	No detectable lumen

Management

In **grade I and grade II** patients who are asymptomatic or with minimal symptoms conservative management or endoscopic dilatation/LASER excision is done.

In symptomatic patients (mainly **grade III and grade IV**) tracheostomy is done till laryngeal reconstruction is planned.

Laryngotracheal reconstruction is done by inserting cartilage graft after splitting the cricoid anteriorly and posteriorly and leaving a stent (**Montgomery T tube**) in the larynx till healing occurs.

Another procedure which is done here is **cricotracheal resection** of the stenotic segment and end to end anastomosis. Cricotracheal resection has higher rate of success than laryngotracheal reconstruction. **Mitomycin C** which is an antineoplastic agent with anti-fibroblastic activity is used here to decrease the chances of adhesions and fibrosis following surgery.

LARYNGOCELE

Any chronic increase in transglottic pressure as in trumpet players, glass blowers or weight lifters or any carcinoma at the site of ventricle that allows entry of air in the saccule but prevents its exit, leads to **enlargement of the saccule** (the lateral extension of mucosa of ventricle) is known as laryngocele (*see* Fig. 37.1).

Clinical Features

The laryngocele can be **intrinsic**, i.e. confined to the larynx. Here it presses on the adjacent structures leading to hoarseness and cough.

When it pierces through the thyrohyoid membrane, it presents as an external swelling in the anterior neck known as **extrinsic** laryngocele. This swelling increases in size on valsalva. On compression of this external swelling there occurs escape of air into the larynx leading to hissing sound. This is known as **Bryce sign.**

Management

Excision is done by an open neck surgery. If excision of extrinsic laryngocele is not possible it can be marsupilised.

LARYNGEAL WEB

Laryngeal webs are formed because of incomplete re-canalisation of the laryngotracheal groove during development. MC site of location of these webs are at the level of glottis and here 90% of them are located anteriorly. The child presents with **weak cry** since birth. Severe cases can also present with stridor. It is managed by division of the web by CO_2 LASER and a silastic keel is secured between the vocal cords at the anterior commissure.

"Points to Ponder/Points for Quick revision"

- Laryngomalacia: MC congenital anomaly of Larynx (*see* "points to ponder" in Chapter 35)
- Diagnosis: DL-inlet large & floppy
- Disappears by 2 years
- Subglottic stenosis: Acquired (MC—prolonged intubation)
- T/t: Excision → Mitomycin C
- Laryngocele: Enlarged saccule → Thyrohyoid membrane (Bryce sign); Excision.

PREVIOUSLY ASKED QUESTIONS

1. Anatomic site of origin of stridor: (*PGI 2000, 2014*)
   a. Larynx
   b. Bronchus
   c. Bronchiole
   d. Trachea
   e. Nasopharynx

2. Stridor is caused by all except: (*AP 96*)
   a. Hypocalcemia
   b. Asthma
   c. Epiglottitis
   d. Laryngeal tumour

3. A one-day-old child presented with weak cry since birth and biphasic stridor. Incomplete canalisation was considered. Most common site of defect would be at: (*AI 2002, Exam 2017*)
   a. Supraglottic
   b. Subglottic
   c. Glottic
   d. Hypopharynx

4. Most common congenital anomaly of larynx:
   (*Delhi 2008, Exam 2015*)
   a. Laryngeal web
   b. Laryngomalacia
   c. Laryngeal stenosis
   d. Vocal cord palsy

5. Congenital laryngeal stridor is also known as:
   (*AI 2001, Exam 2017*)
   a. Laryngomalacia
   b. Quinsy
   c. Laryngotracheobronchitis
   d. Laryngeal web

6. Most common cause of stridor after birth:
   (*UP 2004, Exam 2016*)
   a. Laryngeal papilloma
   b. Laryngeal web
   c. Laryngomalacia
   d. Vocal cord palsy

7. Most common cause of intermittent stridor in a 10 days old child is: (*UP 2007, Exam 2017*)
   a. Laryngomalacia
   b. Foreign body
   c. Vocal nodule
   d. Hypertrophy of turbinate

8. True regarding laryngomalacia: (*PGI 2002, 2015*)
   a. Most common cause of stridor in newborn
   b. Elongated Omega-shaped epiglottis
   c. Inspiratory stridor
   d. Requires immediate surgery
   e. Stridor worsens on lying in prone position

9. All are true regarding laryngomalacia except:
   (*Jharkhand 2004, Exam 2017*)
   a. Poor prognosis
   b. Most common congenital anomaly
   c. Stridor
   d. Gets relieved in prone position

10. About laryngomalacia all are true except:
    (*PGI 2008, 2015*)
    a. MC neonatal laryngeal anomaly
    b. Decreased symptoms during prone position
    c. Self limiting by 2–3 years of age
    d. Large Omega-shaped epiglottis is seen
    e. Surgery is treatment of choice

11. All are true about Laryngomalacia except:
    (*Jharkhand 2004, Exam 2017*)
    a. Most common congenital anomaly of larynx
    b. Stridor disappear on supine position
    c. Manifest many weeks after birth
    d. It needs no treatment in most of the cases

12. Main treatment of congenital laryngeal stridor is:
    (*UP 2007, Exam 2016*)
    a. Tracheostomy
    b. Steroid therapy
    c. Reassurance to the child's parents
    d. Amputating epiglottis

13. An infant is brought with stridor. He is diagnosed as laryngomalacia. The following things will be found in the child except: (*Exam 2013*)
    a. Stridor will be inspiratory
    b. Floppy AE folds
    c. Prominent arytenoids
    d. Hoarse cry

14. About laryngomalacia all are true except:
    (*Bihar 2006, Exam 2016*)
    a. Curled epiglottis, flaccid arytenoids
    b. Curled epiglottis, flaccid aryepiglottic fold
    c. Flaccidity of supraglottic larynx
    d. Treatment is conservative

15. A 25-year-old female presented with gradually increasing respiratory distress since 4 days. She gives history of hospitalisation and mechanical ventilation with orotracheal intubation for 2 weeks. Now she is diagnosed as having severe laryngotracheal stenosis. Next step in the management is:
    (*AIIMS 2001, Exam 2017*)
    a. LASER excision
    b. Steroids
    c. Tracheal dilation
    d. Resection and end to end anastomosis

16. Cotton's grading is used for:
    (*JIPMER 2002, Exam 2017*)
    a. Subglottic stenosis
    b. Laryngeal carcinoma
    c. Superior nerve palsy
    d. Vocal cord misuse

17. A child born with 80% subglottic stenosis should be graded as: (*UP 2003, Exam 2015*)
    a. Grade I
    b. Grade II
    c. Grade III
    d. Grade IV

18. Topical mitomycin C is used to aid the following treatment: (*AIIMS May 2011*)
    a. Endoscopic treatment of angiofibroma
    b. Treatment of laryngotracheal stenosis

Larynx

Section IV

c. Skull base osteomyelitis
d. Tonsillectomy

19. **Laryngocele arises from:**
                    (*AIIMS May 2008, Exam 2012*)
    a. Anterior commissure
    b. Saccule of the ventricle
    c. True cords
    d. False cords

20. **Laryngocele arises as herniation of laryngeal mucosa through the following membrane:**
                    (*AI 2006, Exam 2017*)
    a. Thyrohyoid
    b. Cricothyroid
    c. Cricotracheal
    d. Cricosternal

21. **Bryce sign is seen in:**   (*Exam 2013*)
    a. Laryngocele
    b. Post-cricoids carcinoma
    c. Down's syndrome
    d. Chronic tonsillitis

22. **A 4-year-old child who was operated in infancy for tracheoesophageal fistula came with complaints of cough and expiratory wheeze. Which of the following is likely diagnosis:**   (*Exam 2014*)
    a. Cough variant asthma
    b. Subglottic stenosis
    c. Tracheomalacia
    d. Vocal nodule

23. **Following are the features of laryngo-malacia except:**   (*Comedk 2015*)
    a. Collapse of supraglottic structures on inspiration
    b. Omega-shaped epiglottis
    c. Narrow arytenoid
    d. Aryepiglottic fold mucosal prolapse into airway

24. **Which one of the following conditions does not present with inspiratory stridor in children?**
    a. Laryngomalacia
    b. Acute epiglottitis
    c. Bronchiolitis
    d. None

IMAGE BASED PRACTICE QUESTIONS BY THE AUTHOR

25. **Not true regarding the given condition:**

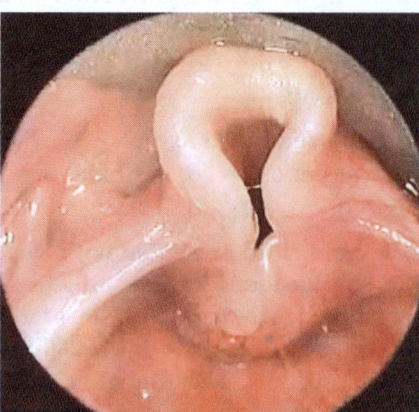

    a. Most common cause of stridor in newborn
    b. Elongated Omega-shaped epiglottis
    c. Inspiratory stridor
    d. Requires immediate surgery

26. **A trumpet player presents as an external swelling in the anterior neck on the left side increasing in size on blowing the trumpet. The following are true about the condition:**

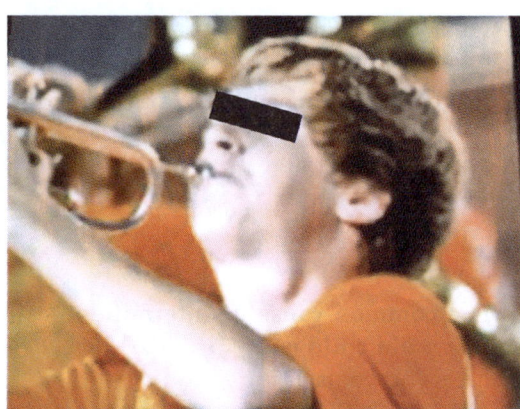

    a. Arises from Saccule of the ventricle
    b. Herniation of laryngeal mucosa through the cricothyroid membrane
    c. Bryce sign is seen here
    d. Elongated Omega-shaped epiglottis
    e. Boyce sign is seen here

ANSWERS AND EXPLANATIONS

1. **(a) (b) and (d)** (*Ref. Current Diagnosis & Treatment Otolaryngology, Lalwani 3rd ed., 481; Scott Brown, 8th ed., Vol 3; 1038*)

Abnormal respiratory sound	Anatomical location
Stertor	Nose, **nasopharynx** and oro-harynx
Stridor	**Larynx, trachea**, primary and secondary **bronchus**
Wheeze	Small tertiary bronchi and **bronchioles**

2. **(b) Asthma** (*Ref. Current Diagnosis & Treatment Otolaryngology, Lalwani, 3rd ed., 481; Scott Brown, 8th ed., Vol 3; 1038*)
   - Asthma involving small tertiary bronchi leads to wheeze.
   - Epiglottitis, i.e. supraglottic laryngitis, laryngeal tumour and hypocalcaemia (causing laryngospasm) all involve larynx and can lead to stridor.

3. **(c) Glottic** (*Ref. Current Diagnosis & Treatment Otolaryngology, Lalwani, 3rd ed., 485; Scott Brown, 8th ed., Vol 2; 335*)
   - In glottic pathologies the cry will not be normal and stridor will be biphasic like in this case. Incomplete canalisation means that the child is having laryngeal web. Laryngeal web is a rare malformation occurring as a result of incomplete canalisation of the larynx. It is present most commonly in the anterior part of glottis.
   - Biphasic stridor will also be present in subglottic pathology but cry will be normal.
   - In supraglottic condition the stridor will be inspiratory and the cry will be normal.
   - Hypopharyngeal pathology presents with dysphagia.

4. **(b) Laryngomalacia** (*Ref. Current Diagnosis & Treatment Otolaryngology, Lalwani, 3rd ed., 480; Scott Brown, 8th ed., Vol 2; 333*)
   - Most common congenital anomaly of larynx is laryngomalacia followed by vocal cord palsy and laryngeal stenosis (subglottic stenosis).

5. **(a) Laryngomalacia** (*Ref. Current Diagnosis & Treatment Otolaryngology, Lalwani, 3rd ed., 481; Scott Brown, 8th ed., Vol 2; 333*)
   - Quinsy is Peritonsillar abscess.
   - Laryngotracheobronchitis also known as croup is a viral infection most commonly caused by para-influenza virus.
   - Laryngeal web is a rare congenital malformation characterised by incomplete canalisation of larynx.

6. **(c) Laryngomalacia** (*Ref. Current Diagnosis & Treatment Otolaryngology, Lalwani, 3rd ed., 481; Scott Brown, 8th ed., Vol 2; 333*)
   - Laryngomalacia, which is the most common congenital anomaly of the larynx, is the most common cause of congenital laryngeal stridor.

- Vocal cord palsy is the 2nd most common cause of congenital stridor. Laryngeal web, a rare malformation can also lead to stridor.
- Laryngeal papilloma is the most common benign tumour of the larynx in children. Here also the child presents with stridor. In laryngeal papilloma there is additionally hoarseness of voice as it involves the vocal cord, whereas in laryngomalacia which is supraglottic the cry of the child is normal. Also laryngeal papilloma is seen in children from 2 to 5 years whereas laryngomalacia disappears by 2 years of age.

7. **(a) Laryngomalacia** (*Ref. Current Diagnosis & Treatment Otolaryngology, Lalwani, 3rd ed., 481; Scott Brown, 8th ed., Vol 2; 333*)
   - Rest of the options are not valid in a 10 days old neonate.

8. **(a) (b) and (c) are true** (*Ref. Current Diagnosis & Treatment Otolaryngology, Lalwani, 3rd ed., 481; Scott Brown, 8th ed., Vol 2; 333*)
   - Management is conservative by reassurance. Stridor improves on making the child lie prone. Refer to the text

9. **(a) Poor prognosis** (*Ref. Current Diagnosis & Treatment Otolaryngology, Lalwani, 3rd ed., 481; Scott Brown, 8th ed., Vol 2; 333*)
   - The prognosis of laryngomalacia is very good; stridor disappears on its own by two years of age. Rest all are true

10. **(e) Surgery is treatment of choice** (*Ref. Current Diagnosis & Treatment Otolaryngology, Lalwani, 3rd ed., 481; Scott Brown, 8th ed., Vol 2; 333*)
    - Reassurance is all that is required.
    - Supraglottoplasty is required to be done only rarely when the stridor is very severe leading to failure to thrive. Kindly refer to the text.

11. **(b) Stridor disappear on supine position** (*Ref. Current Diagnosis & Treatment Otolaryngology, Lalwani, 3rd ed., 483; Scott Brown, 8th ed., Vol 2; 333*)
    - Stridor precipitates in supine position.
    - Rest are true. Kindly refer to text.

12. **(c) Reassurance to the child's parents** (*Ref. Current Diagnosis & Treatment Otolaryngology, Lalwani, 3rd ed., 483; Scott Brown, 8th ed., Vol 2; 334*)

13. **(d) Hoarse cry** (*Ref. Current Diagnosis & Treatment Otolaryngology, Lalwani, 3rd ed., 483*)
    - Laryngomalacia being a supraglottic condition does not lead to hoarseness.
    - Rest all are true refer to the text.

14. **(a) Curled epiglottis, flaccid arytenoids** (*Ref. Current Diagnosis & Treatment Otolaryngology, Lalwani, 3rd ed., 483; Scott Brown, 8th ed., Vol 2; 333*)
    - Arytenoids are prominent in laryngomalacia

15. **(d) Resection and end to end anastomosis** (*Ref. Current Diagnosis & Treatment Otolaryngology, Lalwani, 3rd ed., 487*)

Larynx

Section IV

- Prolonged intubation has resulted in subglottic stenosis. Since it is severe, resection and end to end anastomosis is the treatment of choice. Steroids have no role.
- LASER excision and tracheal dilation are considered in mild subglottic stenosis.

16. **(a) Subglottic stenosis** (*Ref. Cummings, 6th ed., 983*)
- Kindly refer to text.

17. **(c) Grade III** (*Ref. Cummings, 6th ed., 983; Scott Brown, 8th ed., Vol 3; 1083*)

18. **(b) Treatment of laryngotracheal stenosis** (*Ref. Cummings, 6th ed., 985; Scott Brown, 8th ed., Vol 3; 1088*)
- Mitomycin C is an antineoplastic agent with anti-fibroblastic activity. It is used to decrease the chances of adhesions and fibrosis following surgery.
- In ENT it is used for:
  i. Laryngotracheal stenosis (as any fibrosis or adhesion of this area will lead to re stenosis, cricoid being the complete ring),
  ii. Functional endoscopic sinus surgery (FESS) (as any adhesion between the middle meatus and lateral wall of nose will again block the drainage of sinuses)
  iii. After correction of choanal atresia.

- Following surgery for angiofibroma and tonsillectomy, fibrosis and adhesions do not lead to any complications.
- Malignant otitis externa causing skull base osteomyelitis is managed by antipseudomonal antibiotics.

19. **(b) Saccule of the ventricle** (*Ref. Cummings, 6th ed., 918; Scott Brown, 8th ed., Vol 3; 1008*)

20. **(a) Thyrohyoid** (*Ref. Cummings, 6th ed., 919; Scott Brown, 8th ed., Vol 3; 1008*)

21. **(a) Laryngocele** (*Ref. Scott Brown, 8th ed., Vol 3; 1008*)
- Refer to the text

22. **(a) Cough variant asthma** (*Ref. Current Diagnosis & Treatment Otolaryngology, Lalwani, 3rd ed., 486*)
- In rest of the conditions, stridor is seen.

23. **(c) Narrow arytenoid** (*Ref. Current Diagnosis & Treatment Otolaryngology, Lalwani 3rd ed., 481*)

24. **(c) Bronchiolitis** (*Ref. Current Diagnosis & Treatment Otolaryngology, Lalwani, 3rd ed., 481*)
- Bronchiolitis is an acute inflammatory injury of the bronchioles that is usually caused by a viral infection (most commonly respiratory syncytial virus). There will be wheeze in this condition.

25. **(d) and (e)** (*Ref. Current Diagnosis & Treatment Otolaryngology, Lalwani, 3rd ed., 481*)

26. **(a) and (c)** (*Ref. Cummings, 6th ed., 919; Scott Brown, 8th ed., Vol 3; 1008*)

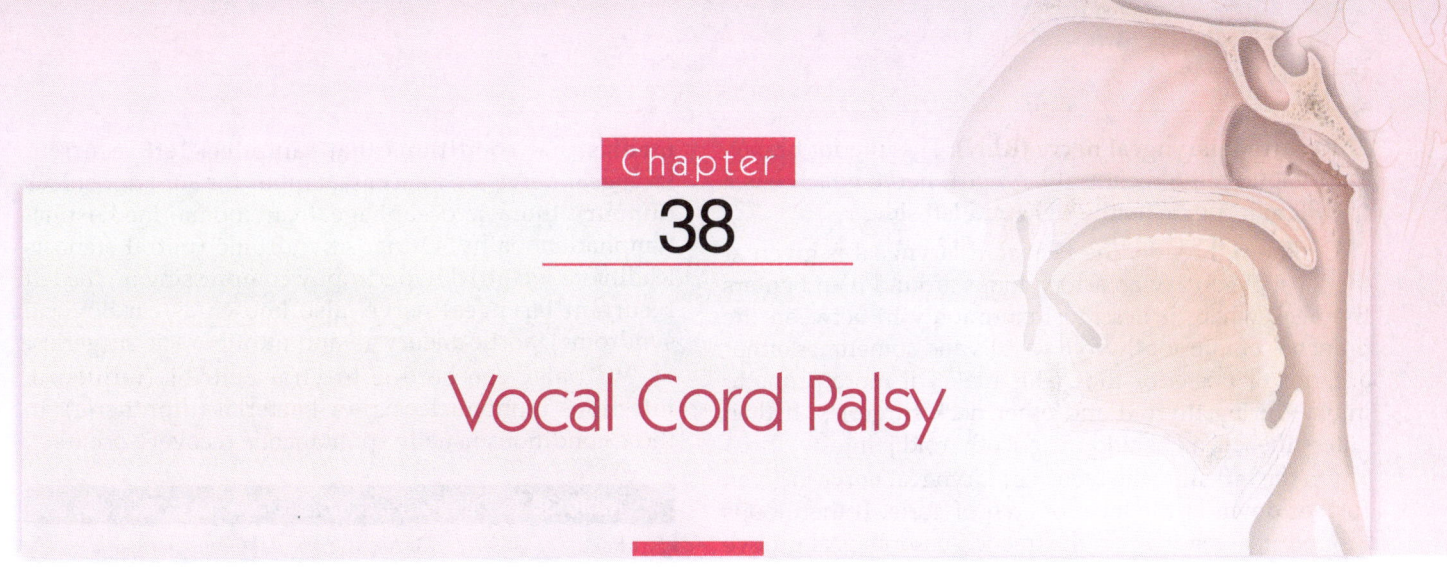

Vocal Cord Palsy

The **larynx is supplied by** the 10th cranial nerve, the **vagus**.

The vagus gives two branches to the larynx—superior laryngeal nerve and recurrent laryngeal nerve:

1. **Superior laryngeal nerve:** After arising from the inferior ganglion of vagus just below the base of skull, the superior laryngeal nerve descends down and in the neck at the level of greater cornu of hyoid gives two branches:
   a. **External laryngeal nerve**
   b. **Internal laryngeal nerve**

External laryngeal nerve: The external laryngeal nerve, as the name, lies externally deep to the **superior thyroid artery** and supplies the **cricothyroid muscle** which is the only intrinsic muscle of the larynx lying externally.

Internal laryngeal nerve: The **internal laryngeal nerve** pierces the thyrohyoid membrane along with the superior laryngeal artery (a branch of superior thyroid artery), passes between the middle and inferior constrictor and gives **sensory supply** to the larynx and hypopharynx **above the level of true vocal cord.** This nerve ends by anastomosing with an ascending branch of recurrent laryngeal nerve. This anastomosis is called **Galen's anastomosis** and is **purely a sensory anastomosis**.

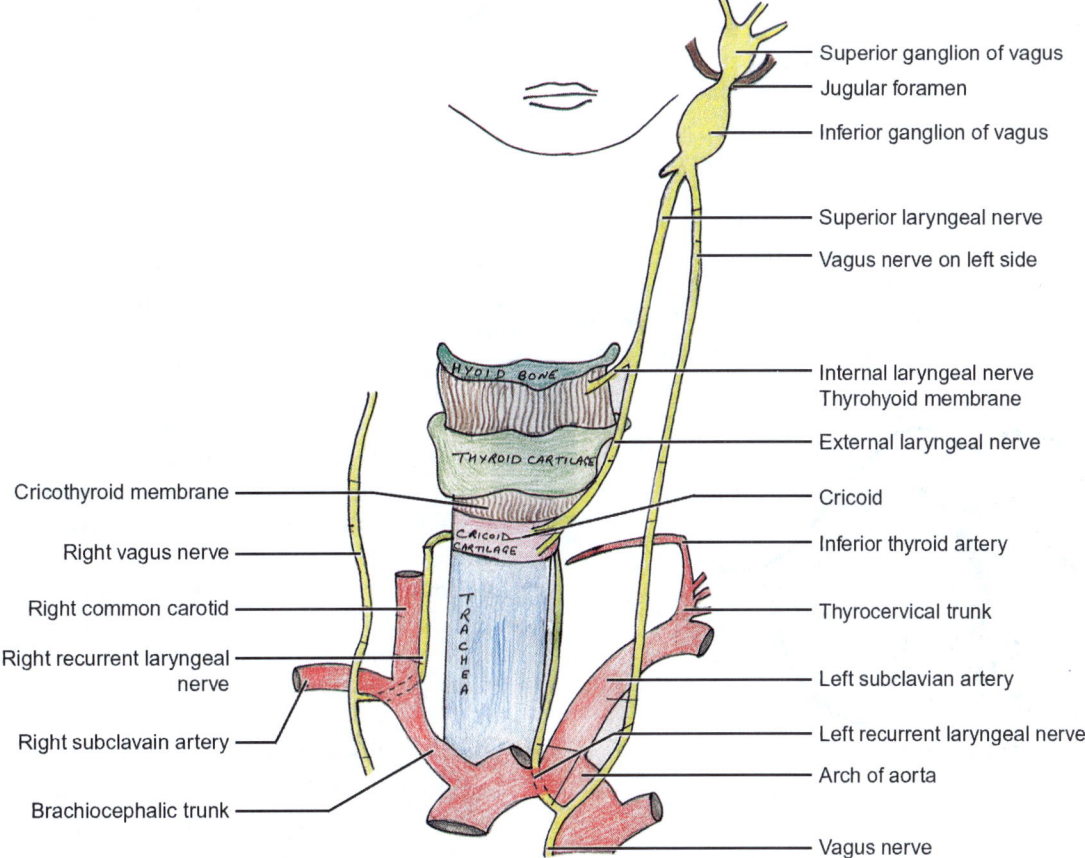

Fig. 38.1: The course of recurrent and superior laryngeal nerves

2. **Recurrent laryngeal nerve (RLN):** The inferior branch of vagus is the recurrent laryngeal nerve which has a different course on the right and left side.

On the **right side,** the recurrent laryngeal is given at the level of subclavian artery, loops around it and enters the neck where it lies most commonly in between the branches of inferior thyroid vessels and sometimes either anterior or posterior to it. This makes it more prone to injury during thyroid and other neck surgeries. It then enters the larynx behind the cricothyroid joint.

On the **left side,** the recurrent laryngeal nerve is given further down at the level of arch of aorta. It then loops around it, ascends up in the tracheo-oesophageal groove reaching the neck where it lies mostly posterior to the **inferior thyroid vessels** and sometimes in between or anterior to them. It then enters the larynx behind the cricothyroid joint.

The recurrent laryngeal nerves give **sensory supply** to the larynx and hypo pharynx **below the level of true vocal cords and motor supply to all the muscles of the larynx** except cricothyroid which, as stated above, is supplied by the external laryngeal branch of superior laryngeal nerve.

Since the **left recurrent laryngeal** nerve has a longer course (in the neck as well as mediastinum), it is **more prone to injury** as compared to the right side (lying in the neck only). **Neck conditions can lead to palsy of both right and left recurrent laryngeal nerve whereas mediastinal pathologies** can lead to the palsy of left recurrent laryngeal nerve only.

In fact the neck conditions can affect not only both the recurrent laryngeal nerves but also the superior laryngeal nerves (e.g. thyroid surgeries, carcinoma of the thyroid, larynx and hypo pharynx, metastatic lymphadenopathy, and penetrating injuries, etc.).

The **most common cause** of **bilateral RLN and external laryngeal nerve** palsy is injury during **thyroid surgery. In thyroid surgeries more prone** to injury is the **right** recurrent laryngeal nerve since it is more often intermingled with the branches of **inferior thyroid vessels**.

The **most common cause** of **left recurrent laryngeal nerve palsy** is **bronchogenic carcinoma**. The other

mediastinal conditions that can affect **left** recurrent laryngeal nerve are Pancoast tumour (or superior sulcus tumour), thoracic oesophageal carcinoma, mediastinal lymphadenopathy, Ortner's syndrome (mitral stenosis leading to left atrial hypertrophy compressing on the left recurrent laryngeal nerve, also known as cardiovocal syndrome), aortic aneurysm and intrathoracic surgeries.

VC palsy can be due to viral neuritis (influenza, infectious mononucleosis) or bacterial (diphtheria). In these conditions usually spontaneous recovery occurs.

Table 38.1: Different positions of vocal cord (VC)		
Position	Distance of vocal cord from midline	Occur normally during
1. Median	Midline	Speech
2. Paramedian	1.5 mm	Whisper
3. Intermediate or cadaveric	3.5 mm	***
4. Gentle abduction	7 mm	Normal respiration
5. Full abduction	9.5 mm	Deep inspiration

***Intermediate or cadaveric:** This is the **neutral position** of vocal cord (VC). Adduction and abduction occur from this position.

As already described in the chapter on anatomy of larynx, all the muscles acting on the vocal cords are adductors except **posterior cricoarytenoid** which is the **only abductor.** Along with adduction **cricothyroid** and **vocalis** have additional function of tensing the vocal cord.

Cadaveric position is the position of vocal cord in **complete palsy** of one sided vagus, i.e. palsy of both the superior and recurrent laryngeal nerve, hence abduction, adduction and tension all are gone. So here the vocal cord is paralysed lying in the neutral position and also appears lax or bowed. This is also the position of vocal cord during general anaesthesia.

So to conclude; if the **recurrent laryngeal nerve gets paralysed** all the intrinsic muscles of the larynx will be paralysed except for cricothyroid (which is supplied by superior laryngeal). The cricothyroid is adductor and tensor and hence will keep the vocal cord in **median or paramedian position (Wagner and Grossman theory).** Another theory **(Semon's theory)** states that since the abductor fibres are phylogenetically newer, they are more susceptible to injury by progressive organic lesions. Hence they are paralysed first compared to adductor fibres. This results in the VC being in median or paramedian position.

In complete palsy of one sided vagus, i.e. palsy of both superior and recurrent laryngeal nerve, abduction, adduction and tension all are gone. So here the vocal cord is paralysed lying in the **cadaveric position.**

VOCAL CORD PALSIES

The **functions of larynx** are mainly respiration, speech, and prevention of aspiration and cough generation. **During respiration** the vocal cords are open, i.e. in **abducted** position; the **remaining three** functions require

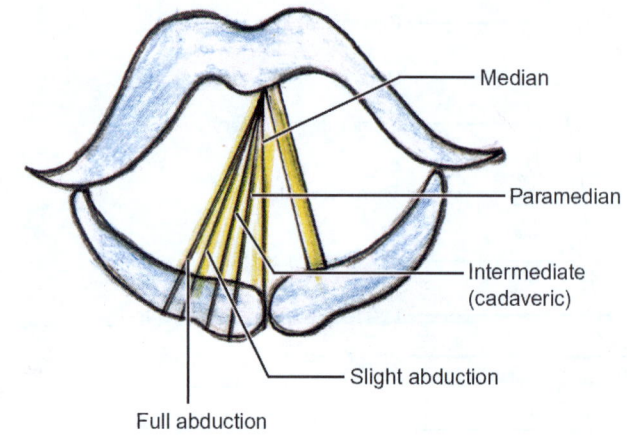

Median

Paramedian

Intermediate (cadaveric)

Slight abduction

Full abduction

Fig. 38.2: Position of vocal cords

the vocal cords to be in **adduction**. The sensory nerve supply of the larynx is also very important in the prevention of aspiration.

These functions need to be evaluated in any vocal cord palsy.

RECURRENT LARYNGEAL NERVE PALSY

The recurrent laryngeal nerve palsy can be unilateral or bilateral:

1. **Unilateral recurrent laryngeal nerve paralysis (RLN):** This is also known as unilateral incomplete palsy (called so since the superior laryngeal nerve is intact). This is also known as U/L abductor palsy as abduction of VC is not possible and the VC remains in median position.

   Position of the involved vocal cord (VC)

   Mostly Median/sometimes Paramedian

   Speech: For phonation both the VC should be in median position, so speech will be **normal** (*see* Fig. 38.3).

   If VC is in paramedian position there might be hoarseness, but since the distance from the midline in paramedian position is only 1.5 mm which the normal VC will be able to compensate over time, this hoarseness will gradually disappear.

   Aspiration: None (since the sensory internal laryngeal nerve supply above the true vocal cord is intact and also there being no gap in between the VC). The patient can cough normally.

   Respiration: Normal as the normal vocal cord is abducting normally (*see* Fig. 38.3).

   Hence patient here is **asymptomatic** or might have **little hoarseness**.

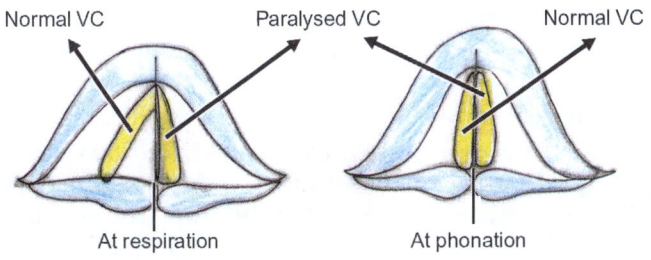

Normal VC   Paralysed VC   Normal VC

At respiration   At phonation

Fig. 38.3

Management: Conservative as the hoarseness will become normal gradually due to compensation by the normal side.

2. **Bilateral recurrent laryngeal nerve palsy:** This is also known as B/L incomplete palsy or B/L abductor palsy (called so as abduction of VC is not possible and VC are in median position as per Wagner and Grossman theory stated above).

   Position of both VC: Mostly median/sometimes paramedian.

   Speech: Largely Normal (If VC is in paramedian position there might be hoarseness).

   Aspiration: None (as explained above). Cough normal

   Respiration: Stridor and dyspnoea. It becomes worse on exertion or other tachypnoeic states, e.g. during

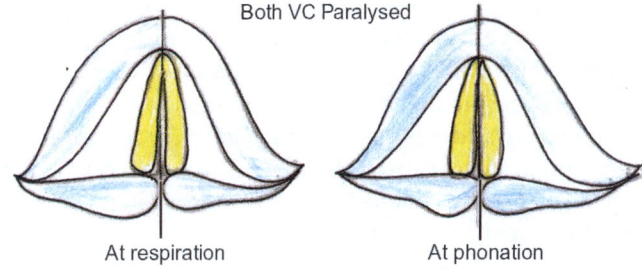

Both VC Paralysed

At respiration   At phonation

Fig. 38.4

acute infection, because here both the VC are paralysed and cannot abduct (*see* Fig. 38.4).

Hence **presentation is stridor** because of which it is also known as life threatening palsy, in fact stridor is seen only in this palsy.

Management: Immediate management is **tracheostomy**.

Later on **vocal cord lateralisation** of usually one vocal cord is done. This will relieve stridor but the voice will become hoarse.

Once the VC is lateralised, patient can be decanulated of the tracheostomy tube.

VC can be lateralised by following procedures

1. **Cordectomy:** A wedge of the vocal cord thickness is excised. The cordectomies have been classified by the European laryngological society as follows:
   a. Type I: Subepithelial cordectomy in which resection of epithelium is done
   b. Type II: Subligamental cordectomy in which resection of epithelium, Reinke's space and vocal ligament is done
   c. Type III: Transmuscular cordectomy which proceeds through the vocalis muscle
   d. Type IV: Total cordectomy
   e. Type V: Extended cordectomy (including arytenoids, subglottis, and/or ventricle)
2. **Thyroplasty type II:** This is thyroid framework surgery for VC lateralisation.
3. **Laryngeal re-innervation procedure:** Nerve muscle implant
4. **Kashima's operation:** It is endoscopic posterior glottic cordectomy. Here a wedge shaped resection is done in the posterior VC for making the airway.
5. **Woodman's operation:** It is lateralisation by Arytenoidectomy through an external approach.

UNILATERAL SUPERIOR LARYNGEAL NERVE (SLN) PARALYSIS

This leads to palsy of both internal laryngeal and external laryngeal nerve of one side therefore leading to anaesthesia above the VC and palsy of cricothyroid of the same side.

Position of VC: Cricothyroid is an adductor and tensor of the VC. Since rest of the adductors are normal, adduction will not be affected, also abduction (which is by posterior cricoarytenoid) will not be affected. So the movement of VC is normal.

But since cricothyroid is a tensor of the VC, so the **VC will be curved/bowed and floppy** producing a gap between the vocal cords during phonation.

To compensate this gap during phonation the affected VC forcefully adducts leading to the anterior commissure being pushed to the healthy side and the posterior commissure in turn points to paralysed side. This is known as **Askew position** of glottis (*see* Fig. 38.5).

Speech: Weakness of voice, voice fatigue and the pitch cannot be raised (due to floppy VC). There is **loss of timbre** or quality of voice.

Aspiration: Occasional aspiration (because the sensation of the other side is normal). Cough is largely effective.

Respiration: Normal (no stridor since VC abduction is preserved).

Management: Conservative.

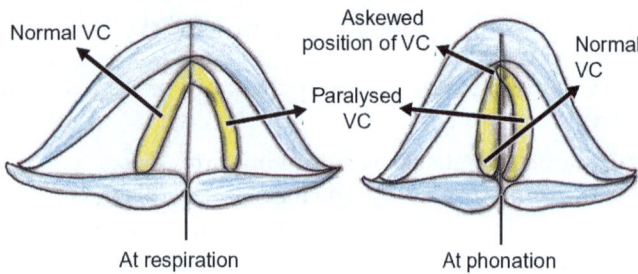

Fig. 38.5

BILATERAL SUPERIOR LARYNGEAL NERVE PARALYSIS

Here both the cricothyroid muscles are paralysed along with anaesthesia of larynx above the true vocal cords.

Position of VC: Both bowed/curved during phonation.

Speech: Weak, husky voice.

Aspiration: Present (total anaesthesia above VC and glottis gap due to bowing of both VC). Weak cough.

Respiration: Normal

Management: Tracheostomy and epiglottopexy (pull down the epiglottis and suture it to the two aryepiglottic folds and arytenoids, i.e. close the inlet of larynx to prevent aspiration).

COMPLETE PARALYSIS/COMBINED SUPERIOR AND RECURRENT LARYNGEAL NERVE PARALYSIS/ ADDUCTOR PARALYSIS

1. **Unilateral complete paralysis:** Injury here is above the origin of superior laryngeal nerve

   Position: Neutral position, i.e. cadaveric/intermediate 3.5 mm from midline.

   Speech: Initially there may be **dysphonia/forced whisper** type of voice or even **aphonia**. Later on when the normal VC tries to compensate the gap there occurs hoarseness of voice, for the normal VC is never able to cover the full 3.5 mm gap.

   Aspiration: Present but **sometimes** as one side sensation is still normal. Another important finding

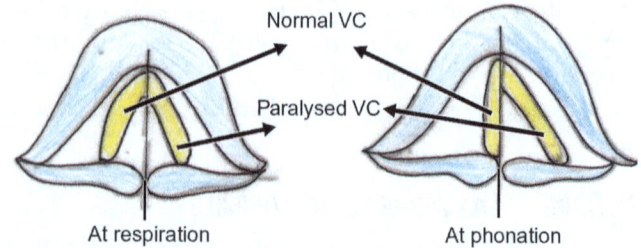

Fig. 38.6

here is that the cough is ineffective due to air wastage because of the gap between VC.

Respiration: Normal (*see* Fig. 38.6)

Management: Medialisation of the affected VC

Once the VC is medialised the voice becomes normal and aspiration is prevented. **Medialisation of VC can be done by the following procedures:**

a. **Injection of Teflon**, collagen or fat lateral to the paralysed vocal cord so that the VC is pushed medially.

b. **Type 1 thyroplasty:** This is a thyroid framework surgery to medialise the vocal cord.

c. Laryngeal re-innervation procedure by nerve muscle implant.

2. **Bilateral complete paralysis:** This is also known as **bilateral adductor paralysis** (as the VC are in cadaveric position and cannot adduct).

   Position: Both the VC in cadaveric position

   Speech: Aphonia

   Aspiration: Present due to anaesthesia of supraglottis and glottic gap. There is also inability to cough. Both of these lead to repeated attacks of bronchopneumonia.

   Respiration: Normal (*see* Fig. 38.7)

   Hence **presentation:** Aphonia and chronic aspiration pneumonias

   Management: Mainly aims at relieving chronic aspiration

   a. **Tracheoesophageal diversion** (*see* Fig. 38.8) with a permanent tracheostome: This is a permanent procedure. This is the **gold standard** surgical procedure for prevention of chronic aspiration. Here the trachea is divided horizontally at the level of 2nd and 3rd tracheal rings. The upper end of the trachea is anastomosed to the cervical oesophagus and the lower end of the trachea is brought out and sutured to the skin making a permanent tracheostome. The voice of the patient will be lost after this procedure.

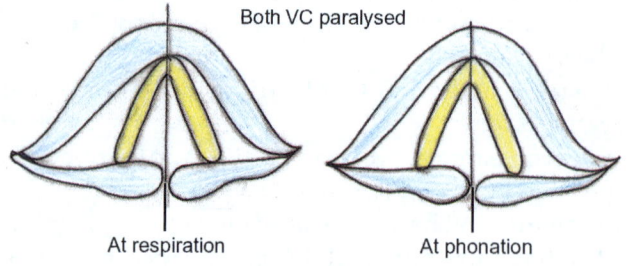

Fig. 38.7

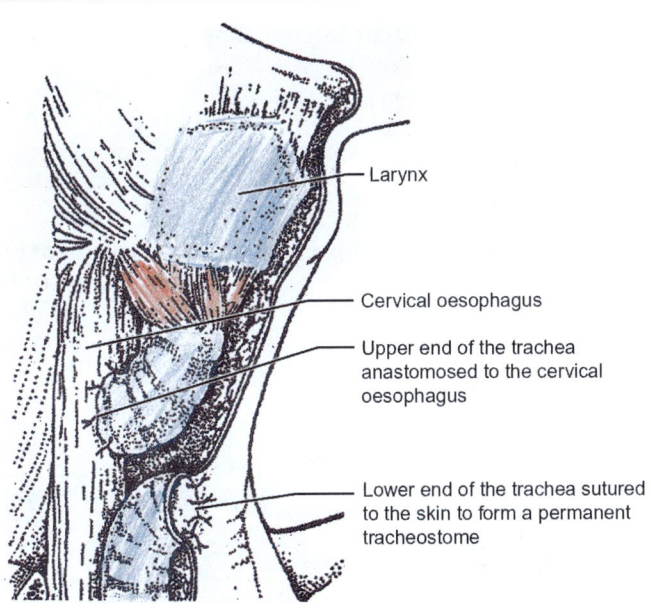

Larynx

Cervical oesophagus

Upper end of the trachea
anastomosed to the cervical
oesophagus

Lower end of the trachea sutured
to the skin to form a permanent
tracheostome

Fig. 38.8: Tracheoesophageal diversion

b. Epiglottopexy or VC plication, i.e. both the VC are sutured in midline (to prevent aspiration) along with tracheostomy (for respiration). This is a reversible procedure.

THYROPLASTY

Thyroplasties are thyroid framework surgeries.

They are of 4 types as described by Isshiki:

1. **Type I:** For medialisation of VC
2. **Type II:** Lateralisation of VC
3. **Type III:** Shortening of VC (relaxing the VC to give a low pitch voice) done to give males (with high pitch female voice) a low pitch male voice, e.g. in puberophonia (a male with high pitch voice) or in gender transformation from female to male.
4. **Type IV:** Lengthening (stretch and tighten the VC to give a high pitch voice). It is used in androphonia (a female with low pitch voice) or in gender transformation to convert male voice to a female voice.

"Points to Ponder/Points for Quick revision"

- In U/L RLN palsy there being largely no consequences, the management is conservative.
- In U/L SLN palsy there is loss of timbre of voice, management is again conservative.
- In U/L complete palsy (RLN + SLN), speech is very poor which can be corrected by medialisation of VC, i.e. type 1 thyroplasty.
- B/L RLN is characterised by stridor and is therefore most life threatening palsy and requires lateralisation of VC, i.e. type 2 thyroplasty.
- B/L SLN and B/L complete are characterised by speech and aspiration problems. Aspiration being life threatening laryngeal closure is required here subsequent to which speech is lost.

Type of palsy	Position of VC	Speech	Aspiration	Respiration	Management
U/L RLN	Mostly median, sometimes paramedian	Normal, Sometimes mild hoarseness initially	None	Normal	Conservative (Therefore this is the palsy with least consequences)
B/L RLN	Mostly median	Largely normal Sometimes mild hoarseness	None	Stridor and dyspnoea on exertion (therefore the most life threatening palsy)	Usually one sided VC lateralisation (by Cordectomy or type II thyroplasty)
U/L SLN	Normally moving curved VC	Weak Voice, voice fatigue, loss of timbre and inability to raise pitch	Occasional	Normal	Conservative
B/L SLN	Normally moving VC but Both are curved	Husky voice	Present	Normal	Tracheostomy and epiglottopexy (To prevent aspiration)
U/L complete	Cadaveric	Initial dysphonia or aphonia subsequently hoarseness	Sometimes	Normal	Teflon/fat injection or Medialisation of VC (type I thyroplasty)
B/L complete	Both VC in cadaveric position	Aphonia	Severe aspiration episodes	Normal	Tracheoesophageal diversion (gold standard)/ Epiglottopexy or VC plication with tracheostomy

- Thyroplasty
  Mnemonic
       Thyro-

Type **I**	**P**	(**P**roximal or medialisation of VC)
Type **II**	**La**	(**La**teralisation of VC)
Type **III**	**S**	(**S**hortening or relaxation of VC)
Type **IV**	**Ty**	(**Ty**ghtening or lengthening of VC)

Larynx

Section IV

PREVIOUSLY ASKED QUESTIONS

1. **Most common nerve injured in ligation of superior thyroid artery:** *(Exam 2013)*
    a. Recurrent laryngeal nerve
    b. Facial nerve
    c. Mandibular nerve
    d. External laryngeal nerve

2. **Recurrent laryngeal nerve is closely related to:** *(Rj 2001, Exam 2016)*
    a. Superior thyroid artery
    b. Middle thyroid artery
    c. Inferior thyroid artery
    d. Superior laryngeal artery

3. **Which of the following muscle is not supplied by recurrent laryngeal nerve?** *(PGI Dec 2008, PGM-CET 2015)*
    a. Post-cricoarytenoid
    b. Thyroarytenoid
    c. Lateral cricoarytenoid
    d. Cricothyroid
    e. Inter arytenoids

4. **Cricothyroid muscle is supplied by:** *(Jharkhand 2003, Exam 2016)*
    a. Internal laryngeal nerve
    b. External laryngeal nerve
    c. Recurrent laryngeal nerve
    d. Glossopharyngeal nerve

5. **Sensory nerve supply of larynx below the level of vocal cord is:** *(AIIMS 98, Exam 2015)*
    a. External branch of superior laryngeal nerve
    b. Internal branch of superior laryngeal nerve
    c. Recurrent laryngeal nerve
    d. Inferior pharyngeal nerve

6. **Recurrent laryngeal nerve has the following course in the neck:** *(PGI 2002, 2015)*
    a. It passes anterior to the inferior thyroid artery
    b. It passes through the sternocleidomastoid
    c. It passes between the branches of inferior thyroid vessels
    d. It passes posterior to inferior thyroid vessels
    e. It is superficial to inferior constrictor muscle

7. **Cadaveric position of vocal cord is:** *(AI 2000, Exam 2016)*
    a. Median   b. Para median
    c. Intermediate   d. Full abduction

8. **On laryngoscopy, vocal cords are described as being in cadaveric position. This means they are:** *(AIIMS 2000, Exam 2017)*
    a. Paralysed and abducted
    b. Paralysed and bowed
    c. Fixed
    d. None of the above

9. **Left sided recurrent laryngeal nerve palsy is most commonly due to:** *(UPSC 2005, Exam 2016)*
    a. Bronchogenic carcinoma
    b. Mitral stenosis
    c. Thyroid malignancy
    d. Thyroid surgery

10. **Most common nerve pressed by an enlargement of left atrium is:** *(AI 96, Exam 2015)*
    a. Phrenic nerve
    b. External laryngeal nerve
    c. Recurrent laryngeal nerve
    d. Sympathetic nerve

11. **Right sided vocal cord palsy is seen in:** *(AIIMS 99, Exam 2016)*
    a. Laryngeal carcinoma
    b. Aortic aneurysm
    c. Mediastinal lymphadenopathy
    d. Right vocal nodule

12. **Bilateral recurrent laryngeal nerve palsy is/are caused by:** *(PGI 2000, 2017)*
    a. Thyroid surgery
    b. Thyroid malignancy
    c. Aneurysm of arch of aorta
    d. Viral infection
    e. Mitral valve surgery

13. **Bilateral recurrent laryngeal nerve palsy is seen in:** *(AI 2004, Exam 2016)*
    a. Thyroidectomy
    b. Carcinoma thyroid
    c. Cancer cervical oesophagus
    d. All of the above

14. **Vocal cord palsy is not caused by:** *(AP 2003, Exam 2017)*
    a. Vertebral secondaries
    b. Left atrial enlargement
    c. Bronchogenic carcinoma
    d. Secondaries in mediastinum

15. **In bilateral palsy of recurrent laryngeal nerves, there is:** *(AIIMS Nov 2003, Exam 2016)*
    a. Complete loss of speech with stridor and dyspnoea
    b. Complete loss of speech but no difficulty in breathing
    c. Preserved speech with severe stridor and dyspnoea
    d. Preserved speech with no difficulty in breathing

16. **Effect of bilateral recurrent laryngeal nerve damage is:** *(MH 2003, Exam 2017)*
    a. Aphonia with stridor
    b. Aphonia without stridor
    c. Stridor
    d. Aspiration

17. **Following total thyroidectomy the patient develops respiratory stridor. The cause is:** *(UPSC 2002, Exam 2016)*
    a. B/L recurrent laryngeal nerve paralysis
    b. B/L complete paralysis
    c. U/L recurrent laryngeal nerve paralysis
    d. U/L complete paralysis

18. **Which one of the following lesions of vocal cord is dangerous to life:** *(UP 2001, Exam 2017)*
    a. Bilateral adductor paralysis
    b. Bilateral abductor paralysis
    c. Combined paralysis of left side superior and recurrent laryngeal nerve
    d. Superior laryngeal nerve paralysis

19. **The voice in a patient with bilateral abductor paralysis of larynx is:** *(AP 2005, Exam 2016)*
    a. Puberophonia
    b. Phonasthenia
    c. Dysphonia plica ventricularis
    d. Normal or good voice

20. **Partial recurrent laryngeal nerve palsy produces vocal cord in which position:** *(UP 96, Exam 2013)*
    a. Cadaveric   b. Abducted
    c. Adducted   d. Paramedian

21. **Injury to superior laryngeal nerve causes:** *(Delhi PG 2009, Exam 2016)*
    a. Hoarseness
    b. Paralysis of vocal cords
    c. No effect
    d. Loss of timbre of voice

22. **Change in pitch of sound is produced by which muscle:** *(Jharkhand 2004, Exam 2017)*
    a. Posterior cricoarytenoids
    b. Lateral cricoarytenoids
    c. Cricothyroid
    d. Interarytenoid

23. **Wagner and Grossman theory is related to:** *(Delhi PG 2009)*
    a. Palatal palsy   b. Vocal cord palsy
    c. Facial palsy   d. Hypoglossal palsy

24. **The voice is not affected in:** *(UP 2008, Exam 2016)*
    a. Unilateral abductor palsy
    b. Unilateral adductor palsy
    c. B/L superior laryngeal palsy
    d. Total adductor palsy

25. **Paralysis of recurrent laryngeal nerve true is:** *(Bihar 2005, Exam 2016)*
    a. More common on left side
    b. 50% idiopathic
    c. Cord will lie laterally
    d. Speech therapy given

26. **Mild hoarseness with stridor is seen in:** *(TN 2008, Exam 2017)*
    a. Unilateral abductor palsy
    b. Bilateral abductor palsy
    c. Laryngomalacia
    d. Tracheal stenosis

27. **Maximum stridor is seen in:** *(Exam 2012)*
    a. U/L incomplete palsy
    b. B/L incomplete palsy
    c. U/L complete paralysis
    d. Bilateral complete paralysis

28. **Aphonia of adductor paralysis can be overcome by:** *(AI 2004, Exam 2017)*
    a. Tracheostomy
    b. Arytenoidectomy
    c. Type II thyroplasty
    d. Teflon injection

29. **In bilateral abductor palsy of vocal cords following is done except:** *(Exam 2015)*
    a. Teflon paste
    b. Cordectomy
    c. Nerve muscle implant
    d. Arytenoidectomy

30. **A 30-year-old female presented with stridor following upper respiratory infection. I/L shows glottic gap is 3 mm. It can be managed by the following except:** *(AIIMS 2002, Exam 2016)*
    a. Tracheostomy   b. Type II thyroplasty
    c. Type I thyroplasty   d. Cordectomy

31. **Type 1 thyroplasty is for:** *(AI 2003, Exam 2016)*
    a. Vocal cord medialisation
    b. Vocal cord lateralisation
    c. Vocal cord shortening
    d. Vocal cord lengthening

32. **In Isshiki thyroplasty type 2, vocal cord is:** *(AP 2004, Exam 2016)*
    a. Lateralised   b. Medialised
    c. Shortened   d. Lengthened

33. **A 10-year-old boy developed hoarseness of voice following an attack of diphtheria. There is no other significant history. On examination his right vocal cord was paralysed. The treatment of choice for paralysed vocal cord will be:** *(AIIMS Nov 2005, Exam 2017)*
    a. Gel foam injection of right vocal cord
    b. Fat injection of right vocal cord
    c. Thyroplasty type 1
    d. Wait for spontaneous recovery of vocal cord

34. **Androphonia can be corrected by doing:** *(AI 2005, Exam 2016)*
    a. Type I thyroplasty b. Type II thyroplasty
    c. Type III thyroplasty d. Type IV thyroplasty

Larynx

Section IV

35. A patient with Pancoast's tumour develops hoarseness of voice after radiation. it is due to:

(*AI 2000, Exam 2016*)

a. Vocal cord infiltration with secondaries
b. Involvement of recurrent laryngeal nerve
c. Irradiation to vocal cords
d. Radiation stenosis of larynx

36. "Gold standard" surgical procedure for prevention of chronic aspiration is:

(*AIIMS Nov 2003, Exam 2017*)

a. Thyroplasty
b. Tracheostomy
c. Tracheal diversion and permanent tracheostome
d. Feeding gastrostomy/jejunostomy

37. True about superior laryngeal nerve, except:

(*Exam 2014*)

a. External laryngeal nerve tenses VC
b. Internal laryngeal branch gives sensory supply to larynx below vocal cords
c. Supplies cricothyroid
d. Internal laryngeal branch gives sensory supply to larynx above vocal cord

38. Stridor is caused by all, except: (*Exam 2014*)

a. Foreign body in left main bronchus
b. Tracheitis
c. Retropharyngeal abscess
d. Unilateral vocal cord palsy

39. Anastomosis of branches of superior laryngeal and Recurrent laryngeal nerves is: (*Exam 2013*)

a. Pure sensory
b. Motor
c. Secretomotor
d. Sympathetic

40. Which one of the following is an intrinsic laryngeal membrane: (*Exam 2015*)

a. Cricotracheal
b. Thyrohyoid
c. Hyoepiglottic
d. Cricovocal

41. All of the following are indication for tracheostomy except: (*Exam 2015*)

a. Fracture mandible with respiratory distress
b. Comatose patient
c. Bilateral abductor palsy
d. Bilateral superior laryngeal nerve palsy

42. What is the treatment of unilateral vocal cord paralysis? (*Exam 2015*)

a. Speech therapy
b. Urgent tracheostomy
c. Total laryngectomy
d. Cordectomy

43. During a thyroid operation, a nerve coursing along with the superior thyroid artery is injured. What can be the possible consequence(s): (*PGI MAY 2013*)

a. Loss of sensation above vocal cord
b. Loss of sensation below vocal cord
c. Paralysis of lateral cricoarytenoid muscle
d. Paralysis of cricothyroid muscle
e. Loss of sensation in pyriform fossa

44. Most common cause of B/L Recurrent laryngeal nerve paralysis: (*PGI MAY 2013*)

a. Thyroid surgery
b. Cancer cervical oesophagus
c. Blow from nasal cavity
d. Thyroid cancer
e. Bronchogenic carcinoma

45. A 30-year-old female patient underwent total thyroidectomy. After surgery patient complained of inability to raise her voice pitch. The most likely cause is injury to: (*COMEDK 2013*)

a. Internal branch of superior laryngeal nerve
b. External branch of superior laryngeal nerve
c. Recurrent laryngeal nerve
d. Ansa cervicalis

46. Cadaveric position of vocal cords is: (*Exam 2015*)

a. Midline
b. 1.5 mm from midline
c. 3.5 mm from midline
d. 7.5 mm from midline

47. In type 4 thyroplasty, vocal cord is: (*Exam 2016*)

a. Medially displaced
b. Laterally displaced
c. Lengthened
d. Shortened

48. True about superior laryngeal nerve except:

(*Exam 2014*)

a. External laryngeal nerve tenses VC
b. Internal laryngeal branch gives sensory supply to larynx below vocal cords
c. Supplies cricothyroid
d. Internal laryngeal branch gives sensory supply to larynx above vocal cord

49. The most likely symptom and laryngeal examination finding in a case of unilateral superior laryngeal nerve palsy are given below. Which is the correct combination: (*Exam 2016*)

a. Aphonia; vocal cord in cadaveric position
b. Weak voice and mild aspiration; bowing of affected vocal cord
c. Severe aspiration without voice change; fully mobile vocal cords
d. Asymptomatic; posterior commissure deviation to normal side

50. Following right hemi-thyroidectomy patient presents with weakness of voice and inability to raise his pitch. On examination the vocal cords moving with respiration and right vocal cord floppy. On phonation there is Askew position of vocal cord. What has probably happened: *(Exam 2016)*
    a. Right superior laryngeal nerve palsy
    b. Right recurrent laryngeal nerve palsy
    c. This is a normal finding after hemi-thyroidectomy
    d. Bilateral recurrent laryngeal nerve palsy

51. In unilateral vocal cord paralysis treatment is:
    (Exam 2016)
    a. Isshiki Type I thyroplasty
    b. Isshiki Type II thyroplasty
    c. Woodman operation
    d. Laser arytenoidectomy

52. Which muscle arises from 4th pharyngeal arch?
    (Exam 2015)
    a. Cricothyroid
    b. Cricoarytenoid
    c. Posterior cricoarytenoid
    d. Thyroarytenoid

53. In bilateral abductor paralysis which of the following is seen: *(PGI 2015)*
    a. Vocal cord is in paramedian position
    b. Voice is affected early
    c. Stridor and dyspnoea occur
    d. Vocal cord lateralisation is done
    e. Hoarseness occurs

54. How many muscles are the tensors of vocal cords?
    (MH CET 2015)
    a. 1   b. 2
    c. 3   d. 4

55. Which one of the following muscles of larynx causes abduction of vocal cords?   *(MH CET 2015)*
    a. Transverse arytenoid
    b. Oblique arytenoid
    c. Posterior cricoarytenoid
    d. Lateral cricoarytenoid

56. Kashima operation done for: *(AIIMS 2015)*
    a. Vocal cord   b. Cholesteatoma
    c. Sinusitis   d. Atrophic rhinitis

57. Tensors of vocal cords includes: *(PGI May 2015)*
    a. Arytenoid   b. Vocalis
    c. Interarytenoid   d. Posterior cricoarytenoid
    e. Cricothyroid

58. Which of the following statements is true regarding vocal cords?   *(APPG 2015)*
    a. Two muscles adduct (close) the vocal cords
    b. One muscle abducts (opens) the vocal cords
    c. One muscle adjusts the length of the vocal cords
    d. One muscle adjusts the tension of the vocal cords

IMAGE BASED PRACTICE QUESTIONS BY THE AUTHOR

59. The marked muscle is supplied by which nerve:

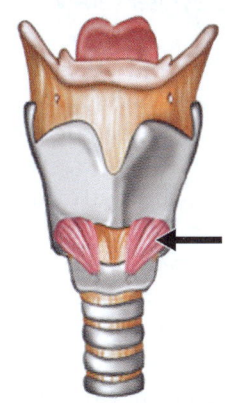

    a. Internal laryngeal nerve
    b. Recurrent laryngeal nerve
    c. External laryngeal nerve
    d. Arnolds nerve

60. Following total thyroidectomy the patient develops respiratory stridor. Endoscopic appearance of the larynx is given (both during inspiration and expiration). He should be managed by:

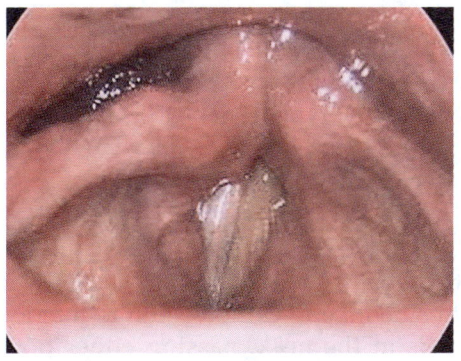

    a. Fat injection   b. Type II thyroplasty
    c. Type I thyroplasty   d. Teflon injection

61. A patient presents with the complaint of aphonia and aspiration. Endoscopic picture of larynx is given (both during inspiration and expiration). What has happened:
    a. Unilateral abductor palsy
    b. Unilateral adductor palsy
    c. B/L superior laryngeal palsy
    d. Total adductor palsy

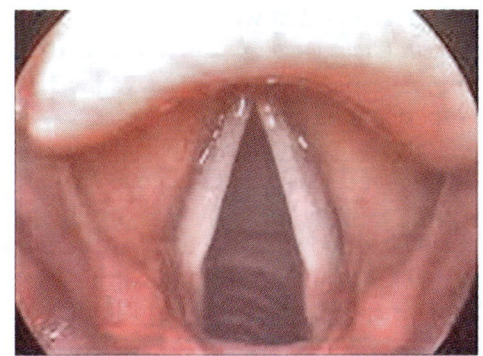

Larynx

Section IV

ANSWERS AND EXPLANATIONS

1. **(d) External laryngeal nerve** (*Ref. Scott Brown, 8th ed., Vol 3; 891*)
   - The superior thyroid artery lies superficial to the external laryngeal nerve, a branch of the superior laryngeal nerve, on the cricothyroid muscle at the upper pole of thyroid. Its ligation here in thyroidectomy can injure the external laryngeal nerve.
   - Recurrent laryngeal nerve is in close relationship with inferior thyroid artery.

2. **(c) Inferior thyroid artery** (*Ref. Scott Brown, 8th ed., Vol 3; 892*)
   - The recurrent laryngeal nerve (RLN) lies either anterior or posterior or intermingled with the branches of the inferior thyroid artery at the lower pole of the thyroid and can be injured here during thyroidectomy.
   - Since right RLN is more often intermingled with the branches of the inferior thyroid artery as compared to left sided RLN, therefore right RLN palsy is more common than left following thyroid surgery. Though overall left RLN palsy is more common (please *refer* to the text).

3. **(d) Cricothyroid** (*Ref. Cummings, 6th ed., 827; Scott Brown, 8th ed., Vol 3; 892*)

4. **(b) External laryngeal nerve** (*Ref. Cummings, 6th ed., 827; Scott Brown, 8th ed., Vol 3; 892*)

5. **(c) Recurrent laryngeal nerve** (*Ref. Cummings, 6th ed., 827; Scott Brown, 8th ed., Vol 3; 892*)

6. **(a), (c) and (d)** (*Ref. Scott Brown, 8th ed., Vol 3; 892*)
   - Both the recurrent laryngeal nerves, particularly the right sided, lie in close relation to inferior thyroid vessels in the neck, passing either posterior or anterior or in between them (please refer to the text).

7. **(c) Intermediate** (*Ref. Current Diagnosis & Treatment Otolaryngology, Lalwani, 3rd ed., 447*)
   - The cadaveric position is so called this is the position in complete palsy of vagus (or in simple language completely dead vagus nerve) i.e. both the superior and recurrent laryngeal nerve palsy hence abduction, adduction and tension all are gone. So here the VC is paralysed lying in the neutral or intermediate position (called so because adduction or abduction occurs from this position).

8. **(b) Paralysed and bowed** (*Ref. Current Diagnosis & Treatment Otolaryngology, Lalwani, 3rd ed., 447*)
   - In complete palsy of one sided vagus i.e. palsy of the superior and recurrent laryngeal nerve abduction (so paralysed and abducted will be wrong choice), adduction and tension all are gone. So here the VC is paralysed lying in the neutral position and also appears lax or bowed (due to loss of tension).
   - Fixed VC indicates restriction of mobility of VC following fixity of cricothyroid joint as in carcinoma.

9. **(a) Bronchogenic carcinoma** (*Ref. Current Diagnosis & Treatment Otolaryngology, Lalwani, 3rd ed., 476*)
   - The most common cause of left sided recurrent laryngeal nerve palsy is bronchogenic carcinoma.
   - Mitral stenosis leading to left atrial hypertrophy can compress on the left recurrent laryngeal nerve leading to its palsy (Ortner's syndrome) but is very rare.
   - Thyroid malignancy, being a condition of neck can affect both the branches of vagus, i.e. superior laryngeal and recurrent laryngeal nerves.
   - The most common cause of bilateral RLN, right sided RLN and external laryngeal nerve palsy is injury during thyroid surgery.

10. **(c) Recurrent laryngeal nerve (left sided)** (*Ref. Scott Brown, 8th ed., Vol 3; 892; Vol 2; 336*)
    Refer the text for Ortner's/Cardiovocal syndrome.

11. **(a) Laryngeal carcinoma** (*Ref. Scott Brown, 8th ed., Vol 3; 892*)
    - Mediastinal conditions, e.g. aortic aneurysm, mediastinal lymphadenopathy etc can lead to only left recurrent laryngeal nerve palsy because of its course in the mediastinum.
    - Vocal nodules do not lead to vocal cord palsy.

12. **(a) (b) and (d)** (*Ref. Current Diagnosis & Treatment Otolaryngology, Lalwani, 3rd ed., 476*)
    - Neck surgeries/conditions can cause bilateral recurrent laryngeal nerve palsy.
    - Mediastinal conditions will involve only the left RLN.

13. **(d) All of the above** (*Ref. Current Diagnosis & Treatment Otolaryngology, Lalwani, 3rd ed., 476*)

14. **(a) Vertebral secondaries** (*Ref. Scott Brown, 6th ed., 1/12/17*)
    - Superior and recurrent laryngeal nerves are not in close proximity to vertebrae.
    - Rest of the given (mediastinal) conditions can cause left recurrent laryngeal nerve palsy.

15. **(c) Preserved speech with severe stridor and dyspnoea** (*Ref. Current Diagnosis & Treatment Otolaryngology, Lalwani 3rd ed., 478; Scott Brown, 8th ed., Vol 2; 336*)
    - In bilateral palsy of recurrent laryngeal nerves both the vocal cords will be in median position, leading to stridor and dyspnoea but speech will be preserved (the most life threatening palsy).
    - Complete loss of speech along with stridor and dyspnoea cannot occur in any of the VC palsies because for speech disturbance to occur VC should be well away from the midline but this will ease respiration. For stridor to happen VC should remain at or near midline but now there won't be speech disturbance.
    - Complete loss of speech but no difficulty in breathing is a feature of bilateral complete paralysis (combined B/L superior and recurrent laryngeal nerve paralysis).

- Preserved speech with no difficulty in breathing is a feature of U/L RLN palsy (palsy with least ill consequences).

16. **(c) Stridor** (*Ref. Current Diagnosis & Treatment Otolaryngology, Lalwani, 3rd ed., 478*)

- Aphonia with stridor cannot occur in any of the VC palsies (kindly see above explanation)

17. **(a) B/L recurrent laryngeal nerve paralysis** (*Ref. Current Diagnosis & Treatment Otolaryngology, Lalwani, 3rd ed., 478*)

- In B/L recurrent laryngeal nerve paralysis the vocal cords will be in median position, leading to stridor. **Note:** This is the only vocal cord palsy with stridor, breathing is normal in the remaining palsies.

18. **(b) Bilateral abductor paralysis** (*Ref. Current Diagnosis & Treatment Otolaryngology, Lalwani, 3rd ed., 478; Scott Brown, 8th ed., Vol 2; 336*)

- In bilateral abductor paralysis or B/L RLN palsy presentation is stridor because of which it is also known as life threatening palsy.
- In bilateral adductor paralysis, i.e. B/L complete paralysis, there will be aspiration bronchopneumonias but the presentation will not be acute life threatening in comparison to stridor in B/L RLN palsy.
- The remaining two options are not life threatening (refer to the text)

19. **(d) Normal or good voice** (*Ref. Current Diagnosis & Treatment Otolaryngology, Lalwani, 3rd ed., 478; Scott Brown, 8th ed., Vol 2; 336*)

- Since the vocal cords are in midline in B/L abductor or RLN paralysis so speech will be normal.
- Puberophonia is persistence of high pitch voice in a boy after puberty.
- Phonasthenia is voice fatigue due to weakness of phonatory muscles
- Dysphonia plica ventricularis is the voice produced by false VC in the absence of functioning true VC (please refer to chapter on speech disorders).

20. **(d) Paramedian** (*Ref. Current Diagnosis & Treatment Otolaryngology, Lalwani, 3rd ed., 476*)

- In VC palsies where the VC is not mobile then the various named positions of VC are used to describe it. Since it is paralysed VC so adduction or abduction terms are not used to describe their position (refer to table on position of the VC).

21. **(d) Loss of timbre of voice** (*Ref. Scott Brown, 8th ed., Vol 3; 892*)

22. **(c) Cricothyroid** (*Ref. Scott Brown, 8th ed., Vol 3; 888*)

- Cricothyroid being a tensor of vocal cord changes the pitch of sound

23. **(b) Vocal cord palsy** (*Ref. Scott Brown, 6th ed., 1/12/17*)

24. **(a) Unilateral abductor palsy** (*Ref. Current Diagnosis & Treatment Otolaryngology, Lalwani, 3rd ed., 476*)

25. **(a) More common on left side** (*Ref. Current Diagnosis & Treatment Otolaryngology, Lalwani, 3rd ed., 476*)

- VC will lie in median/paramedian position so speech being normal, speech therapy not required.

26. **(b) Bilateral abductor palsy** (*Ref. Current Diagnosis & Treatment Otolaryngology, Lalwani, 3rd ed., 478*)

- Laryngomalacia and tracheal stenosis do not affect the VC hence voice remain normal in these though stridor is present.

27. **(b) B/L incomplete palsy** (*Ref. Current Diagnosis & Treatment Otolaryngology, Lalwani, 3rd ed., 478; Scott Brown, 8th ed., Vol 2; 336*)

28. **(d) Teflon injection** (*Ref. Current Diagnosis & Treatment Otolaryngology, Lalwani, 3rd ed., 477; Scott Brown, 8th ed., Vol 2; 336*)

29. **(a) Teflon paste** (*Ref. Current Diagnosis & Treatment Otolaryngology, Lalwani 3rd ed., 478*)

30. **(c) Type I thyroplasty** (*Ref. Current Diagnosis & Treatment Otolaryngology, Lalwani, 3rd ed., 478*)

- Stridor means B/L RLN palsy. Glottic gap being 3 mm so VC are in paramedian position. So the management is tracheostomy followed by lateralisation of the VC by type II thyroplasty or Cordectomy. Type I thyroplasty means doing medialisation of VC which will aggravate the condition.

31. **(a) Vocal cord medialisation** (*Ref. Cummings, 6th ed., 937; Scott Brown, 8th ed., Vol 3; 990*)

- Kindly Refer to text on thyroplasty.

32. **(a) Lateralised** (*Ref. Scott Brown, 8th ed., Vol 3; 990*)

33. **(d) Wait for spontaneous recovery of vocal cord** (*Ref. Current Diagnosis & Treatment Otolaryngology, Lalwani, 3rd ed., 477*)

- Since the patient here has only hoarseness, no stridor, no aspiration it is U/L RLN palsy where the VC are in paramedian position. So conservative management has to be followed. Also since it is following diphtheria chances of spontaneous recovery are present.
- The other choices are for VC Medialisation required in U/L complete palsy where the voice is breathy forced whisper type and there is predisposition to aspiration.

34. **(d) Type IV thyroplasty,** (*Ref. Scott Brown, 6th ed., 5/6/21*) kindly refer to text

35. **(c) Irradiation to vocal cords**

- Pancoast's tumour is an apical (superior pulmonary sulcus) malignant neoplasm of the lung. The symptoms of this tumour are because of compression of adjacent structures, e.g. sympathetic nerves (Horner's syndrome) and brachial plexus (involvement of C8, T1 and T2; leading to shoulder/arm pain and weakness and atrophy of hand muscles). Uncommonly the tumour can also compress the recurrent laryngeal nerve leading to hoarse voice and bovine cough.
- But since the patient has developed hoarseness after radiation, the right answer here is irradiation to vocal

Larynx

Section IV

cords. Radiation to or near the voice box can lead to edema of vocal cords leading to hoarseness. This radiation injury might heal with time after radiation is completed.

- Vocal cord infiltration with secondaries is not seen in Pancoast's or superior sulcus tumour. Similarly laryngeal stenosis has not been described after radiation; moreover laryngeal stenosis will lead to stridor.

36. **(c) Tracheal diversion and permanent tracheostome** (*Ref. Cummings 6th ed., 968*) (*refer to text*)

37. **(b) Internal laryngeal branch gives sensory supply to larynx below vocal cords** (*Ref. Scott Brown, 8th ed., Vol 3; 892*)

38. **(d) Unilateral vocal cord palsy** (*Ref. Current Diagnosis & Treatment Otolaryngology, Lalwani, 3rd ed., 476*)

39. **(a) Pure sensory** (*Ref. Scott Brown, 8th ed., Vol 3; 892*)

40. **(d) Cricovocal** (*Ref. Scott Brown, 8th ed., Vol 3; 887*)

41. **(d) Bilateral superior laryngeal nerve palsy** (*Ref. Scott Brown, 8th ed., Vol 3; 1041*)

42. **(a) Speech therapy** (*Ref. Current Diagnosis & Treatment Otolaryngology, Lalwani, 3rd ed., 476*)

43. **(d) Paralysis of cricothyroid muscle** (*Ref. Scott Brown, 6th ed., 5/9/12*)

- The nerve coursing with the superior thyroid artery is the external laryngeal nerve

44. **(a) Thyroid surgery** (*Ref. Current Diagnosis & Treatment Otolaryngology, Lalwani 3rd ed., 478*)

45. **(b) External branch of superior laryngeal nerve** (*Ref. Scott Brown, 6th ed., 5/9/12*)

46. **(c) 3.5 mm from midline** (*Ref. Scott Brown, 6th ed., 5/9/12*)

47. **(c) Lengthened** (*Ref. Scott Brown, 8th ed., Vol 3; 892*)

48. **(b) Internal laryngeal branch gives sensory supply to larynx below vocal cords** (*Ref. Scott Brown, 8th ed., Vol 3; 892*)

49. **(b) Weak voice and mild aspiration; bowing of affected vocal cord** (*Ref. Scott Brown, 8th ed., Vol 3; 892*)

50. **(a) Right superior laryngeal nerve palsy** (*Ref. Scott Brown, 6th ed., 5/9/12*)

51. **(a) Isshiki Type I thyroplasty** (*Ref. Current Diagnosis & Treatment Otolaryngology, Lalwani, 3rd ed., 476*)

52. **(a) Cricothyroid** (*Ref. Scott Brown, 8th ed., Vol 3; 884*)

- We can remember it as the only muscle supplied by external laryngeal nerve (the 4th pharyngeal arch nerve) is cricothyroid hence derived by 4th arch.
- Rest all the muscles are derived by 6th arch nerve as they are supplied by 6th arch nerve, the recurrent laryngeal nerve.

53. **(a), (c), (d) Vocal cord is in paramedian position, Stridor and dyspnoea occur, Vocal cord lateralisation is done** (*Ref. Current Diagnosis & Treatment Otolaryngology, Lalwani, 3rd ed., 478*)

54. **(b) 2** (*Ref. Scott Brown, 8th ed., Vol 3; 888*)

55. **(c) Posterior cricoarytenoid** (*Ref. Scott Brown, 8th ed., Vol 3; 888*)

56. **(a) Vocal cord** (*Ref. Stell & Maran, 4th ed., 369*)

57. **(b), (e) Vocalis, cricothyroid** (*Ref. Scott Brown, 8th ed., Vol 3; 888*)

58. **(b) One muscle abducts (opens) the vocal cords** (*Ref. Scott Brown, 8th ed., Vol 3; 888*)

- All muscles of VC are adductors except posterior cricoarytenoid which is an abductor.
- The tensors alter the length, hence tension of vocal cords. There are 2 tensors of VC.

59. **(c) External laryngeal nerve** (*Ref. Scott Brown, 8th ed., Vol 3; 892*)

- The marked muscle is cricothyroid

60. **(b) Type II thyroplasty** (*Ref. Current Diagnosis & Treatment Otolaryngology, Lalwani, 3rd ed., 478*)

- As both the vocal cords are in median position, it is bilateral recurrent laryngeal nerve paralysis.

61. **(d) Total adductor palsy** (*Ref. Current Diagnosis & Treatment Otolaryngology, Lalwani, 3rd ed., 479*)

Laryngeal Papillomatosis, Carcinoma Larynx and Occult Primary with Neck Secondary

LARYNGEAL PAPILLOMATOSIS

This is the most common benign tumour of the larynx.

There is bimodal age occurrence for laryngeal papillomas; more common being in children than adults.

1. Juvenile Laryngeal Papillomatosis

The most common benign tumour of the larynx in children is juvenile laryngeal papillomatosis. It is seen at 2 to 5 years of age.

It is caused by human papilloma virus (HPV) subtypes 6 and 11 (**HPV-11** being **more aggressive**).

Transmission to neonate occurs through contact with mother's birth canal during vaginal delivery.

The papilloma starts at the true vocal cords (*see* endoscopic picture) and later on spreads to involve the whole of the larynx. They are multiple (*see* below) and may even reach the mouth, pharynx, oesophagus, trachea and lower respiratory tracts, *see* their advancement in the picture below.

Clinical presentation: Hoarseness and abnormal cry is the presenting feature. Later on stridor occurs.

Laryngoscopy: On examination multiple papillomas are present all over the larynx.

Management: The primary treatment involves **micro-laryngoscopic excision**/de-bulking by microdebrider, CO_2 LASER, cup forceps, or cryosurgery. The most accepted and gold standard means of excision is microdebrider. Microdebrider has the advantage of minimal cutting damage to the surrounding tissues and no thermal trauma.

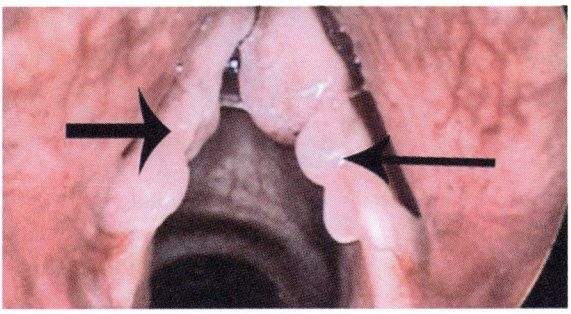

Fig. 39.1

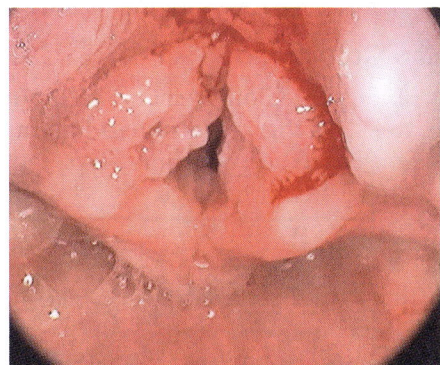

Fig. 39.2

Chances of **recurrence** are **very high** so repeated excisions are required to be done. In the postoperative period alpha-interferon, Bevacizumab, a monoclonal antibody which inhibits angiogenesis, and cidofovir (intralesional) (*Mnemonic:* ABC) has shown to decrease the chances of recurrence.

Tracheostomy should be avoided as it is associated with spread of the papillomas to the distal airways.

Chances of **malignant transformation** as such are rare but are increased post-irradiation to the head and neck and in HPV-11 variant.

Spontaneous remission, though unpredictable, may occur after puberty.

The quadrivalent HPV vaccine by reducing the maternal and paternal HPV reservoir shall prove to be highly efficacious for prevention of laryngeal papillomatosis.

2. Adult Laryngeal Papilloma

Adult papilloma behaves similarly and dissimilarly from juvenile variety as under:

Similarities	• Cause is same, i.e. HPV • Presents with hoarseness • Premalignant though malignant transformation is rare
Dissimilarities	• Adult papilloma is single • Less aggressive (does not present with stridor) • Does not recur after excision • Does not undergo spontaneous resolution

CARCINOMA OF THE LARYNX

Like elsewhere in ENT, most common carcinoma of the larynx is **squamous cell carcinoma**. It is seen more commonly in **males** between **50 and 70 years**.

Risk factors

i. Smoking (most important risk factor)
ii. Alcohol consumption,
iii. Infection with HPV (11, 16, and 18)
iv. Irradiation to neck.

Most common site of involvement is glottis followed by supraglottis and subglottis.

The laryngeal cartilages, ligaments and membranes (hyoepiglottic ligament, thyrohyoid membrane, quadrangular membrane, conus elasticus, Broyle's tendon i.e. the tendon connecting anterior commissure to thyroid cartilage) form **natural barriers** for the spread of tumours.

Supraglottic Carcinoma

Carcinoma of the supraglottis remains asymptomatic for a long time and since this area is **richest in lymphatics** in the whole of the larynx so by the time the patient presents he is already in an advanced stage.

Here the patient **presents with**:

1. Dysphagia
2. Pain throat and referred pain to the ear (vagus supplying both areas).
3. Neck nodes (upper and middle deep cervical lymph nodes)
4. Hoarseness (if spread to glottis has occurred)

Glottis

This is the **most common** site of carcinoma of larynx. Most commonly the carcinoma starts at the edge of the vocal cords.

Patient presents early with hoarseness because of which this is the carcinoma of larynx with **earliest presentation**.

*Note:*

Any male over 50 years of age with a history of smoking, presenting with hoarseness of more than three weeks should be investigated for carcinoma glottis.

Since the glottis literally has no lymphatics, this is the carcinoma of larynx with **least lymphatic metastasis** and hence **best prognosis**.

Subglottis

Here the earliest presentation is **stridor**. The subglottis drains into lower deep cervical and mediastinal lymph nodes either directly or through prelaryngeal and paratracheal lymph nodes.

The prognosis is worst here.

STAGING

Carcinoma in situ or stage 0: This means there are abnormal cells with high mitotic activity which have not invaded through the basement membrane.

Stage	Tumour (T) Node (N) metastasis (M)
Stage I	$T_1 N_0 M_0$
Stage II	$T_2 N_0 M_0$
Stage III	$T_3 N_0 M_0 / T_{1-3} N_1 M_0$
Stage IVa	$T_{4a} N_0 M_0 / T_{1-4a} N2 M_0$
Stage IVb	T_{4b} any N M_0/any T $N_3 M_0$
Stage IVc	**Any T or N, M_1**

Easy to remember stages I to IVb is as per T_1 to T_{4b}. Additional criteria for stages III, IVa and IVb is respectively N_1, N_2, and N_3. Stage IVc means stage with metastasis.

T_1	Tumour limited to one sub site (i.e. only a part) of glottis (T_{1a}–limited to one vocal cord (VC); T_{1b}–involving both VC), supraglottis or subglottis with normal VC mobility.
T_2	Tumour extending to the adjacent sub sites/sites, normal or impaired VC mobility.
T_3	Vocal cord fixation or spread to preepiglottic or paraglottic space or postcricoid area with minor thyroid cartilage (inner cortex) erosion.
T_{4a}	Tumour invades through the thyroid cartilage or tissues beyond larynx locally, e.g. trachea, strap muscles, tongue muscles and oesophagus.
T_{4b}	Tumour invades beyond the larynx to distant places, e.g. prevertebral space, mediastinum, carotid, etc.

N_0	No cervical lymph nodes.
N_1	Single ipsilateral node ≤3 cm without Extra Nodal Extension (ENE –ve).
N_2	Single ipsilateral node 3–6 cm (N_{2a}), multiple ipsilateral (N_{2b}), contralateral or bilateral nodes (N_{2c}) ≤ 6 cm. All without Extra Nodal Extension.
N_{3a}	Single or multiple nodes > 6 cm without Extra Nodal Extension.
N_{3b}	Single or multiple nodes with Extra Nodal Extension (ENE +).

M_0: No metastasis
M_1: Distant metastasis.

Diagnosis: Biopsy is done for diagnosis and histological type of tumour.

For knowing the extent of disease and lymph node metastasis CT and/or MRI are done.

CT vs MRI

CT SCAN	MRI
Multi detector CT (MD CT) is the first line investigation	Very useful adjunct
—	More accurate assessment of cartilage involvement and pre-piglottic, paraglottic extension of tumour.
Unaffected by artefacts caused by breathing or swallowing	Image degradation from artefacts produced by breathing, swallowing or coughing
Faster	Takes longer time
Cost effective	Costlier

Management: During management of carcinoma larynx-**emphasis** is on **preserving the larynx along with the control of the disease**.

Carcinoma in situ or stage 0: This is managed by excision by microlaryngeal surgery (MLS) or TLM (read below) and close follow up.

Stage I and Stage II

Transoral LASER microsurgery (TLM) or Radiotherapy offer equivalent survival outcomes for stage I and stage II.

1. **TLM:** TLM involves tumour resection using microscope, specialised endoscopic instruments and LASER. It is a minimally invasive surgery and aims at functional organ preservation.

   For T_{1a} mid cord lesions of the glottis TLM is the 1st choice. For rest of the early stage tumours TLM or radiotherapy can be given.

   The advantages of TLM over radiotherapy are:

   i. Short treatment period as compared to radiotherapy (radiotherapy requires around 6 weeks).

   ii. Here the side effects of radiotherapy are absent (important side effects being xerostomia, oedema and fibrosis of larynx, chondronecrosis, hypothyroidism, etc.).

2. **Radiotherapy:** External beam radiotherapy has the advantage of organ and voice preservation.

   In case of recurrences after radiotherapy, surgery is the treatment modality (depending upon the stage either conservation surgery or total laryngectomy is done, please *see* below).

3. **Conservation surgeries (voice conservation):** The primary disadvantage of radiotherapy is that it cannot be repeated to the same area, in case there is a recurrence. So if there is a recurrence in patients who have already been given radiotherapy (stages I, II, III, 4a), the only option left is surgical excision, i.e. laryngectomy. But if this recurrence is still in the early stage (stage I or II) we can go for partial laryngectomy aiming at voice conservation hence known as conservation surgeries.

   Important conservation surgeries are:

   a. **Hemi laryngectomy or vertical laryngectomy:** It is done for tumours involving one vertical half of the larynx with subglottic extension not more than 1 cm. Here vocal cord reconstruction, of the resected site, is done with strap muscles.

   b. **Supraglottic laryngectomy:** It is done for **stage I and II** supraglottic tumours not involving the glottis. It can also be done for **T3 carcinomas** of supraglottis which is T3 because of its **preepiglottic spread only**, i.e. without fixity of VC and no involvement of postcricoid area.

   Here the supraglottis is removed. The glottis now lies below the base of tongue hence chances of aspiration are present following this surgery though the voice remains good. Since aspiration is an important side effect of this operation it is done in patients with good pulmonary reserve.

Stage III and Stage IVa

If the **vocal cord is fixed** or there is a **node in the neck** the tumour is stage III and above.

The management here will be by:

1. **Concurrent chemoradiation with cisplatin:** This is the **better management** for stage III and small stage IV a tumours (T4a here is because of local invasion beyond larynx but without thyroid cartilage invasion), as it is organ preserving and hence imparts better quality of life to the patient. Patients with very large stage IV a tumours with thyroid cartilage invasion do not fare well with concurrent chemoradiation. In these as well as patients who cannot tolerate concurrent chemoradiation near total laryngectomy or total laryngectomy can be done depending upon the extent of tumour (please read below). Concurrent chemoradiation is given with Cisplatin or Carboplatin. Both have similar mechanism of action though carboplatin is less toxic than cisplatin. In addition to the myelosuppression primarily thrombocytopenia, these two additionally cause nephrotoxicity, SN deafness and neuropathy. In patients in whom chemotherapy is contraindicated, Cetuximab, which competitively inhibits cell surface epidermal growth factor receptor could be given. (*Mnemonic* all these drugs in Concurrent chemoradiation are starting with the letter 'C').

2. **Total laryngectomy with or without neck dissection followed by radiotherapy (called adjuvant radiotherapy):**

   As discussed above the **indications of total laryngectomy** are:

   1. Stage IV a patients with thyroid cartilage invasion.

   2. Patients with stages III and IVa, who cannot tolerate concurrent chemoradiation.

   3. Patients with recurrences after radiotherapy now presenting with stages III and IVa.

 Note:

Supraglottis is very rich in lymphatics hence both occult and palpable, B/L lymph node metastasis occurs frequently in supraglottic tumours. Hence elective treatment of neck of all except some T_1 supraglottic squamous cell carcinoma should be done. The choice of neck dissection or radiotherapy to the neck depends on how the primary tumour is treated. If the primary tumour is treated with radiotherapy, the neck nodes are also treated with radiotherapy. If the supraglottic carcinoma is treated surgically then the lymph nodes are also treated surgically by neck dissection.

Near total laryngectomy: It is done **for large T_3 and T_{4a} lesions** with **one uninvolved arytenoid**.

Unlike the other partial laryngectomy procedures which are done for radiation failure cases near total laryngectomy is not done for patients whose radiation treatment has failed.

This is done for a selected group of patients who have presented late and who were not the candidates for concurrent chemoradiation due to the thyroid cartilage invasion or side effects of cisplatin and have still an uninvolved arytenoid.

Here the whole of the larynx except for the uninvolved arytenoid is removed and a tracheo-oesophageal pathway for speech is made. The advantage of near total laryngectomy is that it gives better speech than total laryngectomy.

Stage IVb and Stage IVc

Palliative radiotherapy

To summarise

Laryngeal preservation should be the intension at the time of treating carcinoma larynx so as to give a better quality of life to the patient, therefore radiotherapy is given preference over surgical management.

Stage	Treatment
Carcinoma *in situ*	**Excision**
I and II	TLM/External beam **radiotherapy** If radiotherapy fails then conservation surgery
III and IVa without thyroid cartilage invasion	**Concurrent chemoradiation**
IVa with thyroid cartilage invasion	Total laryngectomy along with adjuvant radiotherapy
IVb and c	**Palliative radiotherapy**

PROBLEMS FOLLOWING TOTAL LARYNGECTOMY

i. **Permanent tracheostome:** Following laryngectomy the upper end of the trachea is pulled out and sutured to the skin and the patient breathes through here.

ii. **Speech difficulties:** Speech rehabilitation following laryngectomy can be by the following techniques, all of which employ the pharyngo-oesophageal segment for speech generation:

a. **Oesophageal speech:** Previously the air from the lungs was used to vibrate the vocal cords to produce speech. Now the patient produces speech by **vibration of pharyngo-oesophageal segment** by swallowing small volumes of air during speaking. The intensity of voice produced here is very low.

b. **Tracheo-oesophageal speech:** This is the **most effective** method for voice restoration. In this a small one way valve (**Blom-Singer and Panje valve**) is made between the trachea and oesophagus so that during expiration some air from the lungs enters the pharynx hence vibrating the **pharyngo-oesophageal segment**.

c. **Electrolarynx:** Here an electrical vibrating device held on the skin of neck vibrates the pharyngo-oesophageal segment. The voice produced here is a monotonous robotic voice.

iii. **Loss of smell and decreased taste sensation:** Since the patient cannot respire through the nose, the smell sensation is severely affected after total laryngectomy. Since smell sensation is also responsible to perceive flavour of food hence there also occurs decreased taste sensation.

iv. **Uncoordinated swallowing**.

UNKNOWN/OCCULT PRIMARY WITH SECONDARY LYMPH NODES IN THE NECK

Because of the rich lymphatic network, many carcinomas of head and neck present with neck nodes only without any other symptoms, e.g. nasopharyngeal carcinoma, carcinoma/lymphoma of tonsil, carcinoma base of tongue, pyriform sinus/fossa carcinoma, supraglottic carcinoma and papillary carcinoma thyroid.

Secondary lymph node enlargement of the neck where the primary could not be detected is known as occult primary with neck secondary.

It should be worked up as follows:

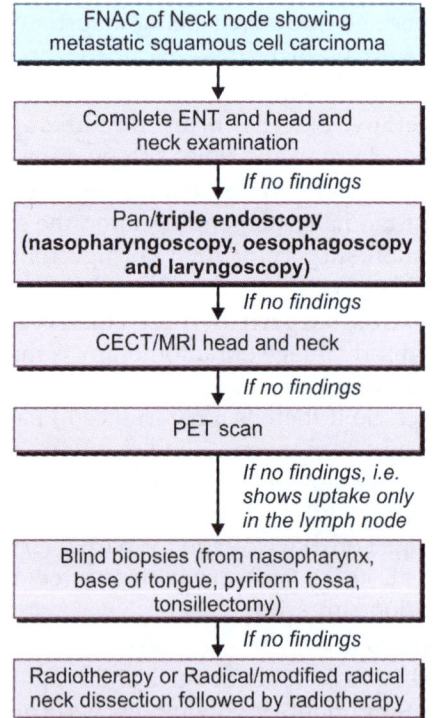

NECK DISSECTION

Neck dissection can be:

1. **Radical neck dissection:** Here there is removal of lymph node groups (levels I to V, *see* below) along with some non lymphatic structures, the important three of which are:
   i. Spinal accessory nerve
   ii. Internal jugular vein
   iii. Sternocleidomastoid muscle

The other non lymphatic structures removed are submandibular salivary gland, parotid salivary gland and omohyoid muscle.

It is not done where the primary tumour or the nodes have become inoperable due to involvement of carotid artery, brachial plexus and base of skull or distant metastasis.

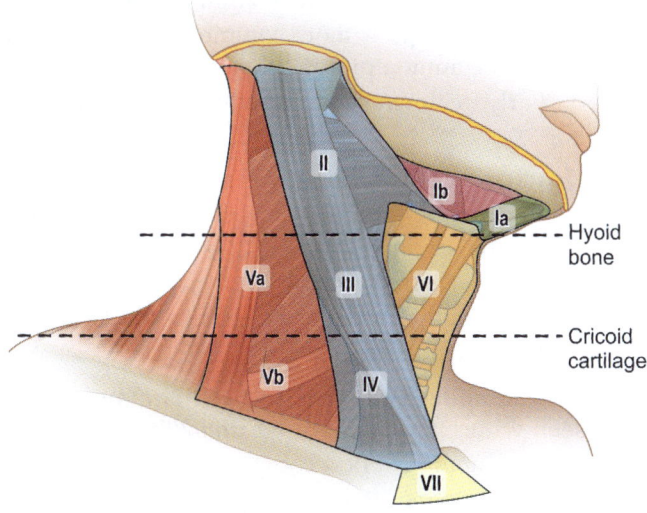

Level Ia: Submental	**Level Va:** Posterior triangle
Level Ib: Submandibular	**Level Vb:** Supraclavicular
Level II: Upper deep cervical	**Level VI:** Anterior compartment lymph nodes
Level III: Middle deep cervical	
Level IV: Lower deep cervical	**Level VII:** Superior mediastinal

Levels of lymph node in the neck

2. **Modified radical neck dissection:** Here we remove lymph node groups I to V with preservation of one or more of the important three non lymphatic structures:

   i. Preservation of spinal accessory nerve (**type I** modified neck dissection).

   ii. Preservation of spinal accessory nerve and internal jugular vein (**type II** modified neck dissection).

   iii. Preservation of spinal accessory nerve, internal jugular vein and sternocleidomastoid muscle (**type III** modified neck dissection/functional neck dissection).

3. **Selective neck dissection:** Here all the non-lymphatic structures are spared and only selective group of lymph nodes draining that particular area is removed:

   i. **Supra-omohyoid neck dissection** removes level I, II and III and is done in oral tumours.

   ii. **Lateral neck dissection** removes II, III and IV. It is done for tumours of oropharynx, larynx and hypopharynx.

   iii. **Posterolateral neck dissection** removes levels II to V. It is done for cutaneous malignant tumours.

   iv. **Anterior compartment neck dissection** removes level VI.

4. **Extended radical neck dissection:** Additional muscles, nerves and lymph nodes of the head and neck along with those removed in radical neck dissection are removed here.

Larynx

Section IV

PREVIOUSLY ASKED QUESTIONS

1. **All of the following are true regarding juvenile papillomas except:** *(AP 2001, Exam 2013)*
   a. Commonly occur in children
   b. LASER surgery is the treatment of choice
   c. Stridor is common
   d. Recurrences are uncommon

2. **Juvenile papillomatosis is caused by:** *(Exam 2013)*
   a. HSV   b. EBV
   c. CMV   d. HPV

3. **True about multiple papillomatosis:** *(PGI Dec 2005, 2015)*
   a. HSV is causative agent
   b. Radiotherapy is treatment of choice
   c. It is premalignant
   d. It is more common in 15–30 years
   e. Its cause is infection during parturition

4. **Of the following statements about recurrent laryngeal papillomatosis, true are all except:** *(AI 2009)*
   a. Caused by human papilloma virus
   b. HPV 6 and HPV 11 are most commonly implicated
   c. HPV 6 is more virulent than HPV 11
   d. Transmission to neonate occurs through contact with mother during vaginal delivery

5. **True about juvenile laryngeal papillomatosis:** *(PGI 2000, 2015)*
   a. Affects children commonly
   b. Lower respiratory tract can be involved
   c. May resolve spontaneously
   d. Microlaryngoscopic surgery is the treatment of choice

6. **Primary treatment of choice in juvenile papilloma is:** *(Delhi 96, Exam 2015)*
   a. Surgical excision   b. Interferon
   c. Antibiotics   d. Radiotherapy

7. **Riddhi 4 years of age presented in emergency with mild respiratory distress. On laryngoscopy she was diagnosed to have multiple juvenile papillomatosis of the larynx. Next line of management is:** *(AIIMS 2001, Exam 2017)*
   a. Tracheostomy
   b. Microlaryngoscopic excision
   c. Steroid
   d. Antibiotics

8. **The most widely used treatment for recurrent respiratory papillomatosis nowadays is:** *(DPG 2009, Exam 2016)*
   a. CO_2 LASER ablation
   b. Diathermy excision
   c. Excision with microdebrider
   d. Wait for spontaneous resolution

9. **True about papilloma is all except:** *(AIIMS 2001, Exam 2017)*
   a. Solitary is more common in adults and most common presentation is change in voice
   b. Solitary type is more aggressive, prognosis is bad and malignant transformation is common
   c. Multiple type is more common in children and most common presentation is hoarse cry
   d. Early treatment leads to better results in multiple type

10. **Hoarseness of voice occurs early in:** *(Rj 2004, Exam 2017)*
    a. Glottic carcinoma
    b. Subglottic carcinoma
    c. Supraglottic carcinoma
    d. Equal incidence in all

11. **Lymph node metastasis in neck is almost never seen with:** *(Exam 2008, Exam 2016)*
    a. Carcinoma of vocal cords
    b. Supraglottic carcinoma
    c. Carcinoma of tonsil
    d. Papillary carcinoma thyroid

12. **Involvement of neck lymph nodes is seen in all of the following except:** *(AI 96, Exam 2011)*
    a. Hodgkin's disease
    b. Vocal cord carcinoma
    c. Tumours of the hypopharynx
    d. Nasopharyngeal carcinoma

13. **Lymphatic drainage of supraglottis is due to:** *(UP 2004, Exam 2016)*
    a. Upper deep cervical
    b. Prelaryngeal
    c. Pretracheal
    d. Lower deep cervical

14. **Highest lymph node involvement is seen in:** *(AIIMS 2005, Exam 2016)*
    a. Glottis carcinoma
    b. Subglottic carcinoma
    c. Supraglottic carcinoma
    d. None

15. **Which of the following carcinomas commonly presents with neck nodes?** *(AI 2004, Exam 2016)*
    a. Cricoid   b. Glottis
    c. Epiglottis   d. Anterior commissure

16. **Supraglottic carcinoma true is:** *(PGI June 2003, 2015)*
    a. Hot potato voice
    b. Aspiration
    c. Smoking is common risk factor
    d. Pain is a manifestation
    e. Lymph node metastasis is uncommon

17. All of the following are true about glottic carcinoma except: *(AI 2003, Exam 2016)*
    a. More common in females
    b. Usually seen over 50 years of age
    c. After laryngectomy esophageal voice can be used
    d. Good prognosis

18. Features of glottic carcinoma: *(PGI June 2005, 2016)*
    a. It is the MC site of carcinoma larynx
    b. Commonly metastasizes to cervical lymph node
    c. Lesions seen at the edge of the vocal cord
    d. Laryngeal ligaments act as barrier
    e. Prognosis is bad

19. True statement about infraglottic carcinoma larynx: *(Exam 2010)*
    a. Commonly spread to mediastinal nodes
    b. Second most common carcinoma
    c. Most common carcinoma
    d. Spreads to submental lymph nodes

20. Select correct statements about carcinoma larynx: *(PGI 2002, 2012)*
    a. Glottic carcinoma is the most common
    b. Supraglottic carcinoma has best prognosis
    c. Lymphatic spread is most common in subglottic carcinoma
    d. T1 tumour is treated by radiotherapy
    e. Smoking predisposes

21. The most common cause of laryngeal stridor in a 60 years old male is: *(JIPMER 2007, Exam 2016)*
    a. Nasopharyngeal carcinoma
    b. Acute severe asthma
    c. Carcinoma larynx
    d. Reinke's edema

22. Laryngeal cartilage involvement, investigation of choice is: *(Bihar 2003, Exam 2016)*
    a. CT   b. MRI
    c. PET scan   d. Biopsy

23. Treatment of carcinoma larynx in stage $T_1 N_0 M_0$ is: *(AI 2000, Exam 2016)*
    a. Radiotherapy
    b. Surgery–total laryngectomy
    c. Partial laryngectomy
    d. Chemotherapy

24. True about carcinoma glottis: *(PGI 2000, 2014)*
    a. It is the most common site
    b. Rarely presents with metastasis
    c. Adenocarcinoma is commonest type
    d. Responds to chemotherapy very well

25. Involvement of anterior commissure in Ca larynx best treatment is: *(Exam 2013)*
    a. Laryngectomy   b. Radiotherapy
    c. Chemotherapy   d. None

26. In a case of glottic carcinoma with fully mobile cords, the treatment of choice is: *(AP 2006, Exam 2016)*
    a. Total laryngectomy
    b. Radiotherapy
    c. Hemilaryngectomy
    d. Chemotherapy

27. LASER most commonly used in laryngeal work: *(AI 2010)*
    a. Argon   b. CO_2
    c. Holmium   d. Nd:YAG

28. Contraindication of supraglottic laryngectomy is/are: *(PGI Nov 2009, 2015)*
    a. Poor pulmonary reserve
    b. Tumour involving pyriform sinus
    c. Tumour involving preepiglottic space
    d. Vocal cord fixation
    e. Cricoid cartilage extension

29. A patient presents with carcinoma of the larynx involving the left false cord, left arytenoids and the left aryepiglottic folds with bilateral mobile true cords. Treatment of choice is: *(AIIMS Nov 2007, Exam 2016)*
    a. Vertical hemilaryngectomy
    b. Horizontal hemilaryngectomy
    c. Radiotherapy followed by chemotherapy
    d. Total laryngectomy

30. Which of the following is not the indication of near total laryngectomy? *(AP 2007, Exam 2016)*
    a. T3 stage
    b. Anterior commissure involvement
    c. Involved of both arytenoids
    d. Supraglottic involvement

31. For carcinoma larynx stage III treatment of choice: *(AIIMS 2005, Exam 2016)*
    a. Total laryngectomy with radiotherapy
    b. Chemotherapy with cisplatin
    c. Partial laryngectomy
    d. Radiotherapy

32. A case of carcinoma larynx with the involvement of anterior commissure and right vocal cord developed perichondritis of thyroid cartilage. Which of the following statements is true for the management of this case: *(AIIMS May 2006, Exam 2017)*
    a. He should be given radical radiotherapy as this can cure early tumours
    b. He should be treated with combination of chemotherapy and radiotherapy
    c. He should first receive radiotherapy and if residual tumour is present, should then undergo laryngectomy
    d. He should first undergo laryngectomy and then postoperative radiotherapy

Larynx

Section IV

33. $T_3N_1M_0$ stage carcinoma larynx is treated by:
    (AI 2010)
    a. Radiotherapy
    b. Concurrent chemoradiation
    c. Chemotherapy
    d. Surgery and radiotherapy

34. A patient of carcinoma larynx with stridor presents in casualty, immediate management is:
    (AIIMS 2002, Exam 2016)
    a. Planned tracheostomy
    b. Immediate tracheostomy
    c. High dose steroid
    d. Intubate, give bronchodilator and wait for 12 hours, if no response, proceed to tracheostomy

35. Radiotherapy is treatment of choice for:
    (AIIMS Nov 2009, Exam 2016)
    a. Nasopharyngeal CaT_3N_1
    b. Supraglottic CaT_3N_0
    c. Glottis CaT_3N_0
    d. Subglottic CaT_3N_0

36. The preferred treatment of small early Verrucous carcinoma of the larynx is: *(UP 2007, Exam 2016)*
    a. Pulmonary surgery b. Electron beam therapy
    c. Total laryngectomy d. Endoscopic removal

37. Laryngofissure is: *(JIPMER 2004, Exam 2016)*
    a. Opening the larynx in midline
    b. Making window in thyroid cartilage
    c. Removal of arytenoids
    d. Removal of epiglottis

38. About total laryngectomy all are correct except:
    (Bihar 2005, Exam 2016)
    a. Loss of smell   b. Loss of taste
    c. Speech difficulty   d. Dyspnoea

39. After laryngectomy dynamic oesophageal voice is produced from: *(AIIMS 2004, Exam 2016)*
    a. Nose
    b. Pharyngo-oesophageal segment
    c. Trachea
    d. Buccal mucosa

40. Structures not removed in radical neck dissection:
    (PGI 2007, 2015)
    a. X nerve   b. XI nerve
    c. Tail of parotid d. Internal jugular vein
    e. Sternocleidomastoid muscle

41. A 50-year-male present with 4 cm hard immobile lymph node in middle deep cervical region. FNAC showing metastatic squamous cell carcinoma. O/E no lesion was found in the head and neck. Further management will be: *(AI 2008, Exam 2016)*
    a. Oesophagoscopy   b. Triple endoscopy
    c. Laryngoscopy   d. Supravital staining

42. Carcinoma larynx T_3N_0 treatment is:
    (AIIMS May 2014)
    a. Radical radiotherapy followed by chemotherapy
    b. Radical radiotherapy without chemotherapy

c. Neoadjuvant chemotherapy followed by surgery
d. Concurrent chemoradiation

43. Which of the following is inappropriate indication for concomitant chemotherapy in case of head and neck cancer?   *(Exam 2014)*
    a. Primary treatment for patient with unresectable disease
    b. As an organ safeguarding method of t/t
    c. Postoperative case of intermediate stage resectable tumour
    d. Metastatic advanced head and neck cancer

44. All are common causes of stridor except:
    (Exam 2010)
    a. Foreign body in larynx and trachea
    b. Laryngomalacia
    c. Multiple papillomas of larynx
    d. Atrophic laryngitis

45. In modified radical neck dissection type I, the structure which is preserved: *(Exam 2015)*
    a. Sternocleidomastoid muscle
    b. Internal Jugular vein
    c. Spinal Accessory nerve
    d. Level I-IV Lymph nodes

46. In modified radical neck dissection type II structures preserved are: *(Exam 2016)*
    a. Spinal accessory nerve + Sternocleidomastoid
    b. Spinal accessory nerve + Internal jugular vein
    c. Sternocleidomastoid + Internal jugular vein
    d. Level I – V lymph nodes + Sternocleidomastoid

47. Carcinoma larynx with fixed vocal cords treatment is: *(Exam 2016)*
    a. Radiotherapy
    b. Total laryngectomy followed by radiotherapy
    c. Neo adjuvant chemotherapy followed by surgery
    d. Concurrent chemoradiation

48. Recurrent papillomatosis is treated by application of: *(Exam 2016)*
    a. Zinc   b. Radiotherapy
    c. Cidofovir   d. Mitomycin-C

49. Which of the following cancers do not usually present with cervical lymph node involvement?
    (Exam 2016)
    a. Glottic cancer
    b. Subglottic cancer
    c. Papillary thyroid cancer
    d. Oral cancer

50. A 55-year-old known smoker presents with a low pitched voice. Endoscopy shows a mass limited to the vocal cord on the left. Biopsy is suggestive of laryngeal cancer type T_1N_0. Treatment of choice would be: *(Exam 2014)*
    a. Concurrent chemoradiation
    b. Radiotherapy

c. Chemotherapy
d. Total laryngectomy with cervical lymph node dissection

51. **Head and neck tumour stage III according to TNM classification involves:**   (*Exam 2015*)
    a. Unilateral mobile lymph nodes <3 cm
    b. Unilateral mobile lymph node >3 cm
    c. Bilateral mobile lymph nodes <3 cm
    d. Bilateral mobile lymph nodes >3 cm

52. **A 55-year-old male came with history of hoarseness of voice for which direct laryngoscopy was done and the lesion was biopsied to detect squamous cell carcinoma. He now requires investigation to detect extent of cartilage involvement, imaging of pre- and paraglottic spaces. Most appropriate investigation of choice would be:**   (*UPSC 2015*)
    a. Endoscopic examination
    b. Repeat direct laryngoscopy under general anaesthesia
    c. MRI
    d. CT scan

53. **A 5-year-old male child presents with 3 month history of hoarseness of voice and 1 week history of stridor. Endoscopic picture is shown below. The diagnosis is:**   (*AIIMS 2016*)

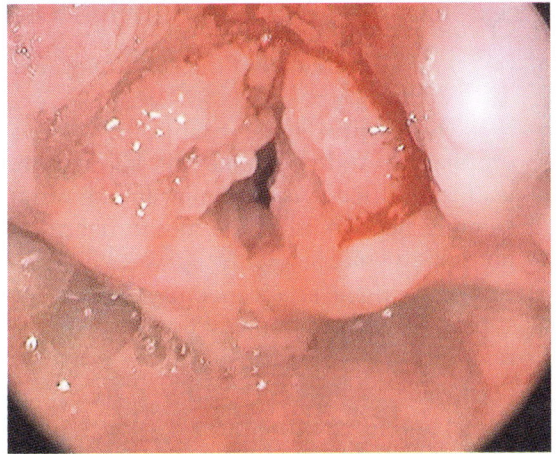

a. Multiple respiratory nodules
b. Respiratory papillomatosis
c. Carcinoma larynx
d. Haemangioma

54. **Blom-Singer prosthesis is used for:**   (*Exam 2016*)
    a. Ossiculoplasty
    b. Thyroplasty
    c. Post-maxillectomy palatal reconstruction
    d. Post-laryngectomy voice

55. **Method of speech communications after laryngectomy include all except:**   (*Exam 2013*)
    a. Electrolarynx
    b. Oesophageal speech
    c. Tracheo-oesophageal puncture
    d. Tracheal speech

56. **A 3-year-old child presents with hoarseness and stridor. Following a normal vaginal delivery, this child received all the routine immunisation. Endoscopic picture of the larynx is given below. Most probable diagnosis is:**   (*Exam 2109*)

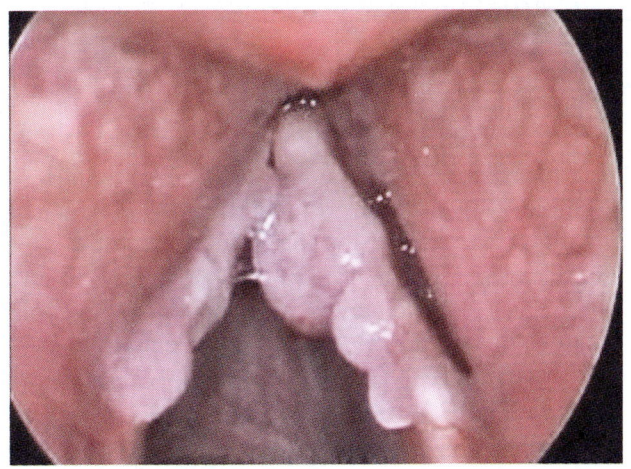

a. Laryngomalacia
b. Epiglottitis
c. Juvenile laryngeal papillomatosis
d. Vocal nodules

Larynx

Section IV

ANSWERS AND EXPLANATIONS

1. **(d) Recurrences are uncommon** (*Ref. Cummings, 6th ed., 922*)

2. **(d) HPV** (*Ref. Cummings, 6th ed., 922*)

3. **(c) and (e)** (*Ref. Scott Brown, 8th ed., Vol 2; 368*)
   - HPV and not HSV is the cause.
   - It is managed by microlaryngoscopic excision. Radiotherapy is not done as it increases the chances of malignant transformation.
   - It is a premalignant condition though chances of malignant transformation as such are rare.

4. **(c)** (*Ref. Cummings, 6th ed., 922*)

5. **(All are true)** (*Ref. Cummings, 6th ed., 923*)
   - At times due to predominant involvement of the lower respiratory tract, laryngeal papillomatosis may mimic asthma in the absence of symptoms of hoarseness, and stridor.
   - Therefore it should be particularly considered in 2 to 4-year-old children with recurrent wheezing that is poorly responsive to aggressive therapy including oral corticosteroids. Rest all are also true please refer to the text.

6. **(a) Surgical excision** (*Ref. Cummings, 6th ed., 923*)
   - Juvenile papilloma is management by excision by CO2 LASER.
   - Chances of recurrence being very high, interferon alpha is given in the postoperative period which has shown to decrease the chances of recurrence.
   - Radiotherapy is not used here as it increases the chances of malignant transformation in the benign juvenile papilloma. Antibiotics have no role.

7. **(b) Microlaryngoscopic excision** (*Ref. Cummings, 6th ed., 923*)
   - Tracheostomy should be avoided as it is associated with spread of the papillomas to the distal airways. Steroids and antibiotics have no role.

8. **(a) CO$_2$ LASER ablation** (*Ref. Cummings, 6th ed., 923*)
   - Spontaneous resolution though may occur after puberty but is unpredictable. Moreover life threatening stridor may occur so CO$_2$ LASER excision is to be done.
   - Various excision techniques, most widely used method is CO$_2$ LASER.

9. **(b)** (*Ref. Cummings, 6th ed., 923*)
   - Solitary type which is more common in adults is less aggressive (no stridor) and malignant transformation is rare.
   - Early treatment will prevent stridor and therefore better results in multiple type in children. Rest are true.

10. **(a) Glottic carcinoma** (*Ref. Cummings, 6th ed., 1612*)
    - Glottic carcinoma, i.e. carcinoma of the vocal cords presents early with hoarseness. In fact hoarseness is its presenting feature.

- Supraglottic and subglottic carcinoma can also lead to hoarseness due to later local spread to glottis.

11. **(a) Carcinoma of vocal cords** (*Ref. Scott Brown, 8th ed., Vol 3; 31*)
    - In carcinoma of vocal cords, i.e. glottic carcinoma, neck node metastasis is almost never seen because of paucity of lymphatics.
    - Rest of the tumours mentioned have rich lymphatics hence neck node metastasis is seen commonly.

12. **(b) Vocal cord carcinoma** (*Ref. Scott Brown, 8th ed., Vol 3; 31, 239*) (please *see* above explanation)
    - Hodgkin's disease is a lymphoid malignancy. Here most patients present with non tender palpable lymphadenopathy in the neck, axilla and mediastinum.
    - Pyriform fossa is the richest in lymphatics in whole of hypopharynx and carcinoma here presents very commonly with upper deep cervical lymph nodes.
    - 70–80% of patients of nasopharyngeal carcinoma present with upper deep cervical lymph nodes.

13. **(a) Upper deep cervical** (*Ref. Scott Brown, 8th ed., Vol 3; 31, 240*)

14. **(c) Supraglottic carcinoma** (*Ref. Scott Brown, 8th ed., Vol 3; 240; 31*)

15. **(c) Epiglottis** (*Ref. Cummings, 6th ed., 1612*)
    - Epiglottis is a part of supraglottis.
    - Anterior commissure is a part of glottis.
    - Cricoid is a part of subglottis.

16. **(a) (c) and (d) are true** (*Ref. Scott Brown, 8th ed., Vol 3; 31, 239*)
    - It is the painful space occupying lesions of the oropharynx and bulky mass in supraglottis which lead to muffled speech similar to one produced by keeping hot potato in the mouth hence known as hot potato voice.
    - There being a space occupying lesion in the supraglottis aspiration will not be seen here. Please refer to the text.

17. **(a)** (*Ref. Cummings, 6th ed., 1610*)

18. **(a), (c) and (d) are true** (*Ref. Cummings, 6th ed., 1612; Scott Brown, 8th ed., Vol 3; 238*)
    - The intrinsic and extrinsic membranes and ligaments of the larynx act as barriers for the spread of laryngeal carcinomas.

19. **(a) Commonly spread to mediastinal nodes** (*Ref. Cummings, 6th ed., 1612*)
    - Most common carcinoma of the larynx is glottic followed by supraglottic.
    - Larynx does not drain into sub mental lymph nodes.

20. **(a), (d) and (e) are correct** (*Ref. Cummings, 6th ed., 1612; Scott Brown, 8th ed., Vol 3; 239*)

21. **(c) Carcinoma larynx** (*Ref. Cummings, 6th ed., 1612*)
    - At this age laryngeal stridor is most commonly caused by carcinoma of the larynx.
    - Patients of nasopharyngeal carcinoma do not have stridor.

- Acute severe asthma will lead to wheeze.
- Patients of Reinke's edema have hoarseness and not stridor (*see* Chapter on infections of larynx).

22. **(b) MRI** (*Ref. Cummings, 6th ed., 1614; Scott Brown, 8th ed., Vol 3;240*)
- Laryngeal cartilage involvement changes the management from organ preserving concurrent chemoradiation to total laryngectomy with adjuvant radiotherapy.
- Accuracy of MRI is higher here, as compared to CT because of more accurate assessment of cartilage involvement and pre-epiglottic, paraglottic extension of tumour.
- CT scan is used for initial staging.
- Biopsy is done to confirm and know the histological type of tumour. It is not done to assess cartilage invasion

23. **(a) Radiotherapy** (*Ref. Cummings, 6th ed., 1615*)
- Radiotherapy is the treatment of choice for carcinoma larynx in stage I (T1 N0 M0).
- Partial laryngectomy can be done for stages I and II tumours where radiation therapy has failed.
- Total laryngectomy followed by radiotherapy is used as the treatment modality for large stage 4a tumours with thyroid cartilage invasion (please refer to the text).
- Chemotherapy alone is not useful for management of carcinoma larynx.

24. **(a) and (b) are true** (*Ref. Cummings, 6th ed., 1612*)

25. **(b) Radiotherapy** (*Ref. Cummings, 6th ed., 1616*)
- Tumour here is involving only a part of the glottis which means it is T1, i.e. stage 1, so the management will be radiotherapy.

26. **(b) Radiotherapy** (*Ref. Cummings, 6th ed., 1616*)
- Fully mobile vocal cords mean it is either stage I or II, where the management is radiotherapy.

27. **(b) CO$_2$** (*Ref. Cummings, 6th ed., 1608*)
- The most common LASER used in ENT surgeries is CO$_2$ LASER.

28. **(a) (b) (d) and (e)** (*Ref. Current Diagnosis & Treatment Otolaryngology, Lalwani 3rd ed., 467*)
- Supraglottic laryngectomy is done for stage I and II carcinoma supraglottis in patients who have failed radiation therapy.
- It can also be done for T$_3$ carcinomas of supraglottis which is T$_3$ because of its pre-epiglottic spread only.
- Since aspiration is an important side effect of this operation it is done in patients with good pulmonary reserve.
- Vocal cord fixation and cricoid cartilage extension means stages 3 and 4a respectively, where supraglottic laryngectomy is not done.
- Involvement of pyriform sinus/fossa, i.e. hypopharynx (meaning beyond the larynx locally) again means stage 4a.

29. **(a) Vertical hemilaryngectomy** (*Ref. Cummings, 6th ed., 1615*)

- Fully mobile vocal cords mean it is either stage I or II, where the management is radiotherapy alone, which is not mentioned in the options given.
- Here we can go for voice conservation surgery. Since the tumour is involving the left half of supraglottis vertical hemilaryngectomy is the treatment as chances of aspiration are high in supraglottic (Horizontal) laryngectomy.

30. **(c) Involved both arytenoids** (*Ref. Current Diagnosis & Treatment Otolaryngology, Lalwani, 3rd ed., 468*)

31. **(a) Total laryngectomy with radiotherapy** (*Ref. Cummings, 6th ed., 1617*)
- This question was asked in 1996 when the treatment of stage III carcinoma larynx used to be total laryngectomy with or without neck dissection followed by radiotherapy.
- But nowadays the best management of carcinoma larynx stage III is concurrent chemoradiation with cisplatin.
- Chemotherapy alone is not given in carcinoma larynx.
- Radiotherapy is used in the management of stage I or II carcinoma larynx.
- Partial laryngectomy is done for stage I and II tumours where radiation therapy has failed.

32. **(d) He should first undergo laryngectomy and then postoperative radiotherapy** (*Ref. Cummings, 6th ed., 1617*)
- Thyroid perichondritis indicates thyroid cartilage invasion making the tumour T4a. Total laryngectomy followed by radiotherapy is used as the treatment modality for stage IV a tumours with thyroid cartilage invasion.

33. **(b) Concurrent chemoradiation** (*Ref. Cummings, 6th ed., 1617*)

34. **(b) Immediate tracheostomy** (*Ref. Scott Brown, 8th ed., Vol 3;1041*)
- Since the patient is in stridor which is due to obstruction caused by laryngeal tumour mass, intubation will not be possible and bronchodilators have no role.

35. **(a) Nasopharyngeal Ca T$_3$ N$_1$** (*Ref. Current Diagnosis & Treatment Otolaryngology, Lalwani, 3rd ed., 464*)
- The best management of nasopharyngeal carcinoma in all the stages is radiotherapy.
- Rest of the tumours mentioned are laryngeal carcinomas stage 3 where the treatment is concurrent chemoradiation.

36. **(d) Endoscopic removal** (*Ref. Cummings, 6th ed., 1626*)
- Verrucous carcinoma is a rare laryngeal malignancy (comprising 1% of laryngeal carcinomas).
- It has a warty papillary surface. Biopsy shows hyperkeratosis and acanthosis.
- Here the tumour being highly differentiated and hence radioresistant, the treatment modality is primarily surgical.

Larynx

Section IV

37. **(a) Opening the larynx in midline** (*Ref. Scott Brown, 8th ed., Vol 3;1031*)

- Opening the larynx by splitting it in the midline of the thyroid cartilage vertically is known as laryngofissure.
- Laryngofissure is done to remove the benign tumours of the larynx which cannot be removed endoscopically.
- Windows are made in the thyroid cartilage in thyroid framework surgeries (e.g. type 1 thyroplasty).

38. **(d) Dyspnoea** (*Ref. Current Diagnosis & Treatment Otolaryngology, Lalwani 3rd ed., 472*)

- Following laryngectomy the patient breathes through the permanent tracheostome. There is no difficulty in breathing. Rest are true, please refer to text.

39. **(b) Pharyngo-oesophageal segment**, (*Ref. Cummings, 6th ed. ,1734*) please refer the text

40. **(a) X nerve** (*Ref. Cummings, 6th ed., 1843*)

41. **(b) Triple endoscopy** (*Ref. Scott Brown, 8th ed., Vol 3;299*)

- Triple endoscopy comprises nasopharyngoscopy, Oesophagoscopy and laryngoscopy, refer to text.
- Supravital staining is staining of living cells outside the body so as to have a better visualisation of cellular structures under the microscope.

42. **(d) Concurrent chemoradiation** (*Ref. Cummings, 6th ed., 1616; Scott Brown, 8th ed., Vol 3;253*)

43. **(d)** (*Ref. Cummings, 6th ed., 1620*)

- Concomitant chemotherapy or Concurrent chemoradiotherapy/chemoradiation maximizes tumour control while maintaining function and quality of life by organ-conservation (e.g. ca larynx), because of which this treatment modality has overtaken surgery as the primary local treatment option for most head and neck cancers.

- It is also the primary mode of treatment for tumours which cannot be treated surgically because of lack of free margins, e.g. nasopharyngeal carcinoma, etc.
- In addition, for those patients whose head and neck cancers are managed with primary surgical resection, patients at high risk of loco regional recurrence (positive margins or extracapsular nodal extension) are often treated with concurrent chemoradiotherapy, for enhancement of loco regional control.
- In metastasis the treatment is palliative radiotherapy.

44. **(d) Atrophic laryngitis** (*Ref. Current Diagnosis & Treatment Otolaryngology, Lalwani, 3rd ed., 481*)

45. **(c) Spinal Accessory nerve** (*Ref. Stell & Maran, 5th ed., 668*)

46. **(b) Spinal accessory nerve + Internal jugular vein** (*Ref. Cummings, 6th ed., 1843*)

47. **(d) Concurrent chemoradiation** (*Ref. Cummings, 6th ed., 1617*)

48. **(c) Cidofovir** (*Ref. Cummings, 6th ed., 3151*)

49. **(a) Glottic cancer** (*Ref. Cummings, 6th ed., 1612; Scott Brown, 8th ed., Vol 3;31*)

50. **(b) Radiotherapy** (*Ref. Cummings, 6th ed., 1615*)

51. **(a) Unilateral mobile lymph nodes <3 cm** (*Ref. Stell & Maran, 5th ed., 668*)

   Stage III–$T_{1-3} N_1 M_0$

52. **(c) MRI** (*Ref. Cummings, 6th ed., 1614; Scott Brown, 8th ed., Vol 3;240*)

53. **(b) Respiratory papillomatosis** (*Ref. Cummings, 6th ed., 3144*)

54. **(d) Post-laryngectomy voice** (*Ref. Cummings, 6th ed., 1733*)

55. **(d) Tracheal speech** (*Ref. Cummings, 6th ed., 1735; Scott Brown, 8th ed., Vol 3; 267*)

56. **(c) Juvenile laryngeal papillomatosis** (*Ref. Scott Brown, 8th ed., Vol 2; 368*)

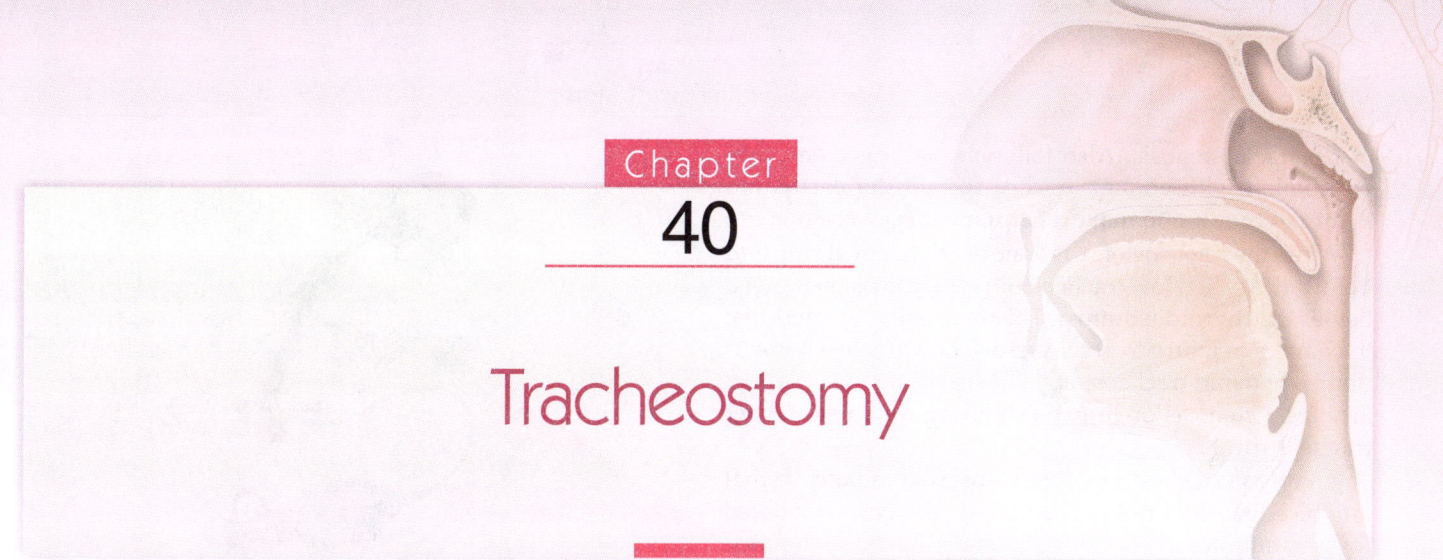

Tracheostomy

Making an opening on the anterior wall of the trachea is known as tracheostomy.

Tracheostomy can be:

a. **Elective**, i.e. planned or

b. **Emergency**

The only difference between the two, other than the haste of doing the procedure, is the skin incision.

Elective tracheostomy	Emergency tracheostomy
Horizontal skin crease incision 2–2.5 cm above the suprasternal notch	**Midline vertical incision on the skin of the neck from the lower border of cricoid to above the suprasternal notch**
Cosmetically better (since it is along the skin crease)	—

While doing tracheostomy the patient is placed in **Rose's position**, *see* Chapter 30. In both types of tracheostomy after the skin incision, the strap muscles and the pretracheal fascia are separated in midline. Finally a vertical incision is made on the 2nd and 3rd or 3rd and 4th tracheal rings.

Please note that mostly the incision is made on the **2nd and 3rd** or **3rd and 4th** tracheal rings and this is described as **mid tracheostomy**, *see* Fig. 40.1. When incision is made on the 1st tracheal ring or below 4th ring it is respectively called high and low tracheostomy.

Overlying the tracheal rings 2, 3 and 4 is the isthmus of thyroid which is retracted up. Then the cricoid is secured and elevated with the help of **cricoid hook** before giving the tracheal incision. Then the cuffed Portex (made up of PVC) tracheostomy tube (which is a **high volume and low pressure tube**, *see* Fig. 40.3) is inserted.

Tracheostomy is usually not done on the **1st tracheal ring** (the only exception is carcinoma larynx, *see* below) as it lies just next to the cricoid and any injury or perichondritis here leading to fibrosis will ultimately result in **laryngeal stenosis**, cricoid being the only complete ring laryngeal cartilage.

When the tracheostomy is done on the 1st tracheal ring it is known as **high tracheostomy**. The only indication of high tracheostomy is **carcinoma of the larynx** because here the larynx any way has to be removed so no complication

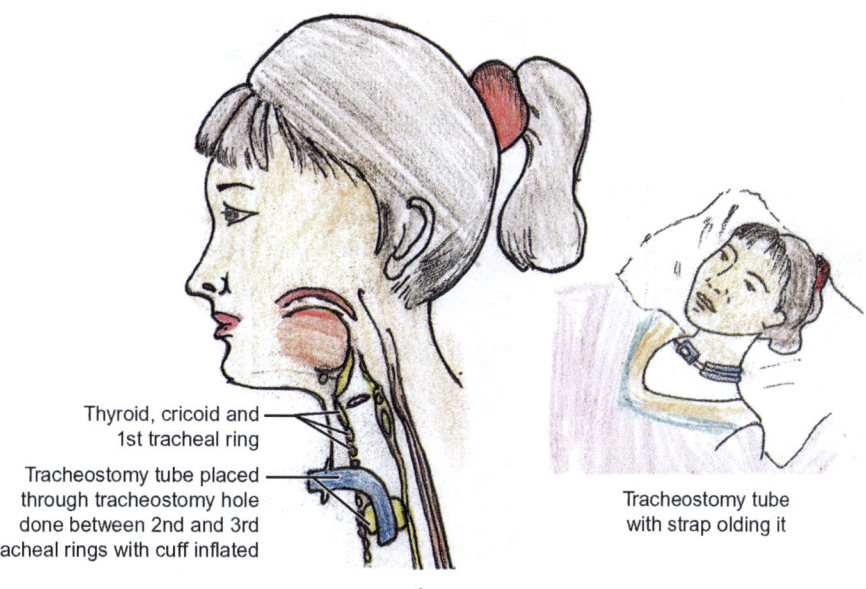

Thyroid, cricoid and 1st tracheal ring

Tracheostomy tube placed through tracheostomy hole done between 2nd and 3rd racheal rings with cuff inflated

Tracheostomy tube with strap olding it

Fig. 40.1

of laryngeal stenosis. Also following laryngectomy, we will be left with enough trachea to pull out easily and suture to the skin to make a permanent tracheostome.

When the tracheostomy is done at **5th tracheal ring and below**, it is called **low tracheostomy** (here incision is given below the thyroid isthmus). This is usually avoided due to chances of injury to great vessels. Low tracheostomy is done when mid tracheostomy (T2–T4) is not possible, e.g. laryngeal stenosis or **injury extending down till upper tracheal rings**.

A cuffed tracheostomy tube is inserted initially so that any bleeding does not get aspirated. The cuff is deflated for few minutes every hour and is permanently deflated after 12 hours to prevent necrosis and stenosis. The inserted cuffed portex tracheostomy tube is then replaced with an uncuffed portex tube after 3 days. Regular suctioning should be done for 5–10 seconds after every 1 to 2 hours. Thereafter this uncuffed tracheostomy tube is **changed every 2–3 days** because it tends to get obstructed from crusting. Any time, however, if there occurs complete obstruction of the tube, it is immediately changed and replaced with a fresh one to maintain the airway.

The tracheostomy tubes can be washed and reused.

Cleaning of the tube with saline and sodium bicarbonate is done frequently in a day as a measure to prevent crusting and delaying obstruction.

MATERIALS USED

The tracheostomy tubes can be either metallic (made up of steel, German silver, titanium silver alloy, etc.) or made from synthetic polymers silicone (Si), polyvinyl chloride (PVC), and polyurethane (PU)).

Metal tubes (e.g. Chevalier Jackson silver tube, see photo below) are **double lumen tubes** of which the inner tube can be easily removed, cleaned and replaced and hence are convenient for home care. The disadvantage of metal tubes is that they are very rigid as compared to polymeric tubes and hence cause mucosal injury to the trachea. They also do not have cuff so cannot prevent aspiration of blood following surgery and also pharyngeal secretions.

Portex (PVC) tracheostomy tube (*see* photo below) is a cuffed and flexible tube. It does not lead to mucosal injury and the cuff prevents aspiration of blood immediately after surgery and also aspiration of pharyngeal secretions.

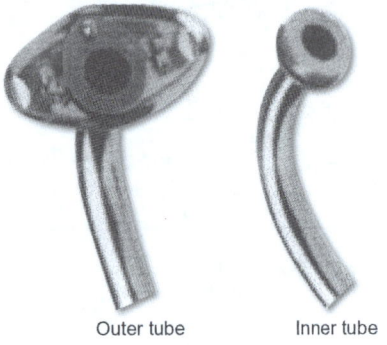

Outer tube   Inner tube

Fig. 40.2: Chevalier Jackson silver tube

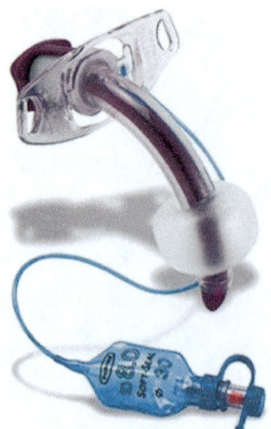

Fig. 40.3: Portex tracheostomy tube with cuff inflated

INDICATIONS OF TRACHEOSTOMY

i. To bypass **respiratory obstruction** above the level of tracheal rings 2, 3 or 4 (this being the site of tracheostomy). The causes of obstruction can be:
   a. Carcinoma larynx or other tumours obstructing airway above larynx.
   b. Trauma (external injury to larynx, maxillofacial injuries)
   c. Infections (e.g. croup, acute epiglottitis, diphtheria)
   d. Foreign body larynx
   e. B/L recurrent laryngeal nerve paralysis

ii. Prolonged mechanical ventilation:

If a patient requires mechanical ventilation for more than 10–14 days, tracheostomy should be done. This is nowadays the most common cause of elective temporary tracheostomy. The conditions that may require prolonged mechanical ventilation are:
- Acute respiratory distress syndrome (ARDS).
- Respiratory insufficiency due to COPD and other obstructive lung diseases.
- Respiratory failure due to Guillain-Barré syndrome, myasthenia gravis, spinal cord injuries, muscular dystrophies, etc.

The **prime indication of tracheostomy in children** is prevention of subglottic stenosis consequent upon conditions requiring prolonged intubation, for example, respiratory distress syndrome and prematurity.

The following are the **advantages of tracheostomy over endotracheal intubation (ETT)** in patients requiring prolonged mechanical ventilation:
a. Tracheostomy tube decreases **dead space by 30–50%**. Work of breathing is significantly less through a 6–12 cm tracheostomy tube than through a 27 cm endotracheal tube. Weaning a patient off mechanical ventilation is greatly facilitated by this decreased work of breathing.
b. Tracheostomy tube provides a more secure airway (it is less likely to be displaced and more readily can be replaced). By improved clearance of airway secretions, there is less likelihood of

tube getting obstructed by inspissated mucus. Also the patient is more comfortable, requiring less sedation and has reduced likelihood of aspiration through improved glottic function).

c. It is more comfortable than endotracheal tube: Pulmonary hygiene as well as oral hygiene is maintained easily. Communication and deglutition are also easily possible.

In patients who require Intermittent Positive pressure ventilation (**IPPV**), **cuffed tracheostomy tube** has to be used to prevent air leak and hence maintain positive pressure. Here a **cuffed ETT** should **not be put for more than 3 days** since it is more likely to cause ulceration, granulation tissue formation and subglottic or laryngeal stenosis.

iii. **For removal of respiratory secretions** when the patient is not able to cough it out, for example, in conditions like comatose states, painful chest injuries, diaphragmatic paralysis in cervical spine injuries (due to phrenic nerve injury) or spasm of respiratory muscles, e.g. tetanus. For the last three, additionally the patient may also require prolonged mechanical ventilation in which case also tracheostomy has to be done.

iv. In **maxillo-facial and head and neck surgeries** where pack has to be put in oropharynx to prevent aspiration while surgery. Instead of tracheostomy a simple endotracheal intubation cannot be considered here because the endotracheal tube will come in the path of the approach of these surgeries.

v. **To prevent aspiration**, e.g. in **B/L superior laryngeal nerve paralysis**, **B/L complete paralysis** (please refer to chapter on vocal cord paralysis).

Mnemonic: Doctors knowing tracheostomy should **O**ccupy **M**ost **S**eats in **M**edical **A**ssociation (**o**bstruction, **m**echanical ventilation, **s**ecretions, **m**axillo-facial surgeries, **a**spiration predisposing conditions).

IMMEDIATE COMPLICATIONS OF TRACHEOSTOMY

i. **Hemorrhage:** This is the most common complication of tracheostomy. It can also be torrential because of injury to **thyroidea ima artery** (a direct branch of the brachiocephalic or innominate artery) which runs in front of trachea to supply thyroid and is present in up to 10% of people.

ii. **Subcutaneous emphysema:** This can occur either because of a large tracheal opening and leakage of air or because of tight skin sutures. It can be managed by loosening/opening the skin sutures.

iii. **Pneumothorax:** This is the most common immediate complication of tracheostomy in children. This occurs because of injury to the apical pleura.

iv. **Injury to adjacent structures:** There may be injury to inferior thyroid vein, isthmus of thyroid and recurrent laryngeal nerve. It is important to note here that the **inferior thyroid artery** does **not** get **injured** as it goes on the under surface of thyroid and as

mentioned above torrential hemorrhage is due to injury to thyroidea ima artery.

v. **Apnoea:** In a patient of prolonged stridor the respiratory stimulant is pent up CO_2. When the trachea is opened during tracheostomy there is sudden washout of CO_2 leading to apnoea.

vi. Tube displacement and obstruction

LATE COMPLICATIONS OF TRACHEOSTOMY

i. Infection: In a patient of tracheostomy, the nasal functions of warming, filtering and humidification of air are lost, making the patient prone to lower respiratory tract infections.

ii. Tracheo-oesophageal fistula

iii. Tracheal stenosis

iv. Difficult decanulation

Difficult decanulation is a very important problem in paediatric tracheostomy. This is usually because the tracheostomy tube, by reducing the dead space, reduces the work of breathing which becomes difficult for children to overcome once the tube has been removed. (Please note that the reduction of dead space was of advantage during weaning off from the ventilator, but the same leads to difficulty during decanulation of tracheostomy tube.) The difficulty in decanulation can also occur due to stomal granulations or subglottic stenosis.

FOREIGN BODIES OF AIR PASSAGES

Accidental foreign body (FB) aspiration is seen most commonly in children of 1–4 years of age.

Nuts and peanuts are the most common and account for half of all the foreign body aspirations in children. Currency coins as FB are also quite commonly seen in clinical practice.

In adults FB aspiration can occur secondary to accidental inhalation during alcoholic intoxication, general anaesthesia or sedation.

Presentation

a. In most of the cases of inhaled F B there is a history of **choking and gagging** followed by paroxysmal coughing. There may be a symptomless interval after the initial process of coughing as the tracheobronchial tree becomes tolerant to the F B. The symptoms may again manifest later due to oedema, ulceration and lung complications.

b. A foreign body **partially obstructing** the larynx may lead to throat discomfort, hoarseness of voice, aphonia, dyspnoea, cough and haemoptysis.

c. A large F B can **totally obstruct** the airway leading to acute respiratory distress.

d. A **tracheal foreign body** not large enough to move into the bronchi will move up and down the trachea with respiration leading to **palpatory thud and audible slap**.

e. A foreign body when clears the trachea is more likely to enter the **right bronchus** which is less angulated and therefore more in line with the trachea. The patient will present with **expiratory stridor** if the foreign body is localised to the main bronchus or is in secondary bronchi.

f. A foreign body small enough to reach **tertiary bronchi** will lead to localised **expiratory wheeze**. The wheeze occurs due to partial blockade of the bronchi.

g. **Sudden onset of a wheeze**, usually unilateral in a child not previously known to have asthma should raise a suspicion of FB inhalation.

h. If there is **complete obstruction** of the **bronchi**, there occurs atelectasis of the involved segment of the lung. This will lead to reduced breath sounds over the involved area.

Identification of location of inhaled/ingested foreign body (a metal coin) on X-ray:

X-ray view	Oesophagus	Trachea
AP	Round	End on/linear
Lateral	End on/linear	Round

The above dissimilar findings on X-ray occur because the transverse diameter of oesophagus is more than its AP diameter and vice versa for trachea.

X-ray AP and lateral views: Coin in the oesophagus, *see* below.

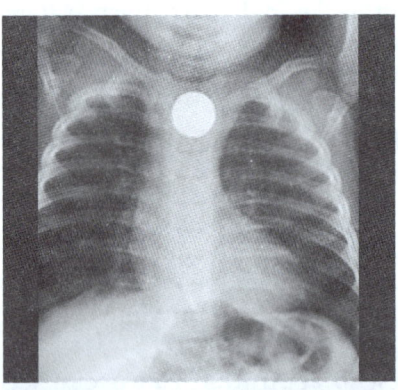

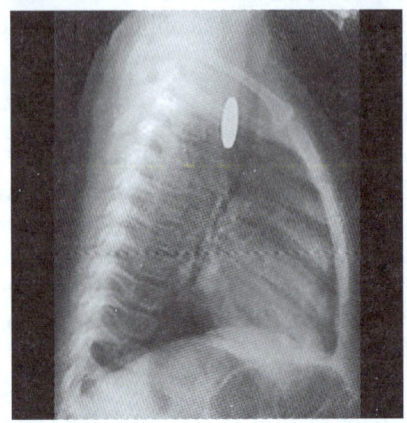

X-ray AP and lateral views: Coin in the trachea, *see* below.

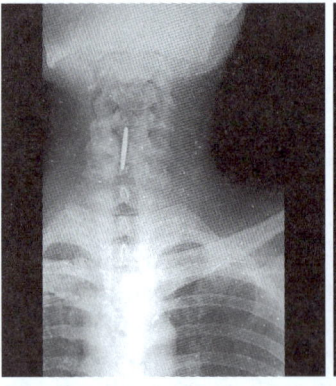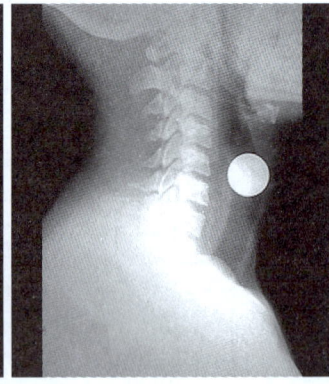

Management

1. The initial immediate management is **Heimlich manoeuvre** where multiple thrusts are given with the wrist in the upper epigastrium while standing behind the patient. This forcefully pushes air out of the lungs pushing the foreign body along. The Heimlich manoeuvre can lead to injury to the abdominal organs and therefore is done only when there is **aphonia** and **severe respiratory distress**.

2. If the patient is able to speak and respiratory distress is not there then the best initial steps will be motivating the patient to **cough and give back slaps**.

3. If the patient becomes unconscious then **finger sweep manoeuvre** is done, i.e. removal of the foreign body with the finger if visible.

4. The above are the first aid measures and when despite these the airway could not have been secured and the patient is into very severe respiratory distress an immediate **Cricothyrotomy** should be done. Cricothyrotomy is an emergency procedure done by making an opening in the Cricothyroid membrane to restore airway where immediate tracheostomy is not possible. Like emergency tracheostomy, the incision in Cricothyrotomy is also vertical, for it causes less bleeding.

   Cricothyrotomy should be changed to a formal **tracheostomy** as early as possible.

   It is faster and easier than tracheostomy but since it carries high risk of tube obstruction and laryngeal injury and stenosis it should be changed to a formal tracheostomy as early as possible.

5. If the patient is not into respiratory distress or once the airway has been secured, then depending upon the site of foreign body, it can be removed either by **direct laryngoscopy** or by **bronchoscopy**.

PREVIOUSLY ASKED QUESTIONS

1. All of the following are true about the tracheostomy tube except: *(Exam 2013)*
   a. Consists of metallic tubes
   b. Consists of silicone and poly vinyl chloride (PVC) material
   c. Portex tube is ideally changed every 15 days
   d. Cuffed tube used for IPPV

2. In emergency tracheostomy the following structures are damaged except: *(AI 2011)*
   a. Isthmus of the thyroid
   b. Inferior thyroid artery
   c. Thyroidea ima artery
   d. Inferior thyroid vein

3. High tracheostomy is done in: *(AI 2008, Exam 2016)*
   a. Laryngeal carcinoma
   b. Vocal cord palsy
   c. Laryngomalacia
   d. Subglottic stenosis

4. Most common complication of high tracheostomy is: *(SGPGI 2004, Exam 2017)*
   a. Laryngeal stenosis
   b. Difficult decanulation
   c. Pneumothorax
   d. Subcutaneous emphysema

5. Best treatment for laceration and crush injury to larynx: *(Exam 2013)*
   a. Cricothyroidotomy
   b. Bag and mask ventilation
   c. Low tracheostomy
   d. None

6. Tracheostomy reduces the dead space by: *(AI 2011)*
   a. 10–20%
   b. 30–50%
   c. 60–70%
   d. 70–100%

7. Which of the following statements is false about tracheostomy: *(AIIMS 2004, Exam 2016)*
   a. Decrease dead space by 30–50%
   b. A frequent problem in infants after tracheostomy is difficult decanulation
   c. In emergency tracheostomy transverse incision is given 2 fingers above sternal notch
   d. A complication of paediatrics tracheostomy is pneumothorax

8. Tracheostomy is not indicated in: *(TN 2004, Exam 2016)*
   a. Emphysema
   b. Bronchiectasis
   c. Atelectasis
   d. Pneumothorax

9. What is the most common indication of tracheostomy in a child? *(UPSC 2010)*
   a. Carcinoma of larynx
   b. Laryngeal diphtheria
   c. Conditions requiring prolonged intubation
   d. Poliomyelitis

10. Tracheostomy done at which level: *(Exam 2013)*
    a. T1
    b. T3
    c. T5
    d. None of the above

11. Late complication of tracheostomy is: *(Bihar 2009, Exam 2016)*
    a. Haemorrhage
    b. Displacement of tube or obstruction
    c. Surgical emphysema
    d. Tracheal stenosis

12. A tracheostomised patient, with Portex tracheostomy tube, in the ward, developed sudden complete blockage of the tube. Which of the following is the best next step in the management: *(AIIMS 2004/MP 2007, Exam 2016)*
    a. Immediate removal of the tracheostomy tube
    b. Suction of tube with sodium bicarbonate
    c. Suction of tube with saline
    d. Transtracheal Jet ventilation

13. Tracheostomy is indicated in all except: *(AI 2003, Exam 2016)*
    a. Carcinoma larynx
    b. Severe bronchial asthma
    c. Diphtheria
    d. Comatose patient

14. All are true about tracheostomy tube except: *(MP 2001, Exam 2016)*
    a. Jackson's tube has 2 lumens
    b. Removal of metallic tubes every 2–3 days
    c. Cuffed tube is used to prevent aspiration of pharyngeal secretion
    d. Made up of titanium silver alloy

15. Complications of tracheostomy are all except: *(AP 2004, Exam 2016)*
    a. Fracture cervical vertebra
    b. Pneumothorax
    c. Subcutaneous emphysema
    d. Apnoea

16. Mid tracheostomy is done over: *(MP 2004, Exam 2016)*
    a. 1st and 2nd tracheal rings
    b. 2nd and 3rd tracheal rings
    c. 4th and 5th tracheal rings
    d. 5th and 6th tracheal rings

17. A double lumen tracheostomy tube all are true except: *(MP 2001, Exam 2016)*
    a. Easy to remove inner cannula
    b. Easy to clean inner cannula
    c. Easy to replace inner cannula
    d. No inner cannula

Larynx

Section IV

18. Maintenance of airway during laryngectomy in a patient with carcinoma of larynx is best done by: (*J & K 2005, Exam 2013*)
    a. Tracheostomy
    b. Laryngeal mask airway
    c. Laryngeal tube
    d. Combi tube

19. Site of emergency needle Cricothyrotomy is: (*AI 2006, Exam 2016*)
    a. Between 1st and 2nd tracheal rings
    b. Between 2nd and 3 rd tracheal rings
    c. Thyrohyoid membrane
    d. Cricothyroid membrane

20. A 2-year-old male child presenting with sudden severe dyspnoea, most common cause is: (*Bihar 2006, Exam 2016*)
    a. Foreign body
    b. Bronchiolitis
    c. Asthmatic attack
    d. None

21. A 5-year-old boy while having dinner suddenly becomes aphonic and develops respiratory distress. What should be the appropriate initial management: (*AI 2011*)
    a. Cricothyrotomy
    b. Emergency tracheostomy
    c. Finger sweep manoeuvre
    d. Heimlich manoeuvre

22. Palpatory thud, audible slap is seen in: (*Exam 2013*)
    a. Tracheal foreign body
    b. Bronchial foreign body
    c. Laryngeal foreign body
    d. None

23. Which one of the following combinations is most appropriate regarding the picture depicted here: (*APPG 2015*)

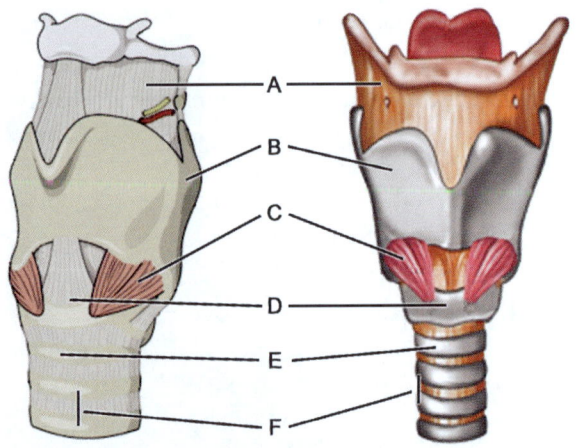

    a. A is cricothyroid membrane and site for cricothyroidotomy and F is site for tracheostomy
    b. A is the thyroid cartilage and B is the hyoid bone
    c. D is the only continuous ring of the trachea and E is the site for tracheostomy
    d. B is Adam's apple and C is the site for cricothyroidotomy

24. Metal coin in the glottis is seen on X-ray as: (*Exam 2016*)
    a. Lateral view—circular
    b. Lateral view—slit
    c. AP view—circular
    d. AP view—globular

25. All are common causes of stridor except: (*Exam 2015*)
    a. Foreign body in larynx and trachea
    b. Laryngomalacia
    c. Multiple papillomas of larynx
    d. Atrophic laryngitis

26. The most common cause of stridor in infant and children is: (*Exam 2015*)
    a. Congenital subglottic stenosis
    b. Laryngomalacia
    c. Vocal cord paralysis
    d. Foreign body in airway

27. Stridor is caused by all except: (*Exam 2014*)
    a. Foreign body in left main bronchus
    b. Bacterial tracheitis
    c. Retropharyngeal abscess
    d. Unilateral vocal cord palsy

28. Which of the following are signs of respiratory obstruction? (*Exam 2015*)
    a. High pitched noise
    b. Hypoxia
    c. Stridor on inspiration
    d. All of the above

29. All of the following are indications for tracheostomy except: (*Exam 2014*)
    a. Coma after head injury
    b. Maxillofacial injury
    c. Bilateral abductor palsy
    d. Superior laryngeal nerve palsy

30. In permanent tracheostome: (*Exam 2015*)
    a. The tracheal remnant is sutured to the strap muscles for safer ventilation of the respiratory tract
    b. The tracheostomy tube is kept permanently with intermittent cleaning of the tube
    c. The chances of tracheal stenosis is high
    d. The remnant of trachea is brought out to the surface as a permanent mouth to the respiratory tract

31. A 40-year-old man who met with a motor vehicle catastrophe came to the casualty with severe maxillofacial trauma. His pulse rate was 120/min, BP was 100/70 mmHg, SpO_2-80% with oxygen. What would be the immediate management? (*Exam 2016*)
    a. Nasotracheal intubation
    b. Orotracheal intubation

c. Intravenous fluid
d. Tracheostomy

32. **What incision is given on skin and cricothyroid membrane during cricothyroidotomy:** (*Exam 2016*)
    a. Transverse
    b. Vertical
    c. Oblique
    d. None

IMAGE BASED PRACTICE QUESTIONS BY THE AUTHOR

33. **Where is the tube shown below put:**

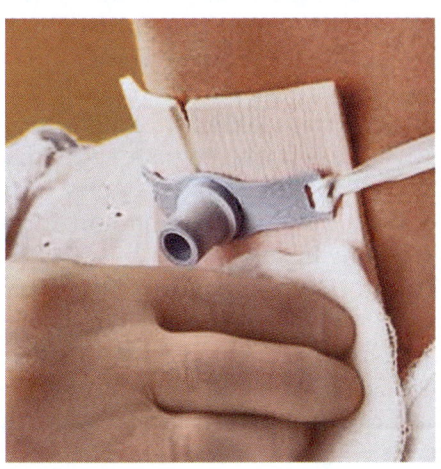

a. 1st tracheal ring
b. 2nd and 3rd tracheal rings
c. 5th and 6th tracheal rings
d. On the cricoid cartilage

34. **A child presents with history of accidentally ingesting/inhaling coin. His X-ray AP view is given below. What is the site of lodgement of this coin:**

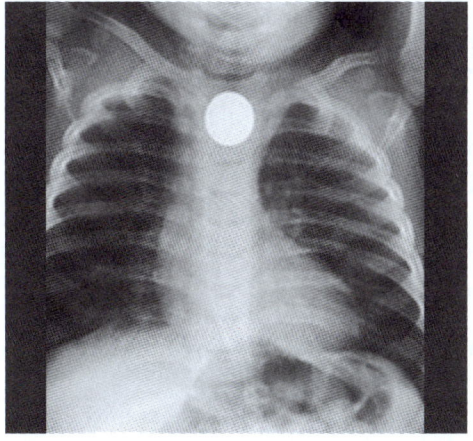

a. Larynx
b. Oesophagus
c. Oropharynx
d. Lungs

ANSWERS AND EXPLANATIONS

1. **(c)** (*Ref. Cummings, 6th ed., 100*)
- The tracheostomy tube is changed every 2–3 days to prevent obstruction from crusting.
- Rest all are true, kindly refer to the text.

2. **(b) Inferior thyroid artery** (*Ref. Cummings, 6th ed., 100*)
- The inferior thyroid artery does not get injured as it goes on the under surface of thyroid.
- Rest all can get damaged. Please refer to the complications of tracheostomy in the text.

3. **(a) Laryngeal carcinoma** (*Ref. Scott Brown, 6th ed., 5/7/9*)
- The only indication of high tracheostomy (i.e. tracheostomy at the 1st tracheal ring) is carcinoma of the larynx.
- In laryngomalacia the management is reassurance. Rarely supraglottoplasty is required but tracheostomy is not done here.
- In vocal cord palsy, it is done at tracheal rings 2 and 3 or 3 and 4.
- In subglottic stenosis, low tracheostomy is done.

4. **(a) Laryngeal stenosis** (*Ref. Scott Brown, 8th ed., Vol 3; 1046*)
- Rest of the options can be the complications of any tracheostomy. Please refer to text.

5. **(c) Low tracheostomy** (*Ref. Scott Brown, 8th ed., Vol 3; 1041*)
- In crush injury to larynx since the obstruction is at the level of larynx, to maintain airway Cricothyroidotomy or bag and mask ventilation will not suffice.
- Here tracheostomy needs to be done. Low tracheostomy is done below T4 level and carries risk to the great vessels. Low tracheostomy is done when mid tracheostomy (T2–T4) is not possible, e.g. laryngeal stenosis or injury extending down till upper tracheal rings.

6. **(b) 30–50%** (*Ref. Scott Brown, 6th ed., 5/7/8*)

7. **(c) is false** (*Ref. Cummings, 6th ed., 97*)
- In emergency tracheostomy a vertical incision is given. Transverse incision is given in elective tracheostomy. Please refer to text.

8. **(d) Pneumothorax** (*Ref. Scott Brown, 8th ed., Vol 3; 1041*)
- Pneumothorax is treated by thoracostomy and subsequently chest tube (or intercostals drain) insertion. This is done in the safe triangle of axilla.
- In emphysema (COPD), bronchiectasis and atelectasis conditions, when the patient goes into respiratory insufficiency and require prolonged mechanical ventilation, tracheostomy is done.
- Please refer text for advantages of tracheostomy over endotracheal intubation in prolonged mechanical ventilation.

9. **(c) Conditions requiring prolonged intubation** (*Ref. Cummings, 6th ed., 96*)
- Previously the tracheostomy in children was used to be done largely for the management of acute severe epiglottitis, laryngotracheobronchitis (croup) and diphtheria.
- But with better antibiotics, medical care and immunisation these days the prime indication of tracheostomy is prevention of subglottic stenosis in infants consequent upon conditions requiring prolonged intubation, for example, respiratory distress syndrome and prematurity.
- Bulbar polio predisposing aspiration used to be an indication of tracheostomy in children but now with intensive pulse polio programmes, India has been declared polio free.
- Carcinoma larynx is a common indication of tracheostomy in an adult.

10. **(b) T3 (3rd tracheal ring)** (*Ref. Scott Brown, 8th ed., Vol 3; 1043*)
- In tracheostomy, i.e. mid tracheostomy a vertical incision is made on the 2nd and 3rd or 3rd and 4th tracheal rings (after retracting the thyroid isthmus upwards).
- T1 is high tracheostomy; incision is made on 1st tracheal ring (above the thyroid isthmus).
- T5 and below is called low tracheostomy (below the thyroid isthmus)

11. **(d) Tracheal stenosis** (*Ref. Cummings, 6th ed., 101*)

12. **(a) Immediate removal of the tracheostomy tube** (*Ref. Scott Brown, 8th ed., Vol 3; 1045*)
- Portex is a PVC tracheostomy tube. In case of complete blockade, the tube needs to be changed immediately.
- Suction with sodium bicarbonate and saline is done frequently in a tracheotomised patient as a preventive measure to avoid obstruction.
- Transtracheal jet ventilation (PTJV: Percutaneous transtracheal jet ventilation) is an emergency technique of providing respiration. This is done by doing a needle Cricothyrotomy (i.e. piercing the cricothyroid membrane). It is a simple, fast and safe access at times during emergency situations when endotracheal intubation or other ventilation methods are not feasible.

13. **(b) Severe bronchial asthma** (*Ref. Cummings, 6th ed., 96*)
- Asthma is a reversible narrowing of lower airways (tertiary bronchi onwards) so tracheostomy which is done at 3rd tracheal ring will not correct this distal obstruction.
- Carcinoma larynx is a common indication of tracheostomy in an adult.
- Diphtheria can cause airway obstruction due to formation of extensive membranes for which tracheostomy is done.
- Tracheostomy is done in comatose conditions to take care of respiratory secretions

14. **(b) Removal of metallic tube in every 2–3 days** (*Ref. Scott Brown, 6th ed., 5/7/10*)
   - The outer metallic tube is left in situ and only the inner tube is removed, cleaned and replaced from time to time. Rest are true.

15. **(a) Fracture of cervical vertebra** (*Ref. Cummings, 6th ed., 100*)
   - All the remaining are complications of tracheostomy, refer the text.
   - In patients of fracture of cervical spine, since the neck cannot be extended tracheostomy has to be done without extension of neck which makes the surgery a little difficult. Fracture cervical vertebra is an indication to do tracheostomy, it is not a complication.

16. **(b) 2nd and 3rd tracheal rings** (*Ref. Scott Brown, 6th ed., 5/7/8*)

17. **(d) No inner cannula** (*Ref. Stell & Maran, 5th ed., 276*)
   - Jacksons and other Metal tracheostomy tubes have a double lumen. The outer tube remains in the trachea while the inner tube can be easily removed, cleaned and replaced.

18. **(a) Tracheostomy** (*Ref. Scott Brown, 8th ed., Vol 3; 1041*)
   - During laryngectomy the intubation tube is kept away from the field of surgery, i.e. the larynx, by doing a tracheostomy in patients not previously tracheotomised. Here intubation is done through the tracheostome.
   - Here oro or nasal intubation is not done, also because the mass in the larynx will not allow doing so.
   - Laryngeal mask airway, Laryngeal tube and Combi tube all deliver oxygen/anaesthesia at or above the larynx and therefore all these will not be of utility in a patient with a mass obstructing the cavity of the larynx. These will also interfere with the field of surgery.

19. **(d) Cricothyroid membrane** (*Ref. Scott Brown, 8th ed., Vol 3; 1041; Stell & Maran 5th ed., 296*)

20. **(a) Foreign body** (*Ref. Current Diagnosis & Treatment Otolaryngology, Lalwani, 3rd ed., 485; Scott Brown, 8th ed., Vol 3; 1039*)
   - Sudden severe dyspnoea in a 2 years old child is indicative of foreign body.
   - Bronchiolitis and asthmatic attack develops acutely, i.e. over a few hours to few days and not suddenly.

21. **(d) Heimlich manoeuvre** (*Ref. Cummings, 6th ed., 485; Scott Brown, 8th ed., Vol 3; 1039*)
   - This child is likely having an accidental inhalation of food. The initial immediate management is Heimlich manoeuvre
   - For rest refer to text.

22. **(a) Tracheal foreign body** (*Ref. Scott Brown, 6th ed., 6/25/3*)
   - A tracheal foreign body not large enough to move into the bronchi will move up and down the trachea with respiration leading to palpatory thud and audible slap.

23. **(d) B is Adam's apple and C is the site for cricothyroidotomy** (*Ref. Scott Brown, 8th ed., Vol 3; 885*)

24. **(a) Lateral view—circular** (*Ref. Dhingra, 6th ed., 438*)

25. **(d) Atrophic laryngitis** (*Ref. Current Diagnosis & Treatment Otolaryngology, Lalwani, 3rd ed., 481*)

26. **(b) Laryngomalacia** (*Ref. Current Diagnosis & Treatment Otolaryngology, Lalwani, 3rd ed., 481*)

27. **(d) Unilateral vocal cord palsy** (*Ref. Current Diagnosis & Treatment Otolaryngology, Lalwani, 3rd ed., 481; Scott Brown, 8th ed., Vol 3; 1038*)
   - Unilateral recurrent laryngeal nerve palsy is asymptomatic
   - Unilateral complete palsy presents with aphonia/dysphonia and occasional aspiration

28. **(d) All of the above** (*Ref. Scott Brown, 8th ed., Vol 3; 1037*)

29. **(d) Superior laryngeal nerve palsy** (*Ref. Cummings, 6th ed., 96*)

30. **(d) The remnant of trachea is brought out to the surface as a permanent mouth to the respiratory tract** (*Ref. Stell & Maran, 5th ed., 656*)

31. **(d) Tracheostomy** (*Ref. Cummings, 6th ed., 96*)
   - In severe maxillofacial trauma, nasotracheal intubation and orotracheal intubation are not possible therefore to maintain the airway tracheostomy should be done.

32. **(b) Vertical** (*Ref. Scott Brown, 8th ed., Vol 3; 1041*)
   - Vertical skin incision for it causes less bleeding

33. **(b) 2nd and 3rd tracheal rings** (*Ref. Scott Brown, 8th ed., Vol 3; 1043*)

34. **(b) Oesophagus** (*Ref. Dhingra, 6th ed., 438*)

Larynx

Section IV

Important Instruments in ENT

Important Instruments in Ear, Nose and Throat Examination and Surgery

Bull's Lamp

It is a source of illumination. It has a 100 watts white bulb. This light is focussed with the plano convex lens placed in front of the bulb. Ideally the Bulls lamp is placed 6 inches above and behind the left shoulder of the patient, at the level of left ear of the patient.

While using a Bull's lamp the examiner must focus the light using a head mirror to illuminate the patient.

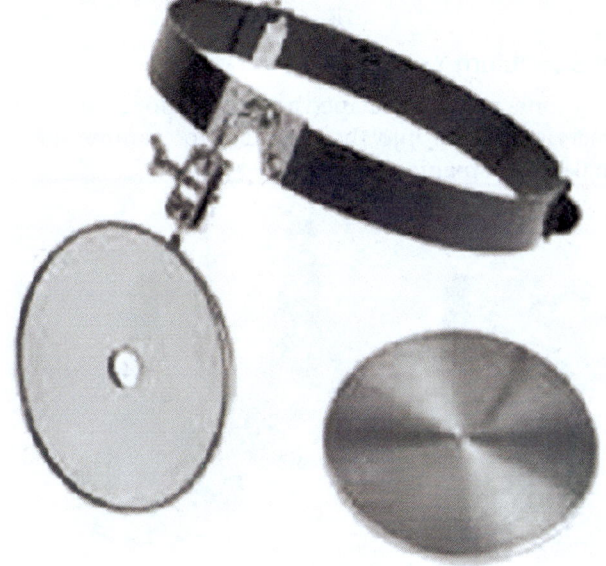

Fig. 41.2

Siegel's Speculum

Please *see* the details of Siegel's speculum in Chapter 4.

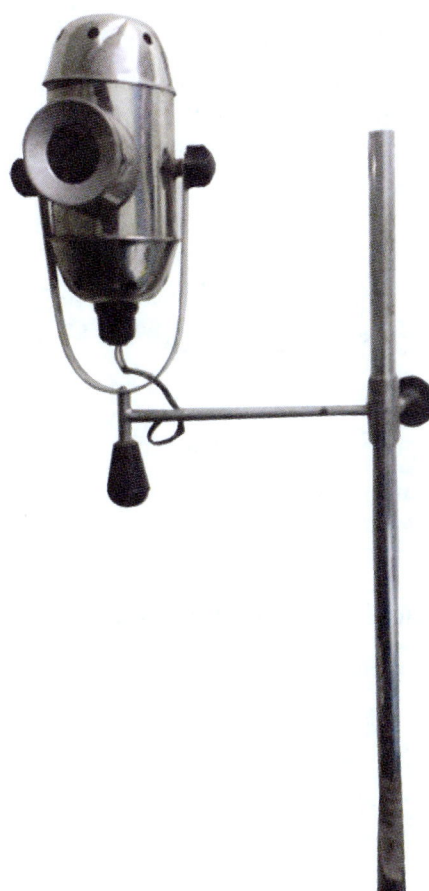

Fig. 41.1

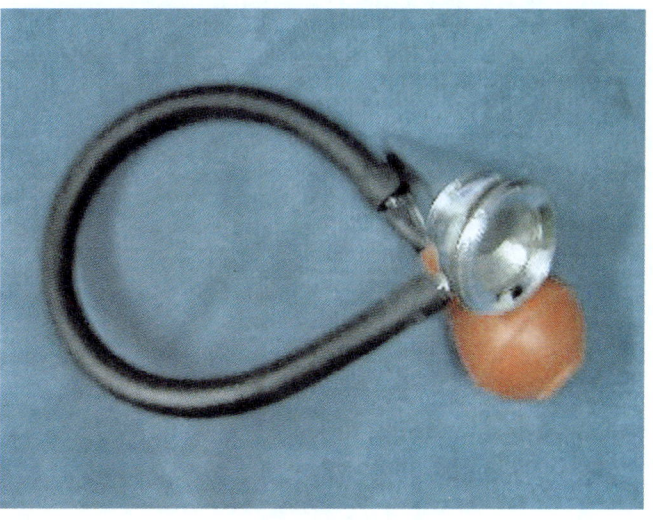

Head Mirror

Please *see* the details of head mirror in Chapter 4.

Fig. 41.3

Otoscope

An otoscope is a device which is used to look into the ears. An otoscope gives a view of the ear canal and tympanic membrane

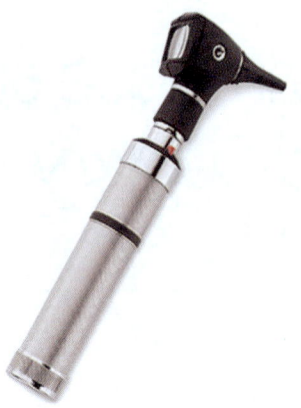

Fig. 41.4

Ear Speculum

It is a cone- or funnel-shaped attachment for an otoscope, which is inserted into the ear canal to examine the ear canal and tympanic membrane.

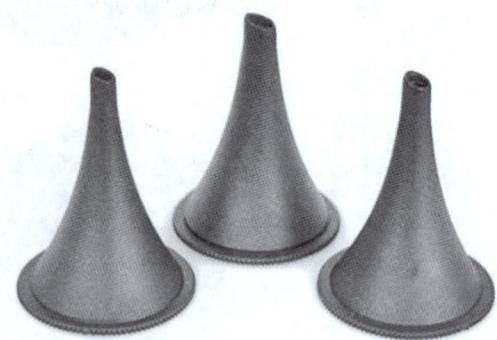

Fig. 41.5

Gardiner-Brown Tuning Fork

In ENT, tuning forks are used to clinically test hearing and identify the type of hearing loss.

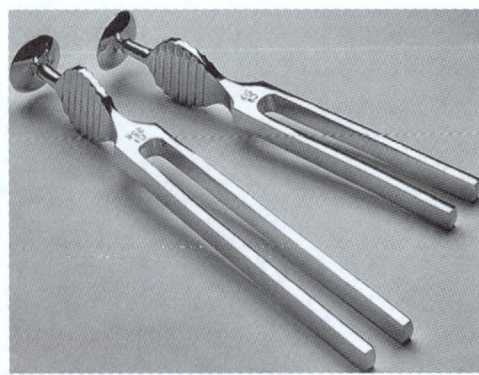

Fig. 41.6

The parts of a tuning fork are:
- Base plate or footplate
- Shaft
- Prongs that vibrate and produce sound

The frequency at which the tuning fork vibrates is denoted in Hertz (Hz). The commonly used tuning forks to test hearing are 256 Hz, 512 Hz and 1024 Hz. These frequencies correspond to the speech frequencies.

- Tuning forks of lower frequencies (like 128 Hz) produce vibrations that are felt more than they are heard, while those higher than 512 Hz frequencies produce more overtones. Therefore, if we have to perform hearing tests with a single tuning fork, we pick the 512 Hz.
- Tests done with these tuning forks include Rinne's, Weber's, absolute bone conduction test, Bing's test, Stenger's, and Gelle's test, etc. *see* Chapter 2.

Cutting and Diamond Burrs

Mastoid exploration involves exposure of the mastoid antrum by removal of the mastoid bone using a cutting burr and diamond burr, *see* Chapter 8.

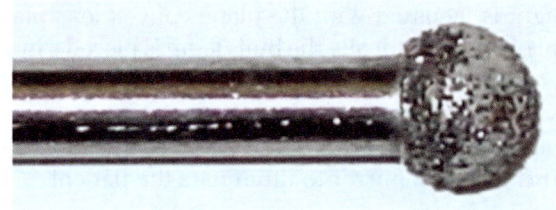

Fig. 41.7

This is the picture of a diamond burr. Diamond burrs are used in approaching vital structures such as the inner ear, facial nerve and the dura as they cut the bone very slowly.

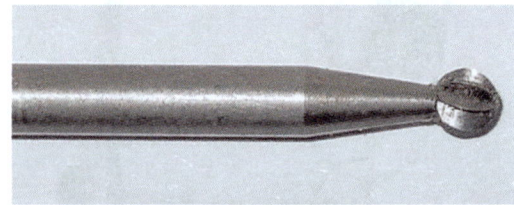

Fig. 41.8

This picture shows a cutting burr. They are sharp and drill away mastoid air cells very fast.

Total Ossicular Replacement Prosthesis (TORP) and Partial Ossicular Replacement Prosthesis (PORP)

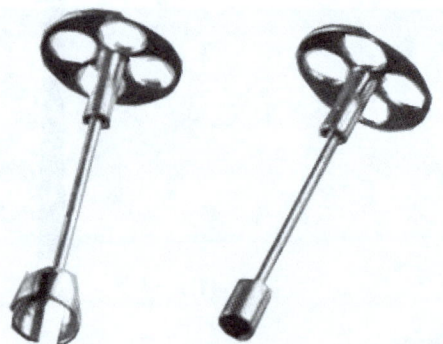

Fig. 41.9

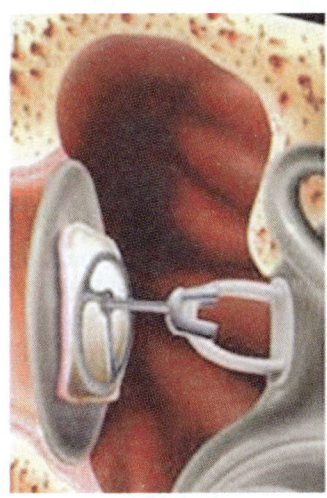

Fig. 41.10

When both the incus and the malleus have been removed, a PORP (partial ossicular replacement prosthesis) is used for repair *see* Chapter 7.

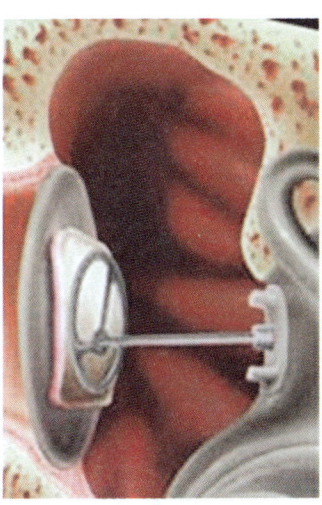

Fig. 41.11

When all the 3 bones have been damaged and removed a TORP (total ossicular replacement prosthesis) is used for repair, *see* Chapter 7.

Grommet

Grommets are used in serous otitis media for ventilation and drainage of middle ear.

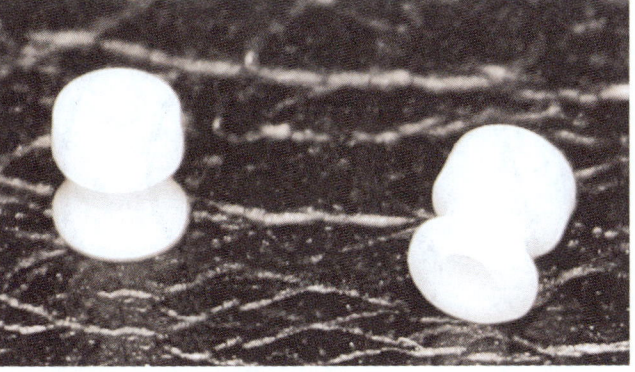

Fig. 41.12

Teflon Piston

Teflon piston is used in stapedotomy to replace the stapes.

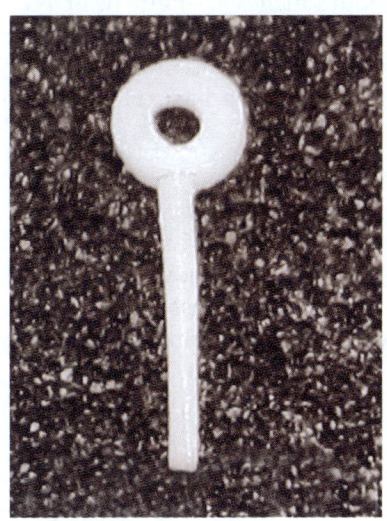

Fig. 41.13

Jobson Horne Probe Double Ended

It is also called the wax hook or ring curette.

One end of the probe is shaped like a ring. This end may be used to hook out wax or foreign bodies from the ear canal. It can also be used to probe an aural polyp or other mass in the ear canal.

The other end of the instrument is sharp and serrated. An ear wick can be fashioned out of this end by rolling cotton on to it and used to mop ear discharge.

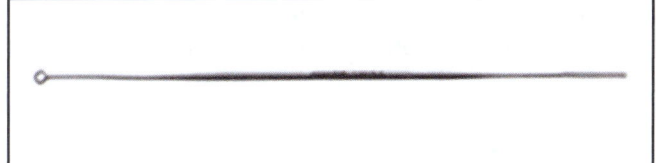

Fig. 41.14

Aural Syringe

This instrument is the metallic aural syringe. The syringe has a nozzle for insertion into the external auditory canal. The syringe is held by inserting fingers into the rings at the back. The third ring is on the piston that forces the water out when pushed.

It is used for removal of wax, foreign body or debris from the ear canal.

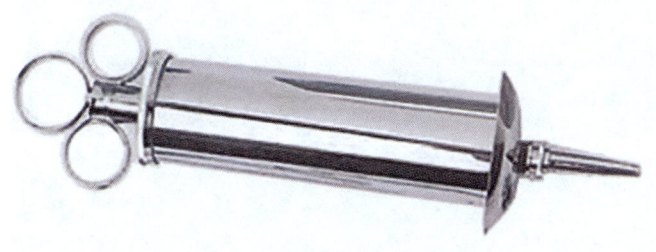

Fig. 41.15

Important Instruments in ENT

Section V

Eustachian Tube Catheter

The Eustachian catheter is a long, thin, metal cannula, measuring about 5 inches in length. Its tip is curved gently downwards. The other end bears a small metal ring in the direction of the curve. This ring serves as a guide to the direction of the curve once the tip is inserted into the nose.

Uses

- Eustachian tube catheterization: used to test Eustachian tube patency, *see* Chapter 6.
- Nasal foreign body removal: The Eustachian catheter is sometimes used for removal of foreign bodies from the nose. It is a sturdy instrument whose curved tip can be used to manoeuvre foreign bodies lodged in the nasal cavity.

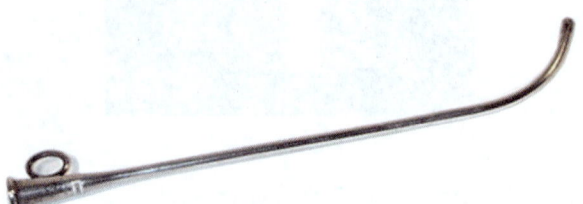

Fig. 41.16

Nasal Speculum—Thudichum

The Thudichum's nasal speculum is an instrument routinely used in the OPD to examine the nose.

The instrument has two flanges that can be inserted into the nostril during anterior rhinoscopy. The flanges widen to open up the nasal cavity, offering a better view of the structures inside the nose.

Uses of the Thudichum's nasal speculum:

- In anterior rhinoscopy
- Foreign body removal from the nose
- Per operatively, for nasal packing
- In septal surgeries (septoplasty and SMR) while making the incision
- Structures seen on anterior rhinoscopy:
  - Nasal septum
  - Lateral wall of the nose including the inferior and middle turbinates and the meatuses
  - Floor of the nasal cavity

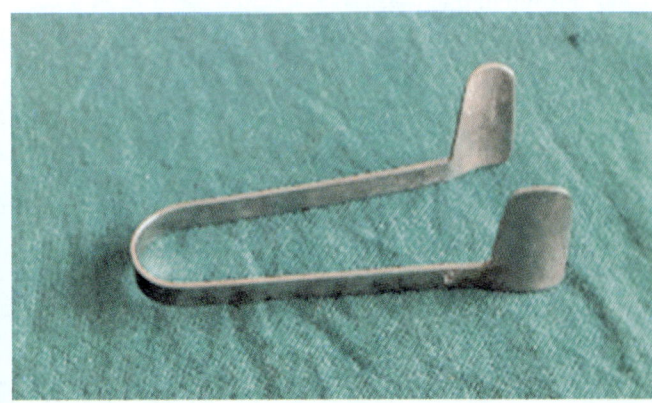

Fig. 41.17

- It is not used to examine the vestibule. Vestibule is examined by lifting up the tip of the nose with finger, using the speculum will only obscure it from vision.

Killian Nasal Speculum

This is a type of nasal speculum.

It comes in several sizes, from small to long-bladed. A screw in the handle can be tightened to hold the blades of the speculum in the open position. This gives the speculum its self-retaining feature, which is very useful during septal surgery.

The Killian's nasal speculum is used for both nasal examination and surgery. Following are its uses:

1. Anterior rhinoscopy
2. Anterior nasal packing
3. Nasal foreign body, rhinolith removal
4. Septoplasty
5. Functional endoscopic sinus surgery
6. Turbinate reduction surgeries

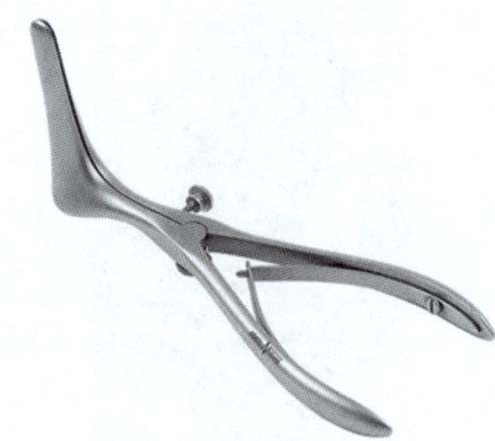

Fig. 41.18

Flexible Fiberoptic Endoscope

Nasal endoscopy involves evaluation of the nasal and sinus passages with direct vision using a magnified high-quality view. Nasal endoscopy may be done with either a flexible fiberoptic endoscope or a rigid endoscope.

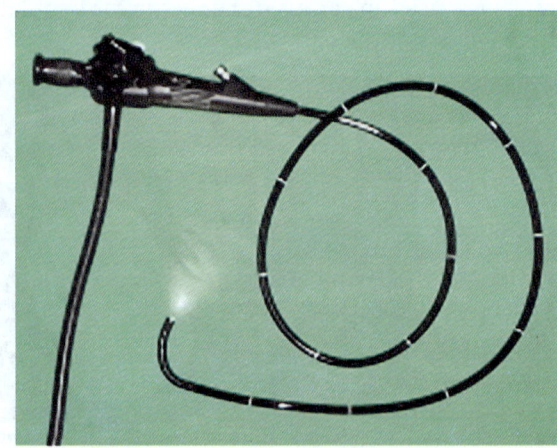

Fig. 41.19

Rigid Nasal Endoscopes

Rigid endoscopes for the nose come in diameters of 2.7 to 4 mm and have tips of different angles (0°, 30°, 45°, 70°), allowing the ENT surgeon to visualize various sinuses and areas within the nasal cavity and sinuses.

Indications for nasal endoscopy include the following:

- Initial identification of disease in patients experiencing sino-nasal symptoms (e.g. mucopurulent drainage, facial pain or pressure, nasal obstruction or congestion, or decreased sense of smell)
- Evaluation of patients' response to medical treatment (e.g. resolution of polyps, purulent secretions, or mucosal edema and inflammation after treatment with topical nasal steroids, antibiotics, oral steroids, and antihistamines)
- Obtaining a culture of purulent secretions
- In performing Functional Endoscopic Sinus Surgery
- Evaluation after FESS
- Evaluation and biopsy of nasal masses or lesions
- Evaluation of the nasopharynx for lymphoid hyperplasia, Eustachian tube problems, and nasal obstruction
- Evaluation of cerebrospinal fluid (CSF) leak
- Evaluation and treatment of epistaxis
- Evaluation of hyposmia or anosmia
- Evaluation and treatment of nasal foreign bodies

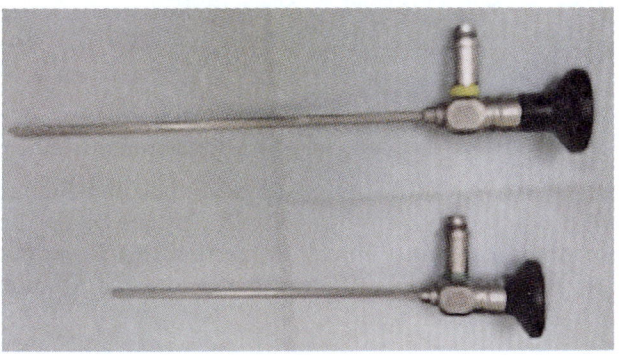

Fig. 41.20

Posterior Rhinoscopy Mirror

This instrument is the St. Clair Thompson postnasal or posterior rhinoscopy mirror.

The mirror side is warmed by keeping it on bulb of bull's eye lamp, flame or warm water and introduced into the oral cavity, while the tongue is depressed with a tongue depressor. The mirror is turned upwards in order to examine the post nasal space, *see* Fig. 41.2A and B.

The shaft of the instrument is bent to achieve a bayonet shape, a feature that helps differentiate it from the indirect laryngoscopy mirror.

- Posterior rhinoscopy is done to look for lesions in the post nasal space—for example, adenoids, tumours of the nasopharynx, etc. however diagnostic nasal endoscopy is the best method to examine this region.

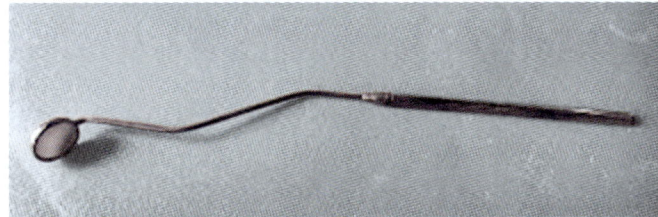

Fig. 41.21

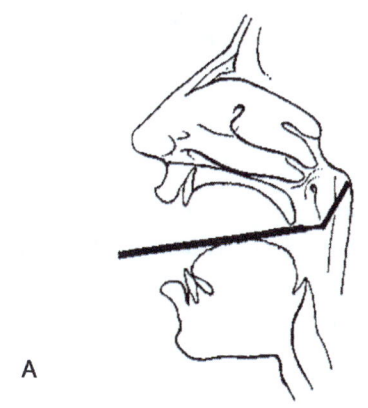

A

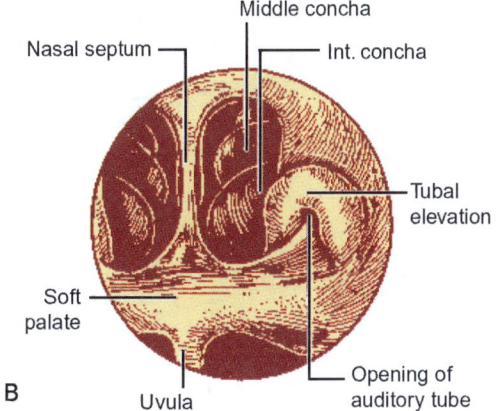

Nasal septum — Middle concha — Int. concha

Tubal elevation

Soft palate

Uvula — Opening of auditory tube

B

Fig. 41.22A and B

Luc Nasal Forceps

It is used in:

1. Caldwell-Luc operation to approach the maxillary sinuses
2. Septoplasty to remove the deviated cartilage and bone.
3. In FESS to remove polyps
4. To take biopsy from nose and oral cavity

The instrument is very similar to the Denis Browne tonsil holding forceps, see instruments of pharynx. To differentiate the two, examine the tips of the forceps. The edges of the tips are smooth in tonsil holding forceps, their job is to just hold tissue, whereas the edges of the tips are sharper in the case of Luc's forceps because they have to do some cutting. Also, the cup-shaped tip of the upper arm fits into the tip of the lower arm in the case of tonsil holding forceps whereas they approximate each other in Luc's forceps.

Important Instruments in ENT

Section V

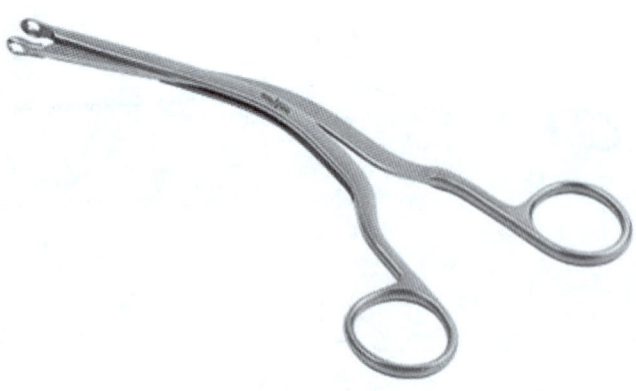

Fig. 41.23

Nasal Fracture Reduction Instruments; (below) Asch Forceps and (above) Walsham Forceps

The Asch's forceps is used to reduce the displaced septum and the Walsham forceps is used to reduce the nasal bones.

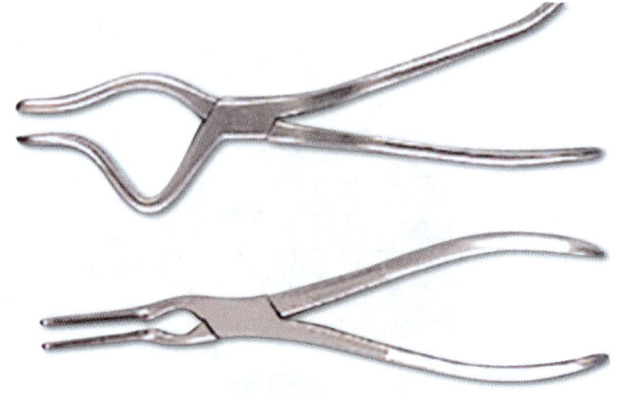

Fig. 41.24

PHARYNX AND LARYNX

Davis-Boyle Mouth Gag Complete Set

1. **Boyles Tongue Depressor**

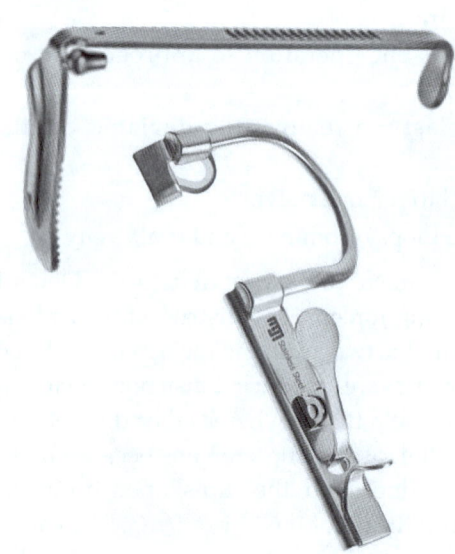

Fig. 41.25

2. **Davis Gag**

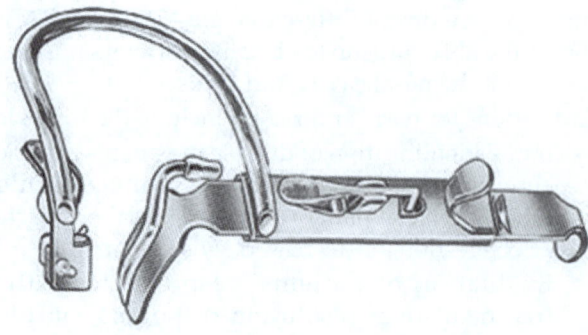

Fig. 41.26

Davis-Boyle mouth gag set arranged

This instrument is part of the tonsillectomy set.

The Boyle Davis mouth gag consists of the Davis gag, a frame that serves to hold the mouth open and the Boyle tongue depressor to hold the tongue down. The tongue depressor comes in several sizes, from paediatric to adult.

Mouth gags are used to keep the patient's mouth open during oral surgery, leaving both hands of the surgeon free to operate.

Uses

Used in oral and oropharyngeal surgeries:
- Adenoidectomy
- Tonsillectomy
- UPPP and other procedures on the soft palate
- Procedures on the hard palate like cyst or tumour excision

It cannot be used to perform procedures on the tongue as it is completely held down by the tongue blade. This instrument can cause injury to the lips and teeth. Care must be taken while applying the mouth gag to avoid getting the lips caught in it.

Eve's Tonsillar Snare

This instrument is part of the tonsillectomy set and is used in the step of removing the dissected tonsil from its final attachment to the fossa.

It consists of a long, thin, hollow tube with a stainless steel wire loop at one end and three large rings at the other. These three rings allow the instrument to be operated using three fingers.

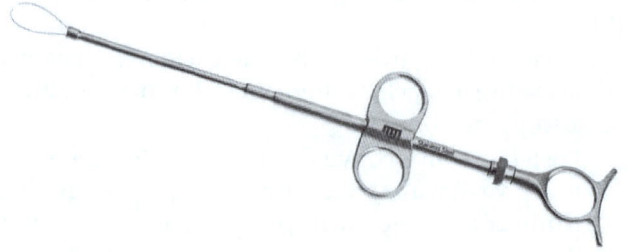

Fig. 41.27

Use: The tonsillar snare is used to both cut and crush the pedicle of the dissected tonsil. Cutting and crushing the pedicle rather than just cutting it helps reduce haemorrhage.

- Earlier, snares were also used to remove ear and nasal polyps, too. Ear polyps should never be avulsed as it may be arising from vital areas, e.g. dehiscent facial nerve, oval window. For managing nasal polyps, FESS is the surgery of choice these days.

Denis Browne Tonsil Holding Forceps

Tonsil holding forceps are long with the shaft bent at an angle to the handle. The tips are cup-shaped with holes. The edges of the tips are smooth to just hold tissue, without cutting.

This instrument is used in tonsillectomy operations.

Uses: Tonsil holding forceps are used to hold the tonsil during tonsillectomy. The tonsil is grasped gently and then pulled medially. This step helps hold the tonsil away from its bed to facilitate dissection and prevent injury to structures in the bed of the tonsil.

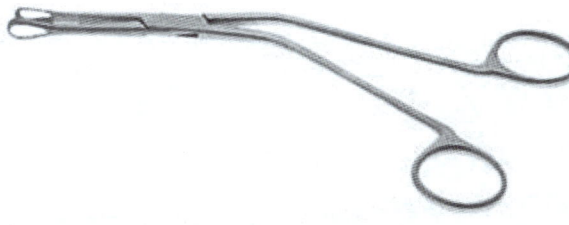

Fig. 41.28

St. Clair Thomson Adenoid Curette

The adenoid curette is used in adenoidectomy operations.

The instrument has a strong handle, a shaft and a curette at the tip. The curette itself is a curved, square window that allows adenoid tissue to engage in it.

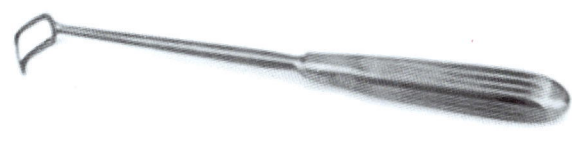

Fig. 41.29

St. Clair Thomson Adenoid Curette with Cage

An adenoid curette with cage comes with a detachable guard that has teeth to hold the removed tissue.

For the adenoidectomy operation, the patient lies in Roses position. The mouth is held open with a mouth gag. Adenoid is palpated to bring the adenoid tissue in midline and also to rule out aberrant vessel overlying the adenoid. The curette is held at the handle like a dagger. The curette is then introduced into the oral cavity, all the way above and behind the soft palate. The adenoid tissue is caught

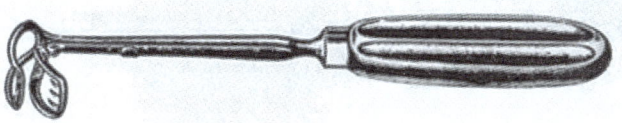

Fig. 41.30

in the curette, the head is flexed and adenoid tissue is removed with a smooth, sweeping movement.

- A nasal endoscope can now be used to visualize the procedure. Endoscopic adenoidectomy achieves better results and lesser complications as the procedure is performed under visualization.

Laryngoscopy

Laryngoscopy may be done in the following ways:
- Indirect laryngoscopy using a laryngeal mirror.
- Laryngoscopy using rigid and flexible endoscopes.
- Laryngoscopy using strobe light (stroboscope).
- Direct laryngoscopy using a laryngoscope.

Indirect Laryngoscopy

Laryngeal Mirror

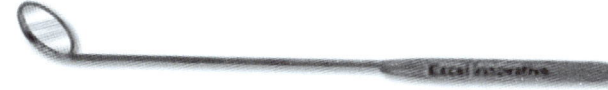

Fig. 41.31

It is an instrument used for viewing the larynx and surrounding area during indirect laryngoscopy.

Direct Laryngoscopy

Curved blade (Macintosh) and straight blade (Miller) laryngoscopes with locking handles.

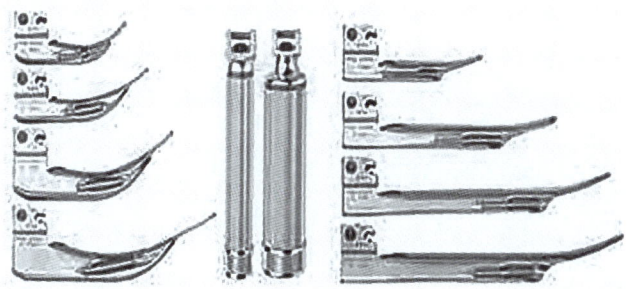

Fig. 41.32

Kleinsasser Suspension Laryngoscope

Kleinsasser suspension laryngoscope with chest stand.

It is used in microlaryngoscopy.

The equipment consists of a short tubular laryngoscope that is locked to a supporting arm that rests on a base plate lying against the anterior chest wall. This arrangement leaves the surgeon's hands free to use instruments and even to position an operating microscope for precise surgery.

Important Instruments in ENT

Section V

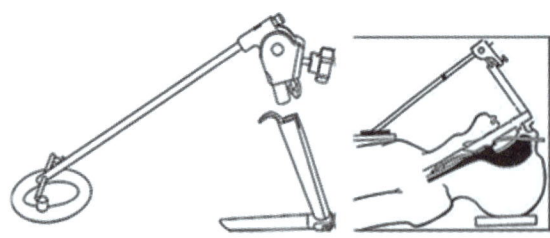

Fig. 41.33

The surgical procedures that can be done with the Kleinsasser suspension laryngoscope include excision of vocal polyps, nodules, laser vaporisation of papillomas, stripping of vocal cord mucosa, taking biopsy, etc.

Stroboscope

A stroboscope, also known as a strobe, is an instrument used to make a cyclically moving object appear to be slow-moving, or stationary. The principle is used for the study of vibrating objects.

Stroboscopes are used to view the vocal cords for diagnosis of conditions producing dysphonia.

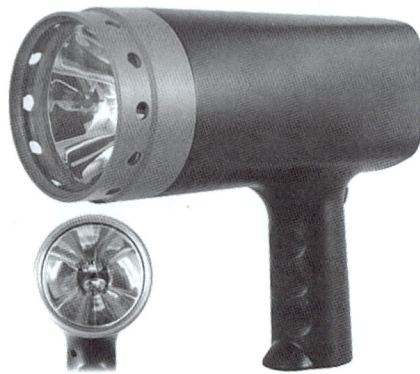

Fig. 41.34

Portex Uncuffed Tracheostomy Tube

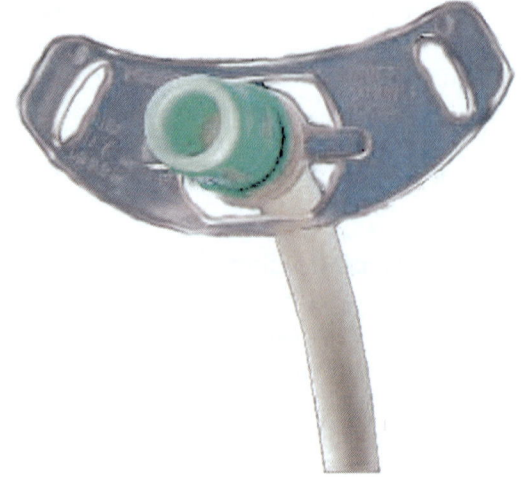

Fig. 41.35

Cricoid Hook

A cricoid hook is used to secure the cricoid cartilage with a hook and elevate it superiorly to facilitate the control of the tracheal entry by pulling up the cricoid cartilage and trachea to a superficial position.

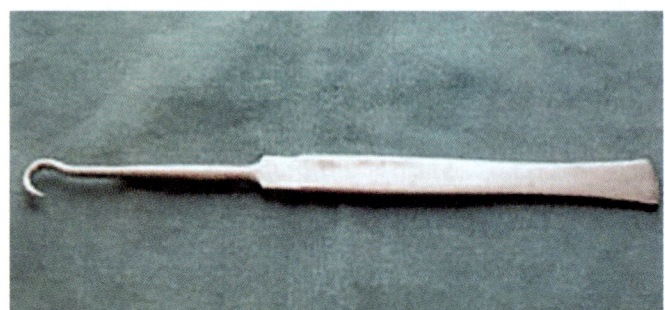

Fig. 41.36

Section V Important Instruments in ENT

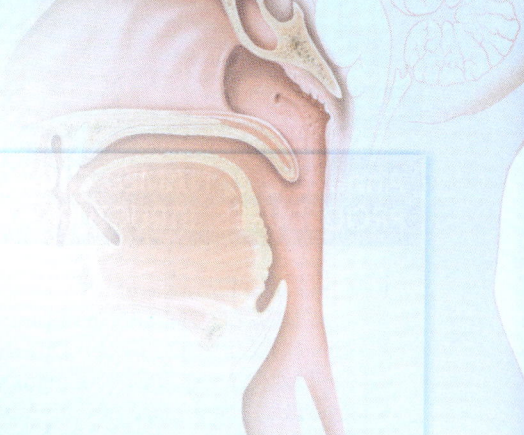

Annexures

Annexure 1: CHILDHOOD HEARING IMPAIRMENT

Congenital causes (66%)

1. *Genetic*
   a. Non-syndromic (70%)
   b. Syndromic (30%)

Syndrome	Inheritance pattern	Features
Usher	Autosomal recessive (AR)	Severe to profound SNHL, vestibular dysfunction, retinitis pigmentosa. This is the most common syndrome among the autosomal recessive syndromes
Pendred	AR	Severe SNHL, goitre
Jervell and Lange-Nielsen	AR	Congenital hearing loss, QT prolongation on ECG
Alport	X: linked dominant (is the most common inheritance pattern)	Hereditary glomerulonephritis, renal failure in males, progressive high frequency SNHL, anterior lenticonus
Waardenburg	Autosomal dominant (AD)	SNHL, pigmentation abnormalities of hairs, eyes and skin, Dystopia canthorum (wide distance between the inner corners of the eyes). This is the most common among the autosomal dominant syndromes
Branchio-oto-renal	AD	Branchial cysts, ear deformities and renal malformations
Stickler	AD	Progressive SNHL, cleft palate, vertebral abnormalities, abnormal development of epiphysis
Neurofibromatosis type 2	AD	B/L vestibular schwannoma

2. *Non-genetic*: Maternal infections like CMV **(MC)**, rubella, syphilis and toxoplasmosis. Use of ototoxic drugs, substance abuse and endocrine disorders during pregnancy.

Acquired Causes (33%)

   i. Infections: Meningitis **(MC)**, measles, mumps, varicella, herpes, toxoplasmosis and chronic otitis media
  ii. Hypoxia
 iii. Hyperbilirubinemia
  iv. Ototoxic drugs
   v. Noise trauma
  vi. Leukaemia and lymphomas

Annexure 2: NAMED CLINICAL/RADIOLOGICAL SIGNS, SYNDROMES, TESTS, FINDINGS, PROCEDURES, STRUCTURES AND ORGANISMS IN ENT

1. *Tragal sign*: Furuncle of EAC
2. *Cauliflower ear*: Hematoma of pinna
3. *Swimmer's or telephonist ear*: Diffuse otitis externa
4. *Skull base osteomyelitis*: Malignant otitis externa
5. *Prussak's space*: Space of epitympanum, medial to pars flaccida, MC site of primary cholesteatoma
6. *Donaldson's line*: Surgical land mark for endolymphatic sac
7. *Trautmann's triangle*: Land mark on medial wall of mastoid antrum for approaching posterior cranial fossa
8. *Macewen's triangle*: Land mark of mastoid antrum
9. *Canal of Huguier*: Opening on anterior wall of middle ear for exit of Chorda tympani
10. *Bill's bar*: Vertical crest in IAM
11. *Korner's septum*: Persistent petro-squamosal suture
12. *Arnold's nerve*: Auricular branch of vagus
13. *Jacobson's nerve*: Tympanic branch of glossopharyngeal
14. *Nerve of Wrisberg/nervus intermedius*: Sensory bundle of facial nerve
15. *Fissures of Santorini*: Deficiency in cartilaginous EAC
16. *Foramen of Huschke*: Deficiency in bony EAC
17. *Hennebert sign*: Congenital syphilis, some cases of Meniere's
18. *Light house sign (pulsatile otorrhoea)*: ASOM, acute mastoiditis
19. *Pulsatile tinnitus*: Glomus
20. *Pulsation/Brown's sign*: Glomus
21. *Phlep's sign*: Glomus
22. *Reservoir sign*: Acute mastoiditis
23. *Reservoir sign/tea-pot sign*: CSF rhinorrhoea
24. *Bezold abscess*: Mastoiditis abscess in relation to sternocleidomastoid
25. *Citelli's abscess*: Mastoiditis abscess in relation to posterior belly of digastric
26. *Citelli's angle*: Sino dural angle
27. *Gradenigo'striad*: Petrositis
28. *Griesinger's sign*: Mastoid emissary vein obstruction in lateral sinus thrombosis
29. *Delta/Empty triangle sign*: Lateral sinus thrombosis
30. *Crowe-Beck sign*: Lateral sinus thrombosis
31. *Tobey Ayer/Queckenstedt's test*: Lateral sinus thrombosis
32. *Schwartze sign/Flammingo pink sign*: Active otosclerosis
33. *Schwartze surgery*: Acute mastoiditis
34. *Cart wheel TM*: ASOM
35. *Red reflex/rising/setting sun appearance*: Glomus
36. *Vanderhoeve syndrome*: Otosclerosis, osteogenesis imperfecta, blue sclera
37. *Carhartz notch*: Dip at 2000 Hz in BC in Otosclerosis
38. *Acoustic dip*: Dip at 4000 Hz in both AC & BC in noise trauma
39. *Tullio's phenomenon*: Meniere's disease
40. *Tumarkin crisis*: Meniere's disease
41. *Lermoyez syndrome*: Reverse Meniere's
42. *Diplacusis*: Meniere's disease
43. *Paracusis Willisii phenomenon*: Otosclerosis
44. *Dix-Hallpike test*: BPPV
45. *Epley's/canal repositioning manoeuvre*: BPPV
46. *Fitzgerald Hallpike test*: Bi-thermal caloric test
47. *Kobrak test*: Cold caloric test
48. *Kernig's sign*: Meningitis
49. *Brudzinski's sign*: Meningitis
50. *Hitzelberger sign*: Acoustic neuroma/vestibular schwannoma
51. *Furstenberg test*: Meningocele, meningoencephalocele
52. *Onodi cell*: Posterior ethmoidal cell lateral to the sphenoid sinus
53. *Haller cell*: Intraorbital anterior ethmoidal cell
54. *Mulberry turbinate/mucosa*: Hypertrophic turbinate
55. *Mulberry/strawberry mass in nose*: Rhinosporidiosis
56. *Cottle's test*: Patency of nasal valve test
57. *Potato nose*: Rhinophyma
58. *Hard/Woody/Hebra/Tapir nose*: Rhinoscleroma
59. *Frisch Bacillus*: Klebsiella rhinoscleromatis
60. *Mikulicz cell*: Rhinoscleroma
61. *Russell bodies*: Rhinoscleroma
62. *CHARGE syndrome*: Choanal atresia
63. *Samter's triad*: Nasal polyps, asthma, aspirin sensitivity
64. *Young's syndrome*: Recurrent sinusitis, bronchiectasis, azoospermia
65. *Kartagener's syndrome*: Recurrent sinusitis, bronchiectasis, situs inversus
66. *Double ring/Halo/Target sign*: Traumatic CSF rhinorrhoea
67. *Double density sign*: Allergic fungal sinusitis
68. *Tear drop sign*: Blow out fracture
69. *Rodent ulcer*: BCC
70. *Ohngren's line*: Maxillary sinus Ca classification
71. *Weber Fergussen incision*: Maxillectomy
72. *Ringertz tumour*: Inverted papilloma
73. *Adenoid facies*: Adenoid hypertrophy
74. *Frog facies*: Angiofibroma
75. *Holman*: Miller/antral -gn-Angiofibroma
76. *Dodd's/crescent sign*: Antrochoanal polyp
77. *Trotter's triad*: Nasopharyngeal Ca
78. *Trotter's/Hippocratic method*: Pinching of nose in epistaxis
79. *Woodruff's plexus*: Venous plexus posterior to inferior turbinate
80. *Kieselbach's plexus*: Arterial plexus at Little's area
81. *Irwin Moore sign*: Chronic tonsillitis
82. *Moure's sign*: Post-cricoid Ca
83. *Plummer Vinson/Patterson Kelly Brown syndrome*: Iron deficiency anemia, hypopharyngeal web, post cricoid dysphagia
84. *Ground glass appearance*: Fibrous dysplasia
85. *Roses position*: Adenoidectomy, tonsillectomy, tracheostomy
86. *Boyce position*: DL, bronchoscopy, oesophagoscopy
87. *Boyce sign*: Zenker's diverticulum
88. *Bryce sign*: Laryngocele
89. *Lushka's/nasopharyngeal tonsils*: Adenoids
90. *Gerlach tonsils*: Tubal tonsils
91. *Thumb sign*: Acute epiglottitis
92. *Steeple/pencil tip sign*: Croup
93. *Elongated omega epiglottis*: Laryngomalacia
94. *Space of Boyer*: Pre-epiglottic space
95. *Space of Tucker*: Paraglottic space
96. *Reinke's space*: Submucosal space of true VC
97. *Turban epiglottis*: TB larynx
98. *Mamillated arytenoids*: TB larynx
99. *Mouse nibbled VC*: TB larynx

Annexures

100. *Styalgia/Eagle's syndrome*: Elongated calcified styloid process
101. *Space of Gillette*: Retropharyngeal space
102. *Nodes of Rouviere*: Lymph nodes in retropharyngeal space
103. *Killian's dehiscence*: Site of Zenker's diverticulum
104. *Dohlman's procedure*: Zenker's diverticulum
105. *Galen anastomosis*: Sensory anastomosis between branches of internal and recurrent laryngeal nerves
106. *Ortner's/Cardiovocal syndrome*: Mitral stenosis, left recurrent laryngeal nerve palsy
107. *Frey's syndrome*: Gustatory sweating due to auriculotemporal nerve injury
108. *Crocodile tears*: Gustatory lacrimation
109. *Sluder's neuralgia*: Anterior ethmoidal neuralgia seen in DNS
110. *Water's view*: X-ray PNS occipito-mental view
111. *Caldwell's view*: X-ray PNS occipito-frontal view
112. *Caldwell Luc's surgery*: Sublabial approach to maxillary sinus
113. *Luc's abscess*: Mastoiditis abscess in relation to posterior wall of EAC

Annexure 3: MICROBES INVOLVED IN ENT INFECTIONS

Microbe	*Conditions*
1. *Pseudomonas aeruginosa*	i. Perichondritis of pinna ii. Diffuse otitis externa iii. Malignant otitis externa iv. CSOM (mixed-MC Pseudomonas)
2. *Streptococcus pneumoniae*	i. ASOM ii. Acute mastoiditis iii. Acute sinusitis iv. Acute pharyngitis v. Myringitis bullosa vi. Meningitis (as a complication of ASOM/CSOM)
3. Group A Beta hemolytic Streptococcus (GABHS)	i. ANOM ii. Acute tonsillitis iii. Acute epiglottitis
4. *Staphylococcus aureus*	i. Furuncle of EAC ii. Chronic sinusitis (mixed, MC-Staph)
5. *Borrelia vincenti* and *F. fusiformis*	• Vincent's angina
6. *Klebsiella ozaenae*	• Atrophic rhinitis
7. *Klebsiella rhinoscleromatis*	• Rhinoscleroma
8. *Rhinosporidium seeberi* (aquatic protozoa)	• Rhinosporidiosis
9. *Aspergillus niger* (MC), others—Candida, *Aspergillus fumigatus*	• Otomycosis
10. *Aspergillus fumigatus*, flavus	i. Fungal ball ii. Allergic fungal sinusitis iii. Invasive fungal sinusitis (immunocompromised)
11. Dermataceous fungi (bipolaris)	• Allergic fungal sinusitis
12. Mucor and Rhizopus	• Mucormycosis (immunocompromised)
13. Influenza (2nd MC)	• Myringitis bullosa
14. Varicella zoster	• Ramsay Hunt syndrome
15. HSV–1	• Bell's palsy
16. Parainfluenza	• Croup
17. Rhinovirus (MC)	• Acute rhinitis
18. HPV-6, 11	• Juvenile laryngeal papillomatosis
19. HPV-16, 18	• Oropharyngeal Ca
20. EBV	• Nasopharyngeal Ca

Annexures

Annexure 4: SURGERIES/PROCEDURES IN ENT

Surgery	Indication
1. Myringotomy in postero-inferior quadrant	• ASOM with impending perforation
2. Myringotomy with Grommet in antero-inferior quadrant	• SOM
3. Myringoplasty	• Mucosal/safe CSOM
4. Tympanoplasty	i. Mucosal/safe CSOM ii. Ossicular discontinuity iii. As a part of MRM
5. MRM/canal wall down mastoidectomy	• Unsafe CSOM with or without complications
6. Posterior tympanotomy/intact canal wall mastoidectomy	i. Unsafe CSOM with limited disease ii. While inserting cochlear implant
7. Schwartze operation	• Acute mastoiditis
8. Microwick	• To insert drugs into inner ear through round window i. Gentamycin in Meniere's ii. Steroids in SSNHL and Meniere's
9. Stapedotomy	• Otosclerosis
10. Endolymphatic sac decompression	• Meniere's
11. Cochlear implant	• B/L severe to profound hearing loss
12. ABI (auditory brainstem implant)	• Following B/L acoustic neuroma excision in NF-type 2
13. BAHA (bone anchored hearing aid)	i. Congenital deformity of Pinna and EAC ii. Discharging cavities following MRM iii. Single deaf ear
14. FESS	i. Chronic rhinosinusitis ii. Allergic fungal sinusitis iii. Fungal ball iv. Nasal polyps and its recurrence v. Fronto-ethmoidal mucocele
15. Septoplasty	• DNS
16. Rhinoplasty	• External deformity of nose
17. Inferior turbinectomy	• Hypertrophic inferior turbinate
18. TESPAL (transnasal endoscopic spheno-palatine artery ligation)	• Epistaxis
19. Septodermoplasty	• Epistaxis in hereditary hemorrhagic telangiectasia/ Osler-Weber-Rendu syndrome
20. Young's operation	• Atrophic rhinitis
21. Vidian neurectomy	• Vasomotor rhinitis
22. Caldwell-Luc operation	• Sub-labial approach to maxillary antrum and sphenopalatine foramen
23. Lynch Howarth procedure	i. To approach frontal sinus for mucocele, pyocele, osteoma excision ii. Anterior ethmoidal artery ligation
24. Adenoidectomy	• Adenoid hypertrophy
25. Marsupialisation	i. Thornwaldt's bursitis ii. Ranula (as 2nd choice, the first being excision of cyst with sublingual gland excision)

(Contd.)

(Contd.)

Surgery	Indication
26. Tonsillectomy	i. Recurrent tonsillitis ii. Obstructive sleep apnoea iii. Chronic tonsillitis iv. Peritonsillar abscess (quinsy) v. Tonsillar malignancy vi. Streptococcal/diphtherial carriers vii. As an approach to styloid process in Eagle's syndrome viii. As an approach to glossopharyngeal nerve in glossopharyngeal neuralgia
27. UPPP (uvulo-palato-pharyngo-plasty)	• Obstructive sleep apnoea
28. Endoscopic diverticulotomy	• Zenker's diverticulum
29. COMMANDO operation	• Radical resection of oral and oropharyngeal Ca
30. Botulinum toxin	i. Crocodile tears ii. Frey's syndrome iii. Spasmodic dysphonia
31. MLS (microlaryngeal surgery)	i. Vocal nodule ii. Vocal polyp
32. Thyroplasty I, II, III, IV	I. Medialisation, U/L complete palsy II. Lateralisation, B/L recurrent laryngeal N palsy III. Shortening, puberophonia IV. Lengthening, androphonia
33. Woodman's procedure	• Lateralisation of vocal cord
34. Kashima's procedure	• Lateralisation of vocal cord
35. Tracheo-oesophageal diversion	• Chronic aspiration following B/L complete palsy
36. Mitomycin C	To reduce synechiae in the following surgeries: i. Nasal packs following nasal surgeries ii. Following choanal atresia repair iii. Following repair of laryngotracheal stenosis
37. Reduction glottoplasty	• Reinke's oedema
38. TLM (transoral LASER microsurgery) with CO_2 LASER	• Stage I and II Ca larynx (1st choice)
39. Partial laryngectomy (horizontal and vertical)	i. Stage I and II Ca larynx (2nd choice after TLM/Radiotherapy) ii. Stage I and II Ca larynx recurrence following radiotherapy
40. Total laryngectomy	i. T4a Ca larynx ii. Stage III, IV Ca larynx recurrence after radiotherapy

Annexures

Recent Exam Questions and New Pattern Questions

1. **Widening cartilaginous part of EAC is known as:**
   a. Myringoplasty
   b. Tympanoplasty
   c. Meatoplasty
   d. Otoplasty

2. **TB otitis media is characterized by all except:**
   a. Ear ache
   b. Multiple perforation
   c. Pale granulation
   d. Ear discharge

3. **Patient presents with U/L proptosis with B/L abducens palsy. Diagnosis is:**
   a. Cavernous sinus thrombosis
   b. Orbital cellulitis
   c. Orbital pseudo-tumour
   d. Orbital lymphoma

4. **On stimulating the outer part of EAC a person gets cough. This is because of stimulation of:**
   a. Auricular branch of vagus.
   b. Auriculotemporal
   c. Greater auricular
   d. Facial

5. **Partial closure of nostril is done in which condition?**
   a. Atrophic rhinitis
   b. Allergic rhinitis
   c. Vasomotor rhinitis
   d. Fungal sinusitis

6. **Saccule develops from:**
   a. Sacculus medius
   b. Sacculus posticus
   c. Pars superior
   d. Pars inferior

7. **Child is brought to the OPD with the history of fever and sore throat. On examination the throat shows the following appearance. Diagnosis is:**

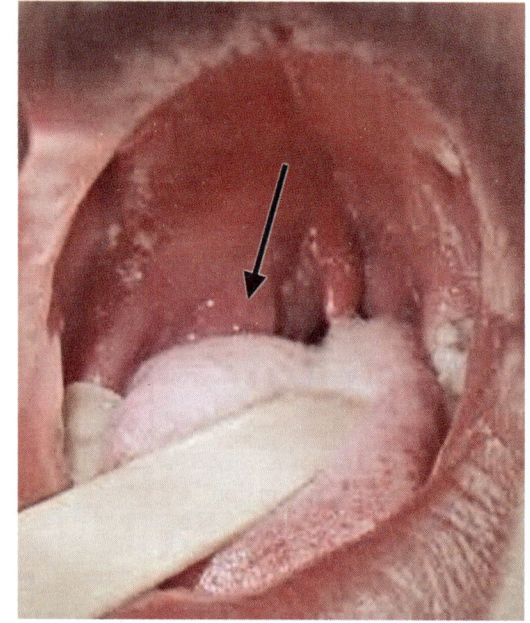

   a. Peritonsillar abscess b. Retropharyngeal
   c. Prevertebral   d. Ludwigs

8. **The sign seen in the given X-ray is:**

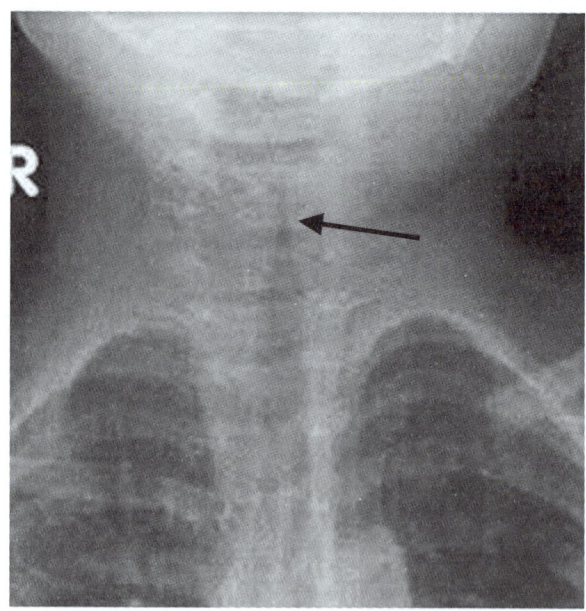

428

a. Thumb sign   b. Steeple sign
c. Halo sign   d. Browns sign

9. **Following car accident, the patient presents with the following appearance. It is known as:**

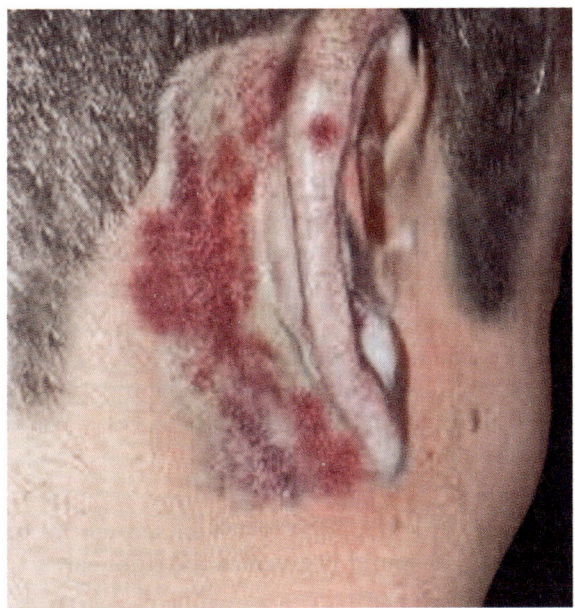

a. Bezold abscess   b. Battle sign
c. Griesinger's sign   d. Raccoon sign

10. **A patient undergoes surgery of the lateral part of the base of skull. Postoperatively the patient presents with aspiration but does not have a change in voice. Which of the following is injured?**
    a. Glossopharyngeal nerve
    b. SLN
    c. RLN
    d. High vagal

11. **Superior semicircular canal dehiscence presents with all except:**
    a. Autophony   b. Tullio phenomenon
    c. Aural fullness   d. SNHL

12. **After a surgery in the carotid triangle a patient presented with weak voice. Which structure is injured?**
    a. Internal laryngeal   b. External laryngeal
    c. Ansa cervicalis   d. Recurrent laryngeal nerve

13. **Occipitomental view of paranasal sinuses with open mouth:**
    a. Waters' view   b. Pierre view
    c. Caldwell view   d. Stenvers view

14. **A patient presents with bilateral hearing loss and hearing better in noisy environment. Rinne's is negative in both the ears and Weber's is centralized. Most probable diagnosis is:**
    a. Meniere
    b. Otosclerosis
    c. Acoustic neuroma
    d. Nasopharyngeal carcinoma

15. **Which of the arteries supplying the septum is not a branch of external carotid artery?**
    a. Sphenopalatine artery
    b. Superior labial artery
    c. Anterior ethmoidal artery
    d. Greater palatine

16. **Following parotidectomy patient had numbness while shaving. The nerve to be involved is:**
    a. Facial
    b. Auriculotemporal
    c. Greater auricular
    d. Maxillary

17. **In radical neck dissection which is spared:**
    a. Submandibular gland
    b. Level II lymph nodes
    c. Sublingual gland
    d. Tail of parotid

18. **Arrange the structures of the auditory pathway in the sequential order of sound transmission:**
    1. Cochlear nerve
    2. Superior olivary complex
    3. Inferior colliculus
    4. Cochlear nuclei
    5. Lateral lemniscus
    6. Medial geniculate body
    a. 1, 4, 2, 5, 3, 6   b. 1, 2, 3, 4, 5, 6
    c. 6, 3, 2, 5, 4, 1   d. 1, 2, 5, 4, 6, 3

RECENT PATTERN QUESTIONS BY THE AUTHOR

19. **Structures passing through the inferior segment of internal acoustic meatus:**
    1. Cochlear nerve
    2. Superior vestibular
    3. Inferior vestibular nerve
    4. Facial nerve
    5. Singular
    a. 1, 3, 5   b. 4, 2
    c. 1, 3, 4   d. 3, 4, 5

20. **Match the following:**
    a. Fistula test positive   1. Hennebert sign
    b. Fistula test false   2. Fenestration operation
       positive   3. Otosclerosis
    c. Fistula test negative   4. Dead labyrinth
    d. Fistula test false   5. Tullios phenomenon
       negative

21. **Arrange the following structures on the posterior of middle ear from lateral to medial:**
    1. Chorda tympani
    2. Facial recess
    3. Vertical segment of facial nerve
    4. Sinus tympani
    a. 1, 2, 3, 4   b. 1, 4, 2, 3
    c. 3, 2, 4, 1   d. 1, 3, 2, 4

22. **Assertion: Myringotomy is done in postero-superior quadrant.**
    Reason: In postero- superior quadrant there are less chances of injury to middle ear structures.
    a. Assertion true: Reason true. Reason is the correct explanation for assertion
    b. Assertion true: Reason true. Reason is not the correct explanation for the assertion
    c. Assertion true: Reason false
    d. Assertion false: Reason true
    e. Aseertion false: Reason false

23. **Arrange the following from lateral to medial:**
    1. MacEwen's triangle
    2. Korners' septum
    3. Mastoid antrum
    4. Trautmann's triangle
    5. Posterior cranial fossa
    a. 1, 4, 2, 5, 3   b. 1, 2, 4, 5, 3
    c. 1, 2, 3, 4, 5   d. 3, 5, 2, 4, 1

24. **The test shown in the given picture measures sound transmission in the following sequence:**

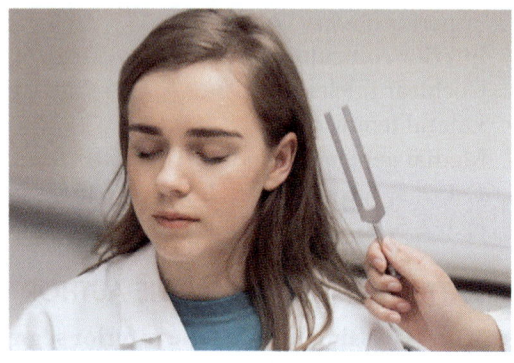

    a. EAC, middle ear, organ of Corti, auditory pathway
    b. Auditory pathway, organ of Corti
    c. EAC, middle ear
    d. EAC, middle ear, auditory pathway, organ of Corti

25. **Match the following:**
    Audiogram diagnosis
    a. Upsloping   1. Ototoxicity
    b. Downsloping   2. Noise trauma
    c. Trough   3. Otosclerosis
    d. Carhartz notch   4. Meniere
    e. Dip at 4k   5. Safe CSOM
        6. Traumatic perforation
        7. Midfrequency hearing

26. **Match the following:**
    1. Increased compliance, normal pressure
    2. Decreased compliance, normal pressure
    3. Decreased compliance, negative pressure
    4. Normal compliance, negative pressure
    a. Otosclerosis
    b. Ossicular discontinuity
    c. Early Eustachian tube obstruction
    d. Nasopharyngeal carcinoma
    e. Meniere
    f. Labyrinthitis

27. **Arrange the stapedial reflex in sequential order when loud sound is given in the right ear.**
    1. Organ of Corti
    2. Superior olivary complex
    3. Bilateral stapedius
    4. Middle ear
    5. Cochlear nerve
    6. Bilateral facial nerve
    a. 4, 1, 5, 2, 6, 3   b. 1, 5, 2, 4, 6, 3
    c. 3, 6, 2, 5, 1, 4   d. 4, 6, 5, 3, 2, 1

28. **A 31-year-old female patient complains of B/L impairment of hearing for the past 5 years. Audiogram shows a B/L conductive deafness. Impedance audiometry is given below. Stapedial reflex is absent in both ears. All constitute part of surgery in this patient:**

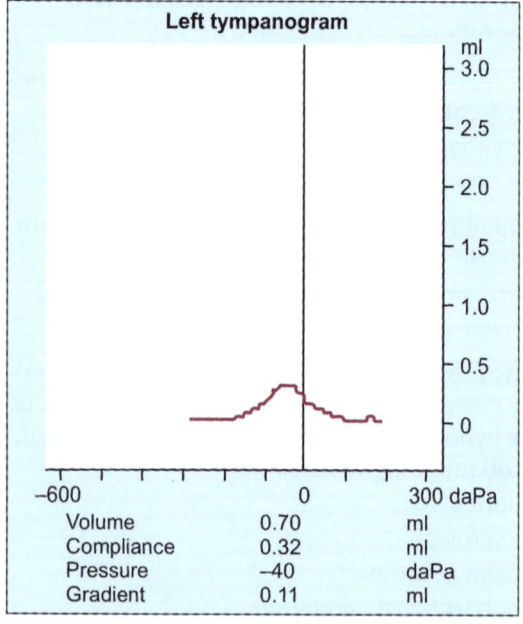

Right tympanogram		
Volume	0.79	ml
Compliance	0.17	ml
Pressure	–12	daPa
Gradient	0.06	ml

Left tympanogram		
Volume	0.70	ml
Compliance	0.32	ml
Pressure	–40	daPa
Gradient	0.11	ml

a. Removal of anterior crura of stapes

b. MRM

c. Sectioning of stapedius tendon

d. Removal of lenticular process of incus

e. Myringotomy

f. Vestibular neurectomy

g. Removal of posterior crura of stapes

1. a, c, d, g   2. a, c, g

3. c, d, e, g   4. a, g

29. **Match the following:**
1. Cauliflower ear
2. Itchy and cotton wool appearance
3. Localised swelling in outer EAC with pain increasing on jaw movement
4. Granulation discharge necrosis of EAC in elderly diabetic

a. Clotrimazole ear drops

b. Ceftazidime

c. Amoxiclav

d. Hematoma

e. Gentamicin

30. **Match the following:**

1. Paracusis Willsii	a. Age related hearing loss
2. Diplacusis	b. Vertigo on loud sounds
3. Presbycusis	c. Normal sounds appearing loud
4. Hyperacusis	d. Double hearing
5. Recruitment	e. Hearing better in noisy surrounding
	f. Loud sounds becoming louder

31. **Match the following:**
Tympanic membrane appearance

1. Red	a. ASOM
2. Flamingo pink	b. Hematoma
3. White patches	c. Normal
4. Red reflex	d. Otosclerosis
5. Blue	e. Tympanosclerosis
	f. Glomus
	g. Acoustic neuroma

32. **Match the following:**

1. Hearing aid	a. Organ of Corti defect
2. BAHA	b. Atresia of external ear
3. Cochlear implant	c. NF2 operated for B/L acoustic neuroma
4. Auditory brainstem implant	d. Otosclerosis

33. **Obstruction in which areas can lead to inspiratory stridor?**
1. Supraglottis   2. Glottis
3. Subglottis   4. Nasopharynx
5. Bronchi

a. 1, 2, 3   b. 1, 2, 4

c. 1, 2   d. 2, 3, 5

34. **In which vocal cord palsy can the voice be normal?**
1. U/L RLN palsy
2. B/L RLN palsy
3. U/L complete palsy
4. B/L complete palsy

a. 1, 2, 3   b. 1, 2

c. 2, 4   d. 1, 2, 4

35. **Assertion: MC sinusitis is maxillary.**
Reason: Maxillary sinus is the largest sinus.

a. Assertion true: Reason true. Reason is the correct explanation for assertion

b. Assertion true: Reason true. Reason is not the correct explanation for the assertion

c. Assertion true: Reason false

d. Assertion false: Reason true

e. Aseertion false: Reason false

36. **Place the following sinuses in their order of development**

1. Maxillary	a. 1, 3, 2, 4
2. Spheroid	b. 1, 2, 3, 4
3. Ethmoid	c. 1, 3, 4, 5
4. Frontal	d. 1, 4, 3, 5

37. **Match the following:**
Presentation
1. U/L nasal polyp in young male
2. U/L polypoidal mass in young male with recurrent epistaxis
3. B/L multiple polyps in middle age
4. U/L multiple polyps in middle age with mucinous secretions and heterogeneous appearance on CT scan
5. U/L polyp mass in elderly
6. U/L polypoidal mass with CT showing pneumatised middle turbinate

Diagnosis

a. Allergic fungal sinusitis

b. Mucormycosis

c. Rhinoscleroma

d. Antrochoanal polyp

e. Ethmoidal polyp

f. Malignancy

g. Concha bullosa

h. Angiofibroma

38. **Assertion: Mucormycosis is life threatening.**
Reason: Mucormycosis is angio-invasive.

a. Assertion true: Reason true. Reason is the correct explanation for assertion

b. Assertion true: Reason true. Reason is not the correct explanation for the assertion

c. Assertion true: Reason false

d. Assertion false: Reason true

e. Aseertion false: Reason false

39. **Assertion: Adenoid hypertrophy leads to rhinolalia-clausa**

Reason: Adenoid hypertrophy leads to velopharyngeal insufficiency.

a. Assertion true: Reason true. Reason is the correct explanation for assertion

b. Assertion true: Reason true. Reason is not the correct explanation for the assertion

c. Assertion true: Reason false

d. Assertion false: Reason true

e. Aseertion false: Reason false

40. **Arrange the spread of angiofibroma in sequential arrangement:**

1. Sphenopalatine foramen
2. Orbits
3. Sphenopalatine fossa
4. Infratemporal fossa

a. 1, 2, 3, 4   b. 1, 3, 2, 4

c. 3, 2, 1, 4   d. 3, 1, 2, 4

41. **Which of the following are lined by ciliated columnar epithelium?**

1. Nasopharyngeal tonsil
2. Faucial tonsils
3. Maxillary sinus
4. True vocal cords
5. Nasal cavity

a. 1, 2, 5   b. 1, 3, 4, 5

c. 1, 3, 5   d. 2, 4, 5

42. **Match the following:**

Symptoms diagnosis

1. Raised floor of mouth
2. U/L paramedian bulge of postpharyngeal wall
3. U/L tonsils pushed medially
4. U/L tonsils pushed medially with bulge at angle of jaw

a. Retropharyngeal abscess

b. Parapharyngeal abscess

c. Quinsy

d. Ludwig's angina

e. Vincent's angina

ANSWERS AND EXPLANATIONS

1. **(c) Meatoplasty**
2. **(a) Ear ache**
3. **(a) Cavernous sinus thrombosis**
4. **(a) Auricular branch of vagus**
5. **(a) Atrophic rhinitis**
6. **(d) Pars inferior**

   The inner ear is separated into two portions: The pars superior and the pars inferior. The semicircular canals and the utricle develop earlier and belong to the pars superior, and the saccule along with the organ of Corti develop later and belong to the pars inferior.
7. **(a) Peritonsillar abscess**
8. **(b) Steeple sign**
9. **(b) Battle sign**
   - Battle sign is present with a basilar skull fracture involving the temporal bone.
   - Battle sign presents as ecchymosis over the mastoid process, located behind the ear. It is typically associated with tenderness of the area as well. Other findings that may be seen that indicate basilar skull fracture include raccoon eyes (periorbital ecchymosis), hemotympanum (which is the presence of blood in the tympanic cavity of the middle ear), facial nerve injury and laceration of the external auditory canal.
10. **(b) SLN**
    - The SLN comprises ILN and ELN. ILN (sensory to supraglottis) injury will result in aspiration. External laryngeal supplies cricothyroid which is for tensing the vocal cords and raising the pitch. If injured will result in inability to raise the pitch of voice, otherwise the voice will be normal.
    - High vagal injury will result in complete palsy of both SLN and RLN and result in aphonia and aspiration.
    - RLN injury will result in stridor.
11. **(d) SNHL**
12. **(b) External laryngeal**
    - External laryngeal supplies cricothyroid which is for tensing the vocal cords and raising the pitch. If

injured will result in inability to raise the pitch of voice.
13. **(b) Pierre view**
    - Occipitomental view of paranasal sinuses is known as Waters' view
    - Occipitomental view of paranasal sinuses with open mouth is known as pierres view
14. **(b) Otosclerosis**
15. **(c) Anterior ethmoidal artery**
16. **(b) Auriculotemporal**
17. **(c) Sublingual gland**
18. **(d) 1, 2, 5, 4, 6, 3**
19. **(a) 1, 3, 5**
20. **a. 2, b. 1, c. 3, d. 4**
21. **a. 1, 2, 3, 4**
22. **(e) Aseertion false: Reason false**
23. **(c) 1, 2, 3, 4, 5**
24. **(a) EAC, middle ear, organ of Corti, auditory pathway**
25. **a. 4, b. 1, c. 7, d. 3, e. 2**
26. **1. b, 2. a, 3. d, 4. c**
27. **a. 4, 1, 5, 2, 6, 3**
28. **2. a, c, g**
29. **1. d, 2. a, 3. c, 4. b**
30. **1. e, 2. d, 3. a, 4. c, 5. f**
31. **1. a, 2. d, 3. e, 4. f, 5. b**
32. **1. d, 2. b, 3. a, 4. c**
33. **c. 1, 2**
34. **b. 1, 2**
35. **(b) Assertion true: Reason true. Reason is not the correct explanation for the assertion**
36. **a. 1, 3, 2, 4**
37. **1. d, 2. h, 3. e, 4. a, 5. f, 6. g**
38. **(a) Assertion true: Reason true. Reason is the correct explanation for assertion**
39. **(c) Assertion true: Reason false**
40. **b. 1, 3, 2, 4**
41. **c. 1, 3, 5**
42. **1. d, 2. a, 3. c, 4. b**

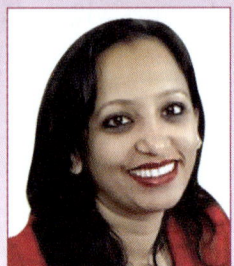
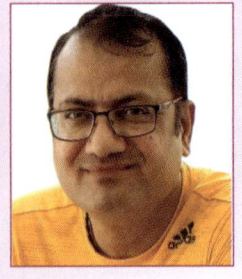
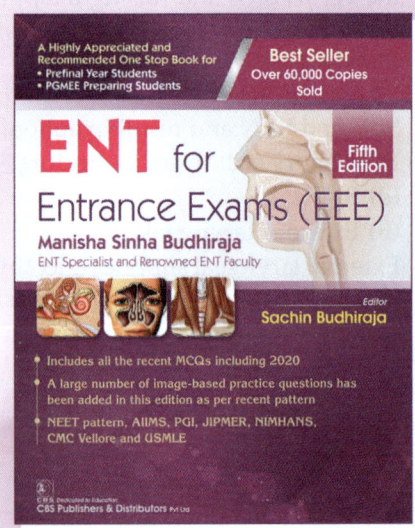